CLINICAL HANDBOOK OF
ANXIETY DISORDERS IN CHILDREN
AND ADOLESCENTS

CLINICAL HANDBOOK OF ANXIETY DISORDERS IN CHILDREN AND ADOLESCENTS

Edited by:

ANDREW R. EISEN, PH.D.
CHRISTOPHER A. KEARNEY, PH.D.
CHARLES E. SCHAEFER, PH.D.

JASON ARONSON INC.
Northvale, New Jersey
London

Production Editor: Elaine Lindenblatt

This book was set in 10 point Goudy by TechType of Upper Saddle River, New Jersey, and printed and bound by Haddon Craftsmen of Scranton, Pennsylvania.

The editors gratefully acknowledge permission to quote from American Psychiatric Association: *Diagnostic and Statistical Manual of Mental Disorders, Fourth Edition (DSM=IV)*. Washington, DC. Copyright © 1994, American Psychiatric Association. Used by permission.

Library of Congress Cataloging-in-Publication Data

Clinical handbook of anxiety disorders in children and adolescents /
  edited by Andrew R. Eisen, Christopher A. Kearney, Charles E.
  Schaefer.
     p. cm.
  Includes bibliographical references and index.
  ISBN 1-56821-294-1
  1. Anxiety in children. 2. Anxiety in adolescence. I. Eisen,
Andrew R. II. Kearney, Christopher A. III. Schaefer, Charles E.
  [DNLM: 1. Anxiety Disorders—in infancy & childhood. 2. Anxiety
Disorders—in adolescence. WM 172 C64175 1995]
RJ506.A58C58 1995
618.92'85223—dc20
DNLM/DLC
for Library of Congress   94-18064

Manufactured in the United States of America. Jason Aronson Inc. offers books and cassettes. For information and catalog write to Jason Aronson Inc., 230 Livingston Street, Northvale, New Jersey 07647.

To my parents
Cynthia and Eric,
my wife Linda,
and my brother Glenn

A. R. E.

To my parents
Jean and Larry,
and to Laurie, Andy, Rick, and Cheryle

C. A. K.

To Anne, Karine, and Eric

C. E. S.

CHILD THERAPY SERIES

A SERIES OF BOOKS EDITED BY
CHARLES SCHAEFER

Cognitive-Behavioral Play Therapy
Susan M. Knell

Play Therapy in Action: A Casebook for Practitioners
Terry Kottman and Charles Schaefer, Eds.

Family Play Therapy
Lois Carey and Charles Schaefer, Eds.

The Quotable Play Therapist
Charles Schaefer and Heidi Kaduson, Eds.

Childhood Encopresis and Enuresis
Charles Schaefer

The Therapeutic Powers of Play
Charles Schaefer, Ed.

Play Therapy Techniques
Donna Cangelosi and Charles Schaefer, Eds.

Children in Residential Care: Critical Issues in Treatment
Charles Schaefer and Arthur Swanson, Eds.

Therapeutic Use of Child's Play
Charles Schaefer, Ed.

Clinical Handbook of Sleep Disorders in Children
Charles Schaefer, Ed.

Clinical Handbook of Anxiety Disorders in Children and Adolescents
Andrew R. Eisen, Christopher A. Kearney, and Charles Schaefer, Eds.

Practitioner's Guide to Treating Fear and Anxiety in Children and
Adolescents: A Cognitive-Behavioral Approach
Andrew R. Eisen and Christopher A. Kearney

CONTENTS

PART III: RELATED INTERVENTION STRATEGIES

PART IV: FUTURE DIRECTIONS

PREFACE

THE PHENOMENON OF ANXIETY is ubiquitous among children, adolescents, and adults. In many instances, however, anxious apprehension intensifies at an early age and produces debilitating effects that necessitate immediate and effective interventions.

Given these instances, literature regarding childhood anxiety and its disorders is accumulating at a rapid and exciting pace. New articles and books are specifically devoted to research and clinical practice in this area. Still, when health professionals look for clinical wisdom and detailed guidelines for treating childhood anxiety disorders, their search can often result in frustration.

With this in mind, the aim of this handbook is to provide comprehensive coverage of all the anxiety and anxiety-related disorders of childhood. To do so, designations in this book reflect current diagnostic criteria. In addition, empirically grounded, state-of-the-art therapeutic techniques are discussed in a step-by-step format by noted authorities in the field. For example, innovative approaches are presented regarding prescriptive treatment strategies, group interventions, and the added role of various family members in treatment. Finally, this handbook has been designed to provide a broad theoretical base that should appeal to most clinicians.

The *Clinical Handbook of Anxiety Disorders in Children and Adolescents* is divided into four parts. Part One is an introductory chapter that carefully examines general issues underlying the diagnosis and treatment of anxiety disorders in youngsters. Part Two contains chapters addressing assessment and treatment strategies for youngsters with specific anxiety disorders as well as those problems with an anxiety component. The format for each chapter is uniform and contains the following headings: Description of Disorder, Differential Diagnosis, Assessment Procedures, Establishing Treatment Goals, Role of the Therapist, Treatment Strategies, Dealing with Common Obstacles to Successful Treatment, Relapse Prevention, Termination, Case Illustration (Typical Treatment), Case Illustration (Overcoming Obstacles), and Summary. Each chapter presents careful assessment and treatment guidelines in a step-by-step format. In addition, most chapters include transcriptions from actual therapy sessions to illustrate the use of specific treatment techniques. The case illustrations are designed to help clinicians understand and confront both typical and difficult cases, and provide ideas about overcoming therapeutic roadblocks that may be encountered. The final chapter in Part Two addresses the issue of comorbidity. The authors of this chapter highlight important conceptual issues and offer suggestions for modifying treatment in cases where several problems overlap.

Part Three examines related intervention strategies that are not disorder- or problem-specific. Part Three includes chapters on Psychodynamic Play Therapy, Family Therapy, Cognitive-Behavioral Group Therapy, and Pharmacotherapy. Last, Part Four is a final chapter that addresses future trends in intervention. The authors of this chapter highlight, among other issues, the increasing role of parents and families in treatment, developmental considerations, and cultural, economic, and ethnic differences in prevention, diagnosis, and intervention.

We hope this handbook will make a wide variety of treatments more accessible to mental health practitioners who work with youngsters with anxiety-related disorders. Moreover, professors and graduate students should find this handbook to be a useful adjunct to courses involving psychopathology and therapy in children and adolescents. We thank the authors for their fine contributions toward these aims.

Andrew R. Eisen
Teaneck, New Jersey

Christopher A. Kearney
Las Vegas, Nevada

Charles E. Schaefer
Teaneck, New Jersey

CONTRIBUTORS

Anne Marie Albano (Ph.D., University of Mississippi, 1991) is the Assistant Director of the Phobia and Anxiety Disorders Clinic of the Center for Stress and Anxiety Disorders, University at Albany, State University of New York (SUNY). She is an adjunct professor of psychology at SUNY-Albany. Her current research is focused on the empirical foundation of diagnostic methods and prescriptive treatment protocols for treating anxiety disorders in youth.

Wesley D. Allan (M.A., University of Nevada, Las Vegas, 1994) is a doctoral student in clinical psychology at the University of Missouri, Columbia. Mr. Allan's research interests include internalizing disorders in children and adolescents, focusing on anxiety and panic disorders.

David H. Barlow (Ph.D., University of Vermont, 1969) is Distinguished Professor of Psychology and Co-director of the Center for Stress and Anxiety Disorders, State University of New York at Albany. In addition, he is a member of the *DSM-IV* Task Force of the American Psychiatric Association and is Co-Chair of the Work Group for revising the anxiety disorder categories.

Donna M. Cangelosi (Psy.D., Pace University, 1988) is Assistant Professor of Counseling Psychology at the University of the Pacific in Stockton, California. She recently completed a postgraduate certificate in Child and Adolescent Psychotherapy at the New Jersey Institute of Psychoanalysis.

Laurie Cashman (B.S., St. Joseph's University, 1993) is a graduate student of the experimental program in health psychology at St. Joseph's University. Her research interests include behavioral pediatrics and behavioral medicine.

Ronald S. Drabman (Ph.D., State University of New York at Stony Brook, 1972) is Professor of Psychiatry and Human Behavior (Division of Psychology) and Director of the Psychology Training Program at the University of Mississippi Medical Center. He has been executive secretary of the

Mississippi State Board of Psychological Examiners and an associate editor of the *Journal of Applied Behavior Analysis*.

Andrew R. Eisen (Ph.D., University at Albany, State University of New York, 1992) is Assistant Professor of Psychology and Director of the Child Anxiety Disorders Clinic at Fairleigh Dickinson University. His current research focuses on prescriptive treatment strategies and the role of family variables in anxious youth.

Linda B. Engler (Ph.D., Binghamton University, 1993) is staff psychologist at the Institute for Child Development, Hackensack Medical Center. Dr. Engler's clinical and research interests include the assessment and treatment of children with head injury, attention deficit hyperactivity disorder, eating disorders, and anxiety disorders.

Michael D. Fetter (M.S., University of Miami, 1994) is an advanced graduate student in the doctoral program in clinical child psychology at the University of Miami. His research interests include children's peer relations and child and adolescent psychopathology.

John R. Freedy (Ph.D., Kent State University, 1990) is Assistant Professor in the Department of Psychiatry and Behavioral Sciences at the Medical University of South Carolina. Dr. Freedy is a clinical psychologist at the Crime Victims Research and Treatment Center, Department of Psychiatry and Behavioral Sciences at the Medical University of South Carolina. He specializes in adult clinical psychology with an emphasis on traumatic stress.

Alice G. Friedman (Ph.D., Virginia Polytechnic Institute and State University, 1985) is Assistant Professor in the Department of Psychology at Binghamton University, State University of New York. Her research focuses on childhood fears and anxiety and psychological factors associated with childhood illness.

Golda S. Ginsburg (Ph.D., University of Vermont, 1990) is Research Associate at Florida International University. She is also the Assistant Director of the Child Anxiety and Phobia program at FIU, where she is involved in the development, implementation, and evaluation of treatment programs for children with anxiety and phobic disorders.

Christopher A. Kearney (Ph.D., University at Albany, State University of New York, 1990) is Assistant Professor of Psychology at the University of Nevada, Las Vegas. Dr. Kearney's research interests include internalizing problems in children and adolescents, as well as environmental variables

affecting adaptive and maladaptive behavior in persons with severe handicaps. Dr. Kearney is the Director of the School Refusal and Panic Disorder
Clinic at the University of Nevada, Las Vegas.

Philip C. Kendall (Ph.D., Virginia Commonwealth University, 1977;
ABPP) is Professor of Psychology, head of the Division of Clinical Psychol-
ogy, and Director of the Child and Adolescent Anxiety Disorders Clinic at
Temple University, Philadelphia, PA. Dr. Kendall is an associate editor of the
Journal of Consulting and Clinical Psychology and is currently on the board of
directors of the Council of University Directors of Clinical Psychology.

Lenna S. Knox (B.A., Ohio University, 1985) is an advanced graduate
student in the doctoral program in clinical psychology at University at
Albany, State University of New York. Her primary research interests focus
on the role of parents in the treatment of anxious children.

David D. Krohn (M.D., University of Michigan, 1984) is currently
Director of the Northwest Michigan Child Guidance Center. Dr. Krohn
completed his residency in psychiatry at Sinai Hospital of Detroit and child
and adolescent training at Hawthorn Center, both affiliated with Wayne
State University. He is a diplomate of the American Board of Psychiatry and
Neurology in both Psychiatry and Child and Adolescent Psychiatry.

William M. Kurtines (Ph.D., The Johns Hopkins University, 1973) is
Professor of Psychology at Florida International University. His current areas
of interest include social, personality, and moral development.

Annette M. La Greca (Ph.D., Purdue University, 1978) is Professor of
Psychology and Pediatrics at the University of Miami, where she also serves
as the Director for the graduate programs in clinical child and pediatric
health psychology. Dr. La Greca is currently the editor of the *Journal of
Pediatric Psychology*, and the associate editor of *Diabetes Spectrum*.

Cynthia G. Last (Ph.D., University at Albany, State University of New
York, 1982) is Professor of Psychology and Director of the Anxiety Treatment
Center in the Department of Psychology at Nova-Southeastern University.
She is editor and founder of the *Journal of Anxiety Disorders*.

Julie A. Lipovsky (Ph.D., University of Florida, 1987) is Associate
Professor in the Department of Psychology at the Citadel in Charleston,
South Carolina, where she is Program Coordinator of The Citadel's Com-
munity Counseling Program. Previously, Dr. Lipovsky was at the Crime
Victims Research and Treatment Center, Department of Psychiatry and
Behavioral Sciences at the Medical University of South Carolina.

Jennifer P. MacDonald, a doctoral candidate in clinical psychology at Temple University, is a senior staff member at the Child and Adolescent Anxiety Disorders Clinic at Temple University, where she has served as diagnostician, therapist, and head therapist. She is currently completing her internship at the Devereaux Foundation in Pennsylvania.

Jodi A. Mindell (Ph.D., University at Albany, State University of New York, 1989) is Assistant Professor of Psychology at St. Joseph's University and Clinical Assistant Professor of Neurology at Medical College of Pennsylvania. She specializes in childhood sleep disorders and maintains a broad-scale clinical research program investigating the assessment and treatment of sleep problems in children and adolescents.

Richelle N. Moen (Ph.D., University of Iowa, 1991) is Clinical Supervisor and Instructor in the Department of Psychiatry at the University of Minnesota Medical School. Dr. Moen is also a licensed psychologist who works with children and their families. She has been involved in research in the areas of school refusal, postdivorce adjustment, and adolescent sex-role development.

Sean Perrin (Ph.D., Nova-Southeastern University, 1994) is an advanced graduate student in the doctoral program in clinical psychology at Nova-Southeastern University. He is currently research coordinator of Dr. Cynthia Last's NIMH-funded investigation of the effectiveness of behavior therapy for the treatment of anxiety-based school refusal.

Donna B. Pincus (B.A., Brandeis University, 1991) is a graduate student in the doctoral program in clinical psychology at Binghamton University, State University of New York. Her research interests include children's fears and anxieties and children's adjustment to medical difficulties.

Edward P. Quinn (M.A., Binghamton University, State University of New York) is an advanced graduate student in the doctoral program at Binghamton University, State University of New York. His research interests include addictions, relapse prevention, and severe emotional problems of childhood.

David P. Ribbe (Ph.D., Virginia Polytechnic Institute and State University, 1993) is Research Associate at the Executive Branch of the National Center for PTSD in White River Junction, Vermont, and Visiting Assistant Professor, Department of Psychiatry at Dartmouth Medical School. Dr. Ribbe is a clinical child psychologist whose research and clinical interests are in the areas of traumatic stress and disaster.

Charles E. Schaefer (Ph.D., Fordham University, 1967) is Professor of Psychology in the doctoral program in clinical psychology at Fairleigh Dickinson University, Teaneck, New Jersey. He is cofounder of the International Association for Play Therapy and founder of the Play Therapy Training Institute. His research interests include parenting skills and creative thinking in children.

Wendy K. Silverman (Ph.D., Case Western University, 1981) is Professor of Psychology at Florida International University and Director of the Childhood Anxiety and Phobia Program at FIU. Dr. Silverman is on the editorial boards of several journals, such as *Journal of Clinical Child Psychology* and *Journal of Anxiety Disorders*.

Jovan G. Simeon (M.D., Zagreb University, Yugoslavia, 1959) is Professor of Psychiatry at the Department of Psychiatry, School of Medicine, University of Ottawa, and Director of Child Psychiatry Research at the Royal Ottawa Hospital. Dr. Simeon completed his training in psychiatry and child psychiatry at Edinburgh University in Scotland. He is a Fellow of the Royal College of Psychiatrists in Great Britian, the American Psychiatric Association, and the Royal College of Physicians in Canada.

Cyd C. Strauss (Ph.D., University of Georgia, 1983) is Visiting Assistant Professor and Clinical Director, Fear and Anxiety Disorders Clinic in the University of Florida Department of Clinical and Health Psychology. She is Co-director of the Center for Children and Families in Gainesville, Florida. She serves on the editorial board of the *Journal of Anxiety Disorders*.

James W. Sturges (Ph.D., University of Alabama, 1994) is Assistant Professor of Psychiatry and Human Behavior (Division of Psychology) and coordinator of the Behavioral Pediatrics rotation at the University of Mississippi Medical Center. Dr. Sturges's clinical and research interests are in health promotion with children, pain management, helping children cope with chronic diseases and disabilities, and the evaluation of cognitive-behavioral interventions in the pediatric population.

Kimberli R. H. Treadwell (Ph.D., Temple University, 1994) completed her internship at Johns Hopkins University in Baltimore. Dr. Treadwell has served as a diagnostician, data manager, and therapist at the Child and Adolescent Anxiety Disorders Clinic at Temple University.

Michael W. Vasey (Ph.D., Penn State University, 1990) is Assistant Professor of Psychology in the clinical psychology doctoral program at The Ohio State University. Dr. Vasey's research focuses on cognitive factors in childhood anxiety with a particular emphasis on information-processing biases, deficiencies in emotion self-regulation skills, and the impact of developmental factors on the content and process of worry in childhood.

Janice R. Wachtel (M.S., University of Florida, 1993) is an advanced graduate student in the doctoral program in clinical psychology at the University of Florida. Her research interests include anxiety in children undergoing invasive medical procedures and internalizing and externalizing behavioral disorders in children.

Sander M. Weckstein (M.D., University of Michigan, 1986) is currently Clinical Director of the Northwest Michigan Child Guidance Center. Dr. Weckstein completed his residency in psychiatry at Detroit Psychiatric Institute, and child and adolescent training at Hawthorn Center, both affiliated with Wayne State University. He is a diplomate of the American Board of Psychiatry and Neurology in both Psychiatry and Child and Adolescent Psychiatry.

Doreen M. Wiggins is a research assistant in child psychiatry at the Royal Ottawa Hospital. She is a qualified elementary school teacher both in England and Canada, and was a research assistant for ten years with the Ottawa Board of Education. Mrs. Wiggins currently works in the area of child and adolescent psychopharmacology for the Director, Child Psychiatry Research, at the Royal Ottawa Hospital.

Harold Wright (M.D., University of Michigan) is currently in part-time private practice. He trained in psychiatry and child and adolescent psychiatry at the University of Michigan and Hawthorn Center, affiliated with Wayne State University. He is a diplomate of the American Boards of Psychiatry and Neurology in Psychiatry, Child and Adolescent Psychiatry, and Pediatrics. Dr. Wright was Director of Hawthorn Center prior to his retirement.

Part I

INTRODUCTION

GENERAL ISSUES UNDERLYING THE DIAGNOSIS AND TREATMENT OF CHILD AND ADOLESCENT ANXIETY DISORDERS

Christopher A. Kearney
Andrew R. Eisen
Charles E. Schaefer

PERHAPS ONE OF THE MOST exciting areas within clinical psychology today is the study of emotional disorders in general and anxiety disorders in particular. Over the past three decades, the classification, assessment, and treatment of adult anxiety disorders have received a substantial amount of research attention, and significant advances in the field are presented in the literature on a regular basis. With respect to anxiety disorders in children and adolescents, however, such rapid-fire advances in conceptual development have only recently been demonstrated. Still, the burgeoning research activity on this topic now mandates a summary of what we know and must continue to pursue. In addition, given the improving technology of the field and the information gap that traditionally exists between researchers and practitioners, accessible presentations of clinical strategies to address this population are needed. These are the purposes of this handbook.

The importance of anxiety disorders in youngsters cannot be understated. The syndromes generally affect 8–11 percent of children and adolescents (Anderson et al. 1987, Costello 1989, Fergusson et al. 1993, Lewinsohn et al. 1993), a figure that almost doubles if one includes anxiety-related disorders such as school refusal behavior or sleep problems. In addition, childhood anxiety is often comorbid with symptoms of depression (e.g., King et al. 1991) and externalizing problems such as hyperactivity and conduct disorder (e.g., Woolston et al. 1989). More important, however, are the debilitating effects that anxiety disorders can produce on a child. Particularly noteworthy are absence from school and poor academic achievement, problematic familial and peer relationships, difficulties maintaining a job or performing in front of others, low self-esteem, chronic fatigue and somatic complaints, and general avoidance of new situations.

Within the past two decades, clinical researchers have focused a substantially greater amount of attention on this population than ever before. As a result, significant improvements have been made in the assessment and treatment of anxiety disorders in youngsters. Specifically, great progress has been made in the design of structured diagnostic interviews, rating systems (especially child self-report measures), and physiological assessment. Indeed, our knowledge about how to assess behavioral, cognitive, and physiological aspects of anxiety is growing at a very rapid pace. In addition, the influence of more sophisticated research designs such as single-subject analysis has promoted the evaluation of various therapeutic techniques. Examples include flooding, self-instruction, and anxiolytics. The study of anxiety-related disorders in children and adolescents may thus be analogous to a fast-flowing river that is constantly being fed by rich tributaries of ideas. The chapters that follow provide the reader with the newest material to help navigate this river. The purpose of this chapter is to alert the reader to the "rocks" in this river, or issues that will need to be resolved in the future if clinicians and researchers are to steer their way toward the best methods of addressing this population.

WHAT LIES AHEAD?

Contributing to the challenge and excitement of addressing youngsters with anxiety disorders is the realization that clinical researchers are at certain "bends in the river" with respect to the future classification, assessment, and treatment of this population. With respect to classification, for example, detailed categorical and dimensional models of anxiety disorders have been made available and extensively researched within the past twenty years. However, both have undergone substantial revision and contain numerous disadvantages when taken alone. One key decision for the future involves which direction, categorical or dimensional, is conceptually best, or whether this dichotomy represents a false choice. With respect to assessment, a variety of measures have been developed to evaluate youngsters with anxiety-related disorders. However, issues of psychometric strength, informant variance, and developmental appropriateness, among others, remain. Key decisions here include the extent to which value should be placed on cognitive, behavioral, and physiological measures as well as those geared toward different sources.

With respect to treatment, one of the most tantalizing aspects of recent literature is the proliferation of data regarding new interventions. However, despite increasing knowledge that treatment is significantly more effective than the lack of treatment, traditional questions remain as to which therapeutic strategy is best for each individual client (Paul 1967). One key decision here involves the extent to which exploration of prescriptive treatments is preferable or justified compared with customary approaches. This chapter will briefly introduce general issues of classification, assessment, and treatment, and outline the primary controversies that mark the study of anxiety disorders in youngsters. The reader is encouraged to carefully consider these issues when reading the following chapters of this handbook.

GENERAL ISSUES OF CLASSIFICATION

The classification of psychopathology is often conceptualized along (1) categorical approaches, which typically involve the presence of clinically derived and discrete diagnostic classes, and (2) dimensional approaches, which typically involve the presence of statistically derived and fluid profiles of behavior. The former is exemplified by the fourth edition of the *Diagnostic and Statistical Manual of Mental Disorders* (*DSM-IV*, American Psychiatric Association, 1994), the primary categorical system used by clinicians and researchers. Currently, only one anxiety disorder is delineated specifically for children and adolescents, that is, separation anxiety disorder. However, youngsters may be diagnosed with adult anxiety disorders if appropriate criteria are met. Examples include panic disorder with or without agoraphobia, specific phobia, social phobia/social anxiety disorder (which subsumes the previous *DSM-III-R* category of avoidant disorder), and obsessive-compulsive, posttraumatic stress, and generalized anxiety disorder (which subsumes the previous *DSM-III-R* category of overanxious disorder).

A major advantage of the *DSM* system is its wide use by clinicians and researchers, which serves to facilitate communication among clients and health professionals. However, this diagnostic system has been criticized for a variety of reasons, some of which are discussed here. First, criteria used to determine whether a person displays an anxiety disorder are not always precisely defined or explicit. For example, one criterion for separation anxiety disorder is a "persistent reluctance or refusal to go to sleep" (*DSM* 1994, p. 113). However, specific guidelines for what constitutes "persistent" are not provided. Second, the psychometric properties (i.e., reliability and validity) of structured interviews based on anxiety disorder criteria are not well established (Silverman 1991). A related criticism concerns the system's content validity, or ability to discern normal from abnormal behavior (Wakefield 1992). Third, the DSM system for anxiety disorders relies heavily on "adultomorphism," or the application of adultlike parameters of behavior to youngsters (Phillips et al. 1975). As a result, the DSM does not consider developmental factors, such as cognitive ability, that potentially differentiate the clinical picture of childhood, adolescent, and adult anxiety (e.g., panic) disorder (Kearney and Silverman 1992).

Another area that needs to be addressed is the DSM's questionable discriminant validity, with diagnostic comorbidity documented in many studies (see Perrin and Last, this volume). Part of this may be due to certain criteria that describe similar behavior across diagnoses. For example, a "persistent reluctance or refusal to go to school" in separation anxiety disorder is similar to "often truant from school" in conduct disorder. Finally, use of the DSM produces a significant loss of taxonomic and clinical information because the only allowable decision about a client is whether he/she "has" or "does not have" a particular disorder (Verhulst and van der Ende 1993). For example, a youngster displaying two criteria for separation anxiety disorder, three panic attack symptoms, and four symptoms of depression may not receive any diagnosis. Despite the presence of problematic behaviors, the DSM regards as significant only those that meet a certain "threshold" for diagnosis (Frances et al. 1990).

Dimensional systems of classification often rely on a quantitative analysis of behavior ratings, such as those provided by clinicians, parents, or teachers. This approach for youngsters is best exemplified by Achenbach's (1991, 1993, Achenbach and Edelbrock 1983) internalizing-externalizing continuum and related measures. On the Child Behavior Checklist for boys, for example, an internalizing "anxious/depressed" factor contains symptoms such as fears, nervousness, and worry. Advantages to this system include its solid psychometric properties, consideration of developmental factors, linkage to standardized assessment techniques, and flexibility in delineating profiles of clinical behavior for specific populations (e.g., Achenbach et al. 1989). Disadvantages, however, include inconsistent usage among clinicians and researchers, a high correlation between internalizing and externalizing factors when psychopathology is broad (Hinshaw 1992), and little research linking specific factors to efficacious treatment strategies (Burke and Silverman 1987).

As mentioned earlier, the question of whether to choose a categorical or dimensional approach for the future classification of childhood anxiety disorders may represent a false choice. Clinicians and researchers are increasingly prone to utilize both approaches, and diagnostic systems such as the *DSM* and *International Classification of Diseases* (*ICD* 1977) are gradually incorporating more categorical and dimensional features (Barlow 1992). In addition, categorical-dimensional approaches have been proposed for specific problems not delineated in the *DSM* (e.g., school refusal behavior, Kearney and Silverman 1993). Such a coalescence may increase the taxonomic flexibility of a classification system while retaining psychometric quality, uniform use among professionals, and linkage to appropriate assessment and treatment strategies. This direction may be particularly beneficial to organizing the often fluid and amorphous nature of the anxiety-related disorders.

GENERAL ISSUES OF ASSESSMENT

The assessment of anxiety-related problems in youngsters is often divided according to information source (i.e., child, parent, teacher, clinician) and/or symptomatology (i.e., cognitive-affective, behavioral, physiological). As the reader will discover when exploring the contents of this handbook, the primary evaluative devices for this population include structured and semi-structured diagnostic interviews, self-report questionnaires of fear/anxiety and other variables, parent/teacher checklists, behavioral observations, and psychophysiological measures. The technology for assessing childhood fear/anxiety and related problems has blossomed in recent years. Such growth, however, has produced key methodological and conceptual issues that must be addressed in the future.

One such issue concerns which evaluative techniques are most appropriate for this population. For example, an overreliance on adult reports during the early period of clinical child psychology has been criticized because parents and teachers are not highly accurate observers of children's behavior (e.g., Kendall et al. 1992a). On the other hand, the utility of self-report or self-monitoring procedures for young children has been questioned because of the children's limited verbal, cognitive, and memory abilities (Ollendick and Meador 1984). In addition, physiological techniques are sometimes impugned for their cost and impracticality in most clinical settings (Silverman and Kearney 1993), and are less necessary for some disorders (e.g., obsessive-compulsive) than others (e.g., generalized anxiety). The reliability and validity of many measures (e.g., behavioral observations) are often unclear as well. As a result, a key task for the future will be to identify which combination of psychometrically sound and clinically useful assessment instruments best evaluate one particular youngster with an anxiety disorder.

A related issue is informant variance, or discrepancies in information gathered from different sources. Much of the research in this area has focused on parent-child agreement, with the general finding that children report more internalizing behaviors than parents, whereas parents report more externalizing behaviors than children (e.g., Kashani et al. 1985). According to Klein (1991), parent-child agreement is poor across diagnostic items on most structured interviews for anxiety disorders. One particular factor that affects such agreement is the child's age. Concordance with parents is lower for younger children (gender and severity of the child or parent's psychopathology are not as influential). Several authors have thus recommended that assessment protocols for youngsters with anxiety-related disorders utilize parents as information sources in addition to children (Klein 1991) or adolescents (Long et al. 1992).

Another key problem is that evaluative devices are not always linked to other clinical processes. For example, not all assessment measures are derived from widely used taxonomic strategies. Exceptions include diagnostic interviews (e.g., Silverman and Nelles 1988) and dimensional rating systems (e.g., Achenbach 1991). However, many self-report measures contain their own idiosyncratic factors (e.g., worry/oversensitivity on the Revised Children's Manifest Anxiety Scale, Reynolds and Paget 1983). In addition, few assessment devices have been linked to effective treatment strategies. Despite an ability to collect a substantial amount of information about a particular child, few investigators have directly assigned treatment on the basis of factors other than diagnosis. Yet even with respect to circumscribed diagnoses, a link to effective treatment has not been fully demonstrated. For example, Last and Strauss (1990) stated that "psychosocial and psychopharmacological outcome studies with 'school phobic' children have . . . not determined whether treatment response is related to diagnosis" (p. 35). Future investigators will likely focus on improving the integration of assessment procedures with standard taxonomic strategies and prevalent treatment practices.

The deemphasis or neglect of developmental factors in some assessment measures must also be addressed in the future. Although many adult measures have been adapted and standardized for children, the implicit assumption that a particular construct (e.g., panic) remains unchanged across the lifespan is debatable. This issue applies primarily to structured diagnostic interviews that were developed for youngsters from adult-oriented instruments (e.g., Schedule for Affective Disorders and Schizophrenia in School-Aged Children, Puig-Antich and Chambers 1978). Also noteworthy is the fact that most interviews specifically designed for youngsters do not contain separate versions for children and adolescents. Other examples where developmental changes are not always considered include youngster self-report (e.g., State-Trait Anxiety Inventory for Children, Spielberger 1973) and physiological measures (e.g., resting heart rate, Beidel and Stanley 1993).

Finally, mental health professionals should be cognizant of the positive correlation among measures of anxiety and depression in children and adolescents. Many investigators in recent years have documented the construct of "negative affectivity," or a coalescence of anxiety- and depressive-related symptoms such as agitation (e.g., King et al. 1991, Ollendick and Yule 1990, Wolfe et al. 1987). Whether negative affectivity is a true personality construct or an artifact of anxiety/depression measures remains to be fully clarified. In the meantime, clinicians and researchers should be aware that determining which disorder (anxiety or depression) is primary can sometimes be difficult given our present assessment technology. Clarifying this issue must receive a high priority, however, given that treatment direction depends considerably on making such a determination (Kendall et al. 1992b).

GENERAL ISSUES OF TREATMENT

Although the disorders discussed in this handbook are quite diverse and heterogeneous in their symptomatology, treatment strategies for those with such disorders can be more succinctly described. Despite substantial variation in their use, primary therapeutic methods for youngsters with fear/anxiety problems include relaxation training and systematic desensitization, exposure to aversive internal and external stimuli, cognitive restructuring, development of coping skills, modeling and role-play, response prevention, parent training and contingency management, family therapy, and pharmacotherapy. Readers should note that many of these are employed in individual as well as group formats. In general, the treatment of youngsters with anxiety disorders has recently concentrated on cognitive-behavioral and/or pharmacological interventions.

Recent meta-analyses, or derivations of effect size for treatment versus no treatment across many outcome studies, reveal some important findings about child/adolescent psychotherapy. Overall, we now know that treatment is a substantially better course of action for psychopathology than little or no treatment (e.g., Casey and Berman 1985, Durlak et al. 1991, Weisz et al. 1987, 1992). This appears to be particularly true for phobic-related disorders and somatic complaints, but less so for problems of social functioning. The conclusion that psychotherapy works, though not exceedingly well, provides clinicians and researchers with a valuable starting point for investigating the next series of questions. Some of these questions are discussed here.

Even if we draw the conclusion that psychotherapy is generally effective for most youngsters with mental disorders, the question remains as to why it is not completely effective for all youngsters with mental disorders. A potential answer lies with some unfortunate developments within the field. First and perhaps foremost is the communication abyss that exists between clinicians and researchers (Kazdin et al. 1990). In essence, clinicians often do not ascribe to trends within the research literature, and researchers often evaluate specific populations that do not correspond to those that most clinicians address. With respect to the latter, for example, Ammerman and colleagues (1993) noted several variables often faced by clinicians but "weeded out" or deemphasized by researchers. These variables include diagnostic comorbidity, familial or societal factors such as abuse or poverty, increased length of treatment, use of multiple treatments and/or therapists, client noncompliance, logistical problems, infrequent client contact, and relapse. As a result, many youngsters with such problems or those treated under such conditions may be inadequately addressed or investigated.

A second problem that may explain less than ideal therapeutic effectiveness is the assignment of a "package" or universal treatment to all youngsters with a particular disorder. An example is a clinical researcher who applies systematic desensitization, contingency management, and teacher-based techniques to treat children and adolescents with a specific phobia. Although such research is invaluable, information is not readily available to answer why a specific percentage did or did not experience behavior change. For example, did some youngsters improve because of a new emphasis on parent involvement with the problem? Conversely, did some youngsters fail to improve because proximal variables such as attention were unaddressed? We cannot be sure.

As a result, current research is expanding beyond this traditional approach and focusing more on comparative and prescriptive outcome strategies. In these methods, individual treatment techniques are compared with each other or assigned on the basis of specific case characteristics. Examples of such characteristics include individual response set (e.g., cognitive versus physiological), developmental status (e.g., concrete versus formal operational), behavior function (e.g., positive versus negative reinforcement), parenting style (e.g., permissive versus authoritative), family environment (e.g., detached versus conflicted), type of referral (e.g., family versus court), and socioeconomic status. Examples of this approach with youngsters are available or ongoing with respect to general anxiety (Eisen and Silverman 1994, Kendall 1994), school refusal behavior (Kearney and Silverman 1990), and specific and social phobia (Albano and Barlow, Silverman, personal communication) as well as severe behavior disorders (Durand 1990). In each case, investigators are able to identify specific characteristics related to treatment outcome and issue recommendations for appropriate, idiographically based therapeutic methods.

Finally, not all youngsters may benefit from treatment because not all youngsters have access to treatment. As Kazdin (1993) noted, many minority groups in the United States are "underserved," or, for cultural, economic, or other reasons, are seen proportionately less in mental health settings than the general population. Because almost one-third of American youngsters will be from a minority group by the year 2000 (Gibbs and Huang 1991), clinical researchers must focus attention on the development of "culturally sensitive" (Kazdin 1993, p. 137) prevention and intervention strategies.

Other general treatment issues must also receive a greater priority among clinical researchers. These include evaluations of (1) gender and etiological factors that affect therapy, including biological and genetic characteristics, (2) pediatric and nonclinical populations with anxiety, (3) treatment integrity, or monitoring whether a specific treatment method was appropriately given, (4) improvements in positive (e.g., social) aspects of functioning, not simply the alleviation of negative aspects, (5) how different combinations of client/family characteristics, therapy techniques, therapists, and settings impinge upon a specific problem, (6) larger sample sizes in treatment outcome studies, (7) nonbehavioral treatment strategies, and (8) long-term treatment effects and longitudinal analyses (Ammerman et al. 1993, Cantwell and Baker 1989, Kazdin 1993, Last 1993, Reynolds 1992, Thyer 1991). In addition, as has been stated for classification and assessment, the incorporation of a developmental perspective should pervade future treatment design. For example, knowing that the utility of cognitive procedures is better for adolescents than children can assist in developing appropriate interventions (e.g., Durlak et al. 1991).

SUMMARY

The classification, assessment, and treatment of psychopathology in children and adolescents represent fast-growing, exciting, and controversial areas of study. Data have emerged to support various models of these clinical processes, although such research also illustrates the substantial work that remains. Specifically, clinicians should be aware that future taxonomic, evaluative, and intervention strategies will probably become more developmentally tailored to youngsters. This statement applies particularly to the anxiety-related disorders, where extrapolation from adult methodology has often been employed. As a result, the field of childhood internalizing disorders is likely to contain fertile ground for many future investigators interested in developing innovative and flexible clinical strategies. The information provided in the following chapters will help to outline the seeds for such growth. In addition, clinicians and researchers must be sensitive to the enlarging information gap between themselves, and cooperate more to provide accessible and realistic assessment-treatment protocols. The ensuing chapters are designed to assist this process.

REFERENCES

Achenbach, T. M. (1991). *Manual for the Child Behavior Checklist/4-18 and 1991 Profile*. Burlington, VT: University of Vermont Department of Psychiatry.

—— (1993). Implications of multiaxial empirically based assessment for behavior therapy with children. *Behavior Therapy* 24:91-116.

Achenbach, T. M., Conners, C. K., Quay, H. C., et al. (1989). Replication of empirically derived syndromes as a basis for taxonomy of child/adolescent psychopathology. *Journal of Abnormal Child Psychology* 17:299-323.

Achenbach, T. M., and Edelbrock, C. (1983). *Manual for the Child Behavior Checklist and Revised Child Behavior Profile*. Burlington, VT: University of Vermont Department of Psychiatry.

Ammerman, R. T., Last, C. G., and Hersen, M. (1993). A prescriptive approach to treatment of children and adolescents. In *Handbook of Prescriptive Treatment for Children and Adolescents*, eds. R. T. Ammerman, C. G. Last, and M. Hersen, pp. 1-8. Boston: Allyn and Bacon.

Anderson, J. C., Williams, S., McGee, R., and Silva, P. A. (1987). *DSM-III* disorders in preadolescent children: prevalence in a large sample from the general population. *Archives of General Psychiatry* 44:69-76.

Barlow, D. H. (1992). Diagnosis, *DSM-IV*, and dimensional approaches. In *Perspectives and Promises of Clinical Psychology*, eds. A. Ehlers, W. Fiegenbaum, I. Florin, and J. Margraf, pp. 13-21. New York: Plenum.

Beidel, D. C., and Stanley, M. A. (1993). Developmental issues in measurement of anxiety. In *Anxiety Across the Lifespan: A Developmental Perspective*, ed. C. G. Last, pp. 167-203. New York: Springer.

Burke, A. E., and Silverman, W. K. (1987). The prescriptive treatment of school refusal. *Clinical Psychology Review* 7:353-362.

Cantwell, D. P., and Baker, L. (1989). Anxiety disorders. In *Recent Developments in*

Adolescent Psychiatry, eds. L. K. G. Hsu and M. Hersen, pp. 162–197. New York: Wiley.

Casey, R. J., and Berman, J. S. (1985). The outcome of psychotherapy with children. *Psychological Bulletin* 98:388–400.

Costello, E. J. (1989). Child psychiatric disorders and their correlates: a primary care pediatric sample. *Journal of the American Academy of Child and Adolescent Psychiatry* 28:851–855.

Diagnostic and Statistical Manual of Mental Disorders. (1994). 4th. ed. Washington, DC: American Psychiatric Association.

Durand, V. M. (1990). *Severe Behavior Problems: A Functional Communication Training Approach.* New York: Guilford.

Durlak, J. A., Fuhrman, T., and Lampman, C. (1991). Effectiveness of cognitive-behavioral therapy for maladapting children: a meta-analysis. *Psychological Bulletin* 110:204–214.

Eisen, A. E., and Silverman, W. K. (1994). *A preliminary examination of matched and mismatched cognitive-behavioral interventions for overanxious disorder.* Manuscript submitted for publication.

Fergusson, D. M., Horwood, L. J., and Lynskey, M. T. (1993). Prevalence and comorbidity of *DSM-III-R* diagnoses in a birth cohort of 15 year olds. *Journal of the American Academy of Child and Adolescent Psychiatry* 32:1127–1134.

Frances, A., Widiger, T., and Fyer, M. R. (1990). The influence of classification methods on comorbidity. In *Comorbidity of Anxiety and Mood Disorders,* eds. J. D. Maser and C. D. Cloninger. Washington, DC: American Psychiatric Association Press.

Gibbs, J. T., and Huang, L. N. (1991). *Children of Color: Psychological Interventions with Minority Youth.* San Francisco: Jossey-Bass.

Hinshaw, S. P. (1992). Externalizing behavior problems and academic underachievement in childhood and adolescence: causal relationships and underlying mechanisms. *Psychological Bulletin* 111:127–155.

International Classification of Diseases. (1977). Geneva: World Health Organization.

Kashani, J. H., Orvaschel, H., Burk, J. P., and Reid, J. C. (1985). Informant variance: the issue of parent-child disagreement. *Journal of the American Academy of Child and Adolescent Psychiatry* 24:437–441.

Kazdin, A. E. (1993). Adolescent mental health: prevention and treatment programs. *American Psychologist* 48:127–141.

Kazdin, A. E., Siegel, T. C., and Bass, D. (1990). Drawing on clinical practice to inform research on child and adolescent psychotherapy: survey of practitioners. *Professional Psychology: Research and Practice* 21:189–198.

Kearney, C. A., and Silverman, W. K. (1990). A preliminary analysis of a functional model of assessment and treatment for school refusal behavior. *Behavior Modification* 14:344–360.

_____ (1992). Let's not push the "panic" button: a critical analysis of panic and panic disorder in adolescents. *Clinical Psychology Review* 12:292–305.

_____ (1993). Measuring the function of school refusal behavior: the School Refusal Assessment Scale. *Journal of Clinical Child Psychology* 12:85–96.

Kendall, P. C. (1994). Treating anxiety disorders in children: results of a randomized clinical trial. *Journal of Consulting and Clinical Psychology* 62:100–110.

Kendall, P. C., Chansky, T. E., Kane, M. T., et al. (1992a). *Anxiety Disorders in Youth: Cognitive-Behavioral Interventions.* Boston: Allyn and Bacon.

Kendall, P. C., Kortlander, E., Chansky, T. E., and Brady, E. U. (1992b). Comorbidity of anxiety and depression in youth: treatment implications. *Journal of Consulting and Clinical Psychology* 60:869–880.

King, N. J., Ollendick, T. H., and Gullone, E. (1991). Negative affectivity in children and adolescents: relations between anxiety and depression. *Clinical Psychology Review* 11:441–459.

Klein, R. G. (1991). Parent-child agreement in clinical assessment of anxiety and other psychopathology: a review. *Journal of Anxiety Disorders* 5:187–198.

Last, C. G. (1993). Conclusions and future directions. In *Anxiety Across the Lifespan: A Developmental Perspective,* ed. C. G. Last, pp. 204–213. New York: Springer.

Last, C. G., and Strauss, C. C. (1990). School refusal in anxiety-disordered children and adolescents. *Journal of the American Academy of Child and Adolescent Psychiatry* 29:31–35.

Lewinsohn, P. M., Hops, H., Roberts, R. E., et al. (1993). Adolescent psychopathology: I. Prevalence and incidence of depression and other *DSM-III-R* disorders in high school students. *Journal of Abnormal Psychology* 102:133–144.

Long, P., Forehand, R., and Wierson, M. (1992). Internalizing problems of adolescents: the role of the informant in identifying family and individual difficulties. *Journal of Child and Family Studies* 1:329–339.

Ollendick, T. H., and Meador, A. E. (1984). Behavioral assessment of children. In *Handbook of Psychological Assessment,* eds. G. Goldstein and M. Hersen, pp. 351–368. New York: Pergamon.

Ollendick, T. H., and Yule, W. (1990). Depression in British and American children and its relation to anxiety and fear. *Journal of Consulting and Clinical Psychology* 58:126–129.

Paul, G. L. (1967). Strategy of outcome research in psychotherapy. *Journal of Consulting Psychology* 31:109–118.

Phillips, L., Draguns, J. G., and Bartlett, D. P. (1975). Classification of behavior disorders. In *Issues in the Classification of Children,* ed. N. Hobbs. San Francisco: Jossey-Bass.

Puig-Antich, J., and Chambers, W. (1978). *The Schedule for Affective Disorders and Schizophrenia for School-aged Children.* New York: New York State Psychiatric Institute.

Reynolds, C. R., and Paget, K. D. (1983). National normative and reliability data for the revised Children's Manifest Anxiety Scale. *School Psychology Review* 12:324–336.

Reynolds, W. M. (1992). Internalizing disorders in children and adolescents: issues and recommendations for future research. In *Internalizing Disorders in Children and Adolescents*, ed. W. M. Reynolds, pp. 311–317. New York: Wiley.

Silverman, W. K. (1991). Diagnostic reliability of anxiety disorders in children using structured interviews. *Journal of Anxiety Disorders* 5:105–124.

Silverman, W. K., and Kearney, C. A. (1993). Behavioral treatment of childhood anxiety. In *Handbook of Behavior Therapy and Pharmacotherapy for Children: A Comparative Analysis*, eds. V. B. Van Hasselt and M. Hersen, pp. 33–53. Boston: Allyn and Bacon.

Silverman, W. K., and Nelles, W. B. (1988). The anxiety disorders interview schedule for children. *Journal of the American Academy of Child and Adolescent Psychiatry* 27:772–778.

Spielberger, C. D. (1973). *Manual for the State-Trait Anxiety Inventory for Children*. Palo Alto, CA: Consulting Psychologists Press.

Thyer, B. A. (1991). Diagnosis and treatment of child and adolescent anxiety disorders. *Behavior Modification* 15:310–325.

Verhulst, F. C., and van der Ende, J. (1993). "Comorbidity" in an epidemiological sample: a longitudinal perspective. *Journal of Child Psychology and Psychiatry* 34:767–783.

Wakefield, J. C. (1992). Disorder as harmful dysfunction: a conceptual critique of DSM- III-R's definition of mental disorder. *Psychological Bulletin* 99:232–247.

Weisz, J. R., Weiss, B., Alicke, M. D., and Klotz, M. L. (1987). Effectiveness of psychotherapy with children and adolescents: a meta-analysis for clinicians. *Journal of Consulting and Clinical Psychology* 55:542–549.

Weisz, J. R., Weiss, B., and Donenberg, G. R. (1992). The lab versus the clinic: effects of child and adolescent psychotherapy. *American Psychologist* 47:1578–1585.

Wolfe, V. V., Finch, Jr., A. J., Saylor, C.F., et al. (1987). Negative affectivity in children: a multitrait-multimethod investigation. *Journal of Consulting and Clinical Psychology* 55:245–250.

Woolston, J. L., Rosenthal, S. L., Riddle, M. A., et al. (1989). Childhood comorbidity of anxiety/affective disorders and behavior disorders. *Journal of the American Academy of Child and Adolescent Psychiatry* 28:707–713.

Part II

INTERVENTION STRATEGIES FOR SPECIFIC PROBLEMS/DISORDERS

2

SCHOOL REFUSAL BEHAVIOR

Christopher A. Kearney

DESCRIPTION OF DISORDER

Of the anxiety-related disorders in childhood and adolescence, perhaps the one most heterogeneous with respect to terminology and symptomatology is school refusal behavior. School refusal behavior is defined here as a refusal to attend classes or difficulty remaining in school for an entire day (Kearney and Silverman 1990). This includes youngsters who resist going to school in the morning but eventually attend, those who go to school but subsequently leave during the course of the day, and those who miss the entire day. School refusal behavior should not be confused with other terms such as *school phobia*, which refers to a smaller set of youngsters who display an excessive, irrational fear of some school-related stimulus (e.g., Waldfogel et al. 1957); *separation anxiety*, which refers typically to very young children who display problems distancing from primary caregivers (Johnson et al. 1941); *truancy*, a multifarious term that often describes persons who refuse school without parental knowledge (e.g., Berg et al. 1988); and *school withdrawal*, a term reserved for parents who deliberately withhold children from school for various reasons (e.g., economic assistance, fear of kidnapping; Kahn and Nursten 1962). The term *school refusal behavior* is preferred here because of its inclusiveness in describing child-motivated problematic absenteeism.

The amorphous nature of school refusal behavior is further demonstrated by its presenting symptoms. Perhaps unique among the disorders discussed in this handbook, school refusal represents a largely unpredictable blend of internalizing and externalizing behavior. Predominant internalizing symptoms include fear, general and social anxiety, depression, somatic complaints, and poor self-esteem (Kearney 1993, Kearney and Silverman 1993, Last 1991, Last and Strauss 1990). Predominant externalizing symptoms include noncompliance, running away from school, and other conduct disorder-related behaviors (Kearney et al. 1989). Although several researchers and taxonomists have attempted to categorize youngsters with school refusal behavior into overcontrolled and undercontrolled subtypes (e.g., Young et al. 1990), the norm for this population remains a hybrid of both. As a result, delineating the epidemiology of this population has been notoriously difficult. Granell de Aldaz and colleagues (1984) found the reported prevalence rate of school refusal behavior to fluctuate between 0.01 and 25.0 percent. The clinical prevalence rate has been noted to be 6.08 percent (Kearney and Beasley 1994), but discrepancies in epidemiology should not obscure the fact that school refusal behavior is a significant social problem. In addition to its close relationship with juvenile delinquency, the long-term consequences of school refusal behavior include psychosocial and marital problems, work-related difficulties, alcoholism and criminal behavior, psychiatric disturbance, and economic dispossession (e.g., Berg 1970, Flakierska et al. 1988, Hibbett and Fogelman 1990, Hibbett et al. 1990, Robins and Ratcliff 1980, Timberlake 1984).

Overall, the classification, assessment, and treatment of school refusal behavior remains highly controversial. Although this chapter will outline the primary evaluative and therapeutic measures for school refusal behavior, the reader is cautioned that this research area is quite fluid and subject to much debate. Given concerns about the level and consequences of problematic absenteeism, however, the study of school refusal behavior deserves substantial attention. This is particularly true for establishing a uniform taxonomy and/or means of differentially diagnosing this population.

DIFFERENTIAL DIAGNOSIS

Another unique feature of school refusal behavior is its omission as a "clinically significant behavioral or psychological syndrome" in the *Diagnostic and Statistical Manual of Mental Disorders* (DSM 1987). Instead, problematic absenteeism is listed as a symptom of two disorders, separation anxiety and conduct disorder (DSM 1994). As a result, a common diagnosis for someone with the singular behavioral problem of school refusal is simple phobia of school. Clinicians and researchers should be aware, however, that this diagnostic structure often misrepresents the true nature of school refusal behavior as one predominated by fear or anxiety. In addition to diagnoses such as simple and social phobia, others commonly ascribed to this population include depression and oppositional defiant and conduct disorder (Bernstein and Garfinkel 1986, Last and Strauss 1990). Approximately 25 percent do not meet criteria for any mental disorder (Kearney 1992). School refusal may be best represented as a specific behavioral problem enveloped by several psychiatric syndromes (Hersov 1985).

Because of difficulties pinpointing a clear diagnostic profile for this population, researchers have relied on alternative methods of organization. Early dichotomists tried to distinguish school phobia from school refusal from truancy, but the discriminant validity of these concepts is questionable (Kearney and Silverman 1995). Another, broader method has been to categorize youngsters with school refusal behavior on the basis of duration. For example, those with acute school refusal behavior may display absenteeism for less than one year, whereas those with chronic school refusal behavior would do so for a longer period of time. However, it should be noted that many youngsters experience "self-corrective" school refusal behavior as well, or a remission of absenteeism within a two-week period. In addition, the classification of youngsters with school refusal behavior based on duration may have implications for determining length of treatment, but its utility for delineating a preferred therapeutic method for a particular case is unclear.

Given the muddied clinical picture usually obtained when organizing this population via symptomatology, recent attention has focused on evaluating the function of school refusal behavior. Kearney and Silverman (1990, 1993) proposed that children and adolescents refuse school for a variety of reasons, including (1) avoidance of stimuli that provoke negative affectivity (e.g., anxiety and depression), (2) escape from aversive social and/or evaluative situations (e.g., peer relationships, oral presentations), (3) attention (e.g., disruptive behavior to stay home with one's parents), and/or (4) positive tangible reinforcement (e.g., finding it more rewarding to be with friends outside rather than inside school). The first two functional conditions describe youngsters who refuse school for negative reinforcement, whereas the latter two describe those who refuse school for positive reinforcement.

Within this functional model, "school phobia" is conceptualized as a branch of the avoidance of negative affectivity dimension. Although few children and adolescents refuse school specifically because of fear of some circumscribed stimulus, a significant amount of research has focused on the assessment and treatment of these youngsters (Graziano and De Giovanni 1979). Subtypes of persons with school phobia most likely include those with a phobic, separation anxiety, and/or affective disorder (Bernstein and Garfinkel 1986, Last and Strauss 1990). Overall, the most complete and useful nosological strategy for persons with school refusal will likely involve the specification of discrete categories with flexible dimensions that allow for variability in behavior (see Kearney and Silverman 1995 for a more thorough discussion). Clinicians and researchers are urged to consider a synthesis of diagnostic-empirical and functional perspectives when conceptualizing this population.

ASSESSMENT PROCEDURES

The most important measurement for school refusal behavior has been and remains actual school attendance. Prior to 1980, however, many researchers also relied on case reports (e.g., Sperling 1967) or archival information (e.g., Waldron et al. 1975) to assess problematic absenteeism. Other authors employed unstructured diagnostic interviews (e.g., Cooper 1966) or rating scales (e.g., Berg and McGuire 1974) specially designed for their samples of youngsters with school refusal behavior. Unfortunately, the psychometric properties of these measures often were not reported.

In the years following the publication of *DSM-III* (*DSM* 1980), researchers of school refusal have tended to rely on a variety of behavioral assessment procedures that possess good reliability and validity. Three sets of illustrative studies are presented here. Granell de Aldaz and colleagues (1984, 1987) employed several child self-report (i.e., fear inventories) and parent/teacher measures (e.g., Child Behavior Checklist, Achenbach and Edelbrock 1983) to determine the prevalence and characteristics of school refusal behavior. Bernstein and Garfinkel (1986, 1988) similarly used a combination of structured and semistructured diagnostic interviews (i.e., Diagnostic Interview for Children and Adolescents, Herjanic and Campbell 1977, Family History Research Diagnostic Criteria, Endicott et al. 1975), child self-report measures (e.g., the Children's Depression Inventory, Kovacs and Beck 1977), and parent ratings of family interaction, personality, and adult diagnosis (i.e., the Family Assessment Measure, Skinner et al. 1983, MMPI, Hathaway and McKinley 1951, NIMH Diagnostic Interview Schedule, Robins et al. 1981) to evaluate youngsters with school phobia and their families. In addition, Last and colleagues (Last et al. 1987, Last and Strauss 1990) implemented the Interview Schedule for Children or the Kiddie-SADS (Puig-Antich and Ryan 1986) to diagnose youngsters with school phobia or refusal. Other measures of familial dynamics (i.e., the Self-Administered Dependency Questionnaire, Berg 1974) and fear/anxiety were also used.

In my work at the School Refusal Clinic at the University of Nevada, Las Vegas, a similar set of procedures is used. During the assessment process, youngsters are interviewed first and separately from their parents. This is done to promptly inform youths of their report's confidentiality (with exceptions, e.g., plans for suicide, running away) and importance equivalent to parental accounts. Such a practice is particularly important for a youngster with school refusal behavior because referral for treatment has likely been made after several authority figures (e.g., parents, school officials) have "targeted" the child as the primary antagonist of the situation. Often, however, treatment targets will more appropriately be the parents or the entire family.

The Anxiety Disorders Interview Schedule for Children (ADIS-C, Silverman and Eisen 1992, Silverman and Nelles 1988) is used to obtain general intake and diagnostic information. The ADIS-C is a semistructured interview designed to identify a variety of behavior problems but with a particular emphasis on anxiety disorders. In addition, the ADIS-C provides a section for school refusal behavior that allows a clinician considerable flexibility in assessing etiology, course, maintaining variables, and severity. The ADIS-C has been found to possess good reliability and validity, and requires approximately 30–60 minutes to complete. Following the interview with the child, the parent version of the ADIS-C is administered. As one party is questioned, the other is asked to separately complete several questionnaires.

The questionnaires utilized in my School Refusal Clinic are designed to assess a range of symptoms and conditions most closely related to school refusal, including fearfulness and negative affectivity, externalizing behaviors (e.g., noncompliance), and problematic family interaction. Specifically, the child is asked to complete the Fear Survey Schedule for Children-Revised (FSSC-R, Ollendick 1983), the Children's Manifest Anxiety Scale-Revised (CMAS-R, Reynolds and Paget 1983), the State-Trait Anxiety Inventory for Children (STAIC, Spielberger 1973), the Social Anxiety Scale for Children-Revised (SASC-R, La Greca and Stone 1993), the Daily Life Stressors Scale (DLSS, Kearney et al. 1993), the Children's Depression Inventory (CDI, Kovacs and Beck 1977), and the Piers-Harris Self-Concept Scale (PHSCS, Piers 1984). Obtaining information on reinforcing activities within the school setting and disruptive behaviors (e.g., via the Youth Self-Report, Achenbach 1991a) is also suggested. In addition, parents are asked to complete the Child Behavior Checklist (CBCL, Achenbach 1991b) and Family Environment Scale (FES, Moos and Moos 1986). Teachers, principals, or school counselors familiar with a particular case are asked to complete the Teacher Report Form (TRF, Achenbach 1991c).

Unfortunately, almost no assessment instruments have been developed specifically for persons with general school refusal behavior. An exception to this was provided by Kearney and Silverman (1993), who devised the School

Refusal Assessment Scale (SRAS). The SRAS is a sixteen-item instrument designed to measure the relative influence of four motivating conditions that serve to maintain absenteeism (i.e., avoidance of stimuli provoking negative affectivity, escape from aversive social/evaluative situations, attention, positive tangible reinforcement). The scale has shown good test-retest and interrater reliability as well as concurrent and construct validity. Similar child and parent versions of the SRAS have been developed. The SRAS is administered to both parties, after which item (four per functional condition) means across each version are calculated. The condition with the highest mean score is considered the primary motivating factor of the child's school refusal behavior. Tie or very closely related scores indicate that multiple functions may need to be addressed. Therefore, the SRAS comprises both categorical and dimensional properties. A primary function may be targeted initially, with other influential functions to be considered additionally as treatment progresses.

Finally, children and parents are asked to complete separate daily logbooks of negative affectivity, overt behavioral problems, and school attendance. The distribution and completion of logbooks serves several purposes, including the enhancement of self-monitoring and parent observation skills (often inadequate in this population), assessment of motivation and likely future compliance of each party, reemphasis that the child's input is highly valued, and, of course, a detailed account of treatment progress and areas of ongoing concern. Frequent contact with school officials is also recommended, particularly school psychologists, teachers, nurses, principals, guidance counselors, or others whose assistance may be crucial during the therapeutic process (e.g., librarians).

In general, the evaluation of school refusal behavior must encompass a variety of information sources to adequately ascertain what mechanisms maintain the problem and how treatment should be focused. The behavior's multifaceted nature mandates that an ongoing assessment process will be painstaking and surprising as new behaviors and avoidant tactics continue to emerge. In addition, given the fluid and crisislike atmosphere in which most cases of school refusal behavior are initially presented, clinicians are encouraged to maintain near-daily contact with children, parents, and school officials.

ESTABLISHING TREATMENT GOALS

As one might expect, when parents of children with school refusal behavior are asked to identify a treatment goal, most choose the resumption of their child's regular attendance. Concurrently, however, many wish for a decrease in their child's negative affectivity and noncompliance and an increase in his/her appropriate social and familial contact. When youngsters with school refusal behavior are asked to identify a treatment goal, most are evasive (i.e., those who wish to maintain the status quo) or choose a reduction in anxiety/depression and/or parental harassment. As a result, I define the primary treatment goal to be a 2-week period of full-time school attendance (excluding legitimate physical illness) without significant levels of distress (or a 75 percent reduction from baseline). Secondary treatment goals usually consist of reducing concurrent problems such as familial conflict and/or increasing desirable behaviors such as extracurricular school activities.

While the goal of treatment for school refusal behavior is often clear, the focus of treatment often is not. Berecz (1980) noted that, across different perspectives of school refusal behavior (e.g., family systems, psychodynamic, behavioral), the focus of treatment often fluctuates between the child, one or both parents, or a combination of these. Unfortunately, a consensus has not been reached as to which party should be targeted for a particular case. As a result, many clinicians likely employ a universal, self-formulated treatment focus for youngsters with school refusal behavior.

Recent research indicates that the focus of treatment could be assigned from knowledge about the function of school refusal behavior and/or current familial interaction patterns. Kearney and Silverman (1990) and Kearney (1992) reported on several cases indicating that the successful treatment of school refusal behavior could be accomplished by tailoring specific therapeutic procedures and foci to specific functions. For example, a child who refuses school to avoid stimuli provoking negative affectivity or aversive social/evaluative situations may require therapy that centers primarily on his/her physiological anxiety or maladaptive thought patterns. For a young child who refuses school for attention, the treatment focus would likely be the parent(s), in which case contingency management procedures could be implemented. For an older child or adolescent who refuses school for positive tangible reinforcement, contracting among all relevant family members may be most beneficial.

Therapists should also consider ongoing familial interaction patterns when making decisions about treatment focus. Data from previous literature (e.g., Mihara and Ichikawa 1986, Remschmidt and Mattejat 1990, Waldron et al. 1975, Weiss and Cain 1964) support the notion that several familial subtypes are characteristic of this population. These include enmeshed, conflictive, detached, isolated, and healthy kinships. Enmeshed families exemplify the conceptualization of school refusal behavior as separation anxiety, in which case clinicians may wish to increase distance between a specific parent and child across several situations. Conflictive and detached families typically involve all family members, so the focus here might be more general. Isolated families, particularly those who resist services to treat a child's absenteeism, may initially require support and encouragement directed toward parents to maintain therapy attendance. Healthy families may display little dysfunctional interaction, yet have a child with a circumscribed problem who would represent the primary focus of treatment. Among other variables, clinicians may wish to consider function and family interaction pattern when differentially assigning treatment focus across cases of school refusal behavior (Kearney and Silverman, in press).

ROLE OF THE THERAPIST

A special challenge to therapists who provide services for youngsters with school refusal behavior is the multiple roles they will be asked to play during the course of assessment and treatment. The primary role, of course, is that of clinician whose choice of technique should enhance school attendance with minimal levels of distress. Because of the arduous nature of the problem, however, therapists in this area should expect to spend a fair amount of time outside the office providing support to family members. This is particularly so during early morning hours and on school days following weekends or holidays (Blagg and Yule 1984). Therapists should note that parents of children with school refusal behavior often require considerable encouragement as well, particularly when they believe that school attendance will aggravate somatic complaints or emotional distress and lead to long-term psychological harm. Also, in some cases, early intervention may be required to resolve marital conflict (Wetchler 1986), a situation often exacerbated by the child's school refusal behavior or one that emerges near the conclusion of the problem.

Another key role played by clinicians in this area is liaison with school officials (Want 1983). Cooperation with psychologists, counselors, teachers, principals, and nurses is essential and will often "make or break" a case. This is particularly true for children who refuse school for negative reinforcement and whose therapy often relies on requests for schedule restructuring, gradual transition from one setting (e.g., nurse's office, library) to the classroom, teacher monitoring of attendance and implementation of behavioral contingencies, and extra time for the child to practice relaxation exercises, receive medication, and/or use the telephone. Supportive psychotherapy and cooperation with school officials often form the basis for the successful treatment of school refusal behavior (e.g., Cooper 1973).

TREATMENT STRATEGIES

Treatment techniques for children and adolescents with school refusal behavior are almost as heterogeneous as the youngsters themselves. Over the past several decades, a variety of tactics from different perspectives have been proposed with different degrees of success. An essential difficulty has been to pinpoint one therapeutic strategy that is effective for most persons with school refusal behavior. This section outlines some primary interventions reported in the literature as well as recommendations for designing a prescriptive approach to address this population.

Among the early psychodynamicists who initially described school refusal behavior as a "phobia" or "separation anxiety," suggested treatment generally involved increasing parent–child distance and providing therapy services for the mother (e.g., Johnson et al. 1941, Rodriguez et al. 1959). With respect to the latter, interventions were designed to modify the mother's repressed hostility, ambivalent emotions, and/or an enmeshed relationship with the child that resulted in erratic school attendance and mutual dependency, guilt, and anger (Coolidge et al. 1957, Frick 1964, Suttenfield 1954). Leventhal and colleagues (1964, 1967) postulated that children with school phobia have a tendency to overestimate their value and possess an unrealistically expanded self-image. Such narcissism is then threatened by events at school (e.g., tests, peer relationships), resulting in an avoidance of the situation with parental indulgence. Suggested treatment included reality testing to modify the child's self-image, decreased privileges at home, and the acquisition of improved social and academic skills. Unfortunately, little empirical data were given to support the efficacy of these interventions.

With the advent of the behavioral approach to clinical psychology, the treatment of children with school refusal behavior (specifically, school phobia) via systematic desensitization became popular. Systematic desensitization, a procedure based on classical conditioning, involves relaxation training, the construction of an anxiety hierarchy, and the association of relaxation with each item on the hierarchy. The procedure was introduced to cases of school phobia by several researchers, including Lazarus and colleagues (1965) who employed in vivo desensitization and a token economy to reduce acute school refusal behavior in a 9-year-old boy. Desensitization procedures were subsequently used to reduce school refusal-related behaviors such as fears of specific stimuli and academic failure as well as speech, separation, and test anxiety (e.g., Johnson et al. 1971, Miller 1972, O'Reilly 1971, Parish et al. 1976, Smith and Sharpe 1970).

Concurrent with the advent of child-focused systematic desensitization was the implementation of a forced school attendance approach suggested by earlier researchers (e.g., Klein 1945). Kennedy (1965) addressed youngsters with "Type I" school phobia, or those with acute absenteeism and characteristic symptoms such as fear and separation anxiety. Parents were instructed to downplay somatic complaints, bring the child to school using "any force necessary" (p. 288), and provide reinforcement for school attendance at night. Exposure to the school setting almost immediately after the onset of school refusal behavior resulted in a 100 percent remission rate. Because most initial absences are temporary and nonproblematic (Hersov 1985), however, it should be noted that Kennedy (1965) may have been addressing youngsters with "self-corrective" school refusal behavior. Still, for instances of new and brief absenteeism, a forced school attendance approach is highly effective.

In addition, a focus on the pharmacotherapy and inpatient treatment of school refusal behavior soon followed. For example, Gittelman-Klein and Klein (1971) treated youngsters with school refusal behavior with either the antidepressant medication imipramine or placebo. After six weeks, 81 percent of the imipramine group had returned to school compared with 47 percent of the placebo group. More recently, Bernstein and colleagues (1990) compared the anxiolytic alprazolam and antidepressant imipramine with placebo in the treatment of twenty-four youngsters with acute school phobia. Those receiving medication showed some improvement in anxiety and depression compared with the placebo group, but improvement in attendance rates were similar across subjects. These studies indicate that the resolution of anxiety *and* depression, particularly in adolescents, is often instrumental for reducing school refusal behavior.

With respect to inpatient/residential treatment, two informative studies are presented here. Berg and Fielding (1978) evaluated thirty-two adolescents with chronic school refusal behavior placed on an inpatient psychiatric unit (Monday through Friday) for a 3- or 6-month period. Treatment consisted of school attendance on the unit, social skills training, and family and supportive-milieu therapy. At 1-year follow-up, 53.1 percent of the sample were rated as well or much improved with respect to symptoms such as fearfulness and social isolation. Longer stays were particularly helpful for girls. Church and Edwards (1984) similarly described a 3- to 18-month inpatient educational treatment program for thirty-five youngsters with severe school refusal behavior. All children under age 13 were successfully integrated into a regular classroom setting, compared with only 25 percent of those over age 13. Degree of parental support was highly predictive of successful integration. These studies illustrate the difficulty of treating persons with chronic school refusal behavior and the importance of resolving the problem at an early stage.

Recent attempts to treat youngsters with school refusal behavior have relied on an individualized approach where various therapies are assigned on a prescriptive, case-by-case basis. For example, Blagg and Yule (1984) evaluated sixty-six youngsters with school refusal behavior. Thirty received behavior therapy consisting of contingency management and in vivo flooding, sixteen were hospitalized and received milieu, educational, occupational, and drug therapy, and twenty received home tuition and outpatient psychotherapy. Full-time school attendance at 1-year follow-up was significantly higher for the behavior therapy group (93.3 precent) compared with the inpatient (37.5 percent) and home tuition (10 percent) groups. Kearney and Silverman (1990) provided preliminary evidence for a prescriptive treatment approach based on the function of school refusal behavior. Youngsters of a particular functional condition (i.e., avoidance of stimuli provoking negative affectivity, escape from aversive social/evaluative situations, attention, positive tangible reinforcement) received systematic desensitization/gradual exposure to the school setting, cognitive therapy/modeling/role-play, parent training, and family contingency contracting, respectively. Results indicated moderate to good improvement in school attendance and related problems such as anxiety and noncompliance.

Given the heterogeneity of this population, clinicians are encouraged to consider the prescriptive assignment of therapy for school refusal behavior. In brief cases of first-time absenteeism, a rapid return to school often reduces the problem quickly and establishes firm parental control. In cases of sporadic or acute school refusal behavior, a short-term, intensive treatment strategy based on function or diagnosis is recommended. In cases of chronic (longer than one year) or extremely severe (longer than two years) school refusal behavior, inpatient/residential treatment, alternative or part-time school enrollment, or home-based tutoring will likely be necessary.

DEALING WITH COMMON OBSTACLES TO SUCCESSFUL TREATMENT

Obstacles to the successful treatment of school refusal behavior will occur as often during the screening and initial assessment process as during therapy itself. The most common problems associated with treating this population are poor family attendance or hostility from one or more members, noncompliance with assigned procedures (e.g., completion of logbooks), child and/or parent depression, marital conflict, and long-term or mixed profile school refusal behavior (where a child refuses school for multiple reasons or with multiple behavior problems or diagnoses). The importance of developing adequate cooperation from school officials was discussed earlier. This section will discuss each obstacle individually.

An ironic aspect of assessing persons with school refusal behavior is that clinicians often never see their clients. Following the initial screening and scheduling of a particular family, the likelihood of cancellation or "no-show" is approximately 25–40 percent (worse as the school year progresses; Kearney and Silverman 1995). Part of this is due to the high spontaneous remission rate characteristic of children with school refusal behavior, and part is the parents' inability to bring the child to the assessment session. In the former case, clinicians are encouraged to inform their clients that a recurrence of school refusal behavior may follow a weekend or extended holiday or change in the child's school routine. In some instances, a sudden rescheduling of the assessment session is necessary. In cases where a family member refuses to attend the assessment session, clinicians are urged to contact the reluctant party and assuage what fears he/she may have. For example, fathers associated with this population are often concerned that they will be blamed for a lack of discipline, whereas adolescents are sometimes upset at the prospect of having to interact with another authority figure (e.g., Rubenstein and Hastings 1980). In these or related cases, clinicians should emphasize themes of acceptance, confidentiality, and willingness to address all points of view. For many persons, this will be sufficient to ensure initial attendance.

During the assessment session itself, common problems are exaggerated accounts of misbehavior about one party as reported by another as well as vague descriptions of behavior. Parents, for example, are often accurate about a child's rate of attendance but misidentify the child's level of discomfort associated with school refusal behavior (e.g., Mansdorf and Lukens, 1987). Youngsters are often accurate about what specific school-related stimuli upset them, but are unable to pinpoint their primary emotion (e.g., depression, panic, anxiety, fear; Friesen 1985). Children are also particularly likely to embellish accounts of parent and teacher harassment (Brulle et al. 1985). Because of the volatile and critical nature of school refusal behavior, clinicians should be aware that family members often amplify the severity and potential consequences of behavior to align themselves with the therapist. A low-key, empathetic, but directive approach during the assessment process often improves this situation.

Following assessment, a primary problem is resistance to the completion of daily logbooks or implementation of recommended treatment procedures (Green 1985). This problem is particularly acute among isolated and detached families who may have a history of inadequate parental monitoring and reciprocal reinforcement. Compliance problems may also indicate a lack of motivation to resolve the school refusal behavior or difficulty understanding ongoing assessments or treatment ingredients. Each possibility should be examined at length. Of particular concern are family members who enthusiastically embrace and subsequently fail to implement an intersession plan of attack. In such cases, clinicians should contact recalcitrant family members on a daily basis to provide encouragement, modify the treatment plan (e.g., a contract) if too difficult, and/or address reasons for noncompliance (e.g., new somatic complaints).

Other problems that can occur at any point of contact with the family are depression and possible suicidal/self-mutilative behavior and marital conflict. With respect to the former, it is not uncommon for school refusal, depression, and related harmful behaviors to be comorbid in nature (Knox 1989). However, such difficulties tend to slow the rate of return to school by expanding treatment goals and foci. For example, an adolescent who refuses school because of difficulty making friends and subsequent depression will require more intensive therapy than one fearful of oral presentations without depression. In many cases, antidepressant medication or inpatient treatment may be necessary before regular school attendance can be sought. Parental psychopathology may also interfere with the design and implementation of therapeutic procedures (Jackson and Sikora 1992) and should be assessed as well.

With respect to marital conflict, it was mentioned earlier that this problem tends to surface near the beginning of an assessment procedure (when parents attempt to blame one another for the child's nonattendance) and/or near the resolution of the behavioral problem (when previous conflicts reemerge following their suppression during treatment). The former is particularly problematic for designing treatment strategies in younger children because parents must provide behavioral contingencies on a regular, unified, and consistent basis (Hsia 1984). Alignment of one parent and the child against the other parent is also damaging to the treatment of adolescent school refusal behavior, where many teens exploit parental permissiveness. In cases where marital conflict appears near the end of treatment, relapse rates are common. For example, a child may have refused school to divert parental attention away from ongoing conflict (Rubenstein and Hastings 1980). With the resolution of the behavioral problem, the parents may resume old disagreements and the child his/her school refusal behavior. As a result, clinicians are urged to closely monitor the presence of spousal conflict, emphasize the importance of uniformity when addressing school refusal behavior, and provide resources for marital therapy when appropriate.

Other obstacles to treatment involve the duration and profile of school refusal behavior. In general, the longer a child is out of school, the more difficult it will be to reinstitute regular classroom attendance (e.g., McDonald and Sheperd 1976). This is due to a variety of factors including the child's anxiety about facing new teachers, peers, school buildings, and class schedules, parents' pessimism regarding the success of reintegration, and potential lack of school resources for providing part-time educational services. With respect to the profile of school refusal behavior, treatment success is likely to be enhanced when the child presents with a singular diagnosis or function. For example, a youngster who displays a circumscribed fear of one school-related stimulus will likely be treated with systematic desensitization more quickly and successfully than one who presents with multiple phobias and types of avoidance (Taylor and Adelman 1990). Similarly, youngsters with mixed functional profiles, such as those who initially avoid school because of negative affectivity and subsequently discover the positive amenities of staying home, will be more resistant to resumed school attendance than those refusing school for one reason. Obstacles to treating school refusal behavior are manifold, but an assessment-intervention approach that additionally focuses on familial attendance and conflict, compliance with evaluative and therapeutic procedures, comorbid behavior problems, and all relevant maintaining variables will serve to alleviate most difficulties.

RELAPSE PREVENTION

Several researchers have indicated that the successful treatment of acute school refusal behavior often results in good long-term functioning (e.g., Berg et al. 1976, Timberlake 1984, Valles and Oddy 1984). However, it is not unusual for minor relapses to occur throughout the school year, particularly following long weekends or extended vacations. Also, some youngsters will occasionally test their parents' resolve to effectively handle school refusal behavior without the immediate assistance of the therapist. Following the termination of a case at my clinic, regular (e.g., twice per month for three months) telephone contact is maintained with the child, parents, and

sometimes school officials to monitor school attendance and distress. In addition, a six-month follow-up of questionnaires and direct contact with family members is conducted to discuss progress and new issues that may contribute to relapse (e.g., schedule changes, academic problems). Parents are also instructed to contact the therapist at any time should school attendance threaten to become problematic or related problems arise.

A crucial time for the therapist to engage in relapse prevention is the onset of a new school year (Ollendick and Mayer 1984). Many children find it difficult to cope with changing social and academic scenarios, especially when advancing to a separate school building (e.g., junior, senior high). Clinicians may wish to provide booster sessions during the summer months to reinforce the efficacy of previous treatment techniques for children (e.g., relaxation training, cognitive restructuring, role-play) and parents (e.g., contracting, contingency management). In addition, many children find it comforting and preparatory to explore the school building prior to the onset of classes. Of special interest are the location of lockers, specific classrooms, cafeteria, libraries, gymnasiums, main and guidance offices, exits, and settings for getting on/off the school bus. Because youngsters with previous school refusal behavior often fear getting lost and looking foolish, such a practice serves to diminish anticipatory anxiety, increase self-efficacy, and prevent relapse.

For youngsters with chronic or extremely severe school refusal behavior, relapse prevention is quite challenging. In general, follow-up of such cases will need to be more frequent, intensive, and encompassing than that usual required for acute school refusal behavior. Relapse prevention in chror cases is likely to depend on several additional variables, including redu familial conflict, modification of parental attitudes, child participation extracurricular activities and appropriate social contact, continued mot tion to attend school, decreased oppositional and conduct problems, maintenance of medical interventions if applicable (e.g., Baker and 1978, Berg and Jackson 1985, Berg et al. 1969, Cooper 1986).

Finally, because youngsters with chronic school refusal behavic often placed into alternative or part-time curricular programs, clin should be aware of upcoming changes that may interrupt attendance. example, a school with financial difficulties was forced to elimin after-school program, then the arrangement of multiple scenarios cruing necessary graduation credits would be beneficial. In addition, sources for related problems (e.g., substance abuse) should be pr Overall, relapse prevention for youngsters with school refusal behav depend on a close monitoring of attendance and related behavior for es

several months. A strong relationship between parents and school officials (e.g., teachers, attendance officers) is also encouraged so that difficulties may be identified and addressed early.

TERMINATION

As mentioned earlier, a recommended criterion for considering the termination of a circumscribed case of school refusal behavior is full-time school attendance for at least two weeks and/or a significant reduction in negative affectivity when going to school. In cases where the child's school refusal is comorbid with externalizing problems (e.g., stealing, aggression), the focus and length of treatment may change and extend the time to termination. In either instance, however, the end of therapy may occur soon after the initial assessment session or up to several months later. Such differences in length will influence the level of therapist-client attachment, an issue that should be addressed prior to termination.

In cases involving adolescents, severe levels of negative affectivity, and/or chronic school refusal behavior, severing the therapist-client relationship can be particularly difficult. With the development of a clear treatment goal following initial assessment, parents and children should be informed that termination will likely occur following the resumption of school attendance. An early introduction to the topic with regular reminders (Thompson and Rudolph 1988) may serve to smooth the transition from therapy-guided school attendance to a more independent status. Difficulty ending a therapeutic relationship in this population is also acute in cases, especially single-parent cases, where dependency toward the therapist has developed (Weiner 1992). Such issues, if applicable, should be addressed intermittently during the therapeutic relationship.

An important aspect of treatment that should precede termination is the presentation of sample problems that clients may face in the future (e.g., Braswell and Kendall 1988). Measurement of the client's response to these hypothetical scenarios should provide some indication of treatment progress as well as steps toward generalization and relapse prevention. For example, youngsters who had refused school to avoid stimuli provoking negative affectivity could be asked to identify muscle groups likely to be tense in a given stressful situation, demonstrate relaxation techniques, and/or provide solutions when feeling uncomfortable in settings like waiting for the school bus or standing in line for lunch. Youngsters who had refused school to escape aversive social/evaluative situations might be required to identify

potential cognitive distortions when speaking with a particular person and create alternative, positive thoughts. Exposure to new social situations could also be practiced via role-play.

Similarly, such scenarios could be created for parents or the entire family. For example, parents trained in contingency management may be asked to develop strategies for reinforcing appropriate and extinguishing inappropriate behavior when faced with a new problem (e.g., exaggerated somatic complaints). Parents and children could also be presented with a sample problem and asked to develop a contract or practice communication skills. In each case, clinicians are encouraged to provide several problems that vary in type, degree, severity, and frequency. Relapses or inadequate responses to sample problems should be discussed at length.

When the time to end treatment is at hand, clinicians may wish to re-administer pretreatment assessment measures to confirm areas of progress. Inconsistencies between questionnaire data and verbal reports should be explored in detail. Family members should be advised to contact the therapist should any further school refusal behaviors surface. In addition, referral to other agencies specializing in severe behaviors related to school refusal (e.g., substance abuse, suicidal ideation, running away) may need to be considered.

CASE ILLUSTRATION (TYPICAL TREATMENT)

Description and History

Eric was a 12-year-old white male referred by a school psychologist and his parents for acute school refusal behavior. Upon entering seventh-grade and a new school building, Eric began to experience a variety of aversive symptoms such as hyperventilation, anxiety, sad mood, and somatic complaints. Although school attendance was not problematic initially, Eric began to report severe headaches in the morning prior to school in mid-September. School attendance then became intermittent. By late September, Eric's aversiveness toward school had worsened and he was staying home on most days. Following several discussions with his parents, Eric was allowed to stay home on a regular basis starting the first week of October.

During an initial interview, Eric appeared moderately tense but also cooperative and verbal. His appearance was somewhat disheveled but his communicative behavior (e.g., eye contact, extended answers) and demeanor were appropriate and pleasant. Eric reported a substantial amount of anticipatory anxiety prior to the beginning of the school year. Much of this was due to his placement in a new building that did not include several of his closest friends from elementary school. In addition, Eric expressed anxiety over meeting new people, moving from class to class, assignments for one course involving public speaking, being late to class, and physical education. With respect to the latter, Eric reported some discomfort with contact sports and a concern over the possibility of getting into fights. He half-heartedly indicated a desire to return to school but only after changes were made in his school schedule (e.g., no English or physical education courses).

Questionnaire data largely confirmed Eric's verbal report. School Refusal Assessment Scale data indicated Eric to be refusing school primarily to escape aversive social/evaluative situations and secondarily to receive attention from his parents. Because Eric's negative affectivity and avoidance of social situations was specific only to school, and because he was not specifically fearful of one particular stimulus, no diagnosis of social/specific phobia was assigned. However, Eric did meet criteria for overanxious disorder.

Eric's parents tended to concentrate more on their son's tendency to challenge their authority. Within the past several weeks, Eric had reportedly become more noncompliant, sullen, and withdrawn from family interaction. This behavior did not seem to affect his close peer relationships, however. Eric's parents indicated that a significant amount of attention was directed toward their son's absenteeism and his mother was considering quitting work to stay home to tutor Eric. Parent questionnaire and School Refusal Assessment Scale data were similar to Eric's report, although attention-getting and externalizing behaviors were emphasized. A diagnosis of overanxious disorder was confirmed.

Conversations with Eric's teachers indicated that the adolescent was timid though likeable in new social situations, but quite averse to assignments that would require him to perform in front of others (e.g., writing, shooting baskets). They reported as well Eric's frequent complaints of headaches and wishes to attend the nurse's office. The nurse stated that Eric displayed no serious symptoms (e.g., fever, vomiting) but that encouragement to return to class was usually ineffective. All indicated a desire to comply with future treatment procedures. Following consultation with the family, specific treatment components with gradual reintroduction to a full-time class schedule were approved. Family members were asked to complete daily logbooks providing ratings of negative affectivity and school attendance.

Synopsis of Therapy Sessions

The treatment of school refusal behavior is likely to be an intensive process that may last days to months. As a result, treatment protocols must be specific enough to deal with circumscribed problems but flexible enough to be useful as a long-term strategy. When a treatment protocol was implemented for this case based on the function of school refusal behavior, the primary interventions were cognitive therapy and modeling/role-play (although it should be noted that contingency management procedures were conducted secondarily). Such a protocol is briefly outlined here on a session-by-session basis.

Session 1

1. Review the completed baseline parent and child logbooks, discussing issues of compliance, problems, or questions (repeated each session).
2. Meet with the child, outline the expected course of therapy. Explain the concept of cognitive restructuring (e.g., substituting positive, rational thoughts for negative, catastrophic ones) and modeling/role-play (e.g., practicing various social interactions with therapist feedback and homework assignments). Introduce how and when the techniques will be used for that particular child.
3. Create an aversive social/evaluative situation hierarchy with the child. Identify ten specific interactions that are most problematic (e.g., speaking in front of a class, meeting someone for the first time, getting lost at school). Rank the interactions from most to least anxiety-provoking. Assign a Subjective Units of Distress Scale (SUDS, Wolpe 1982) score of 0–100 for each.
4. Choose one situation from each of the top, middle, and bottom sections of the hierarchy. Detail problematic and nonproblematic cognitions that occur for each. Identify specific cognitive errors (e.g., overgeneralization, dichotomous thinking, centering). Ask the youngster to practice identifying such errors by maintaining a mental and written record.
5. Outline a schedule for gradually reintegrating the child into school. Solicit feedback from all family members. Preferably, part-time school attendance should begin in 1 week. Between sessions, contact with school officials should be maintained to sanction, coordinate, and/or modify the reintegration.

Session 2

1. Review homework assignments with the child (e.g., identifying negative cognitive distortions and new problematic social interactions). Review the concepts of cognitive therapy and modeling/role-play (repeated each session).
2. Identify a mildly aversive social situation and accompanying negative cognitive distortions. Introduce cognitive techniques to counter irrational or negativistic thinking (e.g., hypothesis testing, thought-stopping, decentering).
3. Discuss specific irrational or negative thoughts/worries and their specific counters or substitutions. Example:

> Client: I know when I stand up in front of the class everyone will laugh at me.
> Therapist: Really? Do you think even your friends and the teacher will laugh?
> Client: No, but some people will.
> Therapist: Has anyone ever laughed at you before when giving a speech?
> Client: No.
> Therapist: That's good. Let's look at what you just said. Your first thought was that everyone would laugh, but when we really looked at that, it wasn't true. Then, a second thought you had was that some people would laugh, but we know that hasn't happened before and you can't be sure it will happen in the future. What might be a better way to think about what could happen?
> Client: Some people might say things, but I don't think my friends will.
> Therapist: Great! By saying "might," you're opening up to more possibilities.

4. Introduce symbolic or participant modeling procedures to practice aversive situations like public speaking. Provide feedback where appropriate and assign homework assignments to practice in real-life settings.
5. If possible, finalize plans to reintegrate the child into a part-time school schedule that is not highly stressful (e.g., non-public-speaking classes, lunch). Maintain frequent contact between sessions with the child, parents, and school officials.

Session 3

1. Assess the homework assignments and current successes and/or problems of school attendance (repeated each session).
2. Role-play again the situation discussed previously. If the child reports feeling comfortable with this situation in and outside the office, then advance to the next aversive social/evaluative situation on the hierarchy. Concentrate on those currently most problematic for full-time school attendance. Introduce countering techniques and positive self-statements where appropriate.
3. Discuss a revised class schedule that includes integration into more diverse classes and extracurricular settings.

Sessions 4 +

1. Generally repeat instructions for Sessions 1–3. Make modifications as necessary and introduce contingency management procedures if applicable. Prompt the child to increasingly provide his/her own solutions to hypothesized social/evaluative scenarios.
2. Continue to maintain contact with school officials regarding the child's attendance, level of distress, and academic performance.
3. Discuss issues related to termination where appropriate.
4. When applicable, schedule posttreatment, follow-up, and relapse prevention sessions. Provide referrals to alternative agencies if necessary.

Following four months of intensive therapy utilizing these procedures, Eric resumed full-time school attendance. In the meantime, his level of noncompliance and social anxiety had diminished considerably, and he was able to participate in several academic and athletic events at school. Eric's parents reported that Eric still exaggerated about somatic symptoms occasionally, but indicated that lessened attention usually decreased such exaggerations. In addition, Eric's parents stated that their son continued to be somewhat withdrawn from family members, and structural family therapy was recommended to address this and related problems (e.g., increased conflict). At 6-month follow-up, however, Eric's school attendance was not problematic.

Comments

This protocol outlines an approach that combines specific therapeutic procedures with a gradual reintroduction to full-time school attendance. It should be noted, of course, that the latter will vary widely from client to client. Some will require little therapy before attempting school attendance, some will begin a part-time schedule almost immediately before resisting the addition of classes, and some will delay any school attendance for long periods of time. In a survey of clinicians who recently treated cases of school refusal behavior (Kearney and Beasley 1994), 12.9 percent reported success within one month, 34.6 percent in one to three months, 22.4 percent in four to six months, 18.4 percent in seven to twelve months, 8.4 percent in thirteen months to two years, and 3.4 percent in longer than two years.

In addition, the protocol outlined above was designed to address the primary function of Eric's school refusal behavior, that is, escape from aversive social/evaluative situations. However, a relatively strong secondary function was attention. In approximately one-quarter of cases of school refusal behavior, a youngster displays absenteeism for two or more reasons (Kearney et al. 1989). In Eric's case, the implementation of contingency management procedures may have increased the efficacy of treatment across time. Clinicians must decide, however, when and to what extent additional therapeutic components will be necessary for a particular client.

Finally, it should be noted that the implementation of cognitive restructuring and modeling/role-play for the case presented here was largely possible given the client's age (12 years). For younger children, an emphasis on positive self-statements and modeling may be more effective given their cognitive functioning. Conversely, older adolescents, particularly those with depression, may respond better to intensive cognitive therapy. The consideration of a client's developmental status during treatment design will likely enhance therapeutic efficacy for this population.

CASE ILLUSTRATION (OVERCOMING OBSTACLES)

Description and History

Linda was a 15-year-old white female referred by her school principal and parents for chronic and severe school refusal behavior. After failing to attend school for most of the previous year (ninth grade) and attain any academic credits toward graduation, Linda displayed similar problems during the current academic year. At the time of her referral in early January, Linda had attended only two weeks of school, that is, the first week of each fall marking period. During days that Linda was supposed to be in school, she generally slept late, watched television, visited with friends who were also missing school, or talked on the telephone.

Following several discussions with school officials and a threat of court action, Linda's parents scheduled the initial assessment session.

During the interview, Linda appeared relaxed but her affect was restricted and her voice monotonal. In addition, her answers and discussion were usually limited to one short sentence at a time. Linda reported feeling depressed and "moody," particularly when the subject of resumed school attendance was discussed. She indicated that her initial school refusal behavior had been motivated by a desire to stay home or be with her friends during the course of the day. Because her parents did not intervene quickly to end the absenteeism, Linda was able to avoid school for extended periods of time. After several weeks, however, she became anxious and depressed at the prospect of having to return to school and face new peers, teachers, and class schedule. She wished to return to school and graduate, but did not feel she could do so on a full-time basis.

Questionnaire data provided more insight into Linda's negative affectivity. She scored near the clinical range on the Children's Depression Inventory (Kovacs and Beck 1977) and very high on fear/anxiety items related to moving about school and potential somatic complaints. School Refusal Assessment Scale data indicated a mixed functional profile of absenteeism, that is, avoidance of stimuli provoking negative affectivity and positive tangible reinforcement. Because Linda's school refusal behavior was her only substantial difficulty, no clinical diagnosis (e.g., conduct disorder) was applicable.

Linda's parents emphasized their daughter's intransigence about returning to school and how school personnel had exacerbated the situation (e.g., failing to notify them of nonattendance, threatening legal action). Linda's mother was particularly adamant about these points whereas her father was passive and withdrawn. Neither was able to provide much insight into Linda's psychological or behavioral functioning, and neither had previously initiated any consistent strategy for returning her to school. Degree of intrafamilial contact was described as poor. Parent School Refusal Assessment Scale data indicated the function of absenteeism to be positive tangible reinforcement. No clinical diagnosis was supported.

Conversations with school officials were not highly informative given their lack of contact with Linda. Instead, data were collected regarding alternative school programs that Linda might be eligible for and enroll in at any time. These included a part-time after-school program, an alternative high school with courses in the afternoon and early evening, and a tutorial that included home-based and supervised in-school laboratory work. Following consultation with the family, a treatment program of contracting and relaxation training with reintegration into a modified school setting was approved. Daily logbooks were assigned as well.

Synopsis of Therapy Sessions

The treatment of chronic school refusal behavior, as noted earlier, presents a special challenge to clinicians because of the many obstacles involved. Obstacles in this case include (1) the equivalent influence of two school refusal behavior functions, i.e., avoidance of stimuli provoking negative affectivity/fear and positive tangible reinforcement, and (2) poor intrafamilial contact. Therefore, primary treatment components should be administered concurrently and procedures for improving communication skills (e.g., Foster and Robin 1989) may be pursued. Such a protocol is briefly outlined here in stages.

Stage 1

1. Review the completed baseline parent and child logbooks, discussing issues of compliance, problems, or questions (repeated each session).
2. Outline the expected course of therapy to the child. Explain relaxation training (e.g., a tension-release system focusing on different muscle groups, Jacobsen 1938) and graduated imaginal and in vivo exposure to new stimuli. Discuss how and when the techniques will be used for that particular child.
3. Introduce the relaxation procedure and proceed with the tension and release of hands, arms, shoulders, face, stomach, legs, and feet. Audiotape and give a copy to the child. Outline a schedule for practice (e.g., once per morning and evening) and ask the child to identify specific muscle groups that are tense in different school-related situations. Create an exposure hierarchy.
4. Outline the concept of contracting to the family, that is, negotiating agreements between parties to increase rewards for school attendance and decrease rewards (or increase punishers) for nonattendance. Ask each party to list desired changes in another party in specific and realistic terms.
5. Meet with the family to create a sample contract initially targeting a minor activity (e.g., financial reward for a chore). Have all family

members read and sign the contract after confirming it is one they fully understand and accept.

6. Outline a schedule for reintegrating the child into school. A meeting with the child, parents, and school officials is desirable to outline options for full- or part-time attendance and/or school district assessment if necessary.

Stage 2

1. Discuss compliance, difficulties, and questions regarding relaxation training with the child. Proceed with relaxation training while the child imagines different scenes from the anxiety hierarchy. If appropriate, describe scenes that are mildly to moderately anxiety-provoking. Instruct the child to practice.

2. Review compliance, difficulties, and questions regarding the sample contract with all family members, making modifications where necessary. When successful, positively reward compliance and create a new contract that incorporates other behaviors and reinforcers. Include provisions from the original contract if applicable and reissue the revised contract.

3. With the contracting procedure, build communication among family members by encouraging a discussion of disagreements. Provide each with uninterrupted time to speak; followed by response from the "targeted" party. Disallow name-calling and focus on procedures that enhance comprehension (e.g., reframing, problem solving). Assign homework (e.g., initiating conversations).

4. Continue to meet with school officials to outline an agenda for gradual school attendance.

Stage 3

1. With respect to the relaxation training procedure, continue imaginal exposure but with items provoking severe anxiety.

2. With respect to the contracting procedure, incorporate aspects of school attendance where applicable. Example:

Therapist: I think now we may like to add Linda's attendance to the contract.

Father: I don't feel comfortable giving her payment for going to school, something she should be doing anyway.

Therapist: That's an understandable point. What if we required initial school attendance for the opportunity to do chores to make money?

Client: You mean if I go to school, I can still make money?

Therapist: Let's put it this way. If you go to school, you earn the privilege of doing some additional chores like cleaning the garage or vacuuming the house for a set amount. If you miss school, though, then you would still have to do your regular chores but without payment. How about that?

Client: That sounds okay, but I want to know exactly what I have to do.

Mother: It sounds okay to me too, but I want her to understand that she will have increased responsibilities when not in school.

Therapist: Those sound like reasonable requests. Let's discuss the details.

3. Issue a new contract and assign homework where applicable. Continue contact with school officials to finalize plans for reintegration.

Stage 4

1. Generally repeat instructions for Stages 1–3. Prompt the child to provide her own solutions to hypothesized fear/anxiety-provoking scenarios. With the advent of school attendance, begin in vivo desensitization.

2. Provide a class schedule that includes integration into basic classes and some extracurricular activities. Engage in frequent monitoring of the child's behavior in preparing for school and any accompanying distress.

3. Continue to maintain contact with school officials regarding the child's attendance, level of distress, and academic performance. Discuss issues related to termination and schedule posttreatment, follow-up, and relapse prevention sessions. Provide referrals to alternative agencies if necessary.

Following four months of sometimes sporadically scheduled therapy, Linda was able to resume school attendance in a special program where she received credit for mathematics, social studies, and reading. Other credits were to be completed during the next summer session. Linda reportedly felt less fearful and "pressured," although she occasionally tried to coerce her parents into letting her stay home. For example, she made several attempts during the next four months to sabotage the changes made during treatment by engaging in acts of vandalism and shoplifting. For their part, Linda's parents reported that (1) their daughter's fearful behavior had improved, (2) they were making a concerted effort to be consistent in their discipline regarding Linda's externalizing behavior, and (3) discussions with school personnel had eased tensions considerably and the parents were now quickly informed about any problems Linda displayed at school. Family therapy and contingency contracting to address remaining issues was recommended and continued.

Comments

Because the treatment of chronic, severe school refusal behavior will require more extensive goals and greater length than acute absenteeism, the preceding therapy synopsis was presented in stages. Most likely, a number of sessions will comprise each stage. This is largely due to the number of obstacles that impede therapeutic progress, including child (e.g., multiple functions/diagnoses), parent/familial (e.g., poor or maladaptive contact), and school (e.g., lack of acceptable placement alternatives) variables. For example, clinicians may find the process of family coercion (Patterson 1982) to be well established following long periods of infighting and pessimistic attitudes. The successful resolution of chronic school refusal behavior may result only after issues such as these are addressed initially.

As mentioned earlier, key challenges to treating school refusal behavior are familial attendance and compliance. In particular, the presence of depression, a condition closely related to therapy nonattendance in adolescents, should be addressed on a continuing basis. In addition, many cases of chronic school refusal behavior involve an acrimonious parent–school official relationship. In some severe cases, the threat of court action is part of a final effort to compel parents to rectify their child's absenteeism. Unfortunately, such circumstances often impede treatment success by fostering poor familial cooperation and enthusiasm. Because long-term cooperation with school officials is imperative for some intervention tactics (e.g., redesign of class schedules, attendance monitoring), however, building rapport among school administrators, teachers, parents, and clients should be given a high priority.

SUMMARY

School refusal behavior is a diverse syndrome marked by varying etiology, symptomatology, course, and outcome. As a result, comprehensive classification, assessment, and treatment strategies remain elusive. With respect to classification, clinicians and researchers may wish to pursue an approach that integrates typological and dimensional features to increase flexibility in organizing this population. With respect to assessment, additional work is required on measures focusing on youngsters with general school refusal behavior and not exclusively on subsets such as school phobia. With respect to treatment, a prescriptive approach based on duration, type of family interaction, developmental status of the child, and relevant diagnoses and functions may be most useful.

In relation to this latter point, clinicians and researchers working with this population may find that the reduction of obstacles to treatment is often as important as the choice of therapy technique. Key obstacles discussed here include variables related to the child (e.g., depression), parents (e.g., marital conflict), family (e.g., compliance, attendance) and school (e.g., resources for alternative curriculum programs). Although the length of treatment for school refusal behavior is variable, the removal or modification of obstacles such as these can significantly enhance therapeutic progress.

Because of the fluid and intensive nature of most cases, the remediation of school refusal behavior in youngsters can be among the most exciting and challenging tasks in clinical child psychology. However, additional research in this area remains crucial. Given that nonattendance is a significant social problem when taken individually, and more so when one considers its comorbidity with many disorders, a coordinated research effort involving educators, psychologists, health professionals, and parents is urged.

REFERENCES

Achenbach, T. M. (1991a). *Manual for the Youth Self-Report and 1991 Profile*. Burlington, VT: University of Vermont Department of Psychiatry.

———— (1991b). *Manual for the Child Behavior Checklist/4–18 and 1991 Profile*. Burlington, VT: University of Vermont Department of Psychiatry.

———— (1991c). *Manual for the Teacher's Report Form and 1991 Profile*. Burlington, VT: University of Vermont Department of Psychiatry.

Achenbach, T. M., and Edelbrock, C. S. (1983). *Manual for the Child Behavior Checklist and Revised Child Behavior Profile*. Burlington, VT: University of Vermont Department of Psychiatry.

Baker, H., and Wills, U. (1978). School phobia: classification and treatment. *British Journal of Psychiatry* 132:492–499.

Berecz, J. M. (1980). Treatment of school phobia. In *Emotional Disorders of Children and Adolescents: Medical and Psychological Approaches to Treatment*, ed. G. P. Sholevar, pp. 563–587. New York: Spectrum.

Berg, I. (1970). A follow-up study of school phobic adolescents admitted to an inpatient unit. *Journal of Child Psychology and Psychiatry* 11:37–47.

_____ (1974). A self-administered dependency questionnaire (S.A.D.Q.) for use with mothers of school children. *British Journal of Psychiatry* 124:1-9.

Berg, I., Brown, I., and Hullin, R. (1988). *Off School, In Court: An Experimental and Psychiatric Investigation of Severe School Attendance Problems.* New York: Springer-Verlag.

Berg, I., Butler, A., and Hall, G. (1976). The outcome of adolescent school phobia. *British Journal of Psychiatry* 128:80-85.

Berg, I., and Fielding, D. (1978). An evaluation of hospital in-patient treatment in adolescent school phobia. *British Journal of Psychiatry* 132:500-505.

Berg, I., and Jackson, A. (1985). Teenage school refusers grow up: a follow-up study of 168 subjects, ten years on average after in-patient treatment. *British Journal of Psychiatry* 147:366-370.

Berg, I., and McGuire, R. (1974). Are mothers of school-phobic adolescents overprotective? *British Journal of Psychiatry* 124:10-13.

Berg, I., Nichols, K., and Pritchard, C. (1969). School phobia: its classification and relationship to dependency. *Journal of Child Psychology and Psychiatry* 10:123-141.

Bernstein, G. A., and Garfinkel, B. D. (1986). School phobia: the overlap of affective and anxiety disorders. *Journal of the American Academy of Child and Adolescent Psychiatry* 25:235-241.

_____ (1988). Pedigrees, functioning, and psychopathology in families of school phobic children. *American Journal of Psychiatry* 145:70-74.

Bernstein, G. A., Garfinkel, B. D., and Borchardt, C. M. (1990). Comparative studies of pharmacotherapy for school refusal. *Journal of the American Academy of Child and Adolescent Psychiatry* 29:773-781.

Blagg, N. R., and Yule, W. (1984). The behavioural treatment of school refusal—a comparative study. *Behaviour Research and Therapy* 22:119-127.

Braswell, L., and Kendall, P. C. (1988). Cognitive-behavioral methods with children. In *Handbook of Cognitive-Behavioral Therapies*, ed. K. S. Dobson, pp. 167-213. New York: Guilford.

Brulle, A. R., McIntyre, T. C., and Mills, J. S. (1985). School phobia: its educational implications. *Elementary School Guidance and Counseling* 20:19-28.

Church, J., and Edwards, B. (1984). Helping pupils who refuse school. *Special Education: Forward Trends* 11:28-31.

Coolidge, J. C., Hahn, P. B., and Peck, A. L. (1957). School phobia: neurotic crisis or way of life? *American Journal of Orthopsychiatry* 27:296-306.

Cooper, J. A. (1973). Application of the consultant role to parent-teacher management of school avoidance behavior. *Psychology in the Schools* 10:259-262.

Cooper, M. (1986). A model of persistent school absenteeism. *Educational Research* 28:14-20.

Cooper, M. G. (1966). School refusal: an inquiry into the part played by school and home. *Educational Research* 8:223-229.

Diagnostic and Statistical Manual of Mental Disorders. (1980). 3rd ed. Washington, DC: American Psychiatric Association.

_____ (1987). 3rd ed. rev. Washington, DC: American Psychiatric Association.

_____ (1994). 4th ed. Washington, DC: American Psychiatric Association.

Endicott, J., Andreasen, N., and Spitzer, R. L. (1975). *Family History Research Diagnostic Criteria*. New York: New York State Psychiatric Institute.

Flakierska, N., Lindstrom, M., and Gillberg, C. (1988). School refusal: a 15–20-year follow-up study of 35 Swedish urban children. *British Journal of Psychiatry* 152: 834–837.

Foster, S. L., and Robin, A. L. (1989). Parent-adolescent conflict. In *Treatment of Childhood Disorders*, ed. E. J. Mash and R. A. Barkley, pp. 493–528. New York: Guilford.

Frick, W. B. (1964). School phobia: a critical review of the literature. *Merrill-Palmer Quarterly* 10:361–373.

Friesen, M. (1985). Non-attendance as a maladaptive response to stress. *School Guidance Worker* 40:9–23.

Gittelman-Klein, R., and Klein, D. F. (1971). Controlled imipramine treatment of school phobia. *Archives of General Psychiatry* 25:204–207.

Granell de Aldaz, E., Feldman, L., Vivas, E., and Gelfand, D. M. (1987). Characteristics of Venezuelan school refusers: toward the development of a high-risk profile. *Journal of Nervous and Mental Disease* 175:402–407.

Granell de Aldaz, E., Vivas, E., Gelfand, D. M., and Feldman, L. (1984). Estimating the prevalence of school refusal and school-related fears. *Journal of Nervous and Mental Disease* 172:722–729.

Graziano, A. M., and De Giovanni, I. S. (1979). The clinical significance of childhood phobias: a note on the proportion of child-clinical referrals for the treatment of children's fears. *Behaviour Research and Therapy* 17:161–162.

Green, B. J. (1985). Systems intervention in the schools. In *Handbook of Adolescents and Family Therapy*, ed. M. P. Mirkin and S. L. Koman, pp. 193–206. New York: Gardner.

Hathaway, S. R., and McKinley, J. C. (1951). *The Minnesota Multiphasic Personality Inventory, Revised*. New York: Psychological Corporation.

Herjanic, B., and Campbell, W. (1977). Differentiating psychiatrically disturbed children on the basis of a structured interview. *Journal of Abnormal Child Psychology* 5:127–134.

Hersov, L. (1985). School refusal. In *Child and Adolescent Psychiatry: Modern Approaches*, ed. M. Rutter and L. Hersov, pp. 382–399. Boston: Blackwell Scientific Publications.

Hibbett, A., and Fogelman, K. (1990). Future lives of truants: family formation and health-related behaviour. *British Journal of Educational Psychology* 60:171–179.

Hibbett, A., Fogelman, K., and Manor, O. (1990). Occupational outcomes of truancy. *British Journal of Educational Psychology* 60:23–36.

Hsia, H. (1984). Structural and strategic approach to school phobia/school refusal. *Psychology in the Schools* 21:360–367.

Jacobsen, E. (1938). *Progressive Relaxation*. Chicago: University of Chicago Press.

Jackson, R. H., and Sikora, D. (1992). Parenting: the child in the context of the family.

In *Handbook of Clinical Child Psychology*, ed. C. E. Walker and M. C. Roberts, pp. 727–747. New York: Wiley.

Johnson, A. M., Falstein, E. I., Szurek, S. A., and Svendsen, M. (1941). School phobia. *American Journal of Orthopsychiatry* 11:702–711.

Johnson, T., Tyler, V., Thompson, R., and Jones, E. (1971). Systematic desensitization and assertive training in the treatment of speech anxiety in middle school students. *Psychology in the Schools* 8:263–267.

Kahn, J. H., and Nursten, J. P. (1962). School refusal: a comprehensive view of school phobia and other failures of school attendance. *American Journal of Orthopsychiatry* 32:707–718.

Kearney, C. A. (1992). *Prescriptive treatment for school refusal behavior.* Symposium presented at the meeting of the Association for the Advancement of Behavior Therapy, Boston, MA, November.

_____ (1993). Depression and school refusal behavior: a review with comments on classification and treatment. *Journal of School Psychology* 31:267–279.

Kearney, C. A., and Beasley, J. F. (1994). The clinical treatment of school refusal behavior: a survey of referral and practice characteristics. *Psychology in the Schools* 31:128–132.

Kearney, C. A., Drabman, R. S., and Beasley, J. F. (1993). The trials of childhood: the development, reliability, and validity of the Daily Life Stressors Scale. *Journal of Child and Family Studies* 2:421–438.

Kearney, C. A., and Silverman, W. K. (1990). A preliminary analysis of a functional model of assessment and treatment for school refusal behavior. *Behavior Modification* 14:344–360.

_____ (1993). Measuring the function of school refusal behavior: the School Refusal Assessment Scale. *Journal of Clinical Child Psychology* 22:85–96.

_____ (1995). *The evolution and reconciliation of taxonomic strategies for school refusal behavior.* Manuscript submitted for publication.

_____ (in press). Family environment of youngsters with school refusal behavior: a synopsis with implications for assessment and treatment. *American Journal of Family Therapy.*

Kearney, C. A., Silverman, W. K., and Eisen, A. R. (1989). *Characteristics of children and adolescents with school refusal behavior.* Paper presented at the meeting of the Berkshire Conference of Behavior Analysis and Therapy, Amherst, MA, October.

Kennedy, W. A. (1965). School phobia: rapid treatment of fifty cases. *Journal of Abnormal Psychology* 70:285–289.

Klein, E. (1945). The reluctance to go to school. *Psychoanalytic Study of the Child* 1:263–279. New York: International Universities Press.

Knox, P. (1989). Home-based education: an alternative approach to school phobia. *Educational Review* 41:143–151.

Kovacs, M., and Beck, A. T. (1977). An empirical-clinical approach toward a definition of childhood depression. In *Depression in Children: Diagnosis, Treat-*

    ment, and Conceptual Models, ed. J. G. Schulterbrandt and A. Raskin, pp. 1–25. New York: Raven.

La Greca, A. M., and Stone, W. L. (1993). Social Anxiety Scale for Children-Revised: factor structure and concurrent validity. *Journal of Clinical Child Psychology* 22:17–27.

Last, C. G. (1991). Somatic complaints in anxiety disordered children. *Journal of Anxiety Disorders* 5:125–138.

Last, C. G., Francis, G., Hersen, M., et al. (1987). Separation anxiety and school phobia: a comparison using *DSM-III* criteria. *American Journal of Psychiatry* 144:653–657.

Last, C. G., and Strauss, C. C. (1990). School refusal in anxiety-disordered children and adolescents. *Journal of the American Academy of Child and Adolescent Psychiatry* 29:31–35.

Lazarus, A. A., Davison, G. C., and Polefka, D. A. (1965). Classical and operant factors in the treatment of a school phobia. *Journal of Abnormal Psychology* 70:225–229.

Leventhal, T., and Sills, M. (1964). Self-image in school phobia. *American Journal of Orthopsychiatry* 34:685–694.

Leventhal, T., Weinberger, G., Stander, R. J., and Stearns, R. P. (1967). Therapeutic strategies with school phobics. *American Journal of Orthopsychiatry* 37:64–70.

Mansdorf, I. J., and Lukens, E. (1987). Cognitive-behavioral psychotherapy for separation anxious children exhibiting school phobia. *Journal of the American Academy of Child and Adolescent Psychiatry* 26:222–225.

McDonald, J. E., and Sheperd, G. (1976). School phobia: an overview. *Journal of School Psychology* 14:291–306.

Mihara, R., and Ichikawa, M. (1986). A clinical study of school refusal with special reference to the classification of family violence. *Japanese Journal of Child and Adolescent Psychiatry* 27:110–131.

Miller, P. M. (1972). The use of visual imagery and muscle relaxation in the counterconditioning of a phobic child: a case study. *Journal of Nervous and Mental Disease* 154:457–460.

Moos, R. H., and Moos, B. S. (1986). *Family Environment Scale Manual*, 2nd. ed. Palo Alto, CA: Consulting Psychologists Press.

Ollendick, T. H. (1983). Reliability and validity of the Revised Fear Survey Schedule for Children (FSSC-R). *Behaviour Research and Therapy* 21:685–692.

Ollendick, T. H., and Mayer, J. A. (1984). School phobia. In *Behavioral Theories and Treatment of Anxiety*, ed. S. M. Turner, pp. 367–411. New York: Plenum.

O'Reilly, P. P. (1971). Desensitization of a fire bell phobia. *Journal of School Psychology* 9:55–57.

Parish, T. S., Buntman, A. D., and Buntman, S. R. (1976). Effect of counterconditioning on test anxiety as indicated by digit span performance. *Journal of Educational Psychology* 68:297–299.

Patterson, G.. (1982). *Coercive Family Process: A Social Learning Approach*. Eugene, OR: Castalia.

Piers, E. V. (1984). *Piers-Harris Children's Self-Concept Scale: Revised Manual 1984*. Los Angeles: Western Psychological Services.

Puig-Antich, J., and Ryan, N. D. (1986). *Schedule for Affective Disorders and Schizophrenia for School-aged Children (6–16) (K-SADS-P)*. Fourth Working Draft.

Remschmidt, H., and Mattejat, F. (1990). Treatment of school phobia in children and adolescents in Germany. In *Why Children Reject School: Views from Seven Countries*, ed. C. Chiland and J. G. Young, pp. 123–144. New Haven, CT: Yale University Press.

Reynolds, C. R., and Paget, K. D. (1983). National normative and reliability data for the revised Children's Manifest Anxiety Scale. *School Psychology Review* 12:324–336.

Robins, L. N., Helzer, J. E., Croughan, J., and Ratcliffe, K. S. (1981). National Institute of Mental Health Diagnostic Interview Schedule: its history, characteristics and validity. *Archives of General Psychiatry* 38:381–389.

Robins, L. N., and Ratcliffe, K. S. (1980). The long-term outcome of truancy. In *Out of School*, ed. L. Hersov and I. Berg, pp. 65–83. New York: Wiley.

Rodriguez, A., Rodriguez, M., and Eisenberg, L. (1959). The outcome of school phobia: a follow-up study based on 41 cases. *American Journal of Psychiatry* 116:540–544.

Rubenstein, J. S., and Hastings, E. M. (1980). School refusal in adolescence: understanding the symptom. *Adolescence* 60:775–782.

Silverman, W. K., and Eisen, A. R. (1992). Age differences in the reliability of parent and child reports of child anxious symptomatology using a structured interview. *Journal of the American Academy of Child and Adolescent Psychiatry* 31:117–124.

Silverman, W. K., and Nelles, W. B. (1988). The Anxiety Disorders Interview Schedule for Children. *Journal of the American Academy of Child and Adolescent Psychiatry* 27:772–778.

Skinner, H. A., Steinhauer, P. D., and Santa-Barbara, J. (1983). The Family Assessment Measure. *Canadien Journal of Community Mental Health* 2:91–105.

Smith, R. E., and Sharpe, T. M. (1970). Treatment of a school phobia with implosive therapy. *Journal of Consulting and Clinical Psychology* 35:239–243.

Sperling, M. (1967). School phobias: classification, dynamics, and treatment. *Psychoanalytic Study of the Child* 22:375–401. New York: International Universities Press.

Spielberger, C. D. (1973). *Manual for the State-Trait Anxiety Inventory for Children*. Palo Alto, CA: Consulting Psychologists Press.

Suttenfield, V. (1954). School phobia: a study of five cases. *American Journal of Orthopsychiatry* 24:368–380.

Taylor, L., and Adelman, H. S. (1990). School avoidance behavior: motivational bases and implications for intervention. *Child Psychiatry and Human Development* 20:219–233.

Thompson, C. L., and Rudolph, L. B. (1988). *Counseling Children*. Belmont, CA: Brooks/Cole.

Timberlake, E. M. (1984). Psychosocial functioning of school phobics at follow-up. *Social Work Research and Abstracts* 20:13–18.

Valles, E., and Oddy, M. (1984). The influence of a return to school on the long-term adjustment of school refusers. *Journal of Adolescence* 7:35–44.

Waldfogel, S., Coolidge, J. C., and Hahn, P. B. (1957). The development, meaning, and management of school phobia. *American Journal of Orthopsychiatry* 27:754–780.

Waldron, S., Shrier, D. K., Stone, B., and Tobin, F. (1975). School phobia and other childhood neuroses: a systematic study of the children and their families. *American Journal of Psychiatry* 132:802–808.

Want, J. H. (1983). School-based intervention strategies for school phobia: a ten-step common sense approach. *Pointer* 27:27–32.

Weiner, I. B. (1992). *Psychological Disturbance in Adolescence.* New York: Wiley.

Weiss, M., and Cain, B. (1964). The residential treatment of children and adolescents with school phobia. *American Journal of Orthopsychiatry* 34:103–112.

Wetchler, J. L. (1986). Family therapy of school-focused problems: a macrosystemic perspective. *Contemporary Family Therapy* 8:224–240.

Wolpe, J. (1982). *The Practice of Behavior Therapy.* New York: Pergamon.

Young, J. G., Brasic, J. R., Kisnadwala, H., and Levin, L. (1990). Strategies for research on school refusal and related nonattendance at school. In *Why Children Reject School: Views from Seven Countries,* ed. C. Chiland and J. G. Young, pp. 199–223. New Haven, CT: Yale University Press.

3

SEPARATION ANXIETY DISORDER

Janice R. Wachtel
Cyd C. Strauss

DESCRIPTION OF DISORDER

Separation anxiety disorder (SAD) is one of three child anxiety disorders identified in the Diagnostic and Statistical Manual of Mental Disorders (*DSM-III*, American Psychiatric Association 1980) and the revised version of the *DSM-III* (*DSM-III-R*, American Psychiatric Association 1987). The defining feature of SAD is an unrealistic and excessive fear of separation from major attachment figures. This anxious reaction must be beyond that expected for the child's developmental level; separation anxiety is normal and common from approximately 6 months of age until 2 to 3 years of age, peaking around 18 months (Rutter 1981, p. 309). For a diagnosis of SAD, the child must experience three of nine criteria defined by the *DSM-III-R*. These criteria include (1) unrealistic and persistent worry about harm to major attachment figures or fear of abandonment, (2) unrealistic and persistent worry that a calamitous event will separate the child from a major attachment figure, (3) school refusal or persistent reluctance to go to school in order to stay with major attachment figures or at home, (4) reluctance to sleep alone or away from home, (5) avoidance of being alone (resulting in "clinging" and "shadowing" attachment figures), (6) nightmares involving the theme of separation, (7) physical complaints upon anticipation of separation from attachment figures, (8) excessive distress in anticipation of separation from home or attachment figures, and (9) excessive distress when separated from attachment figures. For a diagnosis of SAD, symptomatology must occur for at least two weeks, and onset of the disorder must occur before the child is 18 years old (*DSM-III-R* 1987).

SAD remains in *DSM-IV* (American Psychiatric Association 1994) as a separate childhood category, no longer subsumed under a broad category of Anxiety Disorders of Childhood or Adolescence. There are few substantive changes in the specific criteria for this category, with the exception of the following: (1) the child must demonstrate three of *eight* criteria, rather than nine (two criteria have been combined into a single criterion); (2) the duration of the disturbance has been extended from two to four weeks, to be considered clinically significant; and (3) an impairment criterion has been added.

SAD has been diagnosed reliably in numerous recent studies. For instance, adequate diagnostic reliability has been demonstrated in the following studies: (1) Last and colleagues (1987b) reported a Kappa coefficient of .81 for SAD diagnoses using the Interview Schedule for Children (ISC, Kovacs 1983); (2) Silverman and Nelles (1988) reported product-moment correlations of .98 and .99 for interrater agreement of SAD diagnoses using the Anxiety Disorders Interview Schedule for Children, Child and Parent versions (ADIS-C, ADIS-P, Silverman and Nelles 1988), respectively; and (3) Last and colleagues (1987a) reported 90 percent agreement between two clinicians for SAD and school phobia diagnoses using the ISC (Kovacs 1983). Furthermore, numerous descriptive studies have reported epidemiology, comorbidity, assessment methods, and treatment methods for SAD. Findings from these studies will be presented throughout this chapter.

The literature notes consistent findings regarding the onset, precipitants, and course of SAD. The onset of SAD may occur as early as during the preschool years; onset during adolescence is rare (Last et al. 1987b). According to Klein and Last (1989), the onset may be acute or chronic and often occurs after a major stressor, such as the death or illness of a relative, moving to a new school, or moving into a new neighborhood. Onset also has been reported to occur following prolonged vacations or absences from school (e.g., summer vacation, physical illness resulting in missed school) and at certain developmental transitions (e.g., entry into elementary or junior high school). Without intervention, the course of SAD is variable, with symptomatology alternating between periods of exacerbation and remission according to life stressors and developmental transitions (Klein and Last 1989). The prevalence of SAD appears to be greater in younger children than in adolescents in both the general population (Kashani and Orvashel 1988, 1990) and in clinical samples (Last et al. 1987b). The most common disorders for which children are referred to clinics specializing in anxiety disorders appear to be SAD or overanxious disorder (OAD), a second childhood anxiety disorder defined in *DSM-III-R* in which the child worries generally about a range of situations (Last et al. 1987b, Last and Francis 1987c).

Children with SAD have been shown to present with various concurrent childhood disorders. Specifically, children with SAD often present with coexisting specific fears, such as fears of the dark, bumblebees, or ghosts; these fears may or may not be of phobic proportion (Last 1989). Approximately one-third of children with SAD have a concurrent diagnosis of OAD that almost always is secondary to the primary diagnosis of SAD (Last et al. 1987b, Last and Francis 1987c). Furthermore, Last and colleagues (1987b) found that approximately one-third of children with a diagnosis of SAD displayed coexisting major depression. Interestingly, it has been reported that compared with children with a primary diagnosis of OAD, social phobia, and major depression, children with a primary diagnosis of SAD are least likely to receive a concurrent anxiety diagnosis (Last and Francis 1987c). Finally, Last and colleagues (1987b) found that of children diagnosed with SAD or SAD plus OAD, 22–24 percent displayed a coexisting attention deficit disorder, 0–9 percent carried a concurrent diagnosis of conduct disorder, and 14.3–27.2 percent had a coexisting oppositional disorder.

Several studies have examined specific diagnostic symptoms that occur in children with SAD. Last and colleagues (1987a) reported that approximately three-quarters of clinic-referred children diagnosed with SAD showed the diagnostic criterion of school reluctance or avoidance. Furthermore, somatic complaints often accompany school reluctance/avoidance, in which the child complains of symptoms such as headaches or stomachaches prior to attending or while in school. Somatic complaints also occur in other situations where separation from an attachment figure is anticipated. Indeed, in a recent study assessing forty clinic children with SAD, Last (1991) reported that 78 percent of these children reported somatic complaints.

DIFFERENTIAL DIAGNOSIS

Differentiation of SAD from other childhood anxiety disorders generally can be achieved by determining the situational specificity of the anxious symptomatology. In particular, children diagnosed with OAD do not display situation-specific anxiety; the child's anxiety is more pervasive and typically occurs regardless of whether the attachment figure is with the child. Children with OAD display a variety of worries (e.g., about family, social situations, school performance) in a range of situations. Children with a diagnosis of avoidant disorder, the third of the three childhood anxiety disorders found in *DSM-III-R*, demonstrate a specific fear and avoidance of interpersonal contact with strangers, regardless of whether the attachment figure is present.

It is important to distinguish "school phobia" from SAD as well. Reluc tance or refusal to go to school is included as one of the nine symptoms defining SAD and also is characteristic of school phobia. As such, when anxiety about attending school is present, it can stem from separation problems or from an excessive fear about some aspect of going to school, such as anxiety about social contacts at school, test performance, fear of a specific teacher, and so on. Thus, school refusal can be a symptom of various other *DSM-III-R* disorders. For example, if the fear of school is based upon social concerns, such as the possibility of humiliation or embarrassment in front of others, a diagnosis of social phobia is appropriate. When the fear centers on a specific aspect of the school itself (e.g., fear of a specific teacher, fear of vomiting while at school), then simple phobia is diagnosed. In a review of the literature, Burke and Silverman (1987) concluded that a range of *DSM-III* diagnoses can be applied to school refusers, including SAD, OAD, avoidant disorder, simple phobia, panic disorder, depression, and adjustment disorder. Last and colleagues (1987a) further compared forty-eight children with SAD and nineteen children with a phobic disorder of school (either simple or social). Seventy-three percent of the children with SAD and 100 percent of those with school phobia presented with school avoidance. This study found that children with SAD and those with school phobia represented two distinct populations. Children with SAD tended to be female, prepubertal, and from lower SES backgrounds, while children with school phobia generally were male, postpubertal, and from families of higher SES. Additionally, children with SAD more often met criteria for at least one concurrent *DSM-III* diagnosis: 92 percent of children with SAD received an additional *DSM-III* diagnosis, compared with 63 percent of the school phobia group. The authors concluded that this latter difference indicated that children with SAD were more severely disturbed than those with a phobic disorder of school.

Additionally, school refusal due to truancy is sometimes distinguished from school refusal related to anxiety. Children who demonstrate truancy may not exhibit anxiety when in the school setting. These children tend to stay away from the home when absent from school, whereas children with separation anxiety usually remain at home when not in school. Finally, children who are truant often display concurrent conduct disorder behaviors, such as stealing and lying, that rarely are seen in SAD children.

In addition to the previously mentioned reasons for absenteeism from school, excessive absenteeism may be due to genuine physical illness. Whenever a child reports somatic complaints, a thorough physical evaluation should be conducted to rule out medical problems. Assessment of the pattern of somatic complaints also can be helpful in determining the presence of SAD, since SAD children tend to demonstrate physical complaints prior to or in separation situations (e.g., prior to school, when parents are leaving on trips), but not at other times.

Children with SAD may be characterized by their parents as oppositional; however, oppositional behavior most often is restricted to anxiety-provoking situations involving separation from the parents. SAD children may display temper tantrums, disobedience, or argumentativeness when forced to separate from the parent. Therefore, it is important to assess the situations in which the child demonstrates oppositional behavior to differentiate SAD symptoms from those of oppositional disorder.

ASSESSMENT PROCEDURES

Many strategies and measures have been developed to assess the presence, type, and severity of childhood anxiety. Generally, it is recommended that a multimethod strategy be used when assessing a child's anxiety problem. Assessment procedures include structured or semistructured clinical interviews with children and parents, self-report questionnaires, parent and teacher ratings, behavioral observations, and physiological measurements. A complete assessment of childhood anxiety involves collecting data from three separate domains: verbal/cognitive, motoric/behavioral, and physiologic.

The structured or semistructured clinical interview is the only formal assessment instrument currently capable of generating a *DSM-III-R* diagnosis of SAD. Other measures (e.g., self-report questionnaires, behavioral observations) provide a description of symptoms, but do not correspond directly to diagnostic criteria. There are numerous structured and semistructured interviews currently available to evaluate anxiety disorders in children. These include the ADIS-C and ADIS-P (Silverman and Nelles 1988), the ISC (Kovacs 1983), the Schedule for Affective Disorders and Schizophrenia for School-Age Children (K-SADS, Chambers et al. 1985), the Diagnostic Interview Schedule for Children (DISC, Costello et al. 1984), the Diagnostic Interview for Children and Adolescents (DICA, Reich et al. 1982), the Children's Anxiety Evaluation Form (CAEF, Hoehn-Saric et al. 1987), and the Child Assessment Schedule (CAS, Hodges 1987). Each instrument involves interviewing parents and children individually to evaluate the presence and severity of symptoms. As previously noted, research generally has demonstrated adequate reliability and validity for these interview schedules (e.g., Last et al. 1987c, Last et al. 1987b).

Self-report measures can aid in the evaluation of anxiety symptoms that the child experiences. Several such measures commonly are used, including the Revised Children's Manifest Anxiety Scale (RCMAS, Reynolds and Paget 1981), the State-Trait Anxiety Inventory for Children (STAIC, Spielberger 1973), and the Revised Fear Survey Schedule for Children (FSSC-R, Ollendick 1983). Although adequate reliability and validity for these measures generally have been reported, several problems with these measures do exist. Problems with self-report measures include the following: (1) they have high face validity, thereby allowing children to portray themselves as having less severe or fewer problems than they actually experience; (2) many of these measures focus on general symptoms of anxiety and do not identify specific situations that induce anxiety; and (3) these questionnaires have higher age limits than other assessment techniques due to reading requirements, therefore limiting their use with younger children. One relatively new questionnaire that focuses on the specific situation of school refusal (which, as noted earlier, is one symptom of SAD) is the School Refusal Assessment Scale (SRAS, Kearney and Silverman 1993). This questionnaire measures positively and negatively reinforcing factors that may serve to maintain school refusal and is completed by the child, parent, and teacher. Overall, these self-report measures are useful as corroborative sources of data when evaluating the presence and severity of separation anxiety.

The assessment of self-reported cognitions in anxious children is beginning to be used more frequently due to the increased usage of cognitive-behavior therapy in treating childhood anxiety problems. It has been proposed that there is a relationship between cognitions and the acquisition and maintenance of adaptive and maladaptive behavior, making the assessment of cognitions a valuable tool in treatment. Three questionnaires that assess cognitions include the Cognitive and Somatic State and Trait Anxiety Scale (CSSTAS, Fox and Houston 1983), the Children's Cognitive Assessment Questionnaire (CCAQ, Zatz and Chassin 1983), and the Children's Negative Cognitive Error Questionnaire (CNCEQ, Leitenberg et al. 1986). To date, the empirical evaluation of cognitions in anxious children has been limited to nonclinical samples (Francis 1988). Although data provide preliminary support for the use of cognitive techniques in the assessment and treatment of childhood anxiety (e.g., Mansdorf and Lukens 1987, Ollendick et al. 1991), the efficacy of such techniques specifically with SAD children is unknown; considerably more research is needed with clinical samples of anxious children.

Parent and teacher ratings and checklists also are valuable general screening devices in the assessment of SAD. However, like self-report questionnaires, their utility is limited by their failure to identify specific situations that provoke anxiety. The following three questionnaires assess symptomatology particularly related to separation anxiety: the Fear Scale of the Louisville Behavior Checklist (Miller et al. 1971), the Parent Anxiety Rating Scale and the Teacher's Separation Anxiety Scale (Doris et al. 1971), and the Louisville Fear Survey (Miller et al. 1972). In addition to these parent and teacher rating forms that include questions specifically related to separation anxiety, numerous parent and teacher questionnaires assess general anxiety symptomatology (e.g., Child Behavior Checklist, Achenbach and Edelbrock 1983; Conners' Teacher Rating Scale, Conners 1969).

Because interviews and questionnaires may be biased due to their retrospective nature, social desirability, or the child's inability to articulate symptoms, direct observations can offer an informative assessment approach. Nevertheless, this assessment approach has not been utilized commonly in clinical settings. The direct observation method used most often for assessing anxiety in children is the Behavioral Avoidance Test (BAT, Lang and Lazovik 1963). This approach involves exposing the child to a series of controlled and graduated interactions with a feared situation or object. Specifically, children diagnosed with SAD would be observed in situations related to separation from the parent. For example, the child could be observed while touching the parent, with the parent across the room, with the parent in the hall but in sight, and with the parent out of sight. Another more standardized observation measure is the Observation of Separation-Relevant Play (Milos and Reiss 1982). In this procedure, the number of anxiety-relevant responses during play is recorded. Behavioral observations allow verification of parent and child reports and can provide reliable assessments of treatment efficacy.

Currently, there is a growing interest in psychophysiologic assessment of anxiety disorders in children. Recent work has supported the use of measuring heart rate and blood pressure when evaluating anxiety in children and adolescents (Beidel 1988; Matthews et al. 1986). Although physiological assessment has not yet been studied empirically using children with SAD in particular, this method may prove useful given the central role of physiological and somatic symptoms associated with this diagnosis. Since physiological responses are not under voluntary control of the child and are not rated subjectively, they are less susceptible to subject or rater bias. Nevertheless, limitations of physiological assessment include the requirement of expensive equipment and the high level of expertise needed for assessment.

ESTABLISHING TREATMENT GOALS

Establishment of treatment goals requires careful assessment of SAD symptoms, specific situations in which anxiety occurs, behaviors associated with separation anxiety, cognitive and physiological reactions, and precipitants and consequences of separation anxious behavior. Additionally, it is important to assess whether the child presents with pure separation anxiety or has other problem areas that need to be addressed as well. When children present with multiple disorders (e.g., depression, other anxiety disorders), these additional disorders should be included in the treatment plan. Either the disorders could be prioritized, resulting in treatment of disorders one at a time, or a multiple baseline design could be used, in which several problems are treated concurrently.

One important consideration in establishing treatment goals is the child's cognitive and developmental level. For example, young children likely will require greater involvement of parents to facilitate exposure to anxiety-provoking situations. They also are likely to have more difficulty with procedures requiring imagery, so that such approaches would not be chosen for younger children.

Overall, treatment should be aimed at behavioral, cognitive, and psychological aspects of anxiety. First, children with SAD usually display avoidance behavior, such as school refusal and avoidance of leaving parents' presence, so treatment must include procedures to increase approach to the avoided stimulus or situation, such as graduated exposure (i.e., systematic desensitization). Additionally, a child who displays worries in anticipation of or actually in separation-related situations would benefit from cognitive techniques. A child who displays excessive physical tension should be taught relaxation techniques. Most typically, all three modalities will need to be targeted for intervention.

Finally, when establishing treatment goals, the larger system should be considered. Family members may be an important component in the conceptualization and treatment of the child's anxiety. For instance, family members may model or reinforce SAD behavior. Indeed, failure to intervene with family members as well as with the child could lead to ineffectiveness of treatment or result in loss of treatment gains after the child terminates therapy. The incorporation of school or other environmental influences that appear to be important components in the child's anxiety problem should also be included in the treatment plan.

ROLE OF THE THERAPIST

The therapist's role is that of educator and facilitator. The therapist should be supportive, encouraging, and understanding. The therapist educates the child, parents, and school personnel by explaining the symptoms of SAD and the techniques that are helpful in treating this disorder. The therapist instructs parents and/or school personnel regarding how they can be most helpful during treatment. The therapist is a facilitator in the therapy process; he/she assesses the child's problem and plays a primary role in forming the treatment plan. The therapist helps the child (and possibly parent) to construct a hierarchy appropriate to the child's specific problem area(s). The therapist also teaches the child any additional skills that seem appropriate (e.g., relaxation training). The therapist monitors the child's progress with the hierarchy and encourages, but does not pressure, the child throughout treatment. The therapist can reward the child for progress, or can facilitate rewards through the child's environment (e.g., parent, teacher). Finally, the therapist acts as a liaison between the child and the parents, and between the family system and the school system.

TREATMENT STRATEGIES

The treatment of SAD typically includes a behavioral program for increasing independent activities (e.g., returning to school, going to peers' homes) and management of specific anxiety symptoms. Pharmacological treatment also has been used in the treatment of childhood anxiety.

Various behavioral techniques can be used, either individually or in combination, to treat SAD. Systematic desensitization, using a fear hierarchy focused on activities resulting in increasing levels of separation from the attachment figure, is an important component in the treatment of SAD. Systematic desensitization consists of three essential components. First, a response that is incompatible with anxiety, usually muscle relaxation, is taught. Various muscle relaxation techniques exist. For example, progressive relaxation training (Bernstein and Borkovec 1973) is a technique that teaches the patient to tense and release various muscle groups throughout the body, producing relaxation. As skill develops, the number of muscle groups is reduced. Other responses incompatible with anxiety that can be used with children include engaging in a pleasurable activity, imagery, and breathing exercises. The second component of systematic desensitization is the construction of a fear hierarchy. This hierarchy incorporates feared situations ranging from those that elicit very mild levels of anxiety to those provoking extreme anxiety or panic. When the child avoids school as well as other situations that include separation from the home/parents, two hierarchies ordinarily are developed: one consisting of items related to school attendance and the other consisting of items associated with separation from parents in other situations. The hierarchies should cover a wide range of situations that elicit varying degrees of fear and avoidance. Items on a hierarchy explicitly state and vary the duration of time spent in each situation, distance from home/parent, and/or presence of other individuals. The hierarchy is constructed by collaboration among the therapist, child, and parent(s). The items then are arranged in order from least to most anxiety-provoking by having the parent and child rate each item on a Likert scale regarding the amount of anxiety or distress the child would experience in each situation.

The final component in systematic desensitization is implementing the hierarchical exposure. Homework assignments are negotiated by the child, therapist, and parent(s). It is important that the child be in control of the rate at which he/she progresses. The frequency of exposure during the week is dependent on the nature of the particular item, but practice as frequently as possible is encouraged. The child can record the date and level of anxiety actually experienced during each task on the same Likert scale used to develop the hierarchy. The therapist reviews and discusses this record during weekly therapy sessions.

Research suggests that in vivo systematic desensitization is at least equivalent in efficacy to imaginal exposure (Thyer and Sowers-Hoag 1988), if not superior (Ultee et al. 1982), when treating childhood anxiety disorders. Furthermore, the literature with adult agoraphobic patients has demonstrated that in vivo exposure is the central component in the successful treatment of agoraphobia (Barlow 1988, Emmelkamp 1982, Mavissakalian and Barlow 1981). Given the similarities and possible relationship between SAD and panic disorder with agoraphobia (Klein and Last 1989, Moreau and Follett 1993), and since in vivo exposure is at least as effective as imaginal exposure in treating childhood anxiety disorders, it seems advantageous to include in vivo exposure in the treatment of SAD when possible.

Cognitive techniques also can be useful in the treatment of SAD. As noted previously, the assumption is that the child's maladaptive thoughts, beliefs, attitudes, and self-statements lead to or maintain anxiety-related behavior. Cognitive coping strategies can be introduced by first providing a rationale for such procedures. Maladaptive self-statements that the child engages in when anxious should be identified, and then suggestions for more adaptive coping statements to be used when anticipating or confronting anxiety-provoking situations are generated. Such statements for SAD children may include those that stress the child's capability of being independent (e.g., "I can do this on my own"), the fact that the parents will be fine, and self-praise (e.g., how brave the child is when he/she is alone). Cognitive procedures frequently are combined with behavioral procedures, forming a treatment package often referred to as cognitive-behavior therapy.

Mansdorf and Lukens (1987) provided evidence for the efficacy of cognitive-behavioral techniques in a study of two children presenting with school phobia (one also displayed SAD symptomatology). Through the use of cognitive techniques, both children improved by the fourth weekly session of treatment. Follow-up assessments continued for three months after the children reached criterion, with no signs of relapse. Additionally, Ollendick and colleagues (1991) successfully eliminated nighttime fears and other SAD symptomatology in two children through the use of cognitive therapy combined with reinforcement. Interestingly, the addition of reinforcement (e.g., earrings, trips to mall, verbal praise) was a critical factor in treatment success; indeed, the cognitive techniques in the absence of contingent reinforcement produced only slight improvement with one child and no improvement in the second child.

Modeling also can be used in the treatment of SAD. The child may learn to overcome his/her fear of separation by watching other children separate from parents or the home successfully. For example, the child could watch a film of another child saying good-bye to his parents and getting on a bus to go to school. The child can observe a model on tape or a live model. One variant of modeling is participant modeling, which involves having the child attempt to confront the anxiety-provoking situation soon after watching the model. Participant modeling has been shown to be the most effective modeling approach with children, followed by live modeling; taped models appear to be least effective (Ollendick and Cerny 1981). Unfortunately, although investigations have demonstrated the utility of modeling for various childhood fears (Bandura and Menlove 1968, Osborn 1986), to date no studies have tested the efficacy of modeling with SAD children in particular.

Finally, contingency management procedures can be a helpful component in the treatment of SAD. These procedures typically involve modulation of rewards and punishments to increase independence in various situations. In using this approach, it is important to assess the circumstances preceding and/or following separation anxiety that might maintain SAD symptomatology. The child is reinforced with either praise or some tangible reward when he/she separates from the parent or home. Rewards can be used in conjunction with systematic desensitization, so that the child is rewarded for each item gradually accomplished on the hierarchy. Additionally, extinction can be used by removing any consequences that reinforce avoidant behavior, such as the child receiving attention from parents or being allowed to stay home and play when anxious about attending school.

Overall, few controlled empirical studies have evaluated the effectiveness of behavioral treatment for SAD in children. Instead, most research up to this point has focused on interventions for anxiety-based school refusal, which, as noted earlier, is only one feature of SAD and can be related to various anxiety disorders. Mansdorf and Lukens (1987) and Ollendick and colleagues (1991) have provided evidence through the use of case studies for the efficacy of cognitive-behavioral therapy and cognitive-behavioral therapy combined with reinforcement in eliminating school refusal. Additionally, in a review of the literature, Thyer and Sowers-Hoag (1988) found a total of eleven published studies that included behavioral treatment of SAD (eight of these studies were single-subject investigations/case reports). Although these studies suffered from various methodological problems, all eleven studies did obtain positive results through methods of hierarchical exposure to anxiety-provoking stimuli. Exposure therapy was conducted gradually in most cases; however, two studies used rapid exposure. Furthermore, while some studies used real-life exposure therapy, others used imaginal desensitization. Many of the studies reported by Thyer and Sowers-Hoag (1988) also included operant techniques (i.e., tangible or verbal reinforcement) combined with in vivo systematic desensitization. For example, in one study two children were reinforced with M&Ms for behaviors leading to their return to school. Other studies involved teaching the parents to praise their children for specific behaviors, and one study reinforced the child's elimination of anxious behavior by having the absent mother reappear. While these studies suggest that the use of cognitive-behavioral techniques, operant techniques, and systematic desensitization may be useful in the treatment of SAD and/or school refusal, controlled studies are needed to evaluate the efficacy of each individual treatment component.

Research on the efficacy of pharmacological treatment in childhood anxiety disorders is somewhat limited and equivocal. SAD has been the most extensively studied of the childhood anxiety disorders, however, with a few pharmacological studies assessing the efficacy of antidepressant and anxiolytic medications. Only a small number of controlled studies have examined antidepressant drug effects on SAD symptomatology (Berney et al. 1981, Bernstein et al. 1990, Gittelman-Klein and Klein 1971, 1973, 1980, Klein et al. 1992). Unfortunately, all but one of these studies (Klein et al. 1992) were conducted using children with "school phobia" (Berney et al. 1981, Bernstein et al. 1990, Gittelman-Klein and Klein 1971, 1973, 1980). While Bernstein and colleagues (1990) noted that 65 percent of their subjects met criteria for either SAD or OAD, no further delineation regarding disorder type was given.

In the most extensively cited study of this type, Gittleman-Klein and Klein (1971, 1973, 1980) assessed the efficacy of imipramine in treating school refusal. Results indicated that children treated with imipramine showed significantly less school refusal and anxiety symptoms than control groups. However, in a later controlled study of clomipramine involving children with school refusal (Berney et al. 1981), no significant differences were found between the drug and placebo treatments. It is important to note that this study used a much smaller dosage of clomipramine than Gittleman-Klein and Klein's (1971, 1973, 1980) studies using imipramine; thus a therapeutic level may not have been achieved in the Berney (1981) investigation, resulting in no significant effects. Furthermore, interpretation of Berney and co-authors' findings is limited by the small sample size ($N = 5$ to 7 per group) and by the high dropout rate (over 30 percent). Bernstein and colleagues (1990) compared imipramine, alprazolam, and placebo for treatment of school refusers and found no statistically significant differences among treatments. Finally, in the only study examining efficacy of pharmacological intervention in SAD children, specifically, Klein and colleagues (1992) randomly assigned twenty-one children to either an imipramine or placebo group for 6 weeks under double-blind conditions. The authors reported that approximately 50 percent of subjects improved in both imipramine and placebo conditions; no superiority for imipramine was displayed.

Alprazolam (an anxiolytic) has received some attention in the literature as well. Klein and Last (1989) report that their own unpublished data indicated that of eighteen children diagnosed with SAD who were treated with alprazolam, 65 percent rated themselves as improved. Furthermore, over 80 percent of these children were reported to be significantly improved by their parents and psychiatrists. No control group was used in this unpublished study. As noted earlier, Bernstein and colleagues (1990) found that alprazolam did not differ significantly from a placebo in treatment of school refusal.

Important empirical questions remain for all of the treatment procedures discussed. The relative effectiveness of these methods has not yet been verified adequately in controlled experimental designs. Additionally, further research is needed to assess the relationship between type of treatment and long-term therapeutic outcome. Finally, attention needs to be given to the influence of subject characteristics and developmental level on the efficacy of particular treatment approaches. Given the findings in the current literature indicating that SAD symptomatology appears to diminish with behavioral management techniques, and the fact that medications can have various side effects, it is recommended that medication be implemented only when behavioral interventions have not produced satisfactory outcomes (Kutcher et al. 1992). Furthermore, when pharmacological treatment is implemented, it should take place in the context of a comprehensive treatment plan (Kutcher et al. 1992).

DEALING WITH COMMON OBSTACLES TO SUCCESSFUL TREATMENT

Successful treatment is a function of adequacy of assessment, development of the treatment plan, and collaboration among the therapist, the child, the child's family system, and sometimes the school system. A common obstacle to successful treatment of SAD is noncompliance with treatment recommendations on the part of the parent and/or child. Such resistance in the parent or child can interfere with carrying out homework assignments (e.g., practicing items on the hierarchy) or with applying other important aspects of the therapeutic program (e.g., contingency management for the parent, cognitive techniques for the child). Mansdorf and Lukens (1987) report that such noncompliance can be approached using cognitive techniques by examining attitude and belief systems of both the parent(s) and the child. They recommend that once these inappropriate beliefs and attitudes are determined, self-instruction or cognitive disputation can be used to produce changes. Parent resistance highlights the importance of including parents in the treatment plan. Indeed, often treatment is focused on effecting change in both the child and the parent(s).

Parental noncompliance can be a function of various parental characteristics. Two such parental characteristics observed in parents of SAD children include an overprotective parenting style and parental overconcern that the child will experience discomfort. Regarding the former, overprotective parents tend to discourage independence due to their own anxiety regarding separation from their child. Often the parents worry about what might happen to the child if they are not there to "protect" the child. For example, a mother might worry that when her child goes to a friend's home, the parents of the friend might not watch the children carefully, thereby compromising her child's safety. This mother might subtly discourage her child from going to friends' homes by always inviting the child's friends to her home. She may reward the child for having friends over rather than going to their homes (e.g., through extra attention and praise), while at the same time punishing the child when he/she visits friends' homes (e.g., by emotionally rejecting the child at these times). As noted earlier, this can be dealt with by challenging the parent's maladaptive thoughts (cognitive techniques) and having the parents rehearse more adaptive self-statements when in the natural environment. Additionally, systematic desensitization can be used with the parent; this would be done in conjunction with systematic desensitization used to target the child's separation anxiety. The therapist can work with the parent and child together, having both rate anxiety, and leading both to expect anxiety reduction concurrent with practice.

Parents of SAD children sometimes become overconcerned with the child's distress in separation situations and, thus, avoid situations that might cause the child unhappiness. These parents report that they do not "force" their child to separate from themselves or the home (e.g., attend school) because they do not want the child to "suffer." This can be an obstacle to successful treatment because the parent may not encourage the child sufficiently to practice items on the hierarchy, to avoid producing distress in the child. These parents have difficulty tolerating anxiety in the child and often, therefore, acquiesce to child demands/requests that serve to reinforce or increase avoidance behavior. As with parental overprotectiveness, cognitive techniques can be used with these parents by challenging their maladaptive thoughts, teaching coping self-statements, and including the parent in the systematic desensitization hierarchy. It also is important to discuss the long-term goals with the parent and to point out that the long-term adjustment of the child is more important than the immediate desire to reduce the child's discomfort.

Practical issues also can be obstacles to successful treatment. One common issue is the amount of control parents have over specific items in the hierarchy. For example, a child who fears going to other children's homes would benefit from gradual exposure to this situation. While optimally one would gradually increase the time spent at another child's home, practically this may not be possible. Therefore, it is important to assess the practicality of various items included in the hierarchy.

Another common practical obstacle to treatment success can occur when targeting the child's refusal to sleep apart from the parent. The child with SAD often gets into the habit of sleeping in the parents' bedroom or having a parent sleep in the child's bedroom. Graduated exposure would involve having the child gradually return to his/her room or having the parent return to his/her room in a step-by-step manner. Indeed, most parents do not want to wake up in the middle of the night to gradually to decrease the time spent sleeping with the child. Another option is to have the parent gradually move further from where the child sleeps. For example, if the parent is sleeping in the child's bed, the first item on the hierarchy could be to sleep on a separate mattress in the child's room. The second could be to sleep just outside the child's door. With each item the parent could sleep closer to his/her own room until finally sleeping in his/her own bed. A third option is to have the parent remain in the child's room until the child falls asleep and gradually reduce the time spent in the child's room at bedtime. Each of these options involves some level of inconvenience, which may ultimately lead to parent and/or child noncompliance with the hierarchy. Use of potent rewards may facilitate compliance with this segment of treatment.

Finally, secondary gain for the child's separation-anxious behaviors, that is, child gaining additional advantages or reinforcers when remaining with the parent or in the home, can be an obstacle to successful treatment. As noted earlier, secondary gain should be assessed prior to treatment implementation and should be eliminated when possible. For example, does the child who refuses to attend school get to remain home, go on outings with parents, play with toys, and so on, rather than do school work? Does the child get significant attention from the parent or school personnel when anxious about separating? When secondary gain is evident, its elimination should be discussed with the parent(s) and/or school personnel.

RELAPSE PREVENTION

Follow-up studies in the literature (from three months to two years postter-mination) have demonstrated maintenance of treatment improvement (e.g., Bornstein and Knapp 1981, Mansdorf and Lukens 1987, Ollendick et al. 1991), that is, reduction of separation-related fears and behaviors, as well as the elimination of school refusal. However, these studies are limited by the fact that they are case studies, therefore lacking methodological rigor. Nevertheless, these studies provide preliminary evidence regarding mainte-nance of improvement following treatment of SAD symptomatology.

Clinical observations and empirical findings suggest that several factors can enhance maintenance of treatment gains. In particular, continuation of parental encouragement of the child's independence and praise given to the child for engaging in independent activities following treatment termination can result in continuity of gains. Intermittent reinforcement should be used to ensure that such behaviors persist. The parent must be cognizant of any previous secondary reinforcers that contributed to the child's SAD and should be cautious that these reinforcers do not reemerge. Finally, the onset of SAD often occurs after a major stressor, such as moving to a new neighborhood, changing schools, or experiencing the death or illness of a family member; therefore, the parent should be aware that such an event could cause SAD symptomatology to reappear. The parent then can increase praise to the child for independence, can review with the child cognitive self-statements and relaxation skills that he/she can use to cope with the added stress, and can be careful not to reinforce dependent behavior at this time.

An additional relapse prevention technique includes gradual discontinuation of therapist involvement (e.g., biweekly or monthly sessions) and follow-up telephone calls to the family from the therapist. Calls can be made a few weeks to a few months after termination or at the first few major transitions the child makes following termination (e.g., returning to school after summer vacation). Booster sessions also may be useful in ensuring maintenance of treatment gains.

TERMINATION

Following treatment, it is beneficial for assessment measures to be readministered to evaluate presence of *DSM-IV* SAD features, continuation of any avoidance behavior, cognitions, and physiological reactivity. Additionally, it can be useful for the parents to be educated regarding relapse prevention.

It is important to ensure that the termination of therapy not coincide with any critical periods that might be difficult for the child. For example, termination should not take place immediately prior to the child's return to school following a vacation. It is best for termination to be planned at a time when the child's environment is fairly stable. Gradual tapering of sessions may be considered in cases in which the parent or child has become dependent on the therapist or expresses anxiety about abrupt termination.

CASE ILLUSTRATION (TYPICAL TREATMENT)

Description and History

Matthew is a 10-year 5-month-old Caucasian male who was referred by his parents for evaluation and treatment due to separation anxiety and school refusal. Matthew lives with his mother, father, and 2-year-old sister. He currently is in the fifth grade and attends public elementary school.

Matthew's parents reported that he has been extremely fearful of attending school for the past several months and has refused to go to school for the past five weeks. Additionally, Matthew becomes anxious in many situations that involve being separated from his mother (e.g., staying at home with a baby-sitter, going to friends' homes, going to Boy Scout meetings). Should his mother need to go to a neighbor's house for a few minutes, Matthew insists on accompanying her. Matthew reported fearing that something might happen to his mother when he is apart from her, such as his mother being hurt or getting in an accident.

Matthew began to display separation anxiety symptoms nine months prior to the initial interview, following his parents' 1-month marital separation. Matthew's father had moved out of the home at that time due to the separation. Matthew's anxiety regarding separation from his mother gradually became worse in intensity and frequency, resulting in complete school refusal.

Assessment included semistructured diagnostic interviews individually administered to Matthew and his parents. Interview results confirmed a diagnosis of SAD according to *DSM-IV* criteria. Specifically, Matthew displayed the following *DSM-IV* diagnostic criteria: (1) persistent worry about harm befalling his mother, (2) persistent school refusal in order to remain with his mother, (3) recurrent complaints of excessive distress in anticipation of separation from his mother (e.g., cries and pleads with mother not to leave), and (4) recurrent excessive distress when separated from his mother. Matthew did not meet diagnostic criteria for additional anxiety or mood disorders.

In addition to the interview, Matthew completed two self-report measures, the STAIC and the Children's Depression Inventory (CDI, Kovacs 1978). Confirming interview data, results on the STAIC revealed high levels of both state (score = 58) and trait (score = 60) anxiety. Matthew's score on the CDI (score = 6) was consistent with interview data, suggesting that he did not display significant depressive symptomatology at the time of the initial assessment.

Synopsis of Therapy Sessions

Systematic desensitization using graduated in vivo exposure was selected as the primary treatment. Additionally, cognitive self-statements were taught to help Matthew cope with each item of the treatment hierarchy, as well as to eliminate worries regarding his mother's safety. Matthew practiced confronting feared situations on his hierarchy between sessions and recorded his anxiety level (0–8 Likert scale) during each confrontation on a record form provided by the therapist. Matthew was informed that he was in control of the rate at which he proceeded in confronting items on the hierarchy. The therapist, parents, and school personnel provided encouragement and praise throughout treatment.

During the first treatment session the fear and avoidance hierarchies were constructed. Two hierarchies were formed: one for school and another for a combination of other anxiety-provoking separation situations. Each hierarchy consisted of ten situations that provoked increasing levels of anxiety. Treatment first focused on the school hierarchy, since reentry into the school was extremely important. During weekly sessions, Matthew, his parents, and the therapist mutually agreed on the specific homework task that Matthew would practice during the week. Matthew's school hierarchy was as follows:

1. Entering the school building with mother (i.e., no school attendance).
2. Entering the school building alone.
3. Attending class for 15 minutes while mother waits in principal's office.
4. Attending class for 15 minutes with mother absent from school building.
5. Attending class for 30 minutes (mother not in building).
6. Attending class for 1 hour.
7. Attending class for 2 hours.
8. Attending class for 3 hours.
9. Attending class for 4 hours.
10. Attending class entire day.

During therapy sessions, Matthew was taught coping self-statements that he could implement when experiencing anxiety while practicing items on the hierarchy. The following dialogue is a synopsis of one session during which self-statements were generated for use on Matthew's first day returning to school by himself for thirty minutes:

Therapist: What were you thinking when your mother brought you to school today?

Child: I was thinking that she was going to leave me and then I became scared.

Therapist: Why does her leaving you make you scared?

Client: Something might happen to her; she might get hurt and never come back.

Therapist: Has she ever gotten hurt in the past after she dropped you off somewhere?

Client: No, I guess not. But what if she is late picking me up from school?

Therapist: What would happen?

Client: I guess I would wait until she came. I guess she has never been more than a few minutes late.

During this session Matthew's maladaptive self-statements were identified, and more adaptive coping self-statements were taught (e.g., "It is only for a short time. I will be able to handle this." "Mom will be fine. She can take care of herself and has never been hurt before.").

After the sixth week of treatment, Matthew was attending school daily for half of each day. His progress with school had generalized to some extent to other anxiety-provoking separation situations, such as attending Boy Scout meetings. By the end of twelve weeks, Matthew was able to attend full days of school and also had completed his second fear and avoidance hierarchy (begun during third week of treatment). Examples of items on this second hierarchy included allowing mother to leave the home for gradually longer periods of time, staying with a baby-sitter while parents go out for gradually increasing lengths of time, and attending Boy Scout meetings. The completion of this second hierarchy was much more rapid than the first, given that progress on the school hierarchy had generalized substantially.

Following the completion of treatment, assessment measures were re-administered. Results from parent and child reports on the interview indicated that Matthew no longer demonstrated significant symptoms of SAD. His self-reported anxiety on the STAIC was in the normal range for both state (score = 20) and trait (score = 23) anxiety. His posttreatment score on the CDI (score = 0) indicated an absence of depressive symptomatology. Additionally, Matthew rated his anxiety on all items of the Fear and Avoidance Hierarchies as zero.

The therapist spoke with the parents about relapse prevention. The therapist contacted the family two months posttermination, and Matthew's parents indicated that he displayed no symptoms of separation anxiety, was enjoying school, and was interacting well with other children when separated from his mother.

Comments

This case illustrates a typical presentation of a child with SAD. While therapy consisted of systematic desensitization in conjunction with cognitive techniques, other techniques often are used with SAD children. For example, if Matthew had presented with excessive physical tension, progressive relaxation training would have been implemented. Nevertheless, this case was representative of a typical SAD case in that treatment lasted approximately twelve sessions with immediate, but gradual, improvement displayed. Parents were somewhat overprotective, but cooperative with treatment. Finally, improvement was maintained two months posttreatment.

CASE ILLUSTRATION (OVERCOMING OBSTACLES)

Description and History

Jake is an 11-year 6-month-old Caucasian male referred by his physician for evaluation and treatment due to problems with school refusal and physical complaints of stomachaches for which no medical basis could be found. Jake resides with both biological parents and his 15-year-old sister. His father is a blue-collar worker and his mother is a homemaker. Jake attends the sixth grade in a public school.

A clinical interview conducted with Jake and his mother revealed that Jake has a long-standing history of mild anxiety associated with separation from his mother, particularly related to school attendance. Although Jake previously demonstrated anxiety about school attendance following illnesses or vacations, he did not have difficulties with excessive school absenteeism in the past. During the four months preceding the evaluation, however, Jake increasingly refused to attend school; he missed a total of twenty-two days during that period of time. During the two weeks just prior to the assessment, Jake had attended only two full school days. In addition to problems with separation to attend school, Jake displayed difficulties separating from his mother to go to friends' homes, to go to extracurricular activities, and even to be apart while at home (while the mother showered, while Jake dressed in the mornings, and so on).

A semistructured interview conducted separately with Jake and with his mother indicated that Jake met *DSM-IV* diagnostic criteria for SAD and dysthymic disorder. Specific SAD symptoms endorsed by both Jake and his mother included the following: (1) unrealistic worry about possible harm befalling his mother; (2) refusal to attend school to stay at home with his mother; (3) avoidance of being alone or apart from his mother while at home; (4) somatic complaints, including headaches and stomachaches, on school mornings; (5) excessive distress in anticipation of separation from his mother; and (6) excessive distress when apart from his mother.

Jake also completed the RCMAS and the CDI. He demonstrated significant problems with anxiety on the RCMAS, with elevations on the worry/oversensitivity and physiological factors of this measure. His score of 19 on the CDI indicated moderate problems with depression, which was consistent with the diagnosis of dysthymia reported during the semistructured interviews.

Direct observations of Jake's ability to separate from his mother were conducted informally, when Jake was asked to be apart from his mother for the interview. Jake expressed strong reluctance to allow the mother to remain in the waiting area while he accompanied the clinician to the interview room. He became teary-eyed and refused to walk with the clinician. Jake was able to have the mother sit on a chair outside the interview room, with the door closed, during the one-hour interview, without experiencing significant anxiety (i.e., level of 2 on a 0-8 Likert scale).

Synopsis of Therapy Sessions

Initially, the primary treatment approaches employed included a graduated in vivo exposure procedure, use of cognitive coping statements, and progressive muscle relaxation training. Three treatment hierarchies were developed: one for gradual exposure to school attendance, one for being apart while at home, and one for going places without his mother. The school-attendance hierarchy closely resembled the one devised for the typical treatment case in the previous section. The hierarchy aimed at reducing anxiety while apart from his mother at home included items such as: put Jake's shoes and socks on in his own room while mom is in her room; put pants, shirt, shoes, and socks on in his own room while mom is in her room; sit outside bathroom while mom showers with door halfway closed; sit outside bathroom while mom showers with door fully closed; sit down the hall while mom showers with door fully closed; play in his room while mom showers with door fully closed; and so on. Examples of items on the third hierarchy, involving Jake going places without his mother, included go to a friend's house in the neighborhood for twenty minutes; go to a friend's house in the neighborhood for forty-five minutes; go to a friend's house in the neighborhood for two hours; go to a friend's house outside the neighborhood for one hour; go to soccer practice while mom sits in the car; go to soccer practice while mom stays at friend's house ten minutes away; and so on. Use of coping self-statements (e.g., "Mom is fine and so am I." "I'm going to be brave. It is only for twenty minutes.") and relaxation skills facilitated Jake's progress on each treatment hierarchy.

As treatment progressed, it became evident that the mother became increasingly anxious and, consequently, discouraged Jake's independence. For example, she provided numerous excuses for not complying with hierarchy items requiring Jake to leave the home without her. Upon further inquiry, the mother indicated that she experienced anxiety about separating from Jake. The following is an excerpt from a treatment session with Jake and his mother:

Therapist: What occurred this week that interfered with your practice of your hierarchy item: going to a friend's house in the neighborhood for twenty minutes?

Child: I don't know.

Mother: We were very busy and there just was no opportunity.

Therapist: It seems that there were opportunities to practice items on your other hierarchy. Might there be some other difficulty with this particular item?

Mother: Well... I sometimes worry that Jake will become too nervous at his friend's house and will be unable to stay without me. I also become somewhat anxious myself when I am alone without him.

Therapist: Oh, I see. How long have you felt anxious about being apart from Jake?

Mother: As long as I can remember. I just feel more comfortable having him with me.

Therapist: Perhaps we can work on your anxiety about separating from Jake in much the same way we have been helping Jake overcome his fearfulness. How does that sound to you?

Mother: I would like that.

As a result, a separate treatment hierarchy was developed for the mother, containing items related to the mother's own independent activities (e.g., going to the store alone; engaging in activity while Jake completes his homework, rather than sit next to him). While developing the hierarchy, it was learned that the mother had a history of mild panic disorder with agoraphobia. She had commonly included Jake in most activities outside the home, which had discouraged development of independence in Jake. It also became evident that marital problems existed, which led the mother to depend too heavily on Jake's companionship rather than her husband's company.

Once the mother was more actively involved in treatment and provided with coping strategies similar to those developed for Jake, that is, cognitive coping and relaxation skills, Jake's progress increased dramatically. In addition, the parents were referred for marital therapy.

Treatment extended over a five-month period. Jake was able to attend full days of school on a regular basis after fourteen weeks of graduated exposure. He mastered items on the two remaining hierarchies by the fourth month of treatment as well. Jake became increasingly independent over the course of therapy, in that he was able to complete homework on his own, wash his own hair, go to friends' homes without experiencing anxiety, and participate on a soccer team, all skills that were absent prior to the initiation of therapy.

A posttreatment evaluation using baseline assessment measures revealed that Jake no longer met *DSM-IV* criteria for SAD or dysthymic disorder. His low scores on the CDI (3) and RCMAS (5) also indicated that Jake no longer experienced significant problems with depressive or anxiety symptomatology. Jake easily separated from the mother to talk with the clinician on his own.

Comments

Jake's progress in treatment was hindered by his mother's own anxiety about separation and the parents' marital difficulties. Although systematic desensitization, cognitive-behavior therapy, and relaxation training resulted in some improvements, full success was not achieved until treatment addressed the mother's anxiety and marital problems as well. This case illustrates how it could be beneficial to assess parental psychopathology, marital dysfunction, and life stressors routinely prior to initiation of therapy to enhance treatment success.

SUMMARY

This chapter provides a description of SAD and its diagnosis, and reviews methods of assessment, behavioral and cognitive-behavioral therapy strategies, and pharmacological interventions for SAD. The defining feature of SAD is an unrealistic and excessive fear of separation from a major attachment figure, usually the parent. Avoidance of separation from the parent may take several forms, often with the child showing reluctance to attend school.

Many measures have been developed to assess the presence and severity of SAD and other anxiety disorders. Some of these assessment instruments provide a broad overview of the child's distress, whereas others assess specific aspects of the child's anxiety. Instruments include diagnostic interview schedules, parent checklists, self-report inventories, observational strategies, and physiological measures. It is recommended that these measures be used in conjunction with one another to obtain a thorough clinical assessment.

The literature regarding treatment methods for SAD consists mainly of descriptive case reports of behavioral and cognitive-behavioral methods and a few experimental studies examining the efficacy of pharmacotherapy. Reports assessing the efficacy of behavioral and cognitive-behavioral methods support their use in the treatment of SAD. Research assessing the efficacy of pharmacological treatment of SAD remains equivocal. While some studies indicate that imipramine is effective in the treatment of SAD, others find that it is not beneficial. Preliminary evidence also suggests that alprazolam (an anxiolytic) might be effective in reducing SAD symptomatology. Further research is necessary before conclusions regarding the efficacy of specific behavioral techniques and pharmacotherapy can be made.

Although research in the area of SAD is growing, many questions remain regarding the diagnosis, assessment, and treatment of this disorder. The majority of treatment studies are uncontrolled case studies, which do not allow thorough assessment of treatment efficacy. Nevertheless, these studies do provide important information regarding various treatment options and can serve as models for future research in this area.

REFERENCES

Achenbach, T. M., and Edelbrock, C. (1983). *Manual for the Child Behavior Checklist and Revised Child Behavior Profile*. Burlington, VT: University of Vermont Department of Psychiatry.

Bandura, A., and Menlove, F. (1968). Factors determining vicarious extinction of avoidance behavior through symbolic modeling. *Journal of Personality and Social Psychology* 8:99–108.

Barlow, D. H. (1988). *Anxiety and Its Disorders*. New York: Guilford.

Beidel, D. C. (1988). Psychophysiological assessment of anxious emotional states in children. *Journal of Abnormal Psychology* 97:80–82.

Berney, T., Kolvin, I., Bhate, S. R., et al. (1981). School phobia: a therapeutic trial with clomipramine and short-term outcome. *British Journal of Psychiatry* 138:110–118.

Bernstein, D. A., and Borkovec, T. D. (1973). *Progressive Relaxation Training: A Manual for the Helping Professions.* Champaign, IL: Research Press.

Bernstein, G. A., Garfinkel, B. D., and Borchardt, C. M. (1990). Comparative studies of pharmacotherapy for school refusal. *Journal of the American Academy of Child and Adolescent Psychiatry* 29:773–781.

Bornstein, P. H., and Knapp, M. (1981). Self-control desensitization with a multiphobic boy: a multiple baseline design. *Journal of Behavior Therapy and Experimental Psychiatry* 12:281–285.

Burke, A. E., and Silverman, W. K. (1987). The prescriptive treatment of school refusal. *Clinical Psychology Review* 7:353–362.

Chambers, W. J., Puig-Antich, J., Hirsch, M., et al. (1985). The assessment of affective disorders in children and adolescents by semi-structured interview. *Archives of General Psychiatry* 42:696–702.

Conners, C. K. (1969). A teacher rating scale for use in drug studies with children. *American Journal of Psychiatry* 126:884–888.

Costello, A. J., Edelbrock, C. S., Kalas, R., et al. (1984). *Development and Testing of the NIMH Diagnostic Interview Schedule for Children (DISC) in a Clinical Population: Final Report.* Rockville, MD: Center for Epidemiological Studies, NIMH.

Diagnostic and Statistical Manual of Mental Disorders (1980). 3rd ed. Washington, DC: American Psychiatric Association.

Diagnostic and Statistical Manual of Mental Disorders (1987). 3rd ed., revised. Washington, DC: American Psychiatric Association.

Diagnostic and Statistical Manual of Mental Disorders (1994). 4th ed. Washington, DC: American Psychiatric Association.

Doris, J., McIntyre, J. R., Kelsey, C., and Lehman, E. (1971). Separation anxiety in nursery school children. *Proceedings of the 79th Annual Convention of the American Psychological Association* 79:145–146.

Emmelkamp, P. M. G. (1982). *Phobic and Obsessive-Compulsive Disorders: Theory, Research, and Practice.* New York: Plenum.

Fox, J. E., and Houston, B. K. (1983). Distinguishing between cognitive and somatic trait and state anxiety. *Journal of Personality and Social Psychology* 45:862–870.

Francis, G. (1988). Assessing cognitions in anxious children. *Behavior Modification* 12:267–280.

Gittelman-Klein, R., and Klein, D. F. (1971). Controlled imipramine treatment of school phobia. *Archives of General Psychiatry* 25:204–207.

—— (1973). School phobia: diagnostic considerations in the light of imipramine effects. *Journal of Nervous and Mental Disease* 156:199–215.

—— (1980). Separation anxiety in school refusal and its treatment with drugs. In *Out of School,* ed. R. Gittelman, pp. 188–203. New York: Guilford.

Hodges, K. (1987). Assessing children with a clinical research interview: the Child Assessment Schedule. In *Advances in Behavioral Assessment of Children and Families*, vol. 3, ed. R. J. Prinz, pp. 203–234. Greenwich, CT: JAI Press.

Hoehn-Saric E., Maisami, M., and Wiegand, D. (1987). Measurement of anxiety in children and adolescents using semistructured interviews. *Journal of the American Academy of Child and Adolescent Psychiatry* 26:541–545.

———— (1990). A community study of anxiety in children and adolescents. *American Journal of Psychiatry* 147:313–318.

Kashani, J. H., and Orvashel, H. (1988). Anxiety disorders in midadolescence: a community sample. *American Journal of Psychiatry* 145:960- 964.

Kearney, C. A., and Silverman, W. K. (1993). Measuring the function of school refusal behavior: the School Refusal Assessment Scale (SRAS). *Journal of Clinical Child Psychology* 22:85–96.

Klein, R. G., Koplewicz, H. S., and Kanner, A. (1992). Imipramine treatment of children with separation anxiety disorder. *Journal of the American Academy of Child and Adolescent Psychiatry* 31:21–28.

Klein, R. G., and Last, C. G. (1989). Anxiety disorders in children. In *Developmental Clinical Psychology and Psychiatry*, ed. A. E. Kazdin, pp. 32–34. Newbury Park, CA: Sage.

Kovacs, M. (1978). *Children's Depression Inventory (CDI)*. University of Pittsburgh School of Medicine. Unpublished manuscript.

Kovacs, M. (1983). *The Interview Schedule for Children (ISC): Interrater and Parent-child Agreement*. Pittsburgh: University of Pittsburgh School of Medicine. Unpublished manuscript.

Kutcher, S. P., Reiter, S., Gardner, K. M., and Klein, R. G. (1992). The pharmacotherapy of anxiety disorders in children and adolescents. *Psychiatric Clinics of North America* 15:41–67.

Lang, P. J., and Lazovik, A. D. (1963). Experimental desensitization of a phobia. *Journal of Abnormal and Social Psychology* 66:519–525.

Last, C. G. (1989). Anxiety disorders. In *Handbook of Child Psychopathology*, ed. T. H. Ollendick and M. Hersen, 2nd ed., pp. 219–228. New York: Plenum.

Last, C. G. (1991). Somatic complaints in anxiety disordered children. *Journal of Anxiety Disorders* 5:125–138.

Last, C. G., Francis, G., Hersen, M., et al. (1987a). Separation anxiety and school phobia: a comparison using *DSM-III* criteria. *American Journal of Psychiatry* 144:653–657.

Last, C. G., Hersen, M., Kazdin, A. E., et al. (1987b). Comparison of *DSM-III* separation anxiety and overanxious disorders: demographic characteristics and patterns of comorbidity. *Journal of the American Academy of Child and Adolescent Psychiatry* 26:527-531.

Last, C. G., Strauss, C. C., and Francis, G. (1987c). Comorbidity among childhood anxiety disorders. *Journal of Nervous and Mental Disease* 175:726–730.

Leitenberg, H., Yost, L. W., and Carroll-Wilson, M. (1986). Negative cognitive errors in children: questionnaire development, normative data, and comparisons between children with and without self-reported symptoms of depression, low self-esteem, and evaluation anxiety. *Journal of Consulting and Clinical Psychology* 54:528–536.

Mansdorf, I. J., and Lukens, E. (1987). Cognitive-behavioral psychotherapy for separation anxious children exhibiting school phobia. *Journal of the American Academy of Child and Adolescent Psychiatry* 26:222–225.

Matthews, K. A., Manuck, S. B., and Saab, P. G. (1986). Cardiovascular responses of adolescents during a naturally occurring stressor and their behavioral and psychophysiological predictors. *Psychophysiology* 23:198–209.

Mavissakalian, M., and Barlow, D. H. (1981). *Phobia: Psychological and Pharmacological Treatment*. New York: Guilford.

Miller, L. C., Barrett, C. L., Hampe, E., and Noble, H. (1971). Revised anxiety scales for the Louisville Behavior Checklist. *Psychological Reports* 29:503–511.

———— (1972). Factor structure of childhood fears. *Journal of Consulting and Clinical Psychology* 39:264–268.

Milos, M. E., and Reiss, S. (1982). Effects of three play conditions on separation anxiety in young children. *Journal of Consulting and Clinical Psychology* 50:389–395.

Moreau, D., and Follett, C. (1993). Panic disorder in children and adolescents. *Child and Adolescent Psychiatric Clinics of North America* 2:581–602.

Ollendick, T. H. (1983). Reliability and validity of the Revised Fear Survey Schedule for Children (FSSC-R). *Behaviour Research and Therapy* 21:685–692.

Ollendick, T. H., and Cerny, J. A. (1981). *Clinical Behavior Therapy with Children*. New York: Plenum.

Ollendick, T. H., Hagopian, L. P., and Huntzinger, R. M. (1991). Cognitive-behavior therapy with nighttime fearful children. *Journal of Behavior Therapy and Experimental Psychiatry* 22:113–121.

Osborn, E. L. (1986). Effects of participant modeling and desensitization on childhood warm water phobia. *Journal of Behavior Therapy and Experimental Psychiatry* 17:117–119.

Reich, W., Herjanic, B., Welner, Z., and Gandhy, P. R. (1982). Development of a structured psychiatric interview for children: agreement on diagnosis comparing child and parent interviews. *Journal of Abnormal Child Psychology* 10:325–336.

Reynolds, C. R., and Paget, K. D. (1981). Factor analysis of the Revised Children's Manifest Anxiety Scale for blacks, whites, males, and females with a national normative sample. *Journal of Consulting and Clinical Psychology* 49:352–359.

Rutter, M. (1981). Emotional development. In *Scientific Foundations of Developmental Psychiatry*, ed. M. Rutter. Baltimore: University Park Press.

Silverman, W. K., and Nelles, W. B. (1988). The Anxiety Disorders Interview Schedule for Children. *Journal of the American Academy of Child and Adolescent Psychiatry* 27:772–778.

Spielberger, C. D. (1973). *State-Trait Anxiety Inventory for Children*. Palo Alto, CA: Consulting Psychologists Press.

Thyer, B. A., and Sowers-Hoag, K. M. (1988). Behavior therapy for separation anxiety disorder. *Behavior Modification* 12:205–233.

Ultee, C. A., Griffoen, D., and Schellekens, J. (1982). The reduction of anxiety in children: a comparison of the effects of "systematic desensitization in vitro" and "systematic desensitization in vivo." *Behaviour Research and Therapy* 20:61–67.

Zatz, S., and Chassin, L. (1983). Cognitions of test-anxious children. *Journal of Consulting and Clinical Psychology* 51:526–534.

4

PEER RELATIONS

Annette M. La Greca
Michael D. Fetter

INTRODUCTION

Abundant evidence supports the contention that children who experience interpersonal difficulties with peers are at substantial risk for emotional problems (Kupersmidt and Coie 1990, Parker and Asher 1987). Parker and Asher's (1987) analysis of retrospective and prospective research clearly demonstrates that peer ratings of low acceptance and rejection are excellent predictors of later psychological maladjustment. For example, low levels of peer acceptance during the fifth and sixth grades predict adolescent dysfunction, as indexed by dropping out of school (Barclay 1966, Gronlund and Holmlund 1958, Kupersmidt 1983). Moreover, children who are rejected by their classmates in elementary school have been found to display more mental health problems during late adolescence and early adulthood than their more accepted classmates (Cowen et al. 1973). Findings such as these underscore the important role of peer relations in social and emotional adjustment.

Furthermore, it is noteworthy that deficient peer relations are a common feature of a number of child psychiatric disorders (Dodge 1989). For example, impairments in peer relations are included in the diagnostic criteria for several childhood disorders listed in *DSM-IV* (American Psychiatric Association 1994), such as attention deficit–hyperactivity disorder, conduct disorder, oppositional defiant disorder, avoidant disorder of childhood or adolescence, social phobia, adjustment disorder, and autistic disorder, among others (see Dodge 1989 for a summary).

Because of this linkage between peer relationship problems and psychological maladjustment, there has been considerable interest in recent years in developing interventions for children with peer relationship problems. Most of these interventions have been directed at improving the social status and social skills of low accepted or rejected elementary school children (see Dodge 1989, La Greca 1993, Ladd 1985). These interventions and their clinical applications will be the primary focus of this chapter.

LITERATURE REVIEW

Models Linking Peer Relations with Later Maladjustment

To understand the conceptual model underlying the development of social skills interventions, it is important to appreciate the nature of the linkage between children's peer relations and their later social/emotional functioning. Clinical and developmental researchers interested in children's peer relations have proposed at least three models for linking poor peer relations to later maladjustment (see Kupersmidt et al. 1990, Parker and Asher 1987). Problematic peer relations have been viewed alternatively as (1) a marker for more basic underlying disturbance ("incidental model"), (2) a factor that moderates the outcome between vulnerability and later psychopathology, such that problematic peer relations lead to negative outcomes among individuals who are somehow "vulnerable" due to genetic, biological, or other nonosocial reasons, or (3) a causal factor in the development of maladjustment ("causal model"). Of these possibilities, the causal model holds the most promise, as accumulating evidence suggests that peer rejection contributes to children's negative self-perceptions and further behavioral difficulties (Asher et al. 1990, Coie 1990, Kupersmidt et al. 1990, Parker and Asher 1987). Moreover, this causal model underlies the considerable research on interventions to improve children's social skills and peer relations (cf. Ladd 1985).

Stated in very general terms, the basic assumption inherent in the causal model is that rejected children are excluded from normal socialization experiences that are important for social, affective, and cognitive development. The deviant socialization experiences of these children, in turn, contribute to more maladaptive ways of thinking and behaving and, over time, to adjustment problems (Coie 1990, Kupersmidt et al. 1990, Parker and Asher 1987). See Figure 4–1.

Within this basic causal model, two potential mediating pathways link poor peer relations and later maladjustment (Kupersmidt et al. 1990). In one scenario, peer acceptance provides children with the opportunity to interact with peers in ways that may promote the development of social and affective competencies. Thus, children with low peer acceptance, and those who are

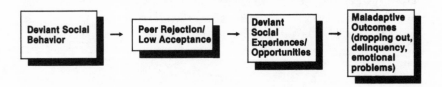

Figure 4-1. Causal Model of Peer Relations and Later Outcome (Adapted from Parker and Asher 1987. Reprinted by permission.)

actively excluded by peers, may develop social-emotional deficiencies that lead to later maladjustment. In a second view, peer rejection may lead to high levels of internal distress (e.g., feelings of loneliness or inadequacy) that in turn foster maladaptive behavior (Kupersmidt et al. 1990). Consistent with the causal model, existing research has consistently linked peer acceptance with positive social skills and adaptive emotional functioning (Coie et al. 1990, La Greca and Stark 1986) as well as linking peer rejection with internal distress (Asher et al. 1990, La Greca et al. 1988) and behavioral problems (Coie et al. 1990).

This model is important to the understanding of social skills interventions. Because of the presumed causal linkages between peer relations and later maladjustment, interventions have focused on strategies for *changing* a child's peer status. In turn, improved peer status should lead to more adaptive social experiences, as well as reductions in subjective distress, with the ultimate benefit of more healthy emotional adaptation over time. Thus, interventions to improve peer status are designed to interrupt a negative chain of events, paving the way for more positive mental health outcomes. In this sense, social skills interventions are perhaps best conceptualized as preventive strategies, although they have also been adapted to clinical situations where peer relationship problems coexist with other behavior problems (e.g., Bornstein et al. 1980, Kolko et al. 1990).

With this conceptual model in mind, the basic assessment strategy has been to first identify *which children are not liked by their peers*; that is, those who may be rejected or left out of peer activities. Once this has been determined, further information on *what the child is like* is necessary to pinpoint the nature of the social problem and develop an intervention plan. In the subsequent sections we will review information pertinent to these two basic assessment and intervention questions.

How Well Is a Child Liked by Peers? Distinctions Between Rejection and Acceptance

In determining a child's peer status, prior research underscores the importance of distinguishing between peer *acceptance* and peer *rejection* as two separate dimensions of peer relations (Coie et al. 1982, Dodge et al. 1982). Peer acceptance (or peer liking) reflects the extent to which a child is liked by classmates. On the other hand, peer rejection (or peer disliking) reflects the extent to which a child is disliked by his or her peers. By examining children's relative standing on the dimensions of peer liking and disliking, various social status classifications have been identified, each with associated characteristics. See Figure 4–2.

The children who appear to have the most interpersonal, emotional, and academic difficulties are those who are actively *rejected* by peers—that is, children who are high on peer disliking and low on peer liking. Rejected children often demonstrate aggressive, disruptive, or inattentive behaviors, in addition to low levels of positive social interaction skills such as cooperation, friendliness, and leadership abilities (Coie and Dodge 1988, Coie et al.

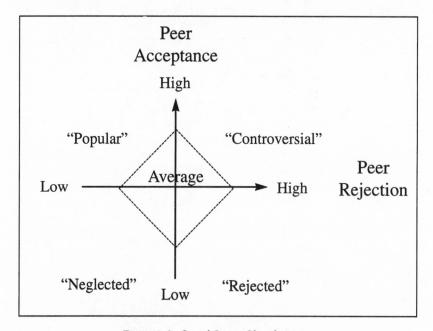

Figure 4–2. Social Status Classifications

1982, Dodge et al. 1982; see Coie et al. 1990 for a review). Furthermore, rejected children often display problems in academic performance (Green et al. 1980, Stone and La Greca 1990), and report feelings of depression, loneliness, and social anxiety at higher rates than their more accepted classmates (Asher and Wheeler 1985, La Greca and Stone 1993). In short, rejected social status has been linked with a host of internalizing and externalizing behavior problems, as well as poor school achievement.

In contrast, children who are *neglected* by peers appear to fare somewhat better. Neglected children are defined as those who are low on peer liking and on peer disliking; they are the students who often go unnoticed by their peers. Unlike rejected youth, neglected children do not typically demonstrate externalizing behavior problems, but have been distinguished from their more socially accepted peers by their low rates of social interaction (Coie and Dodge 1988, Dodge et al. 1982) and their high levels of social anxiety (La Greca et al. 1988, La Greca and Stone 1993). While not as overtly problematic as rejected youth, neglected children who are socially anxious may have difficulty developing supportive friendship ties.

Other social status classifications included *popular* children (i.e., those high on peer liking, low on peer disliking), and *controversial* children (i.e., those high on both peer liking and disliking). While little research has been directed at controversial youth, popular children tend to excel in social relations and display positive interaction skills (e.g., Coie et al. 1982, Coie et al. 1990, Dodge et al. 1982, Hartup 1983).

Following from the above, when a child is experiencing difficulties in peer relations, perhaps the first question to ask is, "How is this child viewed by peers and classmates?" Children who are not well-liked, or have no friends or playmates, may be socially isolated and need some help or support in developing friendship ties. If, in addition to low levels of peer acceptance, children are actively disliked or rejected, then intervention strategies will be needed not only to increase their positive interactions but also to modify the behaviors (or other personal characteristics) that contribute to peers' dislike.

What Is a Child Like? Behavioral and Personal Characteristics of Note

Beyond understanding a child's peer status, an appreciation of a child's behavioral style and personal characteristics will be important for evaluating peer relationship problems and implementing appropriate social interventions. Returning to the causal model of peer relations depicted in Figure 4–1, we are now interested in the question, "What is the child like?" In other words, what behavioral and personal characteristics precede or contribute to peer relationship problems, and how can these be modified?

There are a multitude of factors that may contribute to peer relationship problems. In order to intervene effectively, however, it is imperative to understand the specific nature of peer difficulties for the individual child. Broadly speaking, peer relationship difficulties may fall into one of three categories: (a) deficits in positive interaction skills, (b) the presence of behavior problems that interfere with social interactions, and (c) the presence of other nonbehavioral child characteristics that contribute to peers' dislike. These three categories are highlighted below; however, the reader is referred to several additional sources for more detailed information on factors contributing to poor peer relations (Coie et al. 1990, Dodge 1989, Hartup 1983, Vaughn and La Greca 1988, 1992).

One common factor contributing to peer relationship problems is that some children lack the *social interaction skills* necessary for initiating and maintaining peer friendships and getting along with others. These positive social skills might include cooperating and sharing with others, and knowing how to play with and communicate with others (see Gottman et al. 1975, Hartup 1983, La Greca and Mesibov 1979, Vaughn and La Greca 1988). Children who are lacking in these areas may profit from learning more appropriate ways to interact with peers. Indeed, most social skills intervention programs have been developed for the specific purpose of increasing children's positive social behaviors (e.g., Gresham and Nagle 1980, La Greca and Mesibov 1981, La Greca and Santogrossi 1980, Oden and Asher 1977). Prior to beginning a social skills intervention, it is critical for the children to assess the child's social skills and identify areas of social strength and weakness. Social skills training is likely to have the most impact on children who need to learn or improve their peer interaction skills.

A second consideration for evaluating the nature of a child's peer difficulties is appreciating the child's behavioral style. In many instances, children's behavior problems interfere with successful peer relations. Perhaps the most difficulty can be observed by children with *externalizing* behavior problems. Children who are aggressive, impulsive, or intrusive typically elicit negative reactions from peers (Coie and Kupersmidt 1983, Dodge 1983, Dodge et al. 1982). Because of this, children who have difficulty controlling aversive and intrusive behaviors may need to learn more effective self-control strategies to improve their peer relations (e.g., Bierman et al. 1987, La Greca et al. 1989).

In contrast, although children with *internalizing* behavior problems may not be as prone to peer rejection as their acting-out classmates, evidence suggests that high levels of anxiety interfere with children's initiation of and engagement in peer activities (La Greca and Stone 1993, Strauss et al. 1988, Vernberg et al. 1992). For example, socially anxious children may avoid peer contacts and actively limit their social participation. In such cases, anxiety reduction procedures (e.g., exposure, relaxation) may be necessary components of a social skills intervention program.

Finally, *other child characteristics* may contribute to peers' dislike of an individual child, independent of the child's actual social behavior. These characteristics include low academic achievement, presence of physical disabilities or handicaps, and physical unattractiveness or obesity, among other possibilities. For example, children with poor academic achievement, including those with learning disabilities, have been found to be more rejected and less accepted than their normally achieving classmates (Bryan 1974, 1976, Green et al. 1980, Stone and La Greca 1990). Also, social isolation appears to be a common concomitant of childhood obesity (Wicks-Nelson and Israel 1991). When a problem is evident with academic skills or physical appearance, interventions might take the form of attempting to modify the characteristic (e.g., improving academic performance) and/or modifying children's and teachers' attitudes (e.g., improving classmates' acceptance of handicapped children). For many children, peer relation difficulties cut across multiple categories. In such cases, multiple intervention strategies will be necessary to improve the child's peer functioning and overall adaptation.

Who Are the Child's Friends? A Consideration of Peer Friendships and Peer Support

Although the primary goal of children's social skill interventions has been to improve peer acceptance (or reduce peer rejection), as described above, recent reviews of the social intervention area have argued that this goal is too narrow (cf. La Greca 1993). Current thinking suggests that improving the quality of children's *friendships* is also an important consideration. Even children who are not liked by their peers may have peer friendships that provide support and companionship. In fact, it may be the case that close, supportive peers might help to mitigate the negative psychological impact of peer rejection (Parker and Asher 1987). Although this notion has not been formally evaluated as yet, it appears that supportive peers have been shown to act as a buffer against other life stressors, such as parents' divorce (Sandler et al. 1985) and beginning a new school (Felner et al. 1982, Simmons et al. 1987). Substantial evidence suggests that individuals with strong social support are able to cope more effectively with life stresses than those lacking such resources (Cohen and Wills 1985).

At this point it may be instructive to distinguish peer acceptance and peer-friendship support. Peer acceptance refers to the extent to which a child is liked or accepted by his/her peer group but not the extent or quality of the child's friendships. In contrast, friendship support pertains to the child's perceptions of intimacy, help, and companionship from peer friendships, and these friendships may occur outside the classroom. Getting along with one's classmates is very different from forming close, supportive ties with one or more peers (Furman and Robbins 1985). Furman and Robbins (1985) emphasize that friendships and acquaintanceships serve different emotional needs; friendships provide children with a sense of intimacy, companionship, and self-esteem, whereas group acceptance may give children a sense of social inclusion. Thus, peer acceptance and peer friendship support should be viewed as related but distinct constructs.

Both peer acceptance and peer friendships are likely to be important for a child's emotional health and psychological adjustment. In fact, studies with children and adolescents reveal that peers are significant providers of emotional support and are the main providers of companionship support (Berndt 1989, Cauce et al. 1990, Furman and Buhrmester 1985, Reid et al. 1989). As children progress from preschool through the middle school years, friends take on increasing significance as providers of emotional and companionship support (Furman and Buhrmester 1985, Reid et al. 1989). Furthermore, research with children indicates that emotional support may contribute directly to the development of positive self-appraisals and a sense of competence (Dubow and Tisak 1989). In addition, emotional support is most instrumental in buffering the negative effects of stress (Cohen and Wills 1985), perhaps because emotional support conveys to the stressed individual that he/she is valued, which in turns leads to enhanced self-esteem and more effective coping (Dubow and Tisak 1989). Thus, when evaluating a child's peer relations, one should also consider whether or not the child has close friends and companions, both inside and outside the classroom setting. Developing more supportive friendship ties may be an important goal of children's social interventions.

ASSESSMENT PROCEDURES

As the literature summarized above indicates, multiple areas will be critical for assessing and understanding children's peer relations. Not surprisingly, the assessment of peer relationship problems in children has proven to be difficult and challenging. Although peer ratings are perhaps the most sensitive and ecologically valid means of identifying children who are rejected or not well accepted by their peers (Landau and Milich 1990), such ratings are difficult to obtain in clinical settings. Another disadvantage to peer ratings is that they primarily reflect how well the child is liked, but do not provide clues as to the nature of the child's peer relationship problems, nor do they provide information about friendships or other aspects of supportive relationships. For this reason, professionals will be most interested in using a variety of methods and measures in their assessment of children's peer relations.

The following strategy may facilitate obtaining a comprehensive picture of children's social skills and interpersonal relations. First, some assessment of peers' impressions of the child may be useful. This will provide an indication of how the child is viewed by others, and also may help to identify others who are receptive to the child. Such information will be useful for designing interventions that involve classmates and peers. Although the best strategy for assessing children's social status is through peer reports, these can be difficult to obtain in clinical settings. When peer ratings are not available, teachers' and parents' reports of peer acceptance and rejection may be useful proxies.

Second, it is critical to obtain a picture of the child's current friendships and social contacts, as well as his or her feelings about peer relationships. Feelings of social anxiety, social dissatisfaction, lack of support, or loneliness may help to pinpoint children who are distressed by their current social situation and who may be motivated to change. Also, youngsters' reports of social anxiety may help to explain why some children are avoidant of interactions with peers. Improvements in subjective feelings of social distress may also help to monitor a child's progress through treatment. Information regarding friends and social relations can best be obtained from interviews with the child and parents.

Third, information on the child's level of social skills will be critical for treatment planning. Several methods for assessing social skills currently exist, such as behavioral observations, role-plays, and ratings scales.

Fourth, information on the child's behavior problems (internalizing and externalizing behaviors) that interfere with their peer contacts will be useful. Several parent- and teacher-report measures of behavior problems may prove useful in this regard.

Finally, information on children's special abilities and disabilities, including academic strengths and weaknesses, is also critical. Children's strengths and weaknesses are useful in planning interventions, and may suggest avenues for intervention that complement traditional social skills training (e.g., educational interventions for low-achieving rejected youth).

In the sections below, a representative sampling of measures used to assess children's social functioning is provided. For a more detailed and comprehensive discussion of issues and methods for evaluating children's social functioning and related problems, the reader is referred to several sources (Dodge 1989, Erwin 1993, Hughes 1988, Krehbiel and Milich 1986, La Greca and Stark 1986, Landau and Milich 1990).

Measures of Peer Relations: Acceptance and Rejection

Peer Nominations of Acceptance and Rejection

Peer nominations represent the most widely accepted method for assessing the quality of students' peer relations (Landau and Milich 1990). Typically, youngsters nominate the three classmates they "like the most" (peer acceptance; PA) and the three that they "like the least" (peer rejection; PR). A child's score is the number of nominations received. For research purposes, these nomination scores are then standardized by sex within each classroom or grade. Thus, standardized PA and PR scores are obtained, each with a mean of 0, and standard deviation of 1. Extensive research indicates that peer nominations are stable over time and have good concurrent and predictive validity (Landau and Milich 1990, Roff et al. 1972).

It is important to note that peer nominations of acceptance and rejection are only moderately negatively correlated and represent distinct dimensions of peer status (Landau and Milich 1990). Children's scores on PA and PR have been used to classify children into one of five distinct social status groups: rejected, neglected, popular, controversial, and average (see Coie et al. 1982; also see Figure 4–2).[1] Both rejected and neglected children receive few positive

---

[1]This is accomplished by computing scores for Social Preference (PA minus PR) and Social Impact (PA plus PR), which are again standardized. Social status groups are then derived as follows: (a) *popular*, consisting of youngsters receiving a Social Preference score greater than 1.0, a PA score greater than 0, and a PR score less than 0; (b) *rejected*, consisting of those receiving a Social Preference score less than −1.0, a PA score less than 0, and a PR score greater than 0; (c) *neglected*, consisting of those receiving a Social Impact score less than −1.0, a PA score less than 0, and a PR score less than 0; (d) *controversial*, consisting of those with Social Impact scores greater than 1.0, and PA and PR scores greater than 0; and (e) *average*, consisting of those receiving Social Impact and Social Preference scores between −.5 and .5. In addition, students who do not fit these groups have often been combined with the average students, as recommended by Coie and Dodge (1988).

nominations; however, only rejected youth also receive a high number of negative nominations. Popular children are those who receive a high number of positive nominations, but few or no negative nominations; controversial children receive high numbers of both positive and negative nominations.

Aside from nominations of liked most and liked least, peers have been asked to nominate their classmates for various positive and negative behaviors, such as "starts fights," "acts shy with other kids," or "cooperates with peers" (see Coie et al. 1982), or for roles in a class play that reflect children's interpersonal behaviors (Revised Class Play, Matsen et al. 1985). Such nominations provide an assessment of the child's behavioral characteristics that contribute to peers' impressions of liking and disliking. Reciprocal nominations of best friends have also been used to index children's peer friendships (Berndt 1989, Cauce 1986).

As an alternative to nominations, peer rating scales have been used to obtain ratings for every child in the class or group (e.g., Asher and Dodge 1986). Unlike nominations, for which children typically select only three choices, rating scales require children to rate *each* of their peers or classmates using a Likert-type format. Thus, each child in the group obtains a score on liking, disliking, or behavioral descriptors that represents the average rating received from his or her peers.

In general, peer rating and nomination procedures appear to be moderately stable over time, especially for older elementary-aged children, and for rejected peer status (Hughes 1988, Landau and Milich 1990). This argues for the importance of social interventions during the preadolescent years.

Although peer ratings and nominations provide the best way of assessing a child's peer status, they may be difficult or time-consuming to implement in a clinical setting. If this is the case, interviews with children's teachers and parents may help to determine whether or not the child is accepted or rejected by classmates.

Other Aspects of Social Functioning: Friendships, Social Support, and Subjective Distress

In addition to information on peer status, it is important to know about the child's current friendships and feelings about peer relationships. Most of the measures available in this area are based on children's self-reports. Self-reports have numerous advantages, including their ease and economy of use, and their ability to provide information on the child's perspective (La Greca 1990). Such measures may be supplemented by interviews with the child and parents regarding the child's peer contacts. Several useful measures are delineated below.

Friendship Questionnaire (Bierman and McCauley 1987)

This thirty-two-item questionnaire was designed to evaluate children's friend-ships and peer relations outside the school setting. Youngsters rate the frequency with which they engage in specific peer activities, such as inviting friends to the house, and participating in after-school and weekend activities with peers. A five-point scale is used for these ratings, with $1 = $ not at all, never, and $5 = $ all of the time, every day. This measure has three subscales: Positive Interactions, Negative Interactions, and Extensiveness of Peer Net-work. Bierman and McCauley (1987) provide support for the psychometric properties of this scale with children.

Social Anxiety Scale for Children-Revised (SASC-R)

This revision of the original Social Anxiety Scale for Children (La Greca et al. 1988) is a twenty-two-item scale that assesses children's feelings of social anxiety in situations involving peers. Each item is rated on a five-point scale (three-point scale for those in the early elementary grades) according to how true the item is for the child. Three factors have emerged from factor analytic studies: children's fear of negative evaluations from peers (FNE; e.g., "I worry about being teased"); social avoidance and distress in general (SADG; "I'm shy even around kids I know well"); and social avoidance and distress–new (SADN; "I get nervous when I talk to new kids"). Substantial support for the reliability as well as convergent and discriminant validity have been provided for children in the second through sixth grades (La Greca et al. 1988, La Greca and Stone 1993). For example, internal consistency for the full scale has been .80 or higher in several samples (La Greca 1991). Research with this instrument indicates that girls typically report more social anxiety than boys, and that neglected and also rejected youth report more social anxiety than their more accepted classmates (La Greca et al. 1988, La Greca and Stone 1993, Silverman and La Greca 1992, Vernberg et al. 1992). Vernberg et al. (1992) also reported satisfactory reliability for adolescents, and significant relationships between social anxiety and adolescents' peer relations. Alter-nate versions of this instrument have been developed for adolescents and for parents' reports of their youngsters' social anxiety. The adolescent and parent forms of the SASC-R are contained in the manual for the SASC-R.

Loneliness Scale

In an effort to assess children's feelings of loneliness and dissatisfaction with their peer relations, Asher and colleagues (Asher et al. 1984, Asher and Wheeler 1985) developed the Loneliness Scale. Items from this twenty-four-item questionnaire (sixteen items and eight fillers) are scored on a five-point scale. One version of the scale has wording that pertains to the classroom setting ("I have nobody to talk to in class," "I'm good at working with other children in my class") (Asher and Wheeler 1985). The items on the initial scale are worded more generally (e.g., "I feel alone," "I feel left out of things"). Asher and colleagues (1984) report that the scale has good internal consistency (r = .86). The instrument has been used with third- through sixth-grade children, revealing that rejected children and those with few friends report significantly more feelings of loneliness than those who are more accepted and have more friends (Asher et al. 1984, Asher and Wheeler 1985).

The Social Support Scale for Children and Adolescents (SSSCA) (Harter 1985)

This twenty-four-item scale assesses youngsters' perceptions of support from classmates, close friends, parents, and teachers. Separate scores are obtained for each source of support, and can range from 1 to 4, with higher scores reflecting greater support. Harter (1985) provides extensive data to support the reliability and validity of this instrument for children and adolescents. For example, for several samples of children and adolescents, internal consistencies ranged from .72 to .83 for the various subscales. Of particular interest are the separate subscales for classmates and close friends, which highlight the distinctions between these two sources of peer support.

Measures of Social Skills

After obtaining up-to-date information on peer status and social contacts, it is important to evaluate children's level of skills in social interaction, as such information will be critical for treatment planning. Behavioral observations have proved useful for assessing children's social skills. Major advantages of behavioral observations are the low level of inference required to interpret behavioral data, and the ability of behavioral data to specify target behaviors for interventions (Hughes 1988). Despite their appeal, behavioral observations are costly and time-consuming to gather; for older children, it may not be possible to observe critical peer interactions in an unobtrusive manner (La Greca and Stone 1992). Because of these limitations, other methods for assessing children's social skills, such as role-play assessments, rating scales, and interviews, have also gained favor in clinical settings. Several methods for assessing children's specific social skills are described below.

In each case, the clinician will want to obtain an assessment of the child's social strengths and weaknesses. Social skills training typically focuses on teaching or enhancing the specific social skills needed to initiate and maintain positive interactions with peers. Skills deemed to be important for peer interactions have been gleaned from the literature on behavioral correlates of peer status in children. See Table 4–1. Information regarding children's social strengths and weaknesses will allow the clinician to tailor the intervention to the specific needs of the child. Although the content of the training program may focus on improving children's social weaknesses, knowledge about their social strengths can provide opportunities for recognizing and rewarding appropriate social behaviors. In addition, in a group setting, it is often helpful to have some children with skills in areas that represent weaknesses for others, as they may serve as effective peer models for appropriate social skills.

Table 4–1. Important Social Skills

Skill Area	Key Components
Enjoyment of Interactions	Smiling Laughing
Greeting	Looking at person Smiling Using the person's name Greeting nicely
Joining	Standing near the child Asking to join nicely Acknowledging others when they join Handling refusals (e.g., Don't get mad)
Inviting	Asking other person to do something Accepting invitations nicely Handling refusals (e.g., Ask for another day)
Conversation	Asking conversational questions Talking more/sharing information about self Keeping a conversation going Taking turns in conversation
Sharing/Cooperation	Taking turns in peer activities Following game rules Being a "good sport" (good winner or good loser)
Complimenting/Giving Positive Feedback	Looking at the person, smiling Making a positive statement Accepting compliments from others positively
Conflict Resolution	Compromising Handling name-calling and teasing

Adapted from La Greca and Mesibov 1979, Vaughn and La Greca 1993.

Direct Observations

Direct observation of children's social interactions in the natural environment is usually accomplished by having one or more trained observers record the frequency, duration, and/or quality of certain "target" behaviors, each having a clear, easily observable behavioral description (La Greca and Stark 1986, Michelson et al. 1983). The most commonly assessed behaviors include broad categories, such as children's rate of social interaction, positive social behaviors, and negative social behaviors, although more specific social skills (e.g., cooperation, sharing) have also been assessed (La Greca and Stark 1986). Direct observations have been completed across developmental age groups and in various settings (e.g., classrooms and playgrounds). Observation coding systems that are constructed for direct observations vary, depending on the behaviors targeted for observation and the setting utilized (Michelson et al. 1983). If the coding system takes into account practicality, type of information needed, and social validity, then it is possible to obtain a high degree of external validity, which is often unavailable using other assessment methods (Michelson et al. 1983). (See La Greca and Stark 1986 for a detailed account of behavioral observation codes for children's social skills.)

Behavioral Assessment of Social Skills

Williamson and colleagues (Granberry et al. 1982, Williamson et al. 1983) developed a structured role-play measure to assess children's social skills, called the Social Skills Test (SST). Typically, the SST is videotaped for later review and scoring. It consists of role-play scenes depicting five categories of social behavior: accepting help, accepting praise, giving help, giving praise, and assertiveness. The responses of the student are scored in terms of eight behavioral categories. Williamson et al. (1983) provided psychometric support for this instrument.

Social Skills Rating System (SSRS) (Gresham and Elliot 1990)

The SSRS was developed for use with teachers, parents, and students, and is designed to assess the social skills of youngsters between the ages of 3 and 18 years. Gresham and Elliot (1990) provide extensive data to support the psychometric properties of the test. There are three major scales on the SSRS: Social Skills Scale, Problem Behaviors Scale, and the Academic Competence Scale. To provide a further breakdown of social skills, there are five subscales within the Social Skills Scale: cooperation, assertion, responsibility, empathy, and self-control. The cooperation and assertion subscales cover the kinds of skills that are most typically covered in social skills training programs, and may be of most interest clinically.

Matson Evaluation of Social Skills with Youngsters
(MESSY, Matson et al. 1983)

This measure has child-report (sixty-two items) and teacher-report (sixty-four items) forms. Items are rated on a five-point scale, and pertain to social skills, assertiveness, jealousy, and impulsiveness, all in relation to interpersonal interactions. The MESSY has been used with children between the ages of 4 and 18 years. Matson et al. (1983) have provided psychometric support for this instrument.

Measures of Behavioral Problems
(Internalizing/Externalizing Behaviors)

As noted previously, information on a child's behavioral style will help to identify specific behaviors that interfere with peer interactions and need remediation. Externalizing behaviors (e.g., aggression, impulsivity) are often annoying and intrusive to peers, and may need to be controlled in social situations. On the other hand, high levels of anxiety may contribute to a child's avoidance of social contacts; efforts to minimize such anxiety could facilitate increased peer interactions.

Among the available methods, behavioral rating scales and children's self-reports are perhaps the most common strategies for assessing children's behavior problems. Ratings from classroom teachers are especially useful as they see children in the same contexts as do peers. Teacher rating scales are economical and easy to score, and demonstrate good concurrent validity with behavioral observations. Teacher ratings are limited, however, because of their potential for rater bias, and because teachers often have inadequate opportunities to observe children's interactions in the upper grades (Hughes 1988). Parents are a good source of information regarding children's behavior problems across a broad age spectrum (Loeber et al. 1990).

Among the most widely used teacher rating scales are the Revised Behavior Problem Checklist (RBPC, Quay and Peterson 1987), and the Teacher Report Form (TRF) of the Child Behavior Checklist (Achenbach 1991b), although other scales have been used with young children (e.g., the Social Competence Schedule, Kohn 1977). The RBPC and the TRF cover the age range from the preschool years through adolescence. Teachers typically rate each child on a list of behavior problems, using a scale to indicate the presence and severity of each problem behavior (e.g., 0 = not present, 1 =

present some of the time, 2 = present most of the time). Although the specific subscales vary by instrument, each of these measures provides separate ratings for behaviors that are considered externalizing (e.g., conduct problems) and internalizing (e.g., anxiety-withdrawal), as well as extensive normative information.

Parent ratings of behavior problems can also be obtained from a number of standardized instruments, perhaps most notably the Child Behavior Checklist (CBCL, Achenbach 1991a) and the RBPC (noted above). The CBCL yields separate scores for externalizing and internalizing behavior problems, and has the added advantage over other instruments of providing information on children's Social Competence, as reflected in school and social activities.

Children's self-reports may be valuable adjuncts to parent and teacher reports for assessing internalizing behaviors, as adults are not always good informants of children's internalizing problems (cf. La Greca 1990, Loeber et al. 1990). Thus, self-report measures of anxiety and depression may be useful in clinical settings when assessing factors contributing to (or resulting from) children's social difficulties. (The reader should also consult other chapters in this volume for detailed information on the assessment of anxiety in children and adolescents.)

Measures to assess children's feelings of anxiety include the Revised Children's Manifest Anxiety Scale (RCMAS, Reynolds and Richmond 1978), the State-Trait Anxiety Inventory for Children (STAIC, Spielberger 1973), and the Fear Survey Schedule for Children-Revised (FSSC-R, Ollendick 1983). (See Barrios and Hartmann 1988, Finch and McIntosh 1990, and Kendall et al. 1992 for reviews.) Of these instruments, perhaps the RCMAS is the most widely used.

The RCMAS (or "What I Think and Feel") is a revision of the Children's Manifest Anxiety Scale, and consists of twenty-eight items (plus nine Lie Scale items) that describe anxious symptomatology, to which the child responds "yes" or "no." Considerable psychometric support for this instrument is provided in the manual (Reynolds and Richmond 1985), including normative information for children in grades one through twelve. Factor analysis has revealed three factors (Physiological, Worry/Oversensitivity, and Concentration), in addition to the Lie Scale. Typically, anxiety scores have been higher for girls than boys (Reynolds and Richmond 1978). Although this instrument is not as consistently related to children's social status as are measures of social anxiety and loneliness (cf. La Greca et al. 1988), it represents one of the best self-report methods for evaluating children's general feelings of worry and anxiety.

Aside from anxiety, children's reports of depressive symptoms may also be valuable to assess. The most widely used instrument in this area is the Children's Depression Inventory (CDI, Kovacs 1979). This twenty-seven-item scale assesses depressive symptomatology in children between the ages of 6 and 17. Extensive research supports the reliability and validity of this measure (see Kazdin 1988, 1990 and Kovacs 1979). For reviews of other instruments to assess children's feelings of depression, the reader is referred to several sources (Hughes 1988, Kazdin 1988, 1990).

In addition to specific measures of anxiety and depression, the Youth Self Report (Achenbach 1991c) can be used to evaluate internalizing and externalizing problems. This child-report version of the CBCL can be used with youngsters between the ages of 11 and 18 years. Extensive psychometric support for this instrument is provided by the authors (Achenbach 1991c).

Summary

Because no single method is sufficient, the assessment of children's social difficulties requires a multimethod approach that draws information from a variety of sources and settings. Initial interviews with children, parents, and teachers help to identify the areas of social difficulty and plan further assessment strategies. Assessment should include, at a minimum, an evaluation of the child's (a) social skills and social behaviors, (b) feelings of social anxiety, social inadequacy, and loneliness, (c) friendships and supportive relationships, (d) degree of internalizing and externalizing behavior problems that may contribute to peer difficulties, and (e) existence of academic problems, physical handicaps, or other nonbehavioral problems that may contribute to negative peer interactions.

Once this information is gathered, the next step is to identify appropriate treatment goals (i.e., reducing peer rejection, establishing more friendship ties), and then translate the treatment goals and assessment information into a reasonable intervention plan. The next section deals with the issue of treatment goals, prior to a presentation and discussion of social intervention strategies.

TREATMENT STRATEGIES

Establishing Treatment Goals

A comprehensive assessment of children's social skills and peer relations should provide the clinician with the information necessary to design and implement an appropriate intervention. Table 4–2 lists the type of problems children may have, as well as corresponding strategies for intervention.

Before beginning an intervention, in addition to knowing the nature of the child's social problems, the clinician must keep in mind the primary objectives or goals for the intervention. In many cases, children are seen for treatment because they are disliked or rejected by their classmates. When this happens, one goal of intervention will be to increase peer acceptance or reduce peer rejection; this means that some aspect of the intervention will need to involve the child's classmates and teachers. On the other hand, if the primary problem is that the child has no or few friends, a major goal of intervention would be to increase peer contacts and friendships, and this may be done inside and/or outside the classroom situation. Thus, the ultimate goals of the intervention may dictate the settings and types of intervention strategies used (see Table 4–2 for an illustration).

Because children may have multiple problems (peer rejection, few friends, few positive social skills, presence of intrusive behaviors), interventions that incorporate multiple strategies and goals may be needed. Although current research is limited in terms of designing and evaluating multicompo-

Table 4–2. Summary of Social Intervention Strategies Pertinent to Different Types of Social Problems and Intervention Goals

	Relevant Intervention Strategy
Type of Social Problem	
• Low Levels of Positive Social Skills	Social Skills Training (e.g., coaching, modeling)
• High Levels of Intrusive Behaviors (e.g., inattention, aggression)	Contingency Management; Incentives for Reducing Aversive Behavior
• Presence of Internalizing Problems (e.g., anxiety, social withdrawal)	Gradual Exposure to Peers; Anxiety Reduction Procedures
• "Problematic" Child Characteristics (e.g., learning problems, obesity)	Modifying Peers' Perceptions; Modifying the Characteristics (e.g., educational interventions)
• Few Peer Contacts/Opportunities	Extracurricular Activities that Involve Peers (e.g., scouts, sports activities)
Intervention Goals	
• Increase Peer Acceptance/Reduce Rejection	Work with classmates to modify perceptions of child; Develop peer-pairing or buddy system in school
• Increase Number/Quality of Friendships	Develop peer buddy in school; Develop contacts outside the school setting
• Reduce Subjective Distress Resulting from Negative Peer Contacts	Inoculation training; Find positive peer contacts; Positive reframing

nent interventions, numerous case examples can be found (e.g., La Greca et al. 1989, Matson et al. 1980, Vaughn et al. 1991).

Interventions for Improving Peer Relations

Once the child's social problems have been precisely pinpointed, and the goals for intervention are clear, the clinician is ready to move toward the selection of appropriate treatment strategies. In many cases, children may need a combined treatment approach that includes social skills training, efforts to increase or enhance friendships, and strategies for reducing competing behavior problems (e.g., anxiety, aggression).

One additional consideration to bear in mind is that, because social interventions are trying to improve a child's interactions with peers, it is critical to consider *both* sides of the interaction equation—that is, both the child and his/her peers (La Greca 1993). It is clear that social skills interventions need to incorporate elements of the child's social environment to have an impact on peers and to maintain treatment gains. Indeed, the intervention studies that have involved nonproblem peers in the intervention process have met with greater success than those that did not (Bierman and Furman 1984, Oden and Asher 1977, Vaughn and Lancelotta 1991).

Based on the foregoing discussion, the sections below will describe each of the main intervention strategies used to improve children's social functioning with peers. The primary focus will be on social skills training procedures. To a lesser extent, attention will be devoted to behavior management strategies for reducing intrusive/negative behaviors and methods to enhance children's social networks and peer contacts.

Social Skills Training

Although social skills training programs have been diverse, three broad approaches to intervention can be identified: modeling, coaching, and shaping (Combs and Slaby 1977, Erwin 1993, Ladd 1985, Ladd and Mize 1983). Modeling of appropriate social skills has been used both as an independent treatment strategy (e.g., Keller and Carlson 1974, O'Connor 1972) and as part of a comprehensive program that additionally involves coaching and behavioral rehearsal of social skills (e.g., Bierman and Furman 1984, La Greca and Santogrossi 1980, Oden and Asher 1977). Shaping, or gradually modifying a child's behavior by contingently rewarding increasingly closer approximations to the desired social behavior, has been used primarily with preschoolers, and youngsters with cognitive limitations, such as those with mental retardation. In fact, in a meta-analysis of social skills intervention studies, Schneider (1989) concluded that techniques such as modeling or shaping, that require less cognitive mediation, are more effective with young preschoolers, whereas older children and adolescents are more likely to profit from the more complex, multistrategy interventions. Because of their wide applicability, this section will focus on the multicomponent strategies for social skills interventions; however, the reader is referred to several additional sources for further detailed information on social skills interventions (Combs and Slaby 1977, Erwin 1993, La Greca 1993, Ladd 1985, Ladd and Mize 1983, Vaughn and La Greca 1993).

The most common approach to social skills training involves the combination of *modeling* of appropriate social behavior, *coaching* or instruction in how to behave with peers, *behavioral rehearsal* of social skills, usually through role-plays or actual social interactions, *corrective feedback*, and *reinforcement* for appropriate social skills. This combined approach has been used with rejected and low-accepted elementary school students (e.g., Bierman and Furman 1984, Gresham and Nagle 1980, La Greca and Santogrossi 1980, Oden and Asher 1977), with learning disabled youth (e.g., Hazel et al. 1982, La Greca and Mesibov 1981, Vaughn et al. 1991), and with behaviorally disordered children (Bornstein et al. 1980, Kolko et al. 1990). Applications of this approach for individual children (Bierman et al. 1987, Oden and Asher 1977) as well as for small groups (La Greca and Mesibov 1981, La Greca and Santogrossi 1980) can be found.

Prior to beginning an intervention, the clinician must first identify the specific social skills to be taught or emphasized (see Table 4–1); these may be based on one child's needs, or the collective needs of group members. Once the skills for training have been identified, a standard format is used to teach the skills (cf. Jackson et al. 1983, La Greca 1981, McGinnis and Goldstein 1984).

First, the desired social behavior is described, discussed, and modeled (Introduction). A critical aspect of introducing a specific social skill is making sure the children understand what is expected, and the social contexts that are appropriate and inappropriate for the behavior (e.g., talking with others on the playground or during lunch, but not during quiet work activities in the classroom). In a group format, children may provide many examples of how the skills can be used.

Second, children are provided with opportunities to practice the skills—with the clinician and also with other children (Behavioral Rehearsal). For individually based treatments, the child may practice with the therapist or trainer; in group situations, other group members provide ideal practice partners. Ideas for role-plays and practice may come from actual social situations generated by the children, or be suggested by the therapist.

Third, the behavioral practice is critiqued by the trainer and, for group interventions, by the other group members (Coaching/Feedback). This critique should include pointing out the good aspects of the behavior, as well as areas for improvement (e.g., "You asked good questions, and showed enthusiasm and interest in your tone of voice, but you should try looking at John more when you talk to him"). Typically, further practice and feedback is provided, until children master the skills. To make the training fun and rewarding, generous use of praise and/or contingent reinforcement for appropriate social skills is important (cf. La Greca et al. 1989). Social skills games (see Cartledge and Milburn 1980 for descriptions) have also been developed to guide the practice of appropriate social skills and enhance the enjoyable aspects of treatment.

Finally, once skills have been practiced sufficiently, opportunities to use the skills in naturalistic settings with peers should be provided. This typically entails specific homework assignments to use the skills with classmates or neighborhood children. Although parents and teachers have rarely been involved in studies of social skills interventions (La Greca 1993), in clinical practice these adults can be useful partners in helping children to identify receptive peers and implement their social homework (e.g., inviting peers to play at home, sitting next to a classmate during lunch). At the next meeting, this homework assignment should be reviewed and discussed, with appropriate feedback and reinforcement provided, prior to beginning a new skills area.

The above description provides a brief overview to social skills training. For further details, the reader is referred to several treatment studies and reviews (Bierman and Furman 1984, Bierman et al. 1987, Combs and Slaby 1977, La Greca and Santogrossi 1980, Ladd 1985, Vaughn and La Greca 1993) as well as treatment manuals (Jackson et al. 1983, La Greca 1981, McGinnis and Goldstein 1984) that focus on social skills interventions.

Reducing Concomitant Behavior Problems

A second main strategy for dealing with children's social difficulties involves reducing the types of behavior problems that interfere with children's peer relationships. When children are referred for treatment due to social difficulties it is, therefore, essential to assess concomitant behavior problems and plan a treatment component to address these problems. In most clinical settings, however, the reverse situation will likely occur; that is, a child may be referred for behavior problems (e.g., anxiety, aggressive behavior), rather than social difficulties (cf. La Greca 1993). In this case, the clinician will want to treat the referred behavior problems, but additionally assess the child's peer relations and social skills and include social interventions in the overall treatment plan.

Considerable clinical investigation has been devoted to the treatment of externalizing behavior problems, such as conduct problems and attention deficits (see Barkley 1989, McMahon and Wells 1989), as well as internalizing difficulties, like anxiety-based problems and depression (see Barrios and O'Dell 1989, Kazdin 1989; also see Chapter 5 in this text). A description of these major child-intervention areas are beyond the scope of this chapter. However, some attention will be devoted to the ways in which externalizing and internalizing problems interfere with social contacts, and how these problems might be addressed in the context of a social skills intervention.

In many cases of social rejection, children show inappropriate levels of aggressive behavior toward their peers, which must be reduced to lower the children's level of rejection and improve their peer acceptance. Some researchers (e.g., Pinkston et al. 1973) have used social reinforcement and extinction techniques to reduce aggressive behavior. For example, it is possible for a trainer to ignore aggressive behavior (except to separate the aggressive child from others) and to provide attention to the victim of the verbal or physical attention. The aggressive child is rewarded later for nonaggressive behavior. Pinkston et al. (1973) determined that such a procedure reduced aggressive behavior. Once aversive behavior is reduced, then appropriate interactions with peers can be directly encouraged and reinforced.

Another excellent example of methods for reducing aversive behaviors that interfere with peer relations is provided by Karen Bierman (Bierman 1989, Bierman et al. 1987). Bierman advocates two strategies for reducing children's negative behaviors: (a) the use of contingency management procedures to consequate the negative behaviors of target children and (b) efforts to manipulate peers' responses to the negative behavior of the target child (see Bierman 1989). For example, Bierman and colleagues (1987) effectively used response cost (punishment) procedures to reduce the aggressive behaviors of rejected children who participated in social skills training. Adapting this procedure to a clinical setting means that clinicians should be prepared to use contingency management during individual or group social skills treatment (e.g., La Greca et al. 1989; also see the case description below). Teaching parents and teachers skills for behavior management would also be advisable. Although efforts to manipulate peers' reactions to negative behaviors has proved to be another useful strategy in classroom settings (see Bierman 1989), this type of strategy may be more difficult to implement in a clinical setting, as it involves training classmates to ignore negative behaviors in the target child.

Less attention has been devoted to children who have internalizing problems that interfere with peer relations than to those with externalizing difficulties. In the case of a child whose anxiety interferes with social interactions, the social skills treatment model described above may help to address socially anxious behaviors by providing gradual exposure to peers in social settings, with contingent reinforcement for social engagement. Several case examples illustrate this process (e.g., Kirby and Toler 1970, Ross 1978). For example, in a study by Kirby and Toler (1970), children with low levels of social interaction were instructed by their teachers to distribute candy to the other children in the classroom, a task that required them to ask the others for their preferences. When the children completed the task, they received praise, money, and candy (i.e., direct reinforcements) from their teachers. In a free-play period following the task, these children engaged in increased interactions with peers, perhaps due to the combination of teacher reinforcement, exposure to peer contact, and reinforcement from peers (Kirby and Toler 1970). Thus, for children who are anxious or avoidant with peers, gradual exposure in the clinic and in planned activities outside the clinic, with associated reinforcement for social engagement, may facilitate their social skills treatment.

Strategies for Enhancing Peer Networks and Social Contacts

As mentioned earlier, it is important for social skills interventions to include elements of the child's natural social environment in the treatment process, in order to have an impact on peer acceptance and to maintain treatment gains. In fact, interventions that included nonproblem classmates in the treatment program have been more successful than those that did not (cf. Bierman and Furman 1984, Oden and Asher 1977, Vaughn and Lancelotta 1991).

Two ways of increasing a child's peer contacts that have received empirical support are peer-pairing and cooperative peer activities (cf. La Greca 1993). Both types of activities help nonproblem peers to get to know the target child better, and thus may help the target child to gain entry into peer networks that might otherwise exclude him or her. Furthermore, nonproblem peers may serve as good role models for social skills and positive interaction behaviors, and may reward and reinforce these kinds of behaviors in the child or children receiving social skills treatment.

Peer-pairing involves matching a child with social difficulties with another child who has good social skills and is accepted by other peers. These peer-pairs can work together on social skills, friendship making, or even cooperative learning tasks (e.g., Bierman and Furman 1984, Oden and Asher 1977, Vaughn and Lancelotta 1991). When a child is seen in a clinical setting, peer-pairing might be accomplished by working with classroom teachers. For example, teachers could help to identify a "peer buddy" or socially skilled classmate who could be assigned to work with the target child on classroom projects and activities. Parents may also be helpful in identifying appropriate neighborhood children who could be invited to participate in play or other fun activities with their child.

In addition to peer-pairing, classroom-based cooperative activities have also been developed to enhance children's peer networks in the classroom. These types of cooperative activities might also be adapted for clinic settings (e.g., child groups). A supportive environment, such as the one created through cooperative peer activities (Furman and Gavin 1989), should promote friendship development in the classroom. In fact, following cooperative peer interactions, children have reported feeling more friendly toward others in their group and feeling that peers cared more about them (Furman and Gavin 1989).

Cooperative interaction programs involve children in games or activities that have a shared goal, and are designed to promote cooperation and interdependence (Furman and Gavin 1989). Typically, children from the same classroom (or children who are seen in a clinical setting), who are not mutual friends or enemies, work together on a nonacademic activity for which there is a group goal. Reviews of this intervention strategy (Furman and Gavin 1989, Price and Dodge 1989) indicate that cooperative interaction tasks have a positive impact on children's liking for one another, even when the target child was initially disliked by peers. This intervention strategy is thought to be effective because the helping and sharing behaviors displayed during group activities disconfirm peers' negative impressions of disliked others (Price and Dodge 1989), and because peers are provided with an opportunity to discover ways the target child is like them (Vaughn et al. 1991). Getting to know other children may also be a way for the target child to become a part of other social networks.

In treatment settings, cooperative group activities can be established in a clinic through structured group activities. In addition, teachers may be excellent consultants in this process, as they may be able to identify school activities in which target children can work or play cooperatively with peers. Parents may also be helpful in identifying and supporting extracurricular activities, such as scouts, athletic groups, and so on, that bring children together in a cooperative manner (cf. La Greca 1993).

Despite the appeal of peer-pairing and cooperative peer interactions as an intervention strategy, there is good reason to believe that this approach will work best when combined with social skills training and/or contingency management. Although cooperative peer interactions may have a positive effect on children's peer acceptance and friendships, children with poor peer relations may still require specific social skills training to ensure they have the requisite social behaviors to participate in cooperative peer activities and interact appropriately with others (Price and Dodge 1989). In fact, Bierman and Furman (1984) found that peer involvement increased the frequency of low-accepted children's peer interactions and increased their peer acceptance, but these positive gains were maintained at follow-up only when cooperative tasks were combined with specific training in social skills.

Summary

Modeling, coaching, behavioral rehearsal, corrective feedback, and reinforcement are all approaches that can readily be utilized within a clinical setting for social skills training, with either individuals or groups. It is also possible to reduce problematic behaviors (e.g., aggression or anxiety) in a treatment situation, using reinforcement and extinction techniques. In terms of enhancing social contacts, efforts should be made to increase the child's contacts with nonproblem peers. Parents and teachers can be invaluable resources for extending the child's peer network in an adaptive manner, both in the classroom and in community settings.

CLINICAL ISSUES

The Role of the Therapist

In social skills interventions, the role of the therapist may vary, depending on whether individual, dyadic, or group treatment is used. When the therapist works with the individual child, he/she serves as the direct trainer by providing instruction, serving as a model, giving feedback, and reinforcing the child (Michelson et al. 1983). In this mode, the therapist can provide immediate reinforcement following the child's display of appropriate behavior, since the therapist can focus complete attention on the skills of the individual child.

When an additional child is added to the treatment modality, the clinician still provides initial instruction and serves as the primary model. At the same time, he/she is also able to better simulate situations that the children will encounter outside of the therapeutic setting with other children (Michelson et al. 1983). For example, the therapist can assign "roles" to the two children and serve as an observer, while the children perform the role-play (Jackson et al. 1983). The therapist can then intervene if necessary and provide feedback to the dyad at any time. In addition, through the use of simulated situations, the therapist can get a more accurate picture of the problematic behaviors each child typically exhibits in real-life encounters with peers, especially if naturalistic observations are not feasible (Michelson et al. 1983).

Behavioral rehearsal and more intimate discussion are also possible with small groups (typically made of four to six children). The clinician should have a cotherapist for larger groups, since it is hard to provide praise and positive feedback for each individual member of larger groups and manage the increased noise and interaction with larger numbers of children (Michelson et al. 1983). With smaller groups, the therapist first collects data to determine the appropriateness of group treatment for each child and to decide the composition of the group (Rose 1973). In the first phase, the therapist provides much reinforcement and attempts to build group cohesiveness; at this phase, the therapist takes a directive role (Rose 1973). In the next phase, the therapist transfers some of the responsibility of the direction (i.e., decision making) of the group to the individual members (Rose 1973). The therapist suggests role-plays for the group and monitors each child's progress. In the final phase, the therapist reduces most forms of reinforcement and attempts to reduce the desirability of the group, in order to increase the desirability of outside peer groups (Rose 1973). Meetings become less frequent, and the therapist focuses discussion on termination issues. After the group terminates, the therapist contacts parents and teachers to determine if the changes achieved in the group are being maintained outside of the therapeutic setting (Erwin 1993, Rose 1973, Ross 1978).

Practical Considerations

Once a treatment plan has been developed for an individual child or group, some further practical considerations will shape the actual treatment program. These considerations include the number, length, and frequency of the treatment sessions; the use of individual or group treatment; constraints in setting up groups; involvement of parents or others (e.g., teachers, peers) in the intervention process; and plans for treatment maintenance (La Greca et al. 1989).

The format of sessions should be decided based on the special needs of the individual child. For example, if a child has attentional difficulties, adaptations such as shorter sessions, frequent changes in activity to maintain interest level, and additional "structure" (e.g., a token reinforcement system) should be considered (La Greca et al. 1989). The use of individual or group treatment also depends on the needs of the children participating in therapy, in addition to the motivational level of the children. For instance, some children seem more interested in treatment when other children are involved (La Greca et al. 1989).

Groups of four to six children with two leaders/therapists seem to be ideal for group intervention, depending on the types of problems of the children in the group (La Greca et al. 1989). Smaller groups allow more opportunities for children to practice skills, while larger groups provide more variety in terms of perspective; however, for any group, the children should be similar in age, cognitive level, and physical maturity (La Greca et al. 1989).

Parents and teachers should be involved in the intervention process, since they can provide reinforcement to the child for positive changes seen outside of the clinical setting and help monitor homework assignments that are given to practice skills learned in the training situation (Michelson et al. 1983). Regular contact with parents and teachers, in the form of meetings or phone calls, is crucial in order to collaborate on treatment goals promoted in the clinical setting. Peers should also be involved, to change peers' perception of a given child, especially if the child has other handicaps such as learning disabilities (La Greca et al. 1989).

Common Obstacles to Successful Treatment

Common obstacles in social skills training include resistance, integration of clinic work with ongoing peer relations in school or the community, and maintenance of treatment gains. Resistance is often seen in children who are not concerned about improving their social interactions with others. In such cases, it is important for therapists/group leaders to try to increase the child's level of enthusiasm and interest, to obtain cooperation (La Greca et al. 1989). In more extreme cases, it might also be necessary to construct a contract for a limited number of sessions, to get severely resistant children involved (La Greca et al. 1989).

Other common obstacles are generalizing training to other settings (e.g., school) and preventing a relapse after treatment ends. In the first case, as mentioned earlier, peers can become involved in the intervention process, so that they can better understand the problems of the children who are in treatment. Children can also be trained during sessions in ways to handle negative responses from peers (La Greca et al. 1989). To prevent relapse, it is important to instruct parents and teachers about the treatment and to develop strategies with them to handle any problems that might arise following treatment. Parents can also bring their children back to the clinical setting for "booster" sessions, if necessary.

Termination

As a child in individual treatment reaches his/her treatment goals, the therapist begins to prepare for the child's departure from therapy. At this point, even though the child is behaving more appropriately in the clinical setting and in his/her natural environment, he/she may return to earlier behavioral patterns in an attempt to continue treatment (Plenk 1993). The therapist should discuss the child's successes and the changes he/she has made over the course of therapy, and praise the child for his/her progress. Such a discussion provides a sense of closure to the treatment. In addition, the child should be instructed in ways to handle any setbacks that may occur. The therapist should also talk with parents and teachers to ensure that gains will be maintained away from the clinical setting.

When phasing out a social skills group, several procedures should be carried out to make the ending as comfortable as possible for the children involved. However, the steps taken are dependent on which type of termination is taking place. For example, one individual may leave the group after attaining his or her goals; the group may terminate at the end of the school year; several members may leave because they have been involved with the group longer or have switched groups; or the therapist ends his or her relationship with the group, but a new leader continues the group (Rose 1973).

Rose (1973) recommends that termination should be discussed from the beginning of treatment as part of the introduction to therapy, and at natural opportunities (e.g., when the children begin to plan for summer vacation), to set the stage for the later components of termination. Two months before treatment ends, the issue of termination should be discussed at every meeting, with meetings becoming fewer in number before final termination (Rose 1973). When individuals or certain members are terminating, the terminating members are asked to discuss their posttreatment plans and often become models for the remaining members (Rose 1973). In some cases, the terminating members form a subgroup to discuss termination issues with the therapist.

Rose (1973) outlines several general steps toward termination. The first step is for group members to find friends outside of the group who have fewer behavioral problems than themselves and either bring the other children to the group or spend time usually reserved for group meetings with their new friends. Next, the children in the group are encouraged to join other organizations that involve peers. In the final phase, members come together to talk about their new experiences in brief, more businesslike sessions. Children who meet with success outside the group receive verbal reinforcement from the therapist and the group members (Johnson 1975). The therapist should also prepare the children for setbacks that might occur, by discussing ways to handle such problems. As a final step, the therapist should make sure that teachers, parents, and other significant people in the children's lives are familiar with procedures carried out in treatment, to make sure that the changes are extended to the children's natural environment (Rose 1973).

CASE ILLUSTRATION (TYPICAL TREATMENT)

The following case describes a young boy who exhibited several aversive behaviors (e.g., fighting and talking too much to peers) and had social skills deficits that interfered with his ability to make friends. Intervention consequently focused on his behaviors and social skill deficits, which caused him much distress.

Description and History

Sam T. was an 8-year-old boy in the third grade who was brought for psychological services by his mother, after complaints from his gifted class teacher that he was talking too much and distracting other children from doing their work. This behavior resulted in Sam being actively rejected by peers. His mother was concerned that he had only a few friends and seemed to lack the necessary social skills to make more friends. Ms. T. was also upset with Sam's tendency to get suckered into fights, in which he would retaliate in response to children's teasing. She said that he had talked too much in the classroom and gotten into fights since kindergarten, but only now had the fights become serious, as he had received several detentions and one in-school suspension since the beginning of the school year. Ms. T. felt that Sam needed to learn self-control to avoid these fights and to reduce the amount of talking he did in the classroom.

Sam's parents divorced when Sam was 5, and his father had subsequently remarried and lived in another part of the country. Sam saw his father about twice per year. At the beginning of therapy, Sam lived with his mother and grandmother. Sam had a Big Brother, with whom he did activities on the weekends. Thus, Sam's mother, grandmother, and Big Brother were considered to be the main people who could monitor and reinforce Sam's behavior outside of the clinical setting. At school, Sam seemed closest to his gifted class teacher, so she was also targeted as an adult in his life who could help maintain gains he made in treatment.

In the first phase of treatment, Sam was assessed in terms of his peers' impressions of him, the level of contact he had with other children, the repertoire of social skills he possessed, the specific types of behavior problems (internalizing and externalizing) he exhibited, and the special abilities and disabilities he owned. To assess the first two areas, Sam was interviewed to determine his perceptions of his social status at school and to measure the amount of (and his feelings about the) social contacts he had with children his age in school and at home. Next, he was observed interacting with his mother and was requested to participate in a role-play with the therapist in which he had to engage an unfriendly peer at his school cafeteria, in order to assess his social skills. To assess his behavior problems, Sam's mother completed a Revised Behavior Problem Checklist that pinpointed problematic behaviors at home (RBPC, Quay and Peterson 1987). To look at his functioning at school, his gifted class teacher completed a Teacher Report Form (Achenbach 1991b), to identify problematic behaviors. Both Sam's mother and teacher were also interviewed regarding Sam's peer relations and personal characteristics, in order to verify his self-report of his social functioning and to determine what strengths he would be able to draw upon during social skills training. Ms. T. reported that Sam was very upset about not having more friends. She also said that he was easily angered and stubborn, but also would give up easily on tasks and was quick to blame others for his mistakes. She thought that his irritability and poor treatment of others resulted in his lack of friends. Sam's teacher reported that Sam had difficulties relating to his peers, but wanted to have friends. She said that Sam was "giving" to his classmates and a very bright boy, but he also antagonized them with his excessive talking and disruptive behavior. She thought that his eagerness to make new friends and his cognitive abilities would make him a good candidate for social skills training. Finally, Sam was administered the Social Anxiety Scale for Children, and the Children's Depression Inventory (CDI, Kovacs 1979) to assess levels of social anxiety and depression.

Synopsis of Therapy Sessions

Sam was seen for a total of twenty-eight sessions, four of which were within a group context. At the beginning of therapy, Sam was seen individually, in order to establish rapport and begin to understand the specific behaviors that led to trouble with peers or adults. During the first session, Sam revealed that his teacher had embarrassed him in front of his classmates by asking about his counseling. Three sessions later, Sam reported a specific peer rejection incident that resulted in a detention for him:

> Therapist: Can you tell me why you got a detention this week?
> Client: I don't know.
> Therapist: So, you're not sure why you got in trouble?
> Client: They were calling me names.
> Therapist: Some of the kids were calling you names.
> Client: Yeah. I heard some kids call me a dork.
> Therapist: Someone called you a dork. What did you say?
> Client: I said, "Shut up, you jerks."
> Therapist: Did that help?
> Client: No.
> Therapist: Was there something else you could have said?
> Client: No.
> Therapist: What if you had told the teacher, instead of calling them "jerks"?
> Client: She doesn't care. Anyway, those kids always get detention. I told them to shut up and then the teacher heard me and gave me detention.

In subsequent sessions, the focus was on helping Sam identify instances when he could not control his talking or aggressive behavior (e.g., when he was tired or if someone teased him). In terms of the teasing, the therapist modeled appropriate responses to such comments from peers and then had Sam practice these responses. The therapist then provided feedback to Sam regarding his performance. Also at this point, a social skills group was formed with two other children who were also having difficulty making friends. The group was scheduled biweekly, in order to continue each child's individual treatment. Both of the children were male and approximately the same age as Sam. One (Ricky M.) attended only one group session, due to his parents' inability to bring him for therapy consistently. The other (Hector R.) came for three sessions. Hector's case will be discussed in the next case illustration. For the group sessions, Ricky and Hector's therapist served as a cotherapist.

For the first group meeting, efforts were made to minimize intrusive, aggressive behaviors during group by establishing ground rules (e.g., no hitting, name calling, yelling, or throwing things), especially since it was known from Sam's initial assessment that he was prone to aggressive behavior when he felt rejected by other children. A time-out system was also established to help any child who needed a few minutes to compose himself. In this meeting, the purpose of the group was discussed with the children, and the children were taught how to introduce themselves. Sam had a difficult time with the structured elements of this session (e.g., going over the rules and introducing himself to the other children), and he argued with the therapists as illustrated below:

Client: Why do we need rules? This is stupid.
Therapist 1: We need the rules so that no one gets hurt.
Client: But I already know all this stuff.
Therapist 2: Well, it is still important to make sure that we all know the rules.
Client: Okay, but when do we get to play a game?

At the end of the session, the children and therapists played a social skills game together, which taught the children how to work together toward a shared goal. The next group was not held until three weeks later. In the following individual session, Sam and his therapist continued to practice appropriate ways to handle conflicts with other children. Sam was reinforced whenever he mentioned a suitable solution to a problem (i.e., one not involving aggression).

During the next group session, Sam and Hector were the only children who were able to attend. At first, the two boys could not agree on which game to play, but Sam was able to provide an adequate solution for the dilemma. This reflects the social skill of conflict resolution that he learned, practiced, and was reinforced for by his therapist in individual sessions:

> Sam: I want to play Battleship. (He goes to the game closet to get the game.)
> Hector: Well, I don't. I hate that game.
> Sam: I want to play Battleship, then we can play your game.
> Hector: No. I won't play.
> Sam: How about if we play another game then, like Go to the Head of the Class?
> Hector: That game is not as dumb. I'll play that.

The other group sessions focused on how to join in with others and how to handle name-calling and teasing (cf. Jackson et al. 1983, La Greca 1981, Vaughn and La Greca 1993). At this point in treatment, which was summer vacation for the children, Sam's individual sessions focused on ways to control his intrusive, aggressive behavior while attending summer camp and how to make friends at the camp. Sam was able to identify the feelings he had when another child teased him, and ignored their negative comments, as he was taught to do in his sessions with his therapist. Sam also wanted to talk about his relationship with his father, whom he saw in August. Using a game that addressed issues concerning children of divorce, Sam was able to describe to his therapist how the divorce had affected him. Periodically during the summer, Sam reverted to his old behavior at camp (e.g., pushing another child who had called him a name) as is often the case in social skills training, but his overall behavior improved. In addition, Sam's visit with his father and his stepmother was a difficult one for him, since his father did not spend much time alone with Sam. However, he did not resort to his old behaviors (e.g., excessive talking and physical aggression to peers) following the visit.

Sam was seen for only four more sessions, since his behavior at school improved to the point that his new teacher reported no outbursts or aggressive behavior with his peers, even though he still talked excessively in class. He was also reported to be more accepted by his peers, and he had made a few more friends at school, thus achieving one of his initial goals of therapy. For the last two sessions, Sam was seen together with his mother to talk about the progress Sam had made over the previous 9 months of therapy and to further discuss ways to handle problematic situations with peers once therapy was over.

Comments

Sam's case involved both individual and group components. Individual therapy was necessary at first to establish rapport and to determine if Sam would be a good candidate for group treatment. Even though he showed periods of aggressive behavior, Sam had the cognitive capacity (he was in the gifted program at his elementary school) and the motivation to make more friends. Thus, he was generally receptive to modeling techniques and other forms of instruction from his therapist. Sam's social skills training began with basic techniques (e.g., how to introduce yourself to others), to determine how severe his social deficits were. Later sessions involved more complex social skills (e.g., entering a group and ignoring teasing), as Sam became more proficient at the core skills. Also, social skills were addressed during individual sessions through role-playing (with the therapist taking the role of a peer) and the use of a social skills board game. Individual sessions with Sam were also necessary to discuss problems that occurred periodically in the time between sessions.

Group sessions helped make the social skill lessons more salient for Sam, as they provided him with an opportunity to try out the skills in a protected and reinforcing environment. He was also able to hear some of the possible comments (from the children in the group) that he would later encounter at school. The small number of actual group sessions reflects a common problem when running a group for children in a community-based center. The parents of the other children in the group were unable to consistently bring their children to the center every other week, due to problems with transportation or other stressors in their lives.

CASE ILLUSTRATION (OVERCOMING OBSTACLES)

The following case describes a young boy who exhibited more internalizing-type behaviors, such as anxiety and depression. He was also diagnosed as having social skills deficits and problems with his academic work. Intervention consequently focused on his dysfunctional behaviors and social skill deficits, which caused him much distress.

Description and History

Hector R., an 11-year-old boy in the sixth grade, was brought for psychological services by his mother after her recent divorce and the family's move to Miami from New York. When Hector entered therapy, he lived with his mother, her fiancee, and his younger sister.

According to Hector's mother, Hector, who once excelled in gifted programs, was now struggling to pass his classes. In addition, he seemed to experience difficulty when it came to making friends in general, and particularly in school. Since he did not have friends and often went unnoticed by peers, he could be considered to be neglected (in terms of sociometric status).

In the first phase of treatment, Hector was assessed in terms of his peers' impressions of him, the level of contact he had with other children, the repertoire of social skills he possessed, the specific types of behavior problems (internalizing and externalizing) he exhibited, and the special abilities and disabilities he owned. To assess the first two areas, Hector was interviewed to determine his perceptions of his social status at school and to measure the amount of (and his feelings about the) social contacts he had with children his age in school and at home. Next, he was observed interacting with his mother and was requested to participate in a role-play in which he had to engage an unfriendly peer at his school playground, to assess his social skills. To assess his behavior problems, Hector was administered the Social Anxiety Scale for Children-Revised (La Greca and Stone 1993) to assess his anxiety in social situations involving peers, the Children's Depression Inventory (CDI, Kovacs 1979) to assess his level of depression, the Piers-Harris Children's Self-Concept Scale (Piers and Harris 1969) to measure his self-concept, and the Youth Self Report (Achenbach 1991c) to determine his perceived problematic behaviors. In addition, Hector was administered the Wechsler Intelligence Scale for Children–3rd edition (WISC-III, Wechsler 1991) and Wechsler Individual Achievement Test (WIAT, Wechsler 1992) to determine his true level of intellectual and academic functioning. The results indicated that Hector was experiencing high levels of social anxiety, and moderate levels of depression and anxiety-withdrawal. Hector himself reported that he did not get along with other kids and that he wished he had more friends.

Ms. R. completed a Revised Behavior Problem Checklist that pinpointed behavior problems at home (RBPC, Quay and Peterson 1987), and Hector's teacher completed a Teacher Report Form (Achenbach 1991b), in order to identify problematic behaviors at school. Both Hector's mother and teacher were also interviewed regarding Hector's peer relations and personal characteristics, to verify his self-report of his social functioning and to determine what strengths he would be able to draw upon during social skills training. Ms. R.

reported that she was most concerned with Hector's lack of friends, oppositional behavior at home, inability to accept responsibility, inability to complete homework, and low self-esteem. She also reported that he appeared "sad." However, she did say that he was affectionate, inquisitive, and very intelligent. Hector's teacher reported that Hector had difficulties relating to his peers and was not performing to his true ability. However, both his mother and teacher felt that Hector's desire to have friends and his cognitive ability would make him a good candidate for social skills training. Following the testing, Hector's therapist decided to target Hector's low self-esteem and his high level of social anxiety (which prevented him from making friends), in addition to specific skills (e.g., how to share; how to give and receive positive feedback) that seemed to be absent from his repertoire.

Synopsis of Therapy Sessions

Hector was seen for thirty sessions over ten months in the following modes: individual play therapy (to work on social skills with his therapist acting as a model) and group therapy (to enable Hector to interact with peers under the instruction and with the feedback of two therapists). For the first month, Hector was seen individually by his therapist. Hector was found to exhibit many of the illogical thoughts characteristic of anxious and depressed youngsters, such as overgeneralizing and catastrophizing (Leitenberg et al. 1986). One example of Hector's social anxiety, which demonstrates how fear of negative evaluation from his peers inhibited his behavior, is shown in the following exchange with his therapist.

> Therapist: Can you tell me why you failed that test?
> Client: Don't ask me. I don't know.
> Therapist: So, you don't know why you failed?
> Client: I didn't have a pencil.
> Therapist: You didn't have a pencil.
> Client: Right. I didn't have a pencil, so I couldn't take the test.
> Therapist: What do you mean?
> Client: I didn't have a pencil, and I didn't want to ask anybody for one, or the kids would have laughed.
> Therapist: You think the kids in your class would have laughed if you asked them for a pencil.
> Client: I know they would have.
> Therapist: What about asking your teacher?

Client: She would have made fun of me if I asked her.

Therapist: So, you think that the kids would have laughed and the teacher would have made fun of you.

Client: That's right. So I just sat there.

Hector's therapist also addressed Hector's beliefs about why he didn't have more friends. In one session, Hector was asked what would happen if he were to invite a friend over. His response further indicated a fear of negative evaluation by his peers:

Therapist: Do you ever invite other kids over?

Client: No.

Therapist: Any particular reason?

Client: I would be embarrassed to have them over.

Therapist: You would be embarrassed to have them at your house.

Client: Yes. I think I would do something stupid and they wouldn't like me.

Therapist: Have you had anybody over in the last few weeks?

Client: What's the point? To make a fool of myself?

Hector's therapist also learned that Hector carried a book around with him wherever he went, on the pretense that he was an avid reader. By carrying the book, Hector could avoid engaging others. This was determined to be a way in which he avoided having to make friends. Hector also preferred other solitary activities, such as playing cards by himself and playing golf. Thus, his therapist focused Hector's individual treatment on ways to approach others and engage them in positive ways.

When a social skills group (which included Sam, from the previous case illustration) was organized, Hector still saw his therapist individually every other week. His cognitions concerning his body image (he had a very negative self-image, such as feeling "too chubby") and relations with others were still the focus of these individual sessions. During these later sessions, Hector's therapist created role-plays of scenarios in which Hector had to engage other kids at various places in school and in his neighborhood. When Hector had an appropriate interchange with his therapist, his therapist reinforced his behavior. The group's purpose, on the other hand, was to emphasize skills (e.g., joining a conversation and resolving conflicts) that seemed better suited for being targeted in a group format. However, Hector often seemed resistant to activities of the group, since he didn't feel that it could help him with his problems. An example of his resistance is seen in the following exchange during a group session:

Therapist 1: First we are going to talk about introductions.

Hector: Why bother? This is a dumb thing to do.

Therapist 2: Introductions are important when you meet someone.

Hector: What if I don't want to meet anyone?

Therapist 1: You'll need to be able to introduce yourself in a lot of situations.

Hector: Like what?

Therapist 2: If you are in a new class, or at a party. . .

Hector: I would rather be by myself.

Summer vacation was a difficult time for Hector. He had been to summer camp during previous summers and had had aversive experiences with other children in these camps (e.g., someone put gum in his hair one time). Hector cried when recollecting such incidents. Hector's mother still encouraged him to go to camp again so that he could make new friends, but Hector refused.

During the summer, although his peer contacts were still problematic, Hector's therapist decided to implement family therapy, since she felt that family issues were contributing to his overall problems and interfering with his functioning. She felt that through family sessions she could better boost his self-confidence to communicate not only with his mother, but also with other children. Hector's therapist realized that Hector's mother was very self-critical, as well as critical of her son. This caused Hector to think of himself as a "bad person." The therapist felt that by working with both family members, their patterns of communication could improve. Several sessions were held with both mother and son, which usually resulted in Hector being in tears, due to the emotional nature of these sessions. However, Hector's therapist was able to persuade Hector to try group activities outside of the clinical setting, in which he was able to use skills that were emphasized in his individual sessions with his therapist and in group sessions. Termination occurred at the end of 10 months of treatment, since Hector showed some improvement in terms of participating in group activities outside of the center. The family also encountered other stressors at that point, and Hector's mother requested to end services for her son.

Comments

Hector's case is different from Sam's in several important ways. For example, Hector seemed less motivated (outwardly) to make friends than did Sam.

Even though both boys were anxious about new peer relationships, each had a distinct way of "scaring" other children away. Whereas Sam was often overtly aggressive toward peers, Hector used more indirect techniques (e.g., kicking others under the table, stepping on others' toes, or uttering comments under his breath) that antagonized peers. During group sessions, Hector seemed unmotivated to do group activities, as he often complained about these tasks. Ironically, at his last session, when his therapist asked him which form of therapy he enjoyed most (individual, group, or family), Hector said that he liked group sessions best. Perhaps with some children, even though they do not appear to be benefiting from group sessions, they may still be deriving benefits from the group format (perhaps due to mere exposure to positive peer interactions).

Hector's case also points out the necessity in certain cases to get family members (e.g., parents) directly involved in treatment through family sessions. In such cases, changes will not transfer to the outside world, unless other members also participate. On the other hand, it is also important to make sure that family members respect the child's privacy in individual and group sessions. During several sessions, Hector's mother tried to sit directly outside the playroom door (where individual and group sessions were held), in order to hear what her son was saying. This intrusion interfered not only with her son's treatment but also with the treatment of other children in the group. Hector's therapist dealt with this obstacle by asking Hector's mother to wait for her son in another part of the center.

SUMMARY

As indicated near the beginning of this chapter, children who experience interpersonal difficulties with peers are at substantial risk for emotional problems. Because peer relationship problems are stable over time, are associated with many clinical problems in children, and contribute substantially to children's emotional distress, social interventions should be viewed as an essential aspect of the child treatment process. Peer relations clearly play a significant role in children's social and emotional adjustment.

Drawing from a conceptual model that links peer rejection and problematic peer relations with emotional adaptation over time, interventions to improve peer status have been designed to interrupt this negative chain of events and pave the way for more positive mental health outcomes. Broadly speaking, peer relationship difficulties were described as fitting into one of three categories: (a) deficits in positive interaction skills, (b) the presence of behavior problems that interfere with social interactions, and (c) the presence of other nonbehavioral child characteristics that contribute to peers' dislike. Assessment strategies relevant to these areas were described, and suggestions for appropriate assessment tools were provided. In general, it was advocated that an assessment of children's social functioning should include an evaluation of the child's (a) peer relations, (b) social skills and social behaviors, (c) feelings of social anxiety, social inadequacy, and loneliness, (d) friendships and supportive relationships, (e) degree of internalizing and externalizing behavior problems that may contribute to peer difficulties, and (f) existence of academic problems, physical handicaps, or other nonbehavioral problems that may contribute to negative peer interactions.

Following from this assessment, an intervention program should be planned that incorporates, as needed, social skills training to increase positive interaction skills, behavior management to reduce problematic behaviors that interfere with social functioning, and efforts to involve nonproblem peers in the treatment process to increase a child's social networks and facilitate treatment maintenance. Multiple strategies are likely to be needed for many children, and illustrations of a multicomponent approach to social intervention was illustrated in two case examples. Other treatment considerations, such as the number, length, and frequency of the treatment sessions; the use of individual or group treatment; constraints in setting up groups; the involvement of parents or others (e.g., teachers, peers) in the intervention process; and plans for treatment maintenance were also discussed.

In closing, social skills training has come far in the fifteen or so years since its inception. Future developments in this area are likely to include the development of empirically based strategies for adapting social skills training programs to the needs of the diverse types of cases and problems seen in clinical practice (La Greca 1993). With this important direction in mind, social skills interventions should continue to be an important intervention tool for improving children's social functioning and emotional adaptation.

REFERENCES

Achenbach, T. M. (1991a). *Manual for the Child Behavior Checklist/4-18 and 1991 Profile*. Burlington: University of Vermont Department of Psychiatry.

_____ (1991b). *Manual for the Teacher's Report Form and 1991 Profile*. Burlington: University of Vermont Department of Psychiatry.

_____ (1991c). *Manual for the Youth Self-Report and 1991 Profile*. Burlington: University of Vermont Department of Psychiatry.

Asher, S. R., and Dodge, K. A. (1986). Identifying children who are rejected by their peers. *Developmental Psychology* 22:444–449.

Asher, S. R., Hymel, S., and Renshaw, P. D. (1984). Loneliness in children. *Child Development* 55:1456–1464.

Asher, S. R., Parkhurst, J. T., Hymel, S., and Williams, G. A. (1990). Peer rejection and loneliness in childhood. In *Peer Rejection in Childhood*, ed. S. R. Asher and J. D. Coie, pp. 253–273. Cambridge: Cambridge University Press.

Asher, S. R., and Wheeler, V. A. (1985). Children's loneliness: a comparison of rejected and neglected peer status. *Journal of Consulting and Clinical Psychology* 53:500–505.

Barclay, J. R. (1966). Sociometric choices and teacher ratings as predictors of school dropout. *Journal of Social Psychology* 4:40–45.

Barkley, R. A. (1989). Attention deficit-hyperactivity disorder. In *Treatment of Childhood Disorders*, ed. E. J. Mash and R. A. Barkley, pp. 39–72. New York: Guilford.

Barrios, B. A., and Hartmann, D. P. (1988). Fears and anxieties. In *Behavioral Assessment of Childhood Disorders*, ed. E. J. Mash and L. G. Terdal, 2nd ed., pp. 196–262. New York: Guilford.

Barrios, B. A., and O'Dell, S. L. (1989). Fears and anxieties. In *Treatment of Childhood Disorders*, ed. E. J. Mash and R. A. Barkley, pp. 167–221. New York: Guilford.

Berndt, T. J. (1989). Obtaining support from friends during childhood and adolescence. In *Children's Social Networks and Social Supports*, ed. D. Belle, pp. 308–331. New York: Wiley.

Bierman, K. L. (1989). Improving the peer relationships of rejected children. In *Advances in Clinical Child Psychology*, vol. 12, ed. B. B. Lahey and A. E. Kazdin, pp. 53–84. New York: Plenum.

Bierman, K. L., and Furman, W. (1984). The effects of social skills training and peer involvement on the social adjustment of preadolescents. *Child Development* 55:151–162.

Bierman, K. L., and McCauley, E. (1987). Children's description of their peer interactions: useful information for clinical child assessment. *Journal of Clinical Child Psychology* 16:9–18.

Bierman, K. L., Miller, C. L., and Stabb, S. D. (1987). Improving the social behavior and peer acceptance of rejected boys: effects of social skills training with instructions and prohibitions. *Journal of Consulting and Clinical Psychology* 55:194–200.

Bornstein, M. R., Bellack, A. S., and Hersen, M. (1980). Social skills training for highly aggressive children. *Behavior Modification* 4:173–186.

Bryan, T. H. (1974). Peer popularity of learning disabled children. *Journal of Learning Disabilities* 7:261–268.

_____ (1976). Peer popularity of learning disabled children: a replication. *Journal of Learning Disabilities* 9:307–311.

Cartledge, G., and Milburn, J. F., eds. (1980). *Teaching Social Skills to Children*. New York: Pergamon.

Cauce, A. M. (1986). Social networks and social competence: exploring the effects of early adolescent friendships. *American Journal of Community Psychology* 14:607–628.

Cauce, A. M., Reid, M., Landesman, S., and Gonzales, N. (1990). Social support in young children: measurement, structure, and behavioral impact. In *Social Support: An Interactional View*, ed. B. R. Sarason, I. G. Sarason, and G. R. Pierce, pp. 64–94. New York: Wiley.

Cohen, S., and Wills, T. (1985). Stress, social support, and the buffering hypothesis. *Psychological Bulletin* 98:310–357.

Coie, J. D. (1990). Toward a theory of peer rejection. In *Peer Rejection in Childhood*, ed. S. R. Asher and J. D. Coie, pp. 365–401. Cambridge: Cambridge University Press.

Coie, J. D., and Dodge, K. A. (1988). Multiple sources of data on social behavior and social status in the school: a cross-age comparison. *Child Development* 59:815–829.

Coie, J. D., Dodge, K. A., and Coppotelli, H. (1982). Dimensions and types of social status: a cross-age perspective. *Developmental Psychology* 18:557–570.

Coie, J. D., Dodge, K. A., and Kupersmidt, J. B. (1990). Peer group behavior and social status. In *Peer Rejection in Childhood*, ed. S. R. Asher and J. D. Coie, pp. 17–59. Cambridge: Cambridge University Press.

Coie, J. D., and Kupersmidt, J. B. (1983). A behavioral analysis of emerging social status in boys' groups. *Child Development* 54:1400–1416.

Combs, S. L., and Slaby, D. A. (1977). Social skills training with children. In *Advances in Clinical Child Psychology*, vol. 1, ed. B. B. Lahey and A. E. Kazdin, pp. 161–203. New York: Plenum.

Cowen, E. L., Pederson, A., Babijian, H., et al. (1973). Long-term follow-up of early detected vulnerable children. *Journal of Consulting and Clinical Psychology* 41:438–446.

Diagnostic and Statistical Manual of Mental Disorders. (1994). 4th ed. Washington, DC: American Psychiatric Association.

Dodge, K. A. (1983). Behavioral antecedents of peer social status. *Child Development* 54:1386–1389.

_____ (1989). Problems in social relationships. In *Treatment of Childhood Disorders*, ed. E. J. Mash and R. A. Barkley, pp. 222–244. New York: Guilford.

Dodge, K. A., Coie, J., and Brakke, N. (1982). Behavioral patterns of socially rejected and neglected pre-adolescents: the roles of social approach and aggression. *Journal of Abnormal Child Psychology* 10:389–409.

Dubow, E. F., and Tisak, J. (1989). The relation between stressful life events and adjustment in elementary school children: the role of social support and social problem-solving skills. *Child Development* 60:1412–1423.

Erwin, P. (1993). *Friendship and Peer Relations in Children*. Chichester, England: Wiley.

Felner, R., Ginter, M., and Primavera, J. (1982). Primary prevention during school transition: social support and environmental structure. *American Journal of Community Psychology* 10:227–290.

Finch, A. J., Jr., and McIntosh, J. A. (1990). Assessment of anxieties and fears in children. In *Through the Eyes of the Child: Obtaining Self-Reports from Children and Adolescents*, ed. A. M. La Greca, pp. 234–258. Boston: Allyn and Bacon.

Furman, W., and Buhrmester, D. (1985). Children's perceptions of the personal relationships in their social networks. *Developmental Psychology* 21:1016–1024.

Furman, W., and Gavin, L. A. (1989). Peers' influence on adjustment and development: a view from the intervention literature. In *Peer Relationships in Child Development*, ed. T. J. Berndt and G. W. Ladd, pp. 319–340. New York: Wiley.

Furman, W., and Robbins, P. (1985). What's the point: issues in the selection of treatment objectives. In *Children's Peer Relations: Issues in Assessment and Intervention*, ed. B. H. Schneider, K. H. Rubin, and J. E. Ledingham, pp. 41–56. New York: Springer-Verlag.

Gottman, J., Gonso, J., and Rasmussen, B. (1975). Friendships in children. *Child Development* 46:709–718.

Granberry, S. W., Williamson, D. A., Moody, S. C., and Lethermon, V. R. (1982). *Role play assessment of children's social skills: a standardized procedure and normative data.* Paper presented at the annual meeting of the Association for Advancement of Behavior Therapy, Los Angeles, CA, November.

Green, K. D., Forehand, R., Beck, S. J., and Vosk, B. (1980). An assessment of the relationship among measures of children's social competence and children's academic achievement. *Child Development* 51:1149–1156.

Gresham, F. M., and Elliot, S. N. (1990). *Social Skills Rating System.* Circle Pines, MN: American Guidance Service.

Gresham, F. M., and Nagle, R. J. (1980). Social skills training with children: responsiveness to modeling and coaching as a function of peer orientation. *Journal of Consulting and Clinical Psychology* 84:718–729.

Gronlund, N. E., and Holmlund, W. S. (1958). The value of elementary school sociometric status scores for predicting pupils' adjustment in high school. *Educational Administration and Supervision* 44:225–260.

Harter, S. (1985). *Manual for the Social Support Scale for Children and Adolescents.* Denver: University of Denver.

Hartup, W. W. (1983). Peer relations. In *Handbook of Child Psychology: Vol. 4. Socialization, Personality, and Social Development*, Series ed. P. H. Mussen and Volume ed. E. M. Hetherington, 4th ed., pp. 103–196. New York: Wiley.

Hazel, J. S., Schumaker, J. B., Sherman, J. A., and Sheldon, J. (1982). Applications of a group training program in social skills and problem solving to learning disabled and non-learning disabled youth. *Learning Disabilities Quarterly* 5:398–408.

Hughes, J. N. (1988). *Cognitive Behavior Therapy with Children in Schools.* New York: Pergamon.

Jackson, N. F., Jackson, D. A., and Monroe, C. (1983). *Getting Along with Others: Teaching Social Effectiveness to Children.* Champaign, IL: Research Press.

Johnson, W. G. (1975). Group therapy: a behavioral perspective. *Behavior Therapy* 6:30–38.

Kazdin, A. E. (1988). Childhood depression. In *Behavioral Assessment of Childhood Disorders*, ed. E. J. Mash and L. G. Terdal, 2nd ed., pp. 157–195. New York: Guilford.

_____ (1989). Childhood depression. In *Treatment of Childhood Disorders*, ed. E. J. Mash and R. A. Barkley, pp. 135–166. New York: Guilford.

_____ (1990). Assessment of childhood depression. In *Through the Eyes of the Child: Obtaining Self-Reports from Children and Adolescents*, ed. A. M. La Greca, pp. 189–233. Boston: Allyn and Bacon.

Keller, M. F., and Carlson, P. M. (1974). The use of symbolic modeling to promote social skills in children with low levels of social responsiveness. *Child Development* 45:912–919.

Kendall, P. C., Chansky, T. E., Kane, M. T., et al. (1992). *Anxiety Disorders in Youth: Cognitive-Behavioral Interventions*. Boston: Allyn and Bacon.

Kirby, F. D., and Toler, H. C. (1970). Modification of preschool isolate behavior: a case study. *Journal of Applied Behavior Analysis* 3:309–314.

Kohn, M. (1977). *Social Competence, Symptoms and Underachievement in Childhood: A Longitudinal Perspective*. New York: Holt, Rinehart and Winston.

Kolko, D. J., Loar, L. L., and Sturnick, D. (1990). Inpatient social-cognitive skills training groups with conduct disorders and attention deficit disordered children. *Journal of Child Psychology and Psychiatry and Applied Disciplines* 31:737–748.

Kovacs, M. (1979). *Children's Depression Inventory*. Pittsburgh: University of Pittsburgh.

Krehbiel, G., and Milich, R. (1986). Issues in the assessment and treatment of social rejected children. In *Advances in Behavioral Assessment of Children and Families*, ed. R. J. Prinz, pp. 249–270. Greenwich, CT: JAI Press.

Kupersmidt, J. B. (1983). Predicting delinquency and academic problems from childhood peer status. In J. D. Coie (Chair), *Strategies for identifying children at social risk: longitudinal correlates and consequences*. Biennial meeting of the Society for Research in Child Development, Detroit, MI, April.

Kupersmidt, J. B., and Coie, J. D. (1990). Preadolescent peer status, aggression, and school adjustment as predictors of externalizing problems in adolescence. *Child Development* 61:1350–1362.

Kupersmidt, J. B., Coie, J. D., and Dodge, K. A. (1990). The role of poor peer relationships in the development of disorder. In *Peer Rejection in Childhood*, ed. S. R. Asher and J. D. Coie, pp. 274–305. Cambridge: Cambridge University Press.

La Greca, A. M. (1981). Social skills training with elementary school students: a skills training manual. *JSAS Catalogue of Selected Documents in Psychology*. (No. 2194).

_____ (1990). Issues and perspectives on the child assessment process. In *Through the Eyes of the Child: Obtaining Self-Reports from Children and Adolescents*, ed. A. La Greca, pp. 3–17. Boston: Allyn and Bacon.

_____ (1991). The development of social anxiety in children. Paper presented in T. Ollendick (Chair), *Advances in the assessment and treatment of childhood anxiety and phobic disorders*. American Psychological Association Meeting, San Francisco, CA, August.

_____ (1993). Children's social skills training: where do we go from here? *Journal of Clinical Child Psychology* 22:288–298.

La Greca, A. M., Dandes, S., Wick, P., et al. (198ℰ\. The development of the Social Anxiety Scale for Children (SASC): reliability and concurrent validity. *Journal of Clinical Child Psychology* 17:84–91.

La Greca, A. M., and Mesibov, G. B. (1979). Social skills intervention with learning disabled children: selecting skills and implementing training. *Journal of Clinical Child Psychology* 8:234–241.

_____ (1981). Facilitating interpersonal functioning with peers in learning disabled children. *Journal of Learning Disabilities* 14:197–199, 238.

La Greca, A. M., and Santogrossi, D. A. (1980). Social-skills training: a behavioral group approach. *Journal of Consulting and Clinical Psychology* 48:220–228.

La Greca, A. M., and Stark, P. (1986). Naturalistic observations of children's social behavior. In *Children's Social Behavior: Development, Assessment, and Modification*, ed. P. Strain, M. Guralnick, and H. Walker, pp. 181–213. New York: Academic Press.

La Greca, A. M., and Stone, W. L. (1992). Assessing children through interviews and behavioral observations. In *Handbook of Clinical Child Psychology*, ed. C. E. Walker and M. C. Roberts, 2nd ed., pp. 63–83. New York: Wiley.

_____ (1993). The Social Anxiety Scale for Children-Revised: factor structure and concurrent validity. *Journal of Clinical Child Psychology* 22:17–27.

La Greca, A. M., Stone, W. L., and Noriega-Garcia, A. (1989). Social skills intervention: a case of a learning disabled boy. In *Case Studies in Clinical Child/Pediatric Psychology*, ed. M. C. Roberts and C. E. Walker, pp. 139–160. New York: Guilford.

Ladd, G. W. (1985). Documenting the effects of social skills training with children: process and outcome assessment. In *Children's Peer Relations: Issues in Assessment and Intervention*, ed. B. H. Schneider, K. H. Rubin, and J. E. Ledingham, pp. 243–271. New York: Wiley.

Ladd, G. W., and Mize, J. (1983). A cognitive-social learning model of social skills training. *Psychological Review* 90:127–157.

Landau, S., and Milich, R. (1990). Assessment of children's social status and peer relations. In *Through the Eyes of the Child: Obtaining Self-Reports from Children and Adolescents*, ed. A. M. La Greca, pp. 259–291. Boston: Allyn and Bacon.

Leitenberg, H., Yost, L. W., and Carroll-Wilson, M. (1986). Negative cognitive errors in children: questionnaire development, normative data, and comparison between children with and without self-reported symptoms of depression, low self-esteem, and evaluation anxiety. *Journal of Consulting and Clinical Psychology* 54:528–536.

Loeber, R., Green, S. M., and Lahey, B. B. (1990). Mental health professionals' perceptions of the utility of children, parents, and teachers as informants on childhood psychopathology. *Journal of Clinical Child Psychology* 19:136–143.

Masten, A., Morrison, P., and Pelligrini, D. (1985). A revised class play method of peer assessment. *Developmental Psychology* 21:523–533.

Matson, J. L., Esveldt-Dawson, D., Andrasik, F., et al. (1980). Direct, observational, and generalization effects of social skills training with emotionally disturbed children. *Behavior Therapy* 11:522–531.

Matson, J. L., Rotatori, A. F., and Helsel, W. J. (1983). Development of a rating scale to measure social skills in children: the Matson Evaluation of Social Skills with Youngsters (MESSY). *Behaviour Research and Therapy* 21:335–340.

McGinnis, E., and Goldstein, A. P. (1984). *Skill-Streaming the Elementary School Child: A Guide for Teaching Prosocial Skills.* Champaign, IL: Research Press.

McMahon, R. J., and Wells, K. C. (1989). Conduct disorders. In *Treatment of Childhood Disorders*, ed. E. J. Mash and R. A. Barkley, pp. 73–132. New York: Guilford.

Michelson, L., Sugai, D. P., Wood, R. P., and Kazdin, A. E. (1983). *Social Skills Assessment and Training with Children: An Empirically Based Handbook.* New York: Plenum.

O'Connor, R. D. (1972). Relative efficacy of modeling, shaping, and the combined procedures for modification of social withdrawal. *Journal of Abnormal Psychology* 79:327–334.

Oden, S., and Asher, S. R. (1977). Coaching children in social skills for friendship making. *Child Development* 48:495–506.

Ollendick, T. H. (1983). Reliability and validity of the Revised Fear Survey Schedule for Children (FSSC-R). *Behaviour Research and Therapy* 21:685–692.

Parker, J. G., and Asher, S. R. (1987). Peer relations and later personal adjustment: are low-accepted children at risk? *Psychological Bulletin* 102:357–389.

Piers, E. V., and Harris, D. B. (1969). *The Piers-Harris Children's Self Concept Scale.* Nashville, TN: Counselor Recordings and Tests.

Pinkston, E. M., Reese, N. M., Le Blanc, J. M., and Baer, D. M. (1973). Independent control or a preschool child's aggression and peer interaction by contingent teacher attention. *Journal of Applied Behavior Analysis* 6:115–124.

Plenk, A. M. (1993). *Helping Young Children at Risk: A Psycho-Educational Approach.* Westport, CT: Praeger.

Price, J. M., and Dodge, K. A. (1989). Peers' contributions to children's social maladjustment: description and intervention. In *Peer Relationships in Child Development*, ed. T. J. Berndt and G. W. Ladd, pp. 341–370. New York: Wiley.

Quay, H. C., and Peterson, D. R. (1987). *Manual for the Revised Behavior Problem Checklist.* Longboat Key, FL: H. C. Quay.

Reid, M., Landesman, S., Treder, R., and Jaccard, J. (1989). "My family and friends." 6 to 12 year old children's perceptions of social support. *Child Development* 60:896–910.

Reynolds, C. R., and Richmond, B. O. (1978). What I think and feel: a revised measure of children's manifest anxiety. *Journal of Abnormal Child Psychology* 6:271–280.

—— (1985). *Manual for the Revised Children's Manifest Anxiety Scale.* Los Angeles: Western Psychological Association.

Roff, M., Sells, S. B., and Golden, M. M. (1972). *Social Adjustment and Personality Adjustment in Children.* Minneapolis: University of Minnesota Press.

Rose, S. D. (1973). *Treating Children in Groups*. San Francisco: Jossey-Bass.

Ross, A. O. (1978). Behavior therapy with children. In *Handbook of Psychotherapy and Behavior Change*, ed. S. L. Garfield and E. Bergin. New York: Wiley.

Sandler, I. N., Wolchik, S., and Braver, S. (1985). Social support and children of divorce. In *Social Support: Theory, Research, and Applications*, ed. I. G. Sarason and B. R. Sarason, pp. 371–390. Boston: Martinus Nijhoff.

Schneider, B. H. (1989). Between developmental wisdom and children's social skills training. In *Social Competence in Developmental Perspective*, ed. B. H. Schneider, G. Attili, J. Nadel, and R. P. Weissberg. Dordrecht, Netherlands: Kluwer.

Silverman, W. K., and La Greca, A. M. (1992). *Screening for childhood anxiety: a comparison of test and social anxiety*. Paper presented at the Fourth Annual Meeting of the Society for Research in Child and Adolescent Psychopathology, Sarasota, FL, February.

Simmons, R., Carlton-Ford, S., and Blythe, D. (1987). Predicting how a child will cope with the transition to junior high school. In *Biological-Psycho-Social Interactions in Early Adolescence*, ed. R. M. Lerner and T. T. Foch, pp. 325–375. Hillsdale, NJ: Erlbaum.

Spielberger, C. D. (1973). *Manual for the State-Trait Anxiety Inventory for Children*. Palo Alto, CA: Consulting Psychologists Press.

Stone, W. L., and La Greca, A. M. (1990). The social status of children with learning disabilities: a reexamination. *Journal of Learning Disabilities* 23:32–37.

Strauss, C. C., Lahey, B. B., Frick, P., et al. (1988). Peer social status of children with anxiety disorders. *Journal of Consulting and Clinical Psychology* 56:137–141.

Vaughn, S., and La Greca, A. M. (1988). Social interventions with learning disabled children. In *Learning Disabilities: State of the Art and Practice*, ed. K. Kavale, pp. 123–140. Boston: College Hill Press.

_____ (1992). Beyond greetings and making friends: social skills from a broader perspective. In *Intervention Research with Students with Learning Disabilities: An International Perspective*, ed. B. Wong. New York: Springer-Verlag.

_____ (1993). Social skills training: why, who, what, and how. In *Learning Disabilities: Best Practice for Professionals*, ed. W. N. Bender, pp. 251–271. Boston: Andover Medical Publishers.

Vaughn, S., and Lancelotta, G. (1991). Teaching interpersonal social skills to low accepted students: peer-pairing versus no peer-pairing. *Journal of School Psychology* 28:181–188.

Vaughn, S., McIntosh, R., and Spencer-Rowe, J. (1991). Peer rejection is a stubborn thing: increasing peer acceptance of rejected students with learning disabilities. *Learning Disabilities Research* 6:83–88.

Vernberg, E. M., Abwender, D. A., Ewell, K. K., and Beery, S. H. (1992). Social anxiety and peer relationships in early adolescence: a prospective analysis. *Journal of Clinical Child Psychology* 21:189–196.

Wechsler, D. (1991). *Manual for the Wechsler Intelligence Scale for Children-III*. New York: The Psychological Corporation.

_____ (1992). *Manual for the Wechsler Individual Achievement Test.* New York: The Psychological Corporation.

Wicks-Nelson, R., and Israel, A. C. (1991). *Behavior Disorders of Childhood.* 2nd ed. Englewood Cliffs, NJ: Prentice-Hall.

Williamson, D. A., Moody, S. C., Granberry, S. W., et al. (1983). Criterion-related validity of a role-play social skills test for children. *Behavior Therapy* 14:466–481.

5

SOCIAL ANXIETY DISORDERS

Michael W. Vasey

INTRODUCTION

Diagnostic categories describing social anxiety disorders first appeared over a decade ago with the introduction of social phobia and avoidant disorder in the third edition of the *Diagnostic and Statistical Manual of Mental Disorders* (*DSM-III*, American Psychiatric Association 1980). Unfortunately, despite their presence in the psychiatric nomenclature since 1980, these disorders have only recently begun to receive theoretical and empirical attention. This chapter reviews the small existing literature and the growing body of research in progress to detail the current state of the art in conceptualizing, assessing, and treating social anxiety disorders in young people. The chapter begins with a discussion of the descriptive features of these disorders with special emphasis on the impact of changes appearing in the fourth edition of the *DSM* (*DSM-IV*, American Psychiatric Association 1994). Second, current conceptualizations of social anxiety disorders in young people are reviewed, and their implications for assessment and treatment design are discussed. Third, available assessment techniques are reviewed and fourth, state-of-the-art treatment approaches are discussed. Finally, two case examples are described.

DESCRIPTION OF DISORDERS

Anxiety concerning social evaluation is common among children and adolescents (Ollendick et al. 1985, Orton 1982), becoming increasingly prevalent with age (e.g., Vasey et al. in press). This age-related increase reflects children's developing social-cognitive skills such as the ability to take another's perspective and engage in social comparison (Bauer 1980, Vasey et al. in press). When social anxiety is pervasive or persistent, it has significant potential to interfere with children's social competence, impeding acquisition of social skills and knowledge (Hymel et al. 1985). Consistent with this view, peer ratings show anxious children to be significantly less popular than nonreferred children, and much more likely than either nonreferred or conduct-disordered children to display neglected status on such ratings (Strauss et al. 1988). Furthermore, anxious children are significantly more lonely and withdrawn, and less socially skilled than nonreferred peers. Although the Strauss study did not focus specifically on social anxiety disorders, it seems likely that children with such disorders are especially at risk for social incompetence. There is also evidence that, among adolescents, social anxiety is linked to increased loneliness (Inderbitzen-Pisaruk et al. 1992). Furthermore, social anxiety at the beginning of the second year predicts lower levels of intimacy and companionship several months later (Vernberg et al. 1992).

The potential for social anxiety to interfere with children's developing competence can be thought of as analogous to the notion of "limited shopping" advanced by Patterson to account for the increasing deviance of antisocial youth over time (Patterson et al. 1992). To the extent that children avoid social situations, their opportunities to learn necessary social skills and establish friendships will be limited. Albano and colleagues (1994) point out a clear example of this phenomenon. Many of the socially anxious children seen in their clinic report avoiding a wide range of social situations. Furthermore, they report having unusual interests for their age and frequently justify their social avoidance by saying that they aren't interested in the same things as their peers. In the author's experience, the parents of such children often make similar statements. The cumulative effects of social avoidance clearly have significant potential to produce enduring social incompetence.

Social anxiety is a common feature of several anxiety disorders described in *DSM-III-R* (American Psychiatric Association 1987). The present discussion is focused on social phobia and avoidant disorder, though there are several other disorders in which social anxiety may play a significant role. For example, the *DSM-III-R* criteria for overanxious disorder (OAD) include excessive worry about social evaluation and performance in school, sports, and social relationships (American Psychiatric Association 1987). Similarly, social anxiety is often associated with school phobia or school refusal behavior (Kearney and Silverman 1990). Thus, much of the research concerning such problems and their treatment may have considerable relevance for social anxiety disorders as well.

As defined in *DSM-III-R*, social phobia is primarily characterized by a "persistent fear of one or more situations . . . in which the person is exposed to possible scrutiny by others and fears that he or she may do something or act in a way that will be humiliating or embarrassing" (p. 241). This fear typically leads to avoidance of the phobic situation(s) although social phobics may instead endure feared situations despite intense anxiety. Furthermore, social avoidance and anxiety must interfere significantly with social functioning. *DSM-III-R* specifies two types of social phobia: (1) the specific subtype is characterized by fear of only one type of social situation (e.g., public speaking anxiety); (2) the generalized subtype is characterized by anxiety regarding most social situations.

According to *DSM-III-R* (American Psychiatric Association 1987), the fundamental characteristic of avoidant disorder is excessive avoidance of, or shrinking from, contact with unfamiliar people despite desiring and having warm and satisfying relationships with familiar people. Since its introduction, the validity of avoidant disorder has been questioned because of a lack of empirical support (Kazdin 1983). One of the primary questions is whether avoidant disorder is distinct from social phobia. *DSM-III-R* specified that social phobia should not be diagnosed if avoidant disorder is present, suggesting that avoidant disorder necessarily includes, but is not limited to, the symptoms of social phobia. Recently, Francis and colleagues (1992) formally compared avoidant disorder and social phobia in children and adolescents. Children with avoidant disorder were significantly younger (M = 11.3 years) than those with social phobia (M = 14.2) or both avoidant disorder and social phobia (M = 15.0). Francis and colleagues suggest that this age difference parallels normal development, since "fear of strangers emerges at an earlier age than do social-evaluative fears" (p. 1089). However, other than this age difference, the groups were "indistinguishable in terms of gender, race, and comorbid psychiatric diagnoses" (p. 1088). Therefore, given their similarity, Francis and colleagues recommend that avoidant disorder be considered a subtype of social phobia. Similarly, Beidel (1992) suggested that avoidant disorder and social phobia share much in common and that avoidant disorder may simply be an extreme form of social phobia, since it is characterized by severe disruption of social functioning.

Despite their similarity on some dimensions, it may be that these two disorders differ in ways not yet examined. Further consideration suggests that avoidant disorder may not necessarily capture the essential qualities of social phobia. Avoidant disorder is characterized by anxiety concerning unfamiliar people, but that fear need *not* focus on social evaluation. In contrast, fear of negative social evaluation is clearly the focus of social phobia. Thus, despite the similarity of these two disorders with regard to gender, race, and comorbid conditions, they may differ in other ways that have important implications for treatment and prognosis. Future research should compare these disorders more fully. However, this may prove difficult because avoidant disorder does not appear in *DSM-IV* (American Psychiatric Association 1994). The *DSM-IV* criteria for social phobia have been expanded to include the symptoms of avoidant disorder. Thus, social phobia is no longer exclusively a fear of negative social evaluation. *DSM-IV* now includes a fear of social situations in which the person is exposed to unfamiliar people. The remaining criteria have also been expanded to include specific manifestations in childhood. For example, in children, the anxiety that occurs in such situations may be expressed by crying, tantrums, freezing, or withdrawal from the situation. Furthermore, it is recognized that children may not view their fears as unreasonable.

The prevalence of social phobia in the general population of children appears to be about 1 percent (Anderson et al. 1987, Benjamin et al. 1990, McGee et al. 1990). Few studies have examined the prevalence of avoidant disorder, but available estimates suggest its prevalence to be about 1.5 percent (Benjamin et al. 1990). For both categories, there is some evidence that prevalence rates may be higher for girls than boys. For example, for avoidant disorder, Benjamin and colleagues (1990) reported rates of 0.8 percent for boys and 2.1 percent for girls. For social phobia, Anderson and colleagues (1987) reported a ratio of only one boy to every five girls with the disorder. However, not all studies show such a disparity. Kashani and Orvaschel (1990) report rates of 1 percent for social phobia in both boys and girls. Consistent with developmental expectations, the prevalence of social phobia appears to increase with age. Kashani and Orvaschel (1990) reported rates for 8-, 12-, and 17-year-olds to be 0 percent, 1.4 percent, and 1.4 percent, respectively. Of course, all available estimates are based on *DSM-III* and *DSM-III-R* criteria. Though rates for social phobia should increase with its combination with avoidant disorder, it remains to be seen how this and other changes in *DSM-IV* will affect prevalence rates. For example, the deletion of overanxious disorder (OAD) from *DSM-IV* may mean that prevalence rates for social phobia will increase. Many OAD children have significant anxiety concerning social evaluation that may not be adequately described by a diagnosis of generalized anxiety disorder (GAD). Such children may fit better within the category of social phobia instead of, or in addition to, GAD.

Social anxiety disorders appear to be relatively common among clinically referred anxious children. For example, Albano and colleagues (1994) report that of 156 children ages 7–17 referred to the Center for Stress and Anxiety Disorders at the State University of New York at Albany, 17.9 percent received a primary diagnosis of social phobia based upon structured diagnostic interviews. An additional 16 percent received a secondary diagnosis of social phobia. Unfortunately, Albano and colleagues do not report the percentage of children meeting criteria for avoidant disorder. According to Albano and colleagues (1994), social phobia in young people is often overlooked because shyness is generally accepted as common in our society and, because of the nature of their disorder, such children are unlikely to draw attention to themselves or their problem, even if they recognize it.

Social phobia typically appears to have its onset during adolescence. For example, Thyer and colleagues (1985) found the mean age of onset to be 15.7 years (SD = 8.5). Furthermore, 66 percent of Thyer's subjects reported onset of social phobia in childhood or adolescence. Similarly, comparing samples of 4- to 17-year-old social and simple phobics, Strauss and Last (cited in Strauss 1993) found that social phobics were older at time of intake (14.9 versus 11.1 years) and had a later age of onset (12.3 versus 7.8 years). Furthermore, while simple phobias occurred across the entire age range, social phobia did not appear in children younger than age 10, with virtually all older than age 12. Cognitive developmental limitations make it unlikely that children will present with social phobia before late childhood or early adolescence. However, also in keeping with developmental expectations, avoidant disorder appears to have an earlier age of onset than social phobia (Francis et al. 1992)

DIFFERENTIAL DIAGNOSIS

As defined by *DSM-III-R*, social phobia overlaps considerably with OAD. Both categories include fears of poor performance and negative evaluation. Thus, it is not surprising that it is often difficult to decide which label best describes a given child's problems (Silverman and Eisen 1993). OAD is commonly comorbid with social anxiety disorders (Francis et al. 1992, Last et al. 1987). For example, Francis et al. (1992) found comorbid OAD in 58 percent of children with avoidant disorder, 39 percent of social phobics, and 83 percent of those meeting criteria for both diagnoses. Silverman and Eisen (1993) argue that differentiating between social phobia and OAD is complicated by the failure of *DSM-III-R* to make clear whether the symptoms used to classify a child as socially phobic can also be used as part of the diagnosis of OAD. It is clear that OAD should not be diagnosed if anxiety is limited to social situations, but the converse is not clear. By eliminating the category of OAD and subsuming the problem under the adult label GAD, *DSM-IV* may resolve this difficulty.

In an attempt to identify distinguishing features of social phobia, Beidel

(1991a) compared social phobic, OAD, and normal children on a wide range of measures and found relatively few differences between the anxious groups. The anxious groups reported more test and trait anxiety than normal controls but did not differ from each other. Children completed daily monitoring forms for two weeks and social phobics recorded significantly more anxiety-producing events than normals though they did not differ from the OAD group. However, social phobics did differ from the OAD group in several important ways. They were significantly more likely to react negatively to negative events (46 percent) than either the OAD (26 percent) or normal (21 percent) samples. Thus, social phobia may interfere more with children's daily functioning than OAD. Social phobics also reported significantly lower perceptions of cognitive competence than OAD or normal subjects. Interesting differences also emerged in physiological and cognitive measures during several behavioral tasks. For example, the OAD sample had significantly higher baseline heart rate (HR) than social phobics. In addition, HR changes appeared to follow different patterns in the OAD and social phobic samples. Based upon these data, Beidel concluded that social phobia and OAD are different conditions in childhood and that social phobia in childhood appears to be very similar to the same disorder in adulthood.

Albano and colleagues (1994) provide a number of guidelines for the differential diagnosis of social phobia. First, because social anxiety is such a common problem, particularly in adolescence, social phobia must be distinguished from normal concerns of this sort. Albano and colleagues clearly state the distinguishing features, including intractability of anxiety, pervasiveness of avoidance, and significance of interference with competence. Second, social phobia must be distinguished from simple phobia. This may be done on the basis of the focus of the fear. Third, as noted above, though school refusal behavior is often associated with social phobia, it may be motivated by separation anxiety or other types of anxiety instead. Finally, Albano and colleagues note that depressed or dysthymic young people may exhibit avoidance of social interactions. It is certainly possible for social phobia to be comorbid with such an affective disorder and if so, it is likely to warrant treatment in its own right. However, such social withdrawal may also occur in the absence of social anxiety.

ASSESSMENT PROCEDURES

King (1993) recommends that assessment of social phobia should "begin with broad assessment of the child and his/her environment (e.g., family, school, peers) and move toward gaining more specific information regarding stimulus features, response modes, antecedents and consequences, severity, duration, and pervasiveness of the particular phobias" (p. 311). Thus, treatment decisions are optimally based on a complete functional analysis. This can be most effectively accomplished by acquiring information through as many methods as possible, including interviews, standardized questionnaires, behavioral observations, and physiological measures, from as many sources as possible including the child, parents, and teachers (King 1993). Measures that allow comparison to normative developmental information are especially important given the changing frequency, content, and severity of children's fears (King 1993).

Structured Diagnostic Interviews

Numerous structured diagnostic interviews that cover childhood anxiety disorders are available (see Silverman 1991 for a recent review). However, this discussion will focus on the Anxiety Disorders Interview Schedule for Children (ADIS-C, Silverman and Nelles 1988) because it is among the most widely used and provides extensive coverage of anxiety disorders. The ADIS-C, which is administered to the child, and its companion parent form (ADIS-P) provide detailed coverage of all *DSM-III-R* anxiety disorder categories as well as most other categories relevant to children and adolescents. Several studies have demonstrated that the psychometric characteristics of the ADIS are generally quite good with regard to the identification of anxiety disordered children (Silverman and Eisen 1992, Silverman and Nelles 1988). Though the ADIS appears less able to reliably discriminate among specific anxiety disorders, interrater agreement for most categories is moderate to high, especially when diagnoses are based on the composite of parent and child interviews. For example, for social phobia, Silverman and Eisen (1992) report moderate Kappa coefficients of .46 and .54 for the ADIS-C and ADIS-P respectively but .73 for their composite. Unfortunately, Silverman and Eisen do not report figures for avoidant disorder due to the small numbers of such children in their sample. When the ADIS-C and ADIS-P are revised according to *DSM-IV* guidelines, it seems likely that agreement for social phobia will increase, given the elimination of overlapping categories such as OAD and avoidant disorder.

    Social anxiety and avoidance are covered in four areas of the interview including school refusal behavior, avoidant disorder, social phobia, and OAD. The interview is focused on identifying the stimulus characteristics of situations that produce social anxiety (e.g., size of group, age of people, type of social interaction), the severity of distress, and extent of interference with the child's functioning. It also provides information about the number and quality of children's friendships, ability to make and keep friends, and general level of social involvement. Thus, in summary, the ADIS appears to be an excellent first step in gathering information for purposes of diagnosis and treatment planning.

Child Self-Report Measures

Several studies have used existing adult self-report measures of social anxiety with juvenile samples. For example, Inderbitzen-Pisaruk and colleagues (1992) used Watson and Friend's (1969) adult-based Fear of Negative Evaluation (FNE) and Social Avoidance and Distress (SAD) scales with junior high school students. Though findings in this and similar studies suggest that these scales may be applicable to young people, the wide developmental differences between adults and children make measures developed specifically for use with young people more desirable. Fortunately, a promising child self-report measure of social anxiety, the Social Anxiety Scale for Children (SASC), has been developed by La Greca and colleagues (1988). Like the scales of Watson and Friend (1969), the SASC yields two scales derived from factor analysis: (1) the FNE scale is an index of anxiety regarding social evaluation, and (2) the SAD scale is an index of avoidance of social contacts and level of anxiety while in social situations.

The original SASC appears to have excellent psychometric characteristics (La Greca et al. 1988). However, it has recently been revised and expanded (SASC-R, La Greca and Stone 1993). While the SAD scale of the SASC was focused exclusively on contacts with unfamiliar peers and social situations, the SASC-R yields two SAD scales. The first (SAD-New) reflects avoidance of unfamiliar peers and situations while the second (SAD-G) is focused on generalized social avoidance and distress. La Greca and Stone (1993) argue that the division between SAD-G and SAD-New provided by the SASC-R has important clinical implications. For example, generalized SAD presumably has more potential to interfere with the development of social competence and friendships than SAD that is limited to unfamiliar peers or novel social situations. This view is supported by the findings of Vernberg and colleagues (1992), who studied children entering a new school and found that high SAD-G scores at the start of school predicted lower levels of peer companionship after two months. In contrast, although SAD-New scores were elevated at the start of the school year, they were unrelated to levels of companionship after two months. La Greca and Stone (1993) report adequate reliability and internal consistency for the SASC-R and provide substantial evidence supporting its validity. In summary, the SASC-R appears to be a promising measure. However, future research with clinical populations is necessary.

Social anxiety is associated with loneliness and at least two measures of loneliness are available. Inderbitzen-Pisaruk and colleagues (1992) assessed loneliness using the Revised UCLA Loneliness Scale (Russel et al. 1980), which was originally developed for use with college students. It consists of twenty items rated on a four-point scale. Inderbitzen-Pisaruk and colleagues report satisfactory internal consistency for the scale, and the mean and standard deviation of their ninth grade sample were similar to those of college students. An alternative measure developed specifically for use with children is the Loneliness Questionnaire (Asher et al. 1984). This inventory consists of twenty-four items rated on a five-point scale. Item content is focused on level of social involvement, number and availability of friends, and level of loneliness. Using the Loneliness Questionnaire, Strauss and colleagues (1989) found that clinically anxious children reported significantly more loneliness than nonreferred controls, though no more than clinic controls.

The quality of socially anxious children's friendships is also of interest. Berndt and Perry (1986) developed their Friendship Interview to assess children's self-report levels of companionship and intimacy. This interview yields scales reflecting level of companionship and intimacy with regard to a child's three best friends. The available data show adequate levels of internal consistency for the two scales, though test-retest reliability is only moderate. For example, Vernberg and colleagues (1992) reported Pearson correlations between points separated by two to eight months ranging from .37 to .59. They also reported small but significant correlations ($-.19$ to $-.40$) between Friendship Interview scores and the SASC-R, showing that social anxiety is associated with reduced levels of companionship and intimacy.

Self-perceptions of social competence are also relevant to social anxiety disorders. The Perceived Self Competence Inventory (PSCI, Harter 1982, 1985) is a measure with excellent psychometric characteristics and has been used in at least one study of social phobia in young people (Beidel 1991a). The PSCI is composed of twenty-eight items that make up four scales reflecting cognitive, social, physical, and general competence. The PSCI is appropriate for children ages 8–14. Strauss and colleagues (1989) have shown that clinically anxious children report lower social competence than nonreferred controls, though they did not differ from clinic controls. Furthermore, Beidel (1991a) has reported that low social competence scores on the PSCI distinguish social phobic children from both OAD and normal control groups.

Self-report measures of social skills may be helpful for identifying treatment targets as well as tracking treatment progress. The Matson Evaluation of Social Skills with Youngsters (MESSY, Matson et al. 1983) consists of sixty-two items comprising five scales: (1) Appropriate social skills, (2) Inappropriate assertiveness, (3) Impulsive/recalcitrant, (4) Overconfident, and (5) Jealous/withdrawal. Matson and colleagues developed the MESSY using a sample of children ages 4–18. They report adequate test-retest reliability for the MESSY. There is also evidence supporting its discriminant validity. Strauss and colleagues (1989) found that anxiety-disordered children showed significantly lower levels of appropriate social skills than nonreferred children but did not show high levels of inappropriate assertiveness like clinic controls. Strauss and colleagues also had teachers complete the teacher form of the MESSY and found this same pattern of results.

The social skills necessary to support social competence appear to vary with age (Inderbitzen-Pisaruk and Foster 1990). Consequently, to adequately assess social skills deficits and select appropriate treatment targets, it is important to have age-appropriate measures. Inderbitzen and Foster (1992), arguing there was no adequate measure of adolescents' social skills, recently developed the Teenage Inventory of Social Skills (TISS). As these authors point out, a self-report measure of social skills is particularly essential for adolescents because teachers and parents become decreasingly privy to social behavior during this period. The TISS is a forty-item questionnaire with two twenty-item scales reflecting positive and negative social behaviors. Items are rated on a six-point scale from "does not describe me at all" to "describes me totally." The two scales have excellent test-retest reliability and internal consistency. Inderbitzen and Foster also report evidence of convergent and discriminant validity for both scales. Subjects' self-monitoring records showed that they engaged in significantly more behaviors they rated as describing them well than in behaviors they rated as describing them poorly. Furthermore, positive TISS scores were significantly correlated with sociometric measures and with ratings made by a knowledgeable friend. Negative TISS ratings were correlated with lower rates of positive peer nominations and higher rates of negative behavior reported by a friend. In summary, the TISS has substantial promise as a tool for identifying treatment targets and as a treatment outcome measure. However, further research with clinical groups is needed.

Research on test anxiety has produced several other self-report measures that may prove useful in assessing social anxiety. Zatz and Chassin (1983) developed the Children's Cognitive Assessment Questionnaire (CCAQ), which was subsequently revised and expanded (CCAQ-R, Zatz and Chassin 1985). The CCAQ-R is a fifty-item yes–no inventory of various thoughts children may experience while taking a test. Thoughts include positive and negative self-evaluations, on- and off-task thoughts, and coping self-statements. Data for samples of fifth and sixth graders suggest the measure has adequate internal consistency and test-retest reliability. Both studies by Zatz and Chassin as well as a recent study by Prins and colleagues (1994) show that high test-anxious children report more off-task and negative self-evaluative thoughts than moderate or low test-anxious children. A similar measure called the Cognitive Behavior Questionnaire has been developed by Houston and colleagues (1984).

Finally, a variety of other cognitive assessment techniques are applicable to social anxiety disorders. Among those used with anxious children are think aloud procedures (e.g., Fox et al. 1983) and thought listing (e.g., Prins 1986). However, only one study of socially phobic children has used such a measure. Beidel (1991a) had social phobic, OAD, and normal control groups report their thoughts subsequent to a vocabulary test and an oral reading segment. Thoughts were reliably categorized as positive, negative, or neutral. Only the two anxiety-disordered groups reported any negative thoughts during the vocabulary test but only social phobics and normals reported such thoughts during the oral reading task. It appears that such techniques may prove useful, but further research is clearly warranted. The psychometric characteristics of such techniques with children remain largely open to question. The reader is referred to an excellent discussion of such techniques by Kendall and Chansky (1991).

Self-Monitoring Measures

Beidel and colleagues (1991) have evaluated the feasibility and validity of using daily diaries to assess anxiety among test-anxious children in grades three through six. These authors had children describe anxiety-provoking events and their responses to them. More than half the children completed the procedure for at least ten of fourteen days. The validity of these diaries was assessed in a subsample of children who met criteria for social phobia or OAD compared to age-matched normal controls. Their validity is supported by the fact that, although anxious children reported the same number of negative events as normals, they reported significantly greater distress in response to such events. Also, they more often reported responding with negative behaviors (e.g., crying), avoidance responses, or passivity. It is important to note that no incentive was given to children to complete their daily diaries. It seems likely that use of contingent reinforcement would improve compliance rates. In summary, anxious children appear to be able to provide clinically useful information through daily diaries.

Parent Report Measures

The Child Behavior Checklist (CBCL, Achenbach 1991a) provides several potentially useful measures of social competence. The competence scales of the CBCL include two scores reflecting level of social involvement with friends (e.g., number of friends) and activities (e.g., sports). Achenbach (1991a) reports normative data separately for boys and girls ages 4–18 years and extensive evidence supporting the reliability and validity of these scales. They are particularly useful because there are equivalent forms for children's self report (CBCL-Youth Self Report [YSR], Achenbach 1991b) and teacher report (Achenbach 1991c).

Teacher Report Measures

Because it is often impossible or impractical to obtain sociometric ratings from a child's peers, teacher reports of a child's social competence are often an important alternative source of information regarding children's social functioning in school. There are many teacher report-based measures of children's social skills (see Hops and Greenwood 1988 for a thorough review). One good example is the teacher form of the MESSY (Matson et al. 1983), which is a sixty-four-item measure yielding scale scores reflecting inappropriate assertiveness and appropriate social skills. The teacher MESSY appears to have adequate psychometric characteristics. Preliminary evidence of its validity has been provided by Strauss and colleagues (1989), who found that teacher ratings on the MESSY discriminate clinically anxious children from clinic controls and nonreferred children.

Behavioral Observations

Behavioral observations in the natural setting can be expensive and time consuming. Therefore, it is important to identify specific problem situations through interviews and questionnaires before making such an investment. There are many behavioral observation systems available for assessing social skills deficits. For a thorough review, the reader is referred to Hops and Greenwood (1988). A representative measure of this type is the Consultant Social Interaction Code (CSIC, Hops et al. 1989), which was designed for recording social behavior on the playground. Using 5-second intervals, it provides information about percentage of positive social behavior, percentage of talk, rate of social initiation, rate of responses to peer initiations, rate of interaction, and a sociability ratio (rate of initiations to peer initiations). The Observer Impression Assessment Scale (Weinrott et al. 1981) is an easy-to-use measure that allows observers to rate general impressions of children's free-play interactions on fifteen five-point Likert scale items. These are completed after a 6-minute observation of a child's free-play interactions. The measure yields three scale scores: (1) verbal and social competence, (2) cooperative play, and (3) social participation.

Behavioral observations can be most easily made in analogue settings, role-plays, or standardized behavioral approach tests (BATs). For example, the Behavioral Assertiveness Test for Children (Bornstein et al. 1977) includes nine analogue situations in which the child responds to verbal prompts given by a confederate. Similarly, Beidel (1988, 1991b) has developed two standardized BATs that are appropriate for use with social anxiety disorders. These are 10-minute BATs involving a vocabulary test and oral reading. Using these BATs, Beidel has found clear differences between children with social phobia and those with OAD. Standardized BATs have clear promise but much more research is required to firmly establish their reliability and validity (Albano et al. 1994).

Physiological Measures

Despite the importance of physiological responses to the phenomenon of anxiety, few studies of such responses among anxious children or adolescents are available (Beidel 1989). There is a serious need for research in this domain. Though the collection of such measures from children presents a variety of difficulties, Beidel (1989) concludes that their use is feasible provided a number of guidelines are followed. The reader is referred to Beidel's excellent review for a thorough discussion of guidelines for the collection and use of such measures in children.

In one of the few existing studies, Beidel (1988) collected measures of blood pressure (BP) and heart rate (HR) from twenty-five test-anxious and twenty-five non-test-anxious 8- to 12-year-olds during a baseline period and two standardized BATs: a vocabulary test and an oral reading session. Results showed that test-anxious children had significantly higher HR during both tasks than non-test-anxious children. In addition, the pattern of HR during the tasks differed between groups. Non-test-anxious children tended to show an initial HR increase followed by a return to baseline during each task. In contrast, test-anxious children showed no tendency to return to baseline. Their HR tended to stay elevated throughout each task. Based on these results, Beidel concluded that test-anxious children's patterns of autonomic responses resemble those of socially anxious adults. It should be noted that 60 percent of the test-anxious group met *DSM-III* criteria for an anxiety disorder, most commonly either social phobia or OAD. More recently, Beidel (1991b) has reported evidence that measures of HR and BP are moderately stable over a two-week period. Finally, as described in the discussion of differential diagnosis, Beidel (1991b) has compared the HR responses of social phobic, OAD, and normal control groups. Based on such studies, Beidel concludes that the pattern of autonomic responses of socially phobic young people resembles that of socially phobic adults. However, much more research is needed before clear conclusions can be drawn.

State of the Art

To enhance comparisons across research centers, Albano and Barlow (1993) have recently proposed a standard assessment battery for measuring clinical change in childhood anxiety. They argue that this would increase efficiency in identifying predictors of clinical change and foster increased understanding of the phenomenology of childhood anxiety and the impact of developmental factors. The triple response system model provides the framework for their battery. Within the Verbal/Cognitive domain they advocate (1) thought-listing, (2) daily diaries, (3) standard questionnaire measures such as Revised Children's Manifest Anxiety Scale (Reynolds and Richmond 1978), and (4) individualized fear hierarchy ratings. In the behavioral domain they suggest (1) standardized BATs, (2) individualized BATs, (3) individualized phobic avoidance hierarchy ratings, and (4) behavioral observations in naturalistic settings. Finally, within the physiological domain they advocate the measurement of (1) HR and (2) respiration rate. Wherever possible, multiple sources of information should be sought in each of the three response domains, including (1) clinician ratings of diagnosis and severity (e.g., as in the ADIS-C and ADIS-P), (2) child reports, (3) parent reports, (4) teacher reports, and (5) direct observation. Although individual elements of this battery may be questioned, as a whole it is an excellent framework for assessment.

ESTABLISHING TREATMENT GOALS

Because a variety of factors may be operative in the etiology and maintenance of social anxiety, optimal treatment design relies on conducting a thorough functional analysis. Functional categories similar to those described by Kearney and Silverman (1990) for school refusal behavior can be defined on theoretical grounds. Among the most important factors that may maintain social anxiety disorders are deficient social skills and cognitive factors.

Deficient Social Skills

Theoretically, children who lack knowledge of social situations and appropriate social behaviors are likely to face increased chances of punishment (e.g., teasing or rejection) and reduced changes of reinforcement in social interactions due to inept responding. Thus, such contingencies may produce and maintain social anxiety and avoidance. Furthermore, such avoidance may seriously reduce the rate at which children gain familiarity with social situations and acquire the skills they require to be competent. As noted above, there is mounting evidence that socially anxious children do indeed exhibit a variety of social deficits (e.g., Strauss et al. 1989, Vernberg et al. 1992). Of course, it may be that some socially anxious children are not deficient in social skills. Rather, their use of such skills may be impaired due to anxiety-related cognitive interference.

Cognitive Factors

Cognitive factors are emphasized in most current theories of anxiety disorders (e.g., Barlow 1988, Beck and Emery 1985). For example, Kendall and Ronan (1990) argue that anxious children's information processing is characterized by cognitive distortions that contribute to anxiety. According to this view, socially anxious children are unusually likely to focus on signals of social threat, interpret ambiguous social stimuli as signalling threat, overestimate the likelihood of negative evaluation, and exaggerate its negative consequences. The operation of cognitive distortions in social anxiety calls for the use of cognitive therapy techniques to reduce distortions.

Barlow (1988) argues that anxiety-related cognitive activity interferes with social performance, thereby increasing the likelihood of social failure. Barlow cites a wide range of evidence showing that anxiety is associated with narrowing of attentional focus and redirection of attention inward. In turn, such narrowed, self-focused attention further heightens negative emotional states. As attention is narrowed and drawn inward, social performance is increasingly likely to be impaired. Social performance is assumed to be disrupted by worrisome thoughts and negative self-evaluations that draw attention away from the external cues that guide social behavior.

There is evidence that such attentional disruption does indeed occur in socially anxious young people. Furthermore, it appears to be associated with reduced social skill as perceived by self and others. Johnson and Glass (1989) examined the attentional focus of heterosocially anxious adolescent boys and found that they reported significantly elevated levels of negative self-evaluative attention compared to nonanxious peers. Consistent with Barlow's (1988) theory, boys who reported higher levels of self-focused attention also rated themselves as lower in social skill. Moreover, these social skill deficits were noticed by objective judges who rated such boys lower in social skills, higher in anxiety, and less desirable as a date. In contrast, higher levels of positive and task relevant thoughts (i.e., focused on their conversation and their partner) predicted higher self-ratings of social skill, and ratings of greater social skill and lower anxiety by judges. Based on their findings, Johnson and Glass (1989) recommend clinical interventions that focus on reducing self-focus and increasing task-focus as the best way to reduce subjective anxiety and improve performance. Similar interventions have proved helpful for test-anxious persons (Wigfield and Eccles 1990).

ROLE OF THE THERAPIST

The role of the therapist in most current treatments for social anxiety disorders in young people is consistent with cognitive-behavioral treatments in general (Kendall 1991). The therapist functions to educate clients and their families about social anxiety and to teach techniques for controlling and coping with it to minimize social distress and avoidance. From this perspective, much of a therapist's activities are also focused on facilitating the practice of these new skills in situations designed to enhance generalization and maintenance.

TREATMENT STRATEGIES

King (1993) provides an excellent review of treatment studies relevant to social phobia in young people. These include studies of systematic desensitization, flooding, modeling, operant, and cognitive procedures. Each has been shown to be effective, though such demonstrations have typically focused only on test anxiety or similar problems. None of these studies used adequately standardized diagnostic, treatment, and outcome assessment methods (Albano et al. 1994). In response to this, well-controlled treatment studies are currently under way in several laboratories. This section will focus mainly on the new treatment packages developed in these laboratories. However, past research does warrant brief discussion.

Many studies have evaluated the effectiveness of systematic desensitization (SD) in treating test or speech anxiety (e.g., Barabasz 1973, Deffenbacher and Kemper 1974, Kondas 1967, Laxer et al. 1969, Leal et al. 1981, Mann and Rosenthal 1969). SD rests on the assumption that social anxiety is a classically conditioned emotional response that can be reduced through counterconditioning. Most of these studies have shown SD to be effective, usually compared to an untreated control group (e.g., Barabasz 1973, Deffenbacher and Kemper 1974). However, several have failed to find evidence of effectiveness (e.g., Lazer et al. 1969, Mann and Rosenthal 1969). Unfortunately, because these studies have focused exclusively on test anxiety, their implications for the treatment of clinical social anxiety disorders are unclear. Furthermore, most of these studies have been marred by various methodological problems such as small sample size and questionable methods for selecting test-anxious subjects. Thus, SD may be an effective treatment technique for some forms of social anxiety but its efficacy in clinical populations remains unknown. Given that social anxiety disorders often involve skill deficits that may place such children at risk for social failure (Strauss et al. 1989), it seems unlikely that SD alone could be an effective treatment.

Like SD, imaginal and in vivo exposure methods seek to reduce conditioned fear responses elicited by social stimuli (King 1993). Though very small in number, the available studies suggest that, like SD, such techniques may be effective in treating some forms of social anxiety. For example, Kandel and colleagues (1977) reported two case studies using a combination of in vivo flooding and graduated in vivo exposure with two socially avoidant boys, ages 4 and 8. They found significant reduction in motor fear responses at posttreatment and these gains were maintained at five- to nine-month follow-ups. While promising, at this time there is simply insufficient information available to conclude that exposure treatments are effective in treating social anxiety disorders in childhood.

Even if approaches such as SD or in vivo exposure are effective in reducing social anxiety enough to increase rates of social approach, many socially anxious children lack adequate behavioral skills to avoid punishment during social interactions. The adult literature suggests that social skills training (SST) is essential when treating clients who are both anxious and socially unskilled (Trower et al. 1978). Several studies have evaluated the efficacy of social skills training in treating socially anxious or avoidant children. Unfortunately, there have been no controlled studies of clinically anxious children. For example, Christoff and colleagues (1985) evaluated the effectiveness of social problem solving and conversational skills training using a multiple baseline design with six children ages 12–14. Subjects were selected based on identification by school staff as shy and lacking social skills. Each child received approximately seven 40-minute sessions of training. As a group, participants showed substantial improvements in social problem-solving ability, quality of conversational skills, number of conversations, and self-esteem.

Modeling-based treatments seem well suited to remediating skill deficits and may also provide information that may correct faulty expectations and beliefs about social interaction. Ross and colleagues (1971) reported a case study of a 6-year-old boy with "extreme social withdrawal." Treatment lasted seven weeks with three 90-minute sessions per week. Treatment targeted many variables including frequency of social interaction, physical proximity and contact, and verbal contact with other children. Live and symbolic modeling of each component increased the boy's socially competent behaviors to near the level of his normal peers and significantly reduced his avoidance. Thus, though sparse, available studies suggest that SST and modeling treatments may be effective. Given the growing evidence of social deficits among anxious children (e.g., Strauss et al. 1989), there is a clear need for more thorough evaluation of the use of SST in treating such children.

The adult social phobia treatment literature suggests that the addition of cognitive therapy to exposure treatments significantly enhances their effectiveness (e.g., Mattick et al. 1989). Unfortunately, only a few studies have examined the efficacy of cognitive restructuring and related treatments for social anxiety in childhood (e.g., Craddock et al. 1978, Fox and Houston 1981, Leal et al. 1981, Stevens and Phil 1983). Moreover, all of these studies have limited their focus to nonclinical problems such as test anxiety. Most have shown cognitive techniques to be effective. For example, Stevens and Phil (1983) compared two cognitive treatments with no-treatment in forty-two test-anxious seventh graders. Unfortunately, assignment to treatment groups was done by school and thus was not randomized. The first cognitive treatment trained children in problem solving and cognitive restructuring via verbal self-instructions. The second encouraged students to discuss and develop their own coping strategies. Both treated groups improved significantly compared to the nontreated controls on measures such as the WICS-R Mazes subtest, number of coping strategies generated, and teacher-rated coping ability. Although there are many limitations to this and similar studies, cognitive restructuring techniques appear to be a promising treatment for some forms of social anxiety in young people.

There is a serious need for controlled treatment studies of social anxiety in young people. Fortunately, at least two research groups have treatment outcomes studies under way that have yielded promising preliminary results. Consistent with the current state-of-the-art treatment for social phobia in adulthood (e.g., Hope and Heimberg 1993), both involve group-based treatment programs. The first of these, developed by Albano and her colleagues, is a downward extension of the highly effective Cognitive Behavioral Group Treatment (CBGT) developed by Hope and Heimberg (1993). Albano and colleagues (1994) have reported preliminary data suggesting that CBGT is highly effective with adolescent social phobics. Though group treatment may seem counterintuitive for social anxiety, Hope and Heimberg (1993) argue that it offers several important advantages including opportunities to learn by observing others interact, becoming aware that others have similar problems, and numerous opportunities for exposure and practice.

Albano's version of CBGT is designed for use with adolescents between 13 and 17 years of age in small groups of four to six members. Albano and colleagues stress the importance of assessing the skill levels of each group member so that the group may progress at a pace appropriate for the least skillful member. However, they note that it is also important that the group not be too diverse in terms of skill level. Though the technique is designed for treating social phobia, Albano and colleagues note that with minor modifications CBGT is also appropriate for adolescents with avoidant disorder. For a more detailed description of CBGT, the reader is referred to excellent descriptions of each treatment component in Albano and colleagues' manuals for CBGT (Albano et al. 1991, Marten et al. 1991).

CBGT consists of four basic elements: (1) education about social phobia, (2) skills training, (3) practice, and (4) exposure. The goal of the program is to "teach each group member to minimize their social phobia and concomitant avoidance of social situations by learning to control and cope with anxiety which they experience" (Albano et al. 1991, p. 6). Treatment is composed of sixteen sessions divided into two eight-session phases. The first phase is focused on educating the participants about social phobia and conducting skills training. The second phase expands treatment to include in vivo exposure and practice. Sessions are 90 minutes in length and occur weekly. Assessment takes place at the beginning of each session, with group members completing self-report measures and individualized fear and avoidance hierarchy ratings. This is an important element of treatment as it allows clear tracking of progress or lack of progress. Group members also complete self-monitoring forms each week. These are reviewed at the beginning of each session.

During the first several sessions, group members are instructed in the cognitive-behavior model of social phobia. The three response domains associated with anxiety are emphasized so that members can effectively self-monitor their anxiety responses. The skills training component includes cognitive restructuring, social skills, and problem solving. These skills are taught via modeling, behavioral shaping, and role-playing. Practice of these skills is emphasized in each session during a snack time practice period and between sessions through homework assignments. During snack time practice, therapists model prosocial behavior and coping responses and during later sessions, clients practice specific social behaviors. Practice also occurs during the exposure phase of the program in which clients encounter specific situations drawn from their individual fear and avoidance hierarchies. Albano and colleagues emphasize the benefits of "double exposure" allowed in group sessions by having clients participate in role-plays for the exposure of other group members.

Albano and colleagues (1994) report preliminary evidence that CBGT is effective in treating social phobic adolescents. Five adolescents from 13–16 years of age completed the program. All were initially diagnosed via the ADIS-C/P with social phobia, generalized type, with four at very severe levels. Most had additional diagnoses of anxiety disorders including simple phobias and overanxious disorder. At 3-month follow-up, ADIS-C/P interviews by evaluators naive to pretest diagnoses revealed that the social phobias of four of the five had dropped to subclinical levels. By the 12-month follow-up, four clients were free of any mental disorder, suggesting that the effects of CBGT are durable and generalizable. As a group, these clients also showed dramatic reductions in subjective anxiety during two standardized BATs. The number of negative thoughts reported by clients during the BATs also decreased while neutral thoughts increased. Based on these results, this preliminary study strongly suggests that CBGT is as effective in treating social phobia among adolescents as it has been shown to be among adults. Albano and her colleagues are currently conducting a controlled clinical trial comparing CBGT to a waitlist control condition.

An innovative feature of Albano's program is the inclusion of clients' parents in some treatment sessions. Parents attend sessions one and two so they can be educated about the nature of anxiety and the development, maintenance, and treatment of social phobia. They are also instructed regarding their role as coaches who facilitate their adolescent's application of their new skills between sessions. They also attend the eighth session to review expectations and progress as well as to prepare for the exposure phase of treatment. Finally, parents attend the fifteenth session to discuss progress and the need for continued use of anxiety-management skills after termination. While promising, it remains to be seen whether the inclusion of parents contributes to increased effectiveness of CBGT with adolescents. In their controlled study, Albano and colleagues are currently evaluating this question.

The second group treatment program, developed by Beidel (1992), targets children with avoidant disorder. Beidel (1992) has reported promising preliminary results in case studies of three boys, ages 11–13 years. The initial version of this program was designed based on behavioral observations and social skills assessment of the participants. The boys were placed alone in a room together and observed from behind a one-way mirror. Beidel described the boys as showing significant anxiety merely being in the presence of the others. Therefore, relaxation training was included in the program to help reduce such anxiety. Second, social skills assessment revealed significant deficits in both verbal and nonverbal domains. Therefore, social skills training was also included in the treatment program. Finally, to increase the generalization of newly acquired social skills, the program included in vivo practice. Presumably, in vivo practice also served as an opportunity for exposure.

The program was composed of twelve weekly sessions. The first week was devoted to baseline assessment, followed by relaxation training during weeks two to four. Relaxation was taught in session and children were told to practice at least once daily between sessions using tape-recorded instructions. Weeks five to twelve were devoted to social skills training with one behavior selected each week. Children were trained in "verbal and non-verbal skills designed to promote social engagement." Verbal skills included introducing oneself, asking questions to maintain conversation, and ending conversations. Nonverbal skills included correcting inadequate eye contact and problems of voice (e.g., volume). Weeks seven to twelve also included in vivo practice. Children practiced in vivo only once they mastered skills in session. Practice took place in a museum where the client interacted with other children and adults.

Beidel (1992) reported that this program was generally effective at increasing number of social encounters and decreasing distress during them. For example, one child acquired a best friend for the first time. However, she noted that the relaxation component was only minimally effective and will not be included in future groups. Beidel also suggested that twelve sessions are probably insufficient for severe levels of avoidant disorder (i.e., a lifelong history of social avoidance). She based this conclusion on the most severely and chronically avoidant of her subjects, who made only minimal progress during the twelve-week program. In such cases, Beidel recommends the addition of an in vivo flooding component. The child in question went through an additional four months of flooding sessions and showed significant improvement. Like Albano and colleagues, Beidel also suggests that the inclusion of parents can enhance treatment outcome. The additional exposure sessions described above were carried out partly by the boy's father, who was taught to implement flooding following the basic twelve-week program.

DEALING WITH COMMON OBSTACLES TO SUCCESSFUL TREATMENT

Not surprisingly, given the focus of their anxiety disorder, some clients may resist participation in group-based treatments, fearing they will become too anxious in such a group. Hope and Heimberg (1993) recommend that any potential members who are so anxious that they are unlikely to be able to participate or process the information available in such a treatment should be treated individually. Such clients may become more open to the idea of group treatment after a period of individual treatment.

Comorbid conditions also may present serious obstacles to treatment. For example, Beidel (1992) reported that one of the three boys in her case study was also dysthymic. Because his dysthymia interfered with treatment, he was referred for pharmacotherapy. Beidel notes that behavioral interventions for OCD patients who are also depressed are ineffective until their depression is alleviated and suggests that the situation is similar for children with avoidant disorder. Like Beidel, Albano and her colleagues recommend that clients who have comorbid conditions that are more debilitating than their social phobia should not be treated via CBGT until these other problems have been treated first. For example, they note that it is not uncommon for adolescent social phobics to present with comorbid depression, and clients who are seriously depressed should be treated for their depression before participating in CBGT.

RELAPSE PREVENTION AND TERMINATION

The recovery of fear and the failure of treatment gains to generalize are especially troubling problems when treating social anxiety disorders. Clinically, it is all too common for children to overcome their fear of a specific social situation but remain severely anxious about most other social situations. Bouton (1991) has offered a contextual model of extension that leads to several approaches to increasing generalization and reducing the likelihood of recovery of fear. Bouton argues that fear conditioning generalizes much more easily than extinction of fear. Essentially, extinction makes the meaning of the conditioned stimulus (i.e., social contact) ambiguous and that this ambiguity is resolved largely by attending to contextual features. Thus, the social phobic learns that a small subset of people or situations are safe but all other people or situations may remain anxiety provoking. One implication of this view is that it is important to treat the child in all of the phobic social situations that the child is likely to encounter in the real world. Moreover, interventions that lead children to develop enhanced self-efficacy and coping skills ought to help immunize them against anxiety across contexts (Bouton 1991). Involving parents in treatment may also serve to prevent relapse. For example, Albano and colleagues specifically train parents to help their children continue to apply anxiety-management skills following termination.

CASE ILLUSTRATION (TYPICAL TREATMENT)

Description and History

Barbara was a 14-year-old girl whose social anxiety became a significant concern for her parents following her entry into high school. Her parents reported that she was falling behind in school because she was apparently afraid to ask her teachers for help. Furthermore, she did not join into social activities and seemed excessively shy. Assessment began with the ADIS-C and ADIS-P to gather detailed information about Barbara's anxiety and to screen for the presence of other problems. Based on the combined ADIS-C and ADIS-P, Barbara met criteria for social phobia, generalized type, with a severity rating of 6. CBCLs completed by each parent showed scores in the clinical range on the anxious/depressed and withdrawn scales. Furthermore, CBCL social competence scales suggested that Barbara had few friends and was involved in few social activities. Barbara completed a variety of self-report measures including the SASC-R, CBCL-YSR (Youth Self-Report), the Loneliness Questionnaire, and general measures of anxiety and depression. These provided further evidence that she was markedly anxious, socially withdrawn, lonely, and moderately depressed. Barbara's homeroom teacher also completed a CBCL that confirmed her anxiety and limited social involvement.

Barbara's social skills were assessed in a series of individualized role-play situations. For example, she was required to role-play a telephone call to a friend who was portrayed by her therapist. It quickly became apparent that Barbara exhibited serious deficits in both verbal and nonverbal social skills. She also appeared to be unfamiliar with many social situations and often seemed at a loss regarding how to proceed. She rarely asked questions, did not react with appropriate positive affect, and gave very brief responses to the questions of her partner.

When Barbara was told that treatment would require her to enter into social interactions, she began to deny that her social isolation was as big a problem as it had been. She frequently tried to convince her therapist that she had a number of girlfriends with whom she often talked in school. However, when pressed, she admitted that, since beginning high school, she had few social contacts with friends outside of school and rarely even talked with friends on the telephone. Additionally, checks with her parents confirmed that she rarely visited friends' homes or had friends visit hers and she rarely received or made phone calls. However, discussion with Barbara's teacher supported Barbara's claim that there were several girls with whom she interacted at school, though her teacher described her as taking a passive role in such interactions, rarely seeming to seek out social contacts.

Based on these assessment results, group treatment such as Albano and colleagues' CBGT would normally be the treatment of choice for a client like Barbara. Unfortunately, there were no other socially anxious children of appropriate age available at the time of Barbara's referral. Therefore, Barbara was treated individually. A female graduate student was chosen to be her therapist because formation of friendships with girls was the first goal of treatment and the skills associated with such relationships could be most effectively taught and modeled by a female therapist. Improving Barbara's skill level in telephone and face-to-face interactions was the first target of treatment, mainly through social skills training. Second, exposure-based practice of social skills was used to reduce her anxiety. Third, given that cognitive interventions appear to significantly enhance the effectiveness of social skills and exposure treatments for social anxiety, cognitive restructuring was included.

Synopsis of Therapy Sessions

Patterned after Albano and colleagues' CBGT, Barbara's treatment involved sixteen weekly one-hour sessions, divided into two phases. The first phase of treatment was devoted to psychoeducation, social skills training, and cognitive restructuring. During the first several sessions, Barbara was taught about the development, maintenance, and treatment of social phobia. Sessions one to four also emphasized social skills training via verbal description, modeling, and guided practice through role-playing. Cognitive restructuring and problem solving were emphasized during sessions five to eight. During these sessions, Barbara was taught to identify when she was thinking in distorted, anxiety-producing ways. For example, several cognitive distortions were encountered while discussing why Barbara did not get together with her friends outside of school.

Therapist: It sounds like there are some girls, Mary and Bobbi Jo, who you talk to a lot in school. When do you get to talk to them?

Barbara: Usually at lunch and we're in some of the same classes.

Therapist: Do you ever see them outside of school?

Barbara: Sometimes. Like we might get together at someone's house on the weekend.

Therapist: When was the last time you saw them outside of school?

Barbara: Well . . . Mary had a bunch of us sleep over for her birthday.

Therapist: When was that?

Barbara: Last year right before school let out.

Therapist: That was the last time? How come you haven't gotten together with Mary or the others since then?

Barbara: Well, its hard because we all live out in the country. We can't get together very easily. Our parents don't like to drive us around and it's too far to walk or bike.

Therapist: So Mary and Bobbi Jo don't get together much either?

Barbara: Well, I think they go to the mall together sometimes.

Therapist: Have you ever asked if you could go along?

Barbara: No. They asked me to a few times last year but I couldn't go. We usually visit my sister and her family on the weekend.

Therapist: Did you ever ask your parents if you could go with your friends some weekend?

Barbara: No, but I don't think they'd let me. They don't really know Mary or Bobbi Jo or their parents very well. They probably wouldn't like us being at the mall by ourselves.

Therapist: Sounds like this is a good example of a time when you need to examine the evidence. Right now you believe they wouldn't let you but you don't have any evidence for that belief. How could you get the evidence?

Barbara: I guess I need to ask them, but I know they won't let me. And even if they said I could, I'd have no way to get to the mall. My parents wouldn't drive me all that way.

Therapist: It sounds like you need to test that assumption too. But even if they wouldn't give you a ride, maybe you could ride with Mary or Bobby Jo. Do they ride together?

Barbara: I don't know, but their parents wouldn't want to drive all the way to my house to get me.

Therapist: Maybe not, but do you have any evidence?

Barbara: I guess not.

Therapist: We've talked about how a lot of social avoidance is often due to unrealistic or unfounded beliefs or expectations. We've found several that would be helpful to test out. Let's look for more. What do you think would happen if you ask Mary and Bobby Jo to go to the mall with you?

Barbara: I don't know. They'd probably make some excuse why they couldn't go that weekend.

Therapist: Why would they do that?

Barbara: Because they really wouldn't want me along. And it wouldn't be any fun even if I did go because I'd feel nervous the whole time.

Once identified, such beliefs were challenged repeatedly and Barbara was taught to replace such distortions with rational alternatives. With regard to the example, Barbara learned to recognize such thoughts and label them as catastrophizing. She further learned to challenge the validity of her assumptions and realized that she had little evidence to support her negative expectations. Lists of common cognitive distortions and adaptive alternatives that can be given to clients are provided by Albano and colleagues (1991). Barbara was encouraged to identify cognitive distortions during role-playing and to generate effective responses to dispute such thoughts. For example:

Therapist: Okay, you've learned some ways of challenging your negative expectations. Let's try them out. Last time we were talking about why you never get together with your friends outside of school. For example, you said you knew that your parents wouldn't give you a ride. Look at your list. How can you challenge that?

Barbara: What's the evidence? I haven't asked them in a long time so I don't really know.

Therapist: Very good! What's the worst thing that could happen if you ask?

Barbara: They could say no and yell at me.

Therapist: And if they did, would that be such a big deal? Would you be any worse off in the long run?

Barbara: Not really. Besides, maybe it isn't as likely as I think. Maybe they would take me, at least a few times.

Therapist: Maybe you already have some evidence that says they probably would take you. They brought you to the clinic because they're concerned about you, right? It seems to me that they've already shown that they'd like you to get more involved socially.

Barbara: I guess I hadn't thought about it like that.

Prior to the second phase of treatment, Barbara was helped to select several girls with whom she interacted at school and considered to be her friends. Once she demonstrated proficiency with social skills and cognitive restructuring during role-playing phone conversations, she began weekly homework assignments involving telephone conversations with these girls starting with the ninth session. Barbara consistently completed these homework assignments (confirmed by parent report), though she reported substantial anxiety during the early stages. Self-monitoring records showed that by the sixteenth session Barbara was averaging three telephone conversations per week. These included many that were initiated by her friends. Discussion of phone conversations made it clear that Barbara was discovering that many of her beliefs were erroneous. Self-monitoring records showed that the duration of these conversations and her enjoyment of them increased and anxiety decreased over the course of treatment.

Beginning with the twelfth session, Barbara's homework was expanded to include arranging visits at least once per week with friends (one at a time) outside of school. Barbara practiced using problem-solving techniques to decide what she and her friend could do together. Initially, she discounted many possibilities (e.g., going to the shopping mall together) because she anticipated obstacles (e.g., her parents wouldn't want to take them to the mall and pick them up later or her friend wouldn't want to do that). She was taught to challenge such assumptions and test them before giving up on her ideas. For example, her parents proved only too happy to arrange a trip to the mall provided they had sufficient advance notice. Barbara successfully completed two shopping trips and went to several movies prior to terminating treatment.

Following termination, Barbara's social anxiety was assessed using the battery completed at pretest. Barbara showed improvement on all measures. Based upon the ADIS, she continued to meet criteria for social phobia but at a subclinical level (severity rating of 3). She continued to report mild to moderate anxiety during social interactions, though she also stated that she expected she would become less anxious over time. She and her parents were encouraged to return for booster sessions as she felt necessary. Unfortunately, no follow-up information is available yet for Barbara.

Comments

Barbara's successful progress is representative of treatment with motivated and intelligent young people. Also, while serious, her social anxiety was not severe. Furthermore, though she lacked social skills and had a long history of shyness, her social anxiety had only recently reached serious levels. Other cases, such as the child described by Beidel, who have a lifelong history of generalized social avoidance, may present many challenges not faced with Barbara. For example, though it proved unnecessary in Barbara's case, it is often necessary to rearrange contingencies in the child's environment to support treatment compliance. Such children often strongly resist exposure to social interactions.

CASE ILLUSTRATION (OVERCOMING OBSTACLES)

Description and History

Cyril was a 12-year-old boy who was referred by his school counselor due to severe social withdrawal in school. The initial assessment battery was the same as described for Barbara. Both the ADIS-C and ADIS-P revealed that Cyril met criteria for social phobia, generalized type, at a severe level (severity rating = 7). According to his parents, Cyril had a lifelong history of shyness around unfamiliar people but he did have a small group of friends until his family had moved from out of state early in the previous school year. Cyril had difficulty adjusting to his new school and, when his problems persisted into the following school year, he was referred for services. He was initially seen several months into the new school year because he had made no friends and reacted with intense anxiety and tears when put in situations involving social evaluation (e.g., being asked a question in class). CBCLs completed by both parents showed clinical elevations on the anxious/depressed, withdrawn, and social problems scales. Also, the activities and social competence scales were in the clinical range, indicating that Cyril had no friends and was involved only in solitary activities (e.g., computer games and Lego blocks). Self-report questionnaires also provided evidence of Cyril's social anxiety, depression, withdrawal, and loneliness. Furthermore, the MESSY as completed by Cyril and one of his teachers showed low levels of appropriate social skills. The teacher's report also suggested that Cyril actively avoided most social contacts and showed severe anxiety in social-evaluative situations such as speaking in class. Consequently, she was careful to avoid putting him in such situations unless she was present to provide him with support. During a BAT in which he was to read a passage aloud in front of several graduate students, Cyril showed signs of intense anxiety but was able to complete the task.

Cyril's treatment was impeded by two main obstacles. First, in addition to social phobia, Cyril also met criteria for a diagnosis of dysthymia at the time of his referral. Although his dysthymia was only moderately severe (severity rating = 5), Cyril did exhibit a general malaise that could make it difficult to motivate him to participate in treatment. Furthermore, he showed the type of negative cognitive style that is characteristic of depression. As both Beidel (1991a) and Albano and colleagues (1994) point out, in such cases one must ask whether the child's depressed mood is severe enough that it should be treated prior to treating the social phobia. In Cyril's case, his dysthymia appeared to be less serious than and, to a large extent, secondary to his social phobia. Thus, it seemed unlikely to prevent effective treatment of his social phobia. However, it was serious enough that his chronic sadness and negative cognitive style would have to be addressed in treatment. This might be difficult in a group and might interfere with the treatment of other group members. However, in Cyril's case it seemed equally likely that the other group members might also benefit from treatment directed at depressogenic as well as anxiogenic cognitions. Thus, group treatment appeared to be an appropriate treatment choice despite Cyril's dysthymia.

The second obstacle to Cyril's treatment involved his strong resistance to the idea of group treatment when it was suggested following his pretreatment assessment. Because of his fearful reaction to the idea, Cyril's parents (Mr. and Mrs. P.) were concerned that he would not be able to endure the anxiety aroused by being in such a group. After discussing the issue with Cyril they contacted the author and asked that Cyril instead be treated individually. Such a response on the part of parents is common in the author's experience and parents often must be educated regarding the nature of social anxiety and the advantages of group treatment before they support their child's involvement. However, as Hope and Heimberg (1993) point out, clients who are likely to become intensely anxious in a group should probably be treated individually because they are unlikely to benefit from group treatment. Thus, the possibility that it would indeed be best to treat Cyril individually had to be considered. Pretreatment assessment can be used to determine whether a child is likely to be excessively anxious in the group setting. In Cyril's case, his performance in the BAT showed that, despite exhibiting significant anxiety, he was able to remain in the situation and complete the task. Similarly, Cyril's teacher reported that he was able to tolerate small group activities in school when she remained in the group and provided support. Based on such information, it seemed likely that Cyril could tolerate the group, since demands for participation would be low in early sessions and appropriate levels of adult support could be provided if necessary. Thus, the author met with Mr. and Mrs. P. to explain further the rationale for group treatment and to explain why Cyril seemed likely to be able to tolerate and benefit from group treatment. Discussion of this issue is illustrated briefly below:

> Mrs. P.: Cyril is so upset by the idea of being in the group. I just don't think he's ready for it yet.
>
> Mr. P.: I really think it would be better if he talked to somebody individually instead. I'm afraid that he's going to have a bad experience in the group and then he'll be so embarrassed that he won't be willing to come back.
>
> Therapist: I understand your concern. Many of the parents we see have similar concerns. It's understandable that you want to protect Cyril from a bad experience. But let me assure you that Cyril's nervousness is to be expected. All of the other group members will feel the same way. If given a choice, they would all avoid the group just like they avoid any other social situation. That's the only way they know how to cope with the anxiety those situations produce. But as long as they continue to avoid such situations, they can't learn other better ways to deal with them. They'll stay anxious. The best way for Cyril to learn to be more comfortable around other kids is to be around them. I think it's important that we give Cyril the clear message that we believe this will help and, with our support, that he can do it.

Had Mr. and Mrs. P. continued to express doubts about group treatment for Cyril it is probable that Cyril would have been treated individually instead. This would avoid the possibility that his parents would remove him from the group due to his complaints of anxiety and further reinforce such behavior. Such an event would also be disruptive to the group. However, Mr. and Mrs. P. agreed that perhaps they were too quick to protect Cyril from anxiety-provoking situations and they decided that he should attend the group. Cyril was then invited into the session and they were helped to explain this decision to him. They expressed confidence that he would be able to tolerate the group although he and the other kids in the group would be nervous to start with. The relationship between avoidance and continuing anxiety in social situations was explained to Cyril so that he could understand that his wish to avoid the group would help him be less nervous in the short term but would just make the problem persist in the long term. Finally, Cyril was given an opportunity to ask questions about the group. Once his parents expressed their support for group treatment, Cyril seemed to resign himself to attending.

Synopsis of Therapy Sessions

Cyril was treated in a group with three other 12- and 13-year-old boys who were also socially anxious. In general, the group was similar to the CBGT program of Albano and colleagues (1994). Two advanced graduate students (one male and one female) served as therapists. As in CBGT, treatment was focused on educating clients about factors that produce and maintain social anxiety and avoidance; training in social skills, problem-solving, and cognitive restructuring; and finally, in-session and homework-based in vivo exposure and practice.

During the first session, all four of the boys were visibly nervous but Cyril was perhaps the most anxious. To reduce the pressure on him, Cyril was the last child to be asked to introduce himself. Despite his nervousness, he was able to do so. He seemed surprised to find that other group members shared some of his interests. Similarly, when the group was asked to list situations that made them anxious, Cyril was able to contribute and seemed surprised that others shared his fears. At the end of the first session the therapists were careful to reinforce each member's participation. Cyril and the others all agreed that it hadn't been as bad as they had expected.

During session four, Cyril completed his first discussion of his automatic thoughts. During that discussion, it became apparent that Cyril's thoughts included a variety of depressogenic cognitive distortions as well as those more typical of social phobia. He was not only concerned about things that might go wrong, but also berated himself for his perceived failures and drew conclusions about his personal worth. For example:

Therapist 1: So your thought is something like, "I don't know why I'm even doing this. No one will want to talk to me even if I learn how."

Cyril: Yeah, nobody at school likes me anyway.

Therapist 1: And you think that means you're unlikable?

Cyril: Yeah.

Therapist 2: We've talked about the kind of thinking errors that lead us to feel anxious but other kinds of thoughts can make us feel other ways too . . . like sad. Let's treat your thought the same way we've looked at anxious thoughts. What questions can we ask that might help?

Cyril: You mean like, "What's the evidence?"

Therapist 2: Exactly! What's the evidence that you're unlikable?

Cyril: Nobody at school likes me.

Therapist 2: Do you know that for sure? Have you asked everyone in your class?

Cyril: Well, no, but nobody ever talks to me.

Therapist 2: I suspect that even that's an exaggeration. People probably talk to you more often than you realize. But let's assume it's true for the moment. Are there other explanations for the fact that nobody talks to you? Group, what do you think?

Member 1: [After some discussion] Maybe they don't try because they know it makes you uncomfortable.

Therapist 1: Very good! Does the teacher ever call on you in class? [The therapist knew that the teacher did not because she knew it made Cyril very anxious and he had cried in the past in such situations.]

Cyril: No.

Therapist 1: Would you say that's because she doesn't like you?

Cyril: I guess not. I get along with her pretty good. I guess she just doesn't want me to get upset.

Therapist 1: I've talked to her and I know that's why she doesn't call on you. So you can see that there may be other explanations for the fact that no one talks to you at school.

Cyril: Yeah, I guess so.

Cyril's negative cognitions continued to be the subject of discussion throughout therapy and other group members proved helpful in challenging their validity. Cyril gradually became able to label his depressogenic and anxiogenic automatic thoughts and successfully learned to apply adaptive alternative responses. Posttreatment assessment indicated that Cyril's dysthymia had been reduced to a subclinical level (severity rating = 2). Similarly, his social phobia, though still present, was considerably reduced (severity rating = 4).

Comments

Cyril's ability to benefit from group treatment despite his initial misgivings (and those of his parents) is typical in the author's experience. However, it is impossible to say whether Cyril and others like him might not make greater progress if treated individually. Perhaps it would be best to start treatment individually and move to the group setting as the child progresses. Such questions should be addressed in future treatment studies. Cyril's progress despite his comorbid diagnosis of dysthymia is also not unusual. However, had his dysthymia been more serious or had he presented with a serious major depressive disorder, it would probably have been best to treat Cyril individually or to reduce his depression prior to his entering group treatment.

SUMMARY

Social anxiety is a common and potentially serious problem in childhood and adolescence. Moreover, social anxiety disorders are common among children referred for anxiety problems. Yet only recently have such problems begun to receive the clinical and empirical attention they deserve. Recent years have seen substantial growth in the number and variety of means of assessing social anxiety and its related problems but much more work in this area is needed. More important still is the development of two promising group treatment programs for socially anxious young people. Social anxiety treatment studies such as those of Albano and Beidel and colleagues promise to dramatically expand our knowledge of effective treatment of social anxiety disorders in young people. Particularly if other groups follow the lead of these researchers, the remainder of this decade should prove rich indeed for those young people with such anxiety and for those who treat them.

REFERENCES

Achenbach, T. M. (1991a). *Manual for the Child Behavior Checklist/4-18 and 1991 Profile.* Burlington: University of Vermont Department of Psychiatry.

_____ (1991b). *Manual for the Youth Self-Report and 1991 Profile.* Burlington: University of Vermont Department of Psychiatry.

_____ (1991c). *Manual for the Teacher's Report Form and 1991 Profile.* Burlington: University of Vermont Department of Psychiatry.

Albano, A. M., and Barlow, D. A. (1993). Measurement of clinical change in the treatment of anxiety disorders of children and adolescents. In *The Development and Treatment of Anxiety Disorders in Childhood,* M. R. Dadds (Chair). Symposium conducted at the twenty-seventh annual meeting of the Association for the Advancement of Behavior Therapy, Atlanta, November.

Albano, A. M., Marten, P. A., Heimberg, R. G., and Barlow, D. A. (1994). Children and adolescents: assessment and treatment. Unpublished manuscript, State University of New York at Albany, Center for Stress and Anxiety Disorders, Child and Adolescent Anxiety Disorders Program.

Albano, A. M., Marten, P. A., and Holt, C. S. (1991). *Therapist's Manual for Cognitive-Behavioral Group Treatment of Adolescent Social Phobia.* State University of New York at Albany.

Anderson, J. C., Williams, S., McGee, R., and Silva, P. A. (1987). DSM-III disorders in preadolescent children. *Archives of General Psychiatry* 44:69–76.

Asher, S. R., Hymel, S., and Renshaw, P. D. (1984). Loneliness in children. *Child Development* 55:1456–1464.

Barabasz, A. F. (1973). Group desensitization of test anxiety in elementary school. *Journal of Psychology* 83:295–301.

Barlow, D. A. (1988). *Anxiety and Its Disorders: The Nature and Treatment of Anxiety and Panic.* New York: Guilford.

Beck, A. T., and Emery, G. (1985). *Anxiety Disorders and Phobias: A Cognitive Perspective.* New York: Basic Books.

Beidel, D. C. (1988). Psychophysiological assessment of anxious emotional states in children. *Journal of Abnormal Psychology* 97:80–82.

_____ (1989). Assessing anxious emotion: a review of psychophysiological assessment in children. *Clinical Psychology Review* 9:717–736.

_____ (1991a). Social phobia and overanxious disorder in school-age children. *Journal of the American Academy of Child and Adolescent Psychiatry* 30:545–552.

_____ (1991b). Determining the reliability of psychophysiological assessment in childhood anxiety. *Journal of Anxiety Disorders* 5:139–150.

_____ (1992). The behavioral treatment of avoidant disorder of childhood. In *Recent Advances in Cognitive-Behavioral Treatments of Childhood Anxiety Disorders,* A. M. Albano (Chair). Symposium conducted at the twenty-sixth annual meeting of the Association for the Advancement of Behavior Therapy, Boston, November.

Beidel, D. C., Neal, A. M., and Lederer, A. S. (1991). The feasibility and validity of a daily diary for the assessment of anxiety in children. *Behavior Therapy* 22:505-517.

Benjamin, R. S., Costello, E. J., and Warren, M. (1990). Anxiety disorder in a pediatric sample. *Journal of Anxiety Disorders* 4:293-316.

Berndt, T. J., and Perry, T. B. (1986). Children's perceptions of friendships as supportive relationships. *Developmental Psychology* 22:640-648.

Bornstein, M. R., Bellack, A. S., and Hersen, M. (1977). Social skills training for unassertive children: a multiple baseline analysis. *Journal of Applied Behavioral Analysis* 10:183-195.

Bouton, M. (1991). A contextual analysis of fear extinction. In *Handbook of Behavior Therapy and Psychological Science: An Integrative Approach,* ed. P. R. Martin, pp. 435-453. New York: Pergamon.

Christoff, K. A., Scott, W., Kelley, M. L., et al. (1985). Social skills and social problem-solving training for shy young adolescents. *Behavior Therapy* 16:468-477.

Craddock, C., Cotler, S., and Jason, L. A. (1978). Primary prevention: immunization of children for speech anxiety. *Cognitive Therapy and Research* 2:389-396.

Deffenbacher, J. L., and Kemper, C. C. (1974). Counseling test-anxious sixth graders. *Elementary School Guidance and Counseling* 9:22-29.

Diagnostic and Statistical Manual of Mental Disorders (1980). 3rd ed. Washington, DC: American Psychiatric Association.

_____ (1987). 3rd ed., revised. Washington, DC: American Psychiatric Association.

_____ (1994). 4th ed. Washington, DC: American Psychiatric Association.

Fox, J. E., and Houston, B. K. (1981). Efficacy of self-instructional training for reducing children's anxiety in an evaluative situation. *Behaviour Research and Therapy* 19:509-515.

Fox, J. E., Houston, B. K., and Pittner, M. S. (1983). Trait anxiety and children's cognitive behaviors in an evaluative situation. *Cognitive Therapy and Research* 7:149-154.

Francis, G., Last, C. G., and Strauss, C. C. (1992). Avoidant disorder and social phobia in children and adolescents. *Journal of the American Academy of Child and Adolescent Psychiatry* 31:1086-1089.

Harter, S. (1982). The Perceived Competence Scale for Children. *Child Development* 53:87-97.

_____ (1985). *Manual for the Self-Perception Profile for Children.* Denver: University of Denver.

Heimberg, R. G., and Barlow, D. A. (1991). New developments in cognitive-behavioral therapy for social phobia. *Journal of Clinical Psychiatry* 52(suppl):21-30.

Hope, D. A., and Heimberg, R. G. (1993). Social phobia and social anxiety. In *Clinical Handbook of Psychological Disorders: A Step-By-Step Treatment Manual,* ed. D. H. Barlow, pp. 99-136. New York: Guilford.

Hops, H., and Greenwood, C. R. (1988). Social skill deficits. In *Behavioral Assessment of Childhood Disorders,* ed. E. J. Mash and L. G. Terdal, 2nd ed., pp. 263-314. New York: Guilford.

Hops, H., Walker, H. M., and Greenwood, C. R. (1989). *Procedures for Establishing*

Effective Relationship Skills (PEERS): Manual for Consultants. Delray, FL: Educational Achievement Systems.

Houston, B. K., Fox, J. E., and Forbes, L. (1984). Trait anxiety and children's state anxiety, cognitive behaviors and performance under stress. *Cognitive Therapy and Research* 8:631–641.

Hymel, S., Franke, S., and Freigang, R. (1985). Peer relationships and their dysfunction: considering the child's perspective. *Journal of Social and Clinical Psychology* 3:405–415.

Inderbitzen-Pisaruk, H., Clark, M. L., and Solano, C. H. (1992). Correlates of loneliness in midadolescence. *Journal of Youth and Adolescence* 21:151–167.

Inderbitzen-Pisaruk, H. M., and Foster, S. L. (1990). Adolescent friendships and peer acceptance: implications for social skills training. *Clinical Psychology Review* 10:425–439.

Inderbitzen, H. M., and Foster, S. L. (1992). The Teenage Inventory of Social Skills: development, reliability, and validity. *Psychological Assessment* 4:451–459.

Johnson, R. L., and Glass, C. R. (1989). Heterosocial anxiety and direction of attention in high school boys. *Cognitive Therapy and Research* 13:509–526.

Kandel, H. J., Ayllon, T., and Rosenbaum, M. S. (1977). Flooding or systematic exposure in the treatment of extreme social withdrawal in children. *Journal of Behavior Therapy and Experimental Psychiatry* 8:75–81.

Kashani, J. H., and Orvaschel, H. (1990). A community study of anxiety in children and adolescents. *American Journal of Psychiatry* 147:313–318.

Kazdin, A. E. (1983). Psychiatric diagnosis, dimension of dysfunction, and child behavior therapy. *Behavior Therapy* 14:73–99.

Kearney, C. A., and Silverman, W. K. (1990). A preliminary analysis of a functional model of assessment and treatment for school refusal behavior. *Behavior Modification* 14:340–366.

Kendall, P. C. (1991). Guiding theory for child and adolescent therapy. In *Child and Adolescent Therapy: Cognitive-Behavioral Procedures*, ed. P. C. Kendall, pp. 3–22. New York: Guilford.

Kendall, P. C., and Chansky, T. E. (1991). Considering cognition in anxiety-disordered children. *Journal of Anxiety Disorders* 5:167–185.

Kendall, P. C., and Ronan, K. (1990). Assessment of children's anxieties, fears, and phobias: cognitive-behavioral models and methods. In *Handbook of Psychological and Educational Assessment of Children*, ed. C. R. Reynolds and R. W. Kamphaus, pp. 223–244. New York: Guilford.

King, N. J. (1993). Simple and social phobias. In *Advances in Clinical Child Psychology*, vol. 15, ed. T. H. Ollendick and R. J. Prinz, pp. 305–341. New York: Plenum.

Kondas, O. (1967). Reduction of examination anxiety and 'stage fright' by group desensitization and relaxation. *Behaviour Research and Therapy* 5:275–281.

La Greca, A. M., Dandes, S. K., Wick, P., et al. (1988). Development of the Social Anxiety Scale for Children: reliability and concurrent validity. *Journal of Clinical Child Psychology* 17:84–91.

La Greca, A. M., and Stone, W. L. (1993). Social Anxiety Scale for Children-Revised:

factor structure and concurrent validity. *Journal of Clinical Child Psychology* 22:17–27.

Last, C. G., Strauss, C. C., and Francis, G. (1987). Comorbidity among childhood anxiety disorders. *Journal of Nervous and Mental Disease* 175:726–730.

Laxer, R. M., Quarter, J., Kooman, A., and Walker, K. (1969). Systematic desensitization and relaxation of high test-anxious secondary school students. *Journal of Counseling Psychology* 16:446–451.

Leal, L. L., Baxter, E. G., Martin, J., and Marx, R. W. (1981). Cognitive modification and systematic desensitization with test anxious high school students. *Journal of Counseling Psychology* 28:525–528.

Mann, J., and Rosenthal, T. L. (1969). Vicarious and direct counterconditioning of test anxiety through individual and group desensitization. *Behaviour Research and Therapy* 7:359–367.

Marten, P. A., Albano, A. M., and Holt, C. S. (1991). *Therapist's Manual for Cognitive-Behavioral Group Treatment of Adolescent Social Phobia with Parent Participation.* State University of New York at Albany.

Matson, J. L., Rotatori, A. F., and Helsel, W. J. (1983). Development of a rating scale to measure social skills in children: the Matson Evaluation of Social Skills with Youngsters (MESSY). *Behaviour Research and Therapy* 21:335–340.

Mattick, R. P., Peters, L., and Clarke, J. C. (1989). Exposure and cognitive restructuring for social phobia: a controlled study. *Behaviour Therapy* 20:3–23.

McGee, R., Feehan, M., Williams, S., et al. (1990). *DSM-III* disorders in a large sample of adolescents. *Journal of the American Academy of Child and Adolescent Psychiatry* 29:611–619.

Ollendick, T. H., Matson, J. L., and Helsel, W. J. (1985). Fears in children and adolescents: normative data. *Behaviour Research and Therapy* 23:465–467.

Orton, G. L. (1982). A comparative study of children's worries. *Journal of Psychology* 110:153–162.

Patterson, G. R., Reid, J. B., and Dishion, T. J. (1992). *Antisocial Boys.* Eugene, OR: Castalia.

Prins, P. (1986). Children's self-speech and self-regulation during a fear-provoking behavioral test. *Behaviour Research and Therapy* 24:181–191.

Prins, P., Groot, M., and Hanewald, G. (1994). Cognitions in test-anxious children: the role of on-task and coping cognitions reconsidered. *Journal of Consulting and Clinical Psychology* 62:404–409.

Reynolds, C. R., and Richmond, B. O. (1978). What I think and feel: a revised measure of children's manifest anxiety. *Journal of Abnormal Child Psychology* 6:271–280.

Ross, D. M., Ross, S. A., and Evans, T. A. (1971). The modification of extreme social withdrawal by modeling with guided participation. *Journal of Behavior Therapy and Experimental Psychiatry* 2:273–279.

Russel, D., Peplau, L. A., and Cutrona, C. (1980). The revised UCLA Loneliness Scale: Concurrent and discriminant validity evidence. *Journal of Personality and Social Psychology* 39:472–480.

Silverman, W. K. (1991). Diagnostic reliability of anxiety disorders in children using structured interviews. *Journal of Anxiety Disorders* 5:105–124.

Silverman, W. K., and Eisen, A. R. (1992). Age differences in the reliability of parent and child reports of child anxious symptomatology using a structured interview. *Journal of the American Academy of Child and Adolescent Psychiatry* 31:117–124.

_____ (1993). Overanxious disorder in children. In *Handbook of Behavior Therapy with Children and Adults: A Developmental and Longitudinal Perspective*, ed. R. T. Ammerman and M. Hersen. New York: Allyn and Bacon.

Silverman, W. K., and Nelles, W. B. (1988). The Anxiety Disorders Interview Schedule for Children. *Journal of the American Academy of Child and Adolescent Psychiatry* 27:772–778.

Stevens, R., and Phil, R. O. (1983). Learning to cope with school: a study of the effects of a coping skill training program with test-vulnerable 7th-grade students. *Cognitive Therapy and Research* 7:155–158.

Strauss, C. C. (1993). Developmental differences in the expression of anxiety disorders in children and adolescents. In *Anxiety across the Lifespan: A Developmental Perspective*, ed. C. G. Last, pp. 63–77. New York: Springer.

Strauss, C. C., Lahey, B. B., Frick, P., et al. (1988). Peer social status of children with anxiety disorders. *Journal of Consulting and Clinical Psychology* 56:137–141.

Strauss, C. C., Lease, C. A., Kazdin, A. E., et al. (1989). Multimethod assessment of the social competence of children with anxiety disorders. *Journal of Clinical Child Psychology* 18:184–189.

Thyer, B. A., Parrish, R. T., Curtis, G. C., et al. (1985). Ages of onset of *DSM-III* anxiety disorders. *Comprehensive Psychiatry* 26:113–122.

Trower, P., Yardley, K., Bryant, B., et al. (1978). The treatment of social failure: a comparison of anxiety-reduction and skills acquisition procedures on two social problems. *Behavior Modification* 2:41–60.

Vasey, M. W., Crnic, K. A., and Carter, W. G. (in press). Worry in childhood: a developmental perspective. *Cognitive Therapy and Research.*

Vernberg, E. M., Abwender, D. A., Ewell, K. K., and Beery, S. H. (1992). Social anxiety and peer relationships in early adolescence: a prospective analysis. *Journal of Clinical Child Psychology* 21:189–196.

Watson, D., and Friend, R. (1969). Measurement of social-evaluative anxiety. *Journal of Consulting and Clinical Psychology* 33:448–457.

Weinrott, M. R., Reid, J. B., Bauske, B. W., and Brummett, B. (1981). Supplementing naturalistic observations with observer impressions. *Behavioral Assessment* 3:151–159.

Wigfield, A., and Eccles, J. S. (1990). Test anxiety in the school setting. In *Handbook of Developmental Psychopathology*, ed. M. Lewis and S. M. Miller, pp. 237–250. New York: Plenum.

Zatz, S., and Chassin, L. (1983). Cognitions of test-anxious children. *Journal of Consulting and Clinical Psychology* 51:526–534.

_____ (1985). Cognitions of test-anxious children under naturalistic test-taking conditions. *Journal of Consulting and Clinical Psychology* 53:393–401.

6

ELECTIVE MUTISM

Sander M. Weckstein
David D. Krohn
Harold L. Wright

DESCRIPTION OF DISORDER

Mutism as a presenting clinical symptom in children can be due to several different psychiatric and neurological disorders (Rutter 1977). Elective mutism represents a specific clinical syndrome initially described by Kussmaul in 1877 and named by Tramer in 1934. In this chapter we will describe in detail a treatment approach developed at Hawthorn Center. Elective mutism is a relatively rare and particularly treatment-resistant condition in which children with normal verbal capabilities refuse to speak with people outside the family in most or all unfamiliar social situations, particularly on beginning school. Prevalence rates of 0.3 to 0.8 per 1,000 have been reported (Brown and Lloyd 1975, Fundudis et al. 1979). Although *DSM-IV* (American Psychiatric Association 1994) requires a one-month symptom duration to make the diagnosis, some authors have argued that this diagnosis should be made only in the presence of mutism of at least six months' duration (Kolvin and Fundudis 1981, Wilkins 1985) due to the high rate of transient mutism found in children upon entering school (Brown and Lloyd 1975).

Most authors have reported the electively mute child to be negativistic, oppositional, controlling and manipulative (Browne et al. 1963, Hayden 1980, Kolvin and Fundudis 1981, Krohn et al. 1992, Parker et al. 1960, Wergeland 1979, Wilkins 1985, Wright 1968). They are also described as shy and anxious in public; however, they may be either shy or outgoing around familiar people (Kolvin and Fundudis 1981, Parker et al. 1960, Wright 1968).

The relationship between the mother and child is often described as symbiotic, with the mother overprotecting and overindulging the child (Browne et al. 1963, Hayden 1980, Parker et al. 1960, Wilkins 1985, Wright 1968). Hayden (1980) reported her observation that the mothers appeared jealous of the child's interactions with others. The marital relationship is usually described as conflictual, with the father often uninvolved, and it is hypothesized that this is the reason the mother turns to the child (Browne et al 1963, Parker et al. 1960, Wergeland 1979). Nevertheless, the only two controlled studies have not found family discord to be higher in these families as compared to families of other emotionally disturbed children (Kolvin and Fundudis 1981; Wilkins 1985). Some authors have commented on a general lack of family communication (Hayden 1980, Parker et al 1960). Several authors have noted a general family shyness, history of shyness in the parents, or elevated levels of anxiety in the parents (Hayden 1980, Kolvin and Fundudis 1981, Parker et al. 1960, Wergeland 1979, Wright 1968).

Six studies reporting treatment results for more than ten cases are available in the literature. Browne et al. (1963), reporting ten cases, and Wergeland (1979), reporting eleven, described using a primarily psychodynamic approach and found the treatment long and difficult with a generally poor outcome. Parker et al. (1960), using a treatment approach that involved individual therapy, family work, and school consultation, reported that all twenty-seven of the elective mutes treated in their sample spoke within two years of beginning treatment. Their admission criteria, however, did not control for length of mutism, and success was defined only as "some use of speech" in the classroom. Kolvin and Fundudis's (1981) study of twenty-four electively mute children described 46 percent showing marked to moderate improvement and 54 percent slight to no improvement. The duration of mutism and the treatment technique were not clearly described.

Wright's original (1968) report on nineteen patients found 79 percent to have an excellent or good outcome, whereas 21 percent had a fair to poor outcome (including one schizophrenic). A later additional study of twenty strictly diagnosed elective mutes using the Hawthorn Center approach found a similar high treatment success rate with eighteen (90 percent) having an excellent outcome and two (10 percent) a fair outcome (Krohn et al. 1992).

There are also no larger studies on behavioral therapy of elective mutism, although many of the more recent articles propose this approach (Wright et al. 1985). Behavioral therapy techniques to treat elective mutism are well described (Labbe and Williamson 1984, Sanok and Ascione 1979, Sanok and Striefels 1979). There has been very little written on possible pharmacological interventions in the treatment of elective mutism. One successful case report of the use of Prozac has been reported (Black and Uhde 1992).

DIFFERENTIAL DIAGNOSIS

There has been some disagreement in the field as to whether elective mutism is an anxiety disorder, a specific developmental delay, or part of an oppositional defiant disorder. Previous experience by the present authors suggests that elective mutism is a symptom that must be understood in the context of each individual case history. Any of a number of factors may predispose the child to developing mutism, but the syndrome of elective mutism represents a final common behavioral pathway that develops when mutism becomes entrenched because of the gratification (secondary gain) it brings the child. These children are often anxious when forced to speak, but their anxiety is not pervasive. They are not typically shy or anxious when playing or interacting in other ways, even when being observed, but appear more controlling and oppositional.

Many disorders can also coexist with or present in a manner similar to elective mutism. The evaluator must be cognizant of the nonspecific nature of mutism as a presenting symptom and use the presence or absence of other associated symptoms to rule out possible affective spectrum disorder, anxiety disorder (specifically PTSD and social phobia), speech and language disorder, oppositional-defiant disorder, or psychoses. If the history is suggestive of a diagnosis of elective mutism, the child is nonverbal and does not participate, and other major psychiatric disorders do not appear to be present, a diagnosis of elective mutism can be made.

ASSESSMENT PROCEDURES

A thorough evaluation is the first part of the treatment process. This includes obtaining a complete social history of the child from parents or primary caretakers including the onset, duration, precipitants, and a detailed understanding of the presentation itself as it occurs in different settings (i.e., home, school, and community). A history of the previous interventions or treatments and their results needs to be obtained. In addition, a developmental and medical history should be taken with specific emphasis on possible early speech and language problems or significant physical traumas to the mouth or other areas. A detailed history of the child's motor, language, and social development should also be obtained.

A family history including information about family constellation, relationships, and how the child's mutism is perceived and reacted to by the family is extremely important. It is also useful to ask whether there is a history of elective mutism or use of selective speech in any family members. Information about the current and past stability of the marital relationship should also be obtained. Finally, questions about a family history of psychiatric illness including depression, anxiety disorders, psychosis, and other mental disabilities should be elicited. Observing the child in free play or the family and child interacting in the waiting room is often very useful.

The clinical interview of the child is one of the most important parts of the evaluation process. The interviewer must be extremely cognizant of the child's appearance, cooperativeness, relatedness, and ability to separate from specific family members. If the child is uncooperative and not verbally interactive (as elective mutes often are at first), the interviewer should obtain information nonetheless by attempting to use nonverbal communication through play or art. It is important from the first session to attempt to build a therapeutic alliance, by facilitating interaction between the child and interviewer.

How then can this child, who has been so firmly entrenched in his symptom of silence (a symptom that both controls others and keeps others at a distance) be approached? The child must be drawn into the evaluation and subsequent therapy through play, interpretation, and a pragmatic explanation of the need to give up the symptom so he can make friends and learn. The therapist must be creative in gaining the child's interest and participation. The use of puppets, magic tricks, drawing, playful nonverbal communication such as imitating the child's posture and stance, and supportive interpretation of his feelings can be very useful.

Psychological testing including assessing intellectual functioning, academic achievement, and relevant dynamics is often used as one part of a comprehensive evaluation. However, since when first seen these children are often nonverbal and refuse to participate, more formal psychological testing often must be postponed until later in treatment.

ESTABLISHING TREATMENT GOALS

Helping the child, school, and family extricate themselves from the child's mutism is the main focus of treatment. This usually requires individual therapy for the child, family therapy, and school consultation, initially on at least a weekly basis. The treatment approach can be broadly broken down into nine different stages, all of which must be accomplished for treatment to be successful. These stages should be seen as flexible and they often overlap. They are (1) explaining the proposed technique to the child, family, and school, and acquiring their support of the treatment approach; (2) establishing rapport with the child; (3) the child speaking in response to the setting of the first verbal expectation in a session; (4) generalizing verbal production within the therapy session; (5) continuing exploration of the symptoms and their meaning; (6) generalizing positive verbal and nonverbal behaviors in the school setting simultaneous with generalizing in the community through parental involvement; (7) continuing reinforcement of the child's verbal activities and facilitating of an increased sense of mastery; (8) treating related problems of elective mutism once the symptom remits; and (9) gradually terminating treatment.

ROLE OF THE THERAPIST

The role of the therapist in this approach is a difficult one involving a combination of empathic striving to form an alliance with the child and firm limit setting. It is important to be cognizant of the therapist's possible reactions concerning this approach to the treatment of elective mutism. When faced with treating one of these nonverbal children who can be seen as pathetic, controlling, oppositional, frustrating, overwhelming, anxious, awe-inspiring, depressed, or angry, the therapist must be aware of his evoked feelings. These may run the gamut from anger to helplessness. The therapist must use his own feelings as an ally to help him interpret to the child what it must feel like to be silent, be it frightened or angry, controlling or passive. This helps the child realize that someone is trying to understand his predicament and will do something to help. The therapist must be comfortable with the feelings the child evokes in him as he sets a firm, but appropriate, limit while the child may be crying, whining, standing rigidly in the corner, or trying to escape. Those who come from a more analytic or nonstructured therapeutic background may be uncomfortable with this technique. It has been our experience at Hawthorn Center, using this approach with numerous children, that it is usually effective. This treatment technique does not cause the symptoms of elective mutism to be replaced by others, and will not be harmful to the child when it is carried out by an empathetic therapist with a clear understanding of the symptom, treatment technique, and child development. In fact, the children report and manifest much relief when their symptom is removed. As we previously mentioned, this technique is designed to facilitate ego growth and mastery for those children who are developmentally arrested by their symptom and cannot find a way to extricate themselves from their situation.

TREATMENT STRATEGIES

The first stage of treatment consists of explaining the proposed techniques to the family and actively acquiring the family's assistance in such a way that the family is not threatened. It is further necessary to have the family's assistance in not condoning the child's silence. The therapist's role in this phase of treatment is supportive and psychoeducational. Elective mutism is explained as an extremely detrimental symptom that can seriously impede normal development and, therefore, requires prompt intervention so the child can successfully make friends, progress appropriately in school, and not feel badly about himself because he cannot do what other children are doing. This phase of treatment is usually completed within the first two sessions.

Once the family gives support for the treatment, the therapist must attempt to establish rapport with the child by demonstrating concern and understanding of the child's emotional distress and need for his symptom as well as show the child the importance of giving up his symptom. This is crucial to the ultimate success of the treatment. It is this approach, which combines an insistence that the child give up his silence with the message that the therapist will stick with the child, that provides the basis for sustained progress in treatment. Each therapist has his own style of relating to the child, but this needs to be done in a fairly short period of time over the first two or three sessions with the child. Though one might be tempted to continue this phase of the treatment for a much longer period of time, it is important to let the child know that the therapist (unlike previous adults and children) will not be controlled by the child's symptom and accept continued silence, but will instead help the child to extricate him- or herself.

After rapport has been established, the therapist supportively but firmly conveys to the child that he will be expected to talk in the near future. The child is told that while the therapist understands talking to people outside of the family is difficult, it is something that is necessary. Further, the child is told that there will come a time in the near future (the next one to two sessions) at which the child will be expected to say at least one word before leaving the session. The therapist directly states to the child that he will stay with the child as long as is necessary to accomplish this task. The idea that once he talks he will feel better about himself, that the first few words are the hardest, as well as the fact that it will be more fun for him when he can talk and play like other children, is empathically explained and repeatedly highlighted to the child.

To accomplish the step of setting the first verbal expectation the therapist must schedule a day when he can spend enough time with the child to accomplish the first verbal task of saying at least one word to the therapist. In the majority of cases the session where the verbal expectation is set should occur by the third or fourth session with the child. The therapist should anticipate spending an extended period of time with the child and plan to have food and paperwork available and the resolve to carry through to the goal. Throughout the session the therapist periodically discusses the expectation that in order to end the session the child must say at least one word. The therapist alternates between being supportive, interpreting the child's feelings, attempting to engage the child in play, and seemingly ignoring the child at times. The times when the therapist seemingly ignores the child serve the purpose of allowing the child to go at his own pace, as well as clearly conveying to the child that the therapist will maintain a firm limit and not be controlled by the mutism.

After the child is verbal, the child is praised for his ability to master the situation, is told that he will continue to feel better about himself as he talks more, and is told he will be expected to be increasingly verbal at the next session. Then the child is taken back to his family, who have been instructed to praise the child's accomplishment.

The next stage of treatment consists of attempting to increase the child's verbalizations within the therapy framework while continuing to build a therapeutic alliance. This should be done in such a way that it is enjoyable for the child. It is often helpful to have the child bring in familiar objects, toys, or pictures. The child is encouraged to continue to be verbal by making a verbal response necessary for any activity that the child chooses. In some children this is not necessary, as they talk to the therapist in session fairly normally after they have completed the first verbal hurdle. Further, many children enjoy reading, naming colors or body parts, or talking about pictures that they have brought. We have found it important at this point to ask the child to do only things that he is capable of doing and has done before with family members. As stated before, the sense of mastery and enhancement of self-esteem that the child receives by being increasingly verbal in these ways with a therapist is tremendously reinforcing to the continued use of speech. Nevertheless, the therapist should use praise as well as other tangible reinforcers as needed.

The next phase consists of further exploration of the symptom by using play therapy techniques to help the child gain insight into his fears, fantasies, and concerns. The specific areas that need to be addressed in therapy vary significantly from child to child depending on what treatment discloses as the conflicts that led the child to develop the symptom of elective mutism. Often issues of anger, low self-esteem, passive aggressiveness, and oppositional behavior arise and are dealt with as the treatment continues. As the symptom remits, the child's developmental growth continues and tends to proceed along appropriate developmental lines. The child is happier, feels better about himself, and his anxiety and feelings of inferiority are replaced by feelings of mastery and a sense of self-worth.

The next phase of therapy involves generalization of verbal and nonverbal mastery to the school setting. This phase is begun after a strong therapeutic alliance has been formed and the child is comfortably speaking with the therapist. This can usually be accomplished between two weeks and three months from beginning therapy.

This phase requires the teacher's time and effort and, thus, a good working relationship with the teacher and the school is necessary for success. Shortly after treatment begins, it is important to contact, with parental approval, the child's principal, teacher, and school social worker to develop a dialogue and working relationship with the school staff who will be involved with the child's treatment. Often the school is the source of the referral and will contact the therapist with questions after the initial evaluation. It is helpful to briefly explain your treatment plan to those involved and then suggest to them that in the near future you will be contacting them to enlist their aid in the transfer of the child's verbal ability from the therapy to the school setting.

In preparing the child for this next step, the therapist must focus on the child's newfound verbal industry and self-mastery and side with the child's desire to "talk" and "be like other kids" or "show how smart he is." Further, the child's previous verbal accomplishments in therapy are highlighted and praised. The child's anxieties should be explored and addressed by suggesting that after the child becomes verbal in the school setting, he will feel better about himself, just as he does now in therapy. Then, a specific verbal task should be selected, practiced, and mastered. This may include reading a particular story or naming particular colors or body parts. This task should be repeatedly practiced in the sessions with much positive reinforcement.

Desensitization through role-playing and imagining what it might be like to talk in the school setting can also be very helpful for the child. If the child's ambivalence is expressed through oppositional behavior and refusal, it should be addressed. A pragmatic explanation of why speaking is important, for example, "If you don't speak, the teacher cannot know how smart you are," can be given to the child. At the same time, positive reinforcers of tangible gifts, "I have a secret, special surprise waiting for you when you talk," the family's pride in the child's verbal accomplishments, and the fact that he will feel better about himself can be used.

The next step is to set a day on which the child is expected to speak in school. This is done with the collaboration of school personnel, and the specific details of the process are explained so that the teacher and other staff are able to participate fully.

The child is first given the opportunity to perform the preselected verbal task alone with the teacher. If this is unsuccessful after a few tries, the therapist should consider going to the school to help facilitate the generalization of verbal behaviors to the teacher.

After the child has begun speaking to the teacher alone, the teacher should continue to meet with the child individually on a daily basis for a period of time. The therapist then helps the teacher to generalize the child's verbal behaviors to the rest of the class, using both positive and negative reinforcement. However, as time goes on the reinforcement of being able to speak again, to socialize with peers and teachers, and the rewards of self-mastery should take the place of tangible rewards. Finally, after the child is comfortable with the selected teacher, that teacher may further generalize the child's verbal abilities in school to other teachers using the above described techniques.

Once the child is comfortable in being verbal in the therapy setting and is working on being verbal in the school setting, it is time to further the generalization of the child's verbal behavior in the community through the family. It is important at this time to attempt to explore and understand the child's symptom choice and the dynamics behind it in the family setting. Often, with elective mutism, there is some overenmeshment of the family. In addition, family members may be perpetuating the symptom. Therapeutic work with the family is directed at helping them recognize and acknowledge their symptom-perpetuating behaviors, thus developing a collective observing ego. Further, it is often important to counsel parents on techniques of firm and appropriate limit setting.

At this phase in the treatment a reassessment is indicated. One should determine whether additional interventions are needed such as intensive family therapy or referral of other family members for individual treatment, or whether the treatment of the child and limited family work is sufficient to deal with the specific problems. Further, during this part of therapy, the therapist should continue to explore the child's symptom in individual therapy. He should also reinforce the child's gains, his industry, and his self-mastery through play and verbal means.

DEALING WITH COMMON OBSTACLES TO SUCCESSFUL TREATMENT

One of the common challenges to the successful treatment of elective mutism is maintaining an alliance with the family throughout the treatment. The therapist should anticipate the possibility of a family stopping treatment if the child appears unhappy or angry, because these parents have usually been controlled by the child previously. This issue should be anticipated and addressed by explaining to the parents that during the treatment there may well be times when the child seems unhappy and angry and will not want to come to the sessions. Their child may direct his anger at them in such a way as to make them feel guilty or uncomfortable, but it is important to continue treatment, even if they are uncomfortable with this technique. Parents are told that other parents have felt this way in the past, but with continued treatment, their children improved. It is reiterated that they are the most important people in their child's life and their continued participation in the treatment is paramount. Often families may be noncompliant to treatment suggestions and this must be gently pointed out as evidence of their ambivalence and the issue addressed. Further, introducing techniques of using concrete props such as star charts, lists, or worksheets can be useful. It is important to involve all family members in treatment. If one or another parent is more distant (often the father in elective mute families), he or she should be encouraged to join in the treatment.

We have found that some mothers of elective mutes encourage, covertly or overtly, their child's mutism because of their need to keep the child dependent, often because of their own unresolved dependency needs or dissatisfaction in the marriage (Krohn et al. 1992). This must be evaluated and approached in a sensitive manner. It is important to highlight the child's gains to the family members as well as to give the family members much of the credit for these gains while at the same time discussing the family members' ambivalence about the child's increasing mastery and decreased dependence.

The most difficult part of this treatment (for the therapist as much or more than the child) is the session in which the verbal expectation is set. Children with elective mutism have often had years of practice in bringing family members, teachers, principals, and often therapists to their knees over the issue of mutism. The child's own ambivalence about this symptom and the negative effect it has on a child's development must always be remembered.

It is very important not to allow the child to leave the session in which the limit is set without talking unless both the child and the therapist are both physically and emotionally exhausted. At times, in very difficult cases, it has been useful to tell the child that it is not fair to keep his mother or family waiting any longer. He is told that the family will be sent home and will return later in the day when the child is verbal. This serves to raise the child's anxiety and show that the family will no longer be controlled by the child's mutism. If the child is verbal in any manner (whiny or whispered words), the therapist may choose to accept and reinforce this response with the understanding that next time it must be more audible, or continue to wait for a more audible response.

RELAPSE PREVENTION

Children treated with the Hawthorn Center approach have had a very low rate of relapse. This is in large part due to the work done with the families of the children. The families' commitment to encouraging and reinforcing their child's verbal participation in all settings by establishing appropriate and firm limits when needed is crucial to treatment and to prevention of relapse. During the active phase of the treatment, the families work through the conflicts and understand the dynamics of the role that they usually have played in their child's mutism. The understanding and confidence they have gained and the commitment they have to their child's continued healthy growth and development, which they come to realize requires appropriate speech, allows them to follow through with the treatment plan as described and not fall back into the pattern of giving in to their child's mutism. Along with this, the understanding and commitment of school personnel in requiring the child's verbal participation in the school setting is important. Finally, the child's newfound abilities of being able to speak freely and to socialize with family, peers, and others is tremendously reinforcing. As the child's verbal abilities increase, the child develops an increased sense of mastery over himself and the world around him. This sense of mastery serves to further perpetuate the child's continued growth.

TERMINATION

When the child is functioning at a developmentally appropriate level and his symptoms have resolved, it is time for a gradual termination of treatment. The time between the child's appointments is slowly increased in length, depending on the child's needs, over a 2- to 6-month period of time. A gradual termination allows the child to slowly break the strong bond with the therapist that often develops during the treatment. The issues of loss precipitated by the planned termination of therapy must be approached and worked through before treatment can be successfully ended. The child should be told that he may return to therapy even after termination if ever he feels the need.

During the termination phase, the child may show some regression, such as a recurrence of controlling behaviors. Working with the family or school to set appropriate limits and discussing feelings and fears about control with the child will usually resolve these behaviors.

CASE ILLUSTRATION (TYPICAL TREATMENT)

Description and History

Jonathan was a 7-year-old first grader when initially seen. He had not spoken for the first four months of first grade, had spoken only a few words in the first month of kindergarten before refusing to speak, and had not spoken in day care, which he attended for a year prior to attending kindergarten. His mother said that she was surprised when he began not speaking in school as he was quite animated and outgoing at home and with the family. She did state that he was extremely reluctant to talk in public but that she had thought that this was normal for his age. She said that she was initially not bothered by his mutism and was seeking the evaluation at the teacher's request. Jonathan was described as having no other emotional or behavioral difficulties but as being a somewhat strong-willed and stubborn child.

Jonathan's developmental and medical history were unremarkable. Language milestones were recalled as being normal. Jonathan lived at home with his mother and an older brother. Jonathan's father had left the family somewhat suddenly when Jonathan was 3 years of age. He had little contact with the family after leaving the home.

Jonathan's family history was also unremarkable. There was no family history of mental illness. Jonathan's mother recalled that she herself had been somewhat quiet in school and that it was hard for her to speak in the early grades.

Synopsis of Therapy Sessions

When seen for the initial evaluation, Jonathan refused to speak to the evaluator, although he was observed to speak quietly with his mother in the waiting room. The evaluator was, however, able to initiate animated and interactive play using puppets and allowing him to shoot basketball in the room. His play was very logical and coherent and he appropriately followed the nonverbal social cues of the examiner. The results of Jonathan's evaluation were discussed with his mother.

> Therapist: After going over the information you presented to us and having a chance to spend some time with Jonathan, I feel Jonathan has a problem called elective mutism.
>
> Mother: That's what the teacher said when she said I should call you, but I still don't understand what elective mutism is.
>
> Therapist: Elective mutism is a problem in which a child with normal speech abilities refuses to speak with people outside of the family in most or all unfamiliar situations. So Jonathan is able to speak normally, but he's fallen into a pattern of not talking that needs to stop.
>
> Mother: Is it really anything we have to worry about?
>
> Therapist: It is a serious problem, but fortunately it can be successfully treated. All children's intellectual, social, and emotional growth in the early years is largely based on their ability to verbally interact with other children and adults at home, school, and in the community. Though this can be accomplished to a certain extent by gestures, Jonathan's refusal to speak puts him at a tremendous disadvantage. He will have, and is already having, a very difficult time making and keeping friends, as well as learning and interacting in a normal manner at school. These things will likely lead to him feeling badly about himself as he sees he is not able to do what the other children are doing.
>
> Mother: Why does Jonathan have this problem? Is it my fault?
>
> Therapist: No, it's not a matter of fault. Kids fall into the pattern of being silent for many reasons. Once they do, however, they often get lots of attention for their silence as other people talk and do things for them. That's an easy pattern for families and parents to fall into, as it is natural to want to do anything to help your child or make them feel more comfortable. I think Jonathan and you have gone through a lot, and there are many positive things about Jonathan. I don't know all the reasons Jonathan stopped talking, and we probably won't know for a while, but we need to get Jonathan back on track talking as quickly as possible.

Mother: You know, I think I have gotten into the habit of talking for
Jonathan and doing things for him too. I was only trying to
help. So now what? How can we help my son?

Therapist: Fortunately, as I said before, elective mutism is a very
treatable problem and we have had the chance to successfully
treat many children with elective mutism here at Hawthorn
Center.

The treatment technique was described to Jonathan's mother.
When told of the detrimental effect of not speaking, she described how
she had lately been worried as he was not making friends and that she
had observed him in school being somewhat lonely and isolated. She
was in agreement with the treatment plan. Jonathan was told at the
evaluation that at the next session he would be expected to speak.

An appointment was then scheduled for the next week. The therapist cleared his schedule of patients in the morning and made prior
arrangements to possibly cancel meetings that were planned for the
afternoon. Jonathan came readily to the therapist's office and when
asked how he was doing responded, "Fine," while walking back to the
office. Upon entering the office he stood in a corner and was more
reticent than when previously seen. When asked another question after
entering the office, he refused to speak. After a few minutes, he pointed
at the basketball and indicated nonverbally that he wanted to again
shoot baskets. As a good rapport was felt to have been established during
the evaluation and as Jonathan had spoken coming back to the office,
the therapist made the decision to require Jonathan to name the toy with
which he wished to play. After approximately thirty seconds Jonathan
pointed to the basketball and said, "Basketball." Following this session
he was taken back to the waiting room after being given much praise by
the therapist. His mother also praised him and announced that he would
be taken for ice cream for having spoken during the session.

In the first half of the next session Jonathan spoke very softly and
offered very little speech other than naming the toy with which he
wished to play. During the second half of the session he was required to
speak progressively louder the word *basketball* to have it rebounded for
him. By the end of the session he was yelling the word *basketball* and
appeared to enjoy this.

At the next session, after initially being required to get to the
point of yelling the word *basketball*, he was told that he would have to
say progressively one more word in order to have the basketball

rebounded for him. By the end of the session he was saying strings of twenty-two words.

The following session the same limit was again imposed but by the end of the session, as he ran out of things to name, Jonathan stated that he would rather just talk, and the guideline was set that he had to say a sentence before the ball would be rebounded. The therapist and Jonathan also spoke during that and the next session about what would be the easiest thing for him to say in the classroom. He felt that answering to the attendance roll call would probably be the easiest. This was practiced by having both the therapist and Jonathan practice answering, using a wide range of voices, volumes, and tones. His teacher was called and it was arranged that at a particular roll call he would be expected to answer. Jonathan was able to do this approximately one month after the first limit-setting session. On the same day as answering attendance, he also read a sentence aloud to the class when it was his turn to read without any additional prompting by the teacher. In subsequent sessions we continued to work on reading and increasing his verbal fluency.

In addition to the individual work with Jonathan, Jonathan's mother was seen on a biweekly basis. Four weeks into the treatment she spontaneously stated that she had been wondering if she had given Jonathan a covert message not to speak to others outside of the home because of her own difficulties in handling the abandonment by her husband. She also described how she felt she may have been supporting Jonathan becoming too dependent on her because of her own loneliness.

Six weeks into treatment she stated she had begun on her own to require Jonathan to speak in the community, as she felt he was ready. She described that beginning about a week after Jonathan spoke in the therapy session, they went out to dinner as a family. She told Jonathan prior to going out that he would have to order his own dinner. When he refused to speak in the restaurant, he did not receive dinner. The family afterward went out for ice cream and the same condition was set for Jonathan and she described how Jonathan had no difficulty in ordering ice cream. Since that time he had been able to order in restaurants and had also been able to speak with a librarian at the public library.

By three months after beginning treatment, Jonathan was speaking appropriately in the home, school, and community. His mother indicated that she had resumed dating again and she had sought her own individual therapy to address her difficulties with trust. A planned tapered termination was then instituted in which Jonathan came every two weeks for two sessions, then a month later, and then two months later. Jonathan continued to speak appropriately in all settings. At the final session, when asked, he stated that he did not remember why he had refused to speak in school and described feeling much happier now that he could. He proudly stated that he had made a number of new friends both in school and in his neighborhood.

Comments

Jonathan represents a fairly typical treatment course for elective mutism using this technique. With the therapist's facilitation and appropriate limit setting the child usually is verbal the first session following the explanation of the expectation. While it was somewhat unusual in that he spoke coming back to the therapy room, most children are usually verbal after fifteen minutes to one hour in the session where the verbal expectation is set. After the child is over the first verbal hurdle, increasing speech within each session becomes progressively easier. In most elective mutes the feelings of increased mastery that occur as each fearful hurdle is overcome are tremendously reinforcing and speech becomes generalized in most settings with decreasing difficulty.

CASE ILLUSTRATION (OVERCOMING OBSTACLES)

Description and History

Mark Wilson (a pseudonym) was a 6½-year-old boy who was seven months into first grade when he came to Hawthorn Center for evaluation. Mark's parents related to us that Mark had always had problems talking and "never really talked a lot" and "only to certain people."

The Wilsons told us that in kindergarten Mark initially refused to talk, but in the middle of the year did say single words to the teacher on a few occasions in response to being told by the teacher that he had to speak before he would be allowed to leave school. He returned to being totally mute for the last three months of kindergarten as the teacher did not follow through with her limit setting. In first grade, Mark returned to being totally mute in school. In both kindergarten and first grade, Mark never talked to others, participated spontaneously, ate in school, or used the bathroom. He would often stand in the corner refusing to participate.

The Wilsons downplayed the seriousness of Mark's problems, telling us that they came to Hawthorn Center primarily because the school social worker "thought it would be helpful." The Wilsons further described Mark as a perfectionistic, strong-willed, and moody child. When angry, he would often respond by screaming, kicking, throwing a temper tantrum, or refusing to talk. In the community, Mark was described as a shy, withdrawn, clingy child who would not talk with anyone outside a few select people.

Mark's developmental milestones were described as unremarkable other than Mrs. Wilson stating that Mark was very resistant to toilet training until approximately 3½ years of age, but "when he decided to do it, it was no problem." Mark's past medical and developmental histories were essentially unremarkable.

Mark was in a dynamic insight-oriented therapy for approximately six months before coming to Hawthorn Center. During that period of time, Mark never talked to his therapist.

On first observing the Wilson family in the waiting room, Mark and Mrs. Wilson were noted to be sitting extremely close to one another with Mrs. Wilson's arm encircling him. Mr. Wilson was sitting off to the side.

In the first interview, Mark presented as a small boy who stood rigidly in the corner, with downcast eyes, whimpering, and remaining a silent nonparticipant throughout the interview. Mark further refused to participate in psychological testing that day and in that setting also stood rigidly in the corner unresponsive to attempts to engage him in the testing process.

Synopsis of Therapy Sessions

The treatment technique was explained to the Wilsons, including the fact that after the child becomes comfortable with his therapist and rapport has developed, the therapist would make a morning appointment for the child and set aside the day with the expectation that the child say at least one word in the therapy session. The Wilsons were informed that Mark would be told that he would not be allowed to leave until he spoke. The Wilsons expressed their concern that this might in some way hurt Mark. They said, "The other therapist said she could get Mark to talk, but if she forced him it would hurt him." This issue was explored in depth and the Wilsons were assured that this technique had been used very successfully with many children over a number of years and had not been found to be harmful. In addition, they were told it helps children to feel better about themselves when used by a person who is sensitive to the child's feelings and who understands elective mutism. It was further explained that, for treatment to be successful, family support is imperative, for it is the family and not the therapist who would ultimately make the difference. The Wilsons expressed some skepticism but agreed to the treatment.

Mark's reaction to being told he must say at least one word before leaving the next session was a controlled, rigid, pitiful cry. Nonetheless, an appointment was set with the Wilsons and the therapist cleared his schedule for the day. The Wilsons were told to bring Mark in the morning and expect to spend a portion or all of the day at Hawthorn Center.

Mr. and Mrs. Wilson arrived as scheduled with Mark at 8:00 A.M. on the day of the appointment. Mark was tearful and rigid and refused to go with the therapist. Mr. Wilson picked Mark up in a warm but firm manner (with the therapist's prompting) and carried him to the therapist's office. He then succeeded in disentangling himself from Mark and left. Mark stood rigidly in the corner, whimpering. The therapist asked Mark why he was crying but Mark did not answer. The therapist told Mark that he knew it was scary for him to be in the therapist's office and he was probably feeling angry and frightened about talking, but nonetheless, today was the day and the therapist would be willing to stay all day with him if needed for Mark to talk.

The therapist initially tried to engage Mark by asking him if he might want to talk now and tell the therapist with which game or toy he wanted to play. Mark was silent. The therapist got out some animal figures and played with them near Mark in an attempt to involve him, but he would not participate. Playfully, the therapist made a small dog figure crawl up Mark's leg and his stomach to his shoulder and finally to talk to Mark. Mark stood with his arms rigidly at his sides and tried to push the figure away with his body but would not use his hands to accomplish this task. The therapist created a voice for the dog figure, which told Mark that it was scared and then ran down Mark's body and hid in Mark's sock. This effort produced a small smile, which he quickly tried to hide. Then the dog figure (with some of his animal friends) attempted to get Mark to play with the animals or talk to them. Mark remained silent. An interpretation of how scary it must be to have to be the boss all the time was made to Mark through the dog figure.

The therapist told Mark that he had helped many other children with this problem and that Mark would feel better about himself after talking. The therapist then told Mark that if he wanted to do anything or play anything, he had but to ask, but if not, the therapist would then go and work on some paperwork at his desk. However, Mark would not be allowed to go home until he said at least one word. This statement caused Mark to cry once again.

This approach, which involved alternating between being supportive, clarifying feelings, encouraging Mark to participate, setting firm limits, and at times pretending to ignore Mark and do paperwork, continued for approximately four hours. Lunch was eaten in the room. Food and drink for Mark were placed on a table, but Mark stood rigidly in the corner, whimpering. Finally, much to the therapist's relief, Mark began quietly, with a closed mouth, to attempt to whine something. The therapist reacted to this by coming over to Mark to ask him what he said. Mark became silent once again. The therapist tried engaging Mark and encouraging him but to no avail. The therapist then returned to his paperwork. Mark started crying again and whining something. Again, the therapist attempted to respond to this, with the same result. This was repeated for approximately one hour until, in a barely audible, whiny whisper, Mark said, "Mommy." The therapist praised Mark's accomplishment, told him next time it would be easier to talk, and rewarded Mark by immediately taking him to his mother, who had been instructed ahead of time to praise his actions. Mark was further told that he would be seen in two days and, at that time, he would need to say more than one word in the session.

Mark was slow to become more verbal in subsequent sessions. Initially, each new word was difficult for Mark, was barely audible, and was produced only in response to therapeutic interventions. Mark brought in pictures and toys but at first would not tell the therapist about them or what he wanted to do. The therapist finally told him that if he couldn't say yes or no about doing something, they wouldn't be able to play. The therapist took out a toy Mark had brought and asked if he wanted to play with it. Mark shook his head no. The therapist told Mark he could not understand him unless Mark could verbally tell the therapist. Mark very quietly said "no." The therapist quickly decided to use humor to further the therapeutic alliance. He acted as if he were horrified and said in a humorous way, "You stubbed your toe? Where?!" The therapist then proceeded to grab one of Mark's feet. Mark laughed and said "no" much louder. The therapist would continue to find using humor a useful technique in treating Mark. Humor allowed Mark to interact in a playful, childlike manner and, thus, abandon his guarded, controlling silence. Humor further allowed Mark to enjoy being with the therapist while firm expectations were being set.

As Mark became more comfortable with talking during sessions, oral reading was introduced using a book he was studying in school, and which he had already been able to read aloud to his mother. Again, this started out slowly and almost inaudibly. His efforts and abilities were praised and he appeared proud of himself. It was useful to introduce reading early on in the therapy, as it was planned to use reading as a logical extension to verbal behavior at school.

As the therapist continued treating Mark, his mother reported that he told her he had bad guys in his head and they were keeping him from talking. When the therapist initiated a discussion of the mother's report with Mark, he confirmed this fantasy. As therapy continued, Mark began to tell the therapist that the bad guys in his head were disappearing and being replaced by good guys who allowed him to be comfortable with talking.

Mark enjoyed coming to the sessions and Mrs. Wilson reported improvement in the home and community with a decrease in Mark's temper tantrums and an improved capacity to enjoy himself. She further reported that Mark said, "I like my doctor. He is an adult who can act like a child." This appeared to confirm that Mark was comfortable in the sessions and enjoyed interacting in a less controlled, more childlike manner.

In Mark's case, he required the therapist's direct participation in the school setting. The therapist planned to speak with Mark initially alone and then to have Mark speak with the teacher and classmates. Initially, Mark refused to accompany the therapist out of the classroom. He was then informed of his choices in the situation, which were that he either accompany the therapist on his own initiative, or the therapist would intervene to the extent of physically carrying him out of the classroom, if necessary.

Mark would not come with the therapist, so the therapist followed through and picked Mark up and carried him out of the room. Once out of the room Mark said, "Put me down, I'll walk." He then showed the therapist to a private room where he talked and played for a short period of time. He read his particular practice story for the therapist and then the therapist told him that it was time to read it for the teacher, but to pretend that she was not there at first. The teacher then entered the room but Mark would not read the story. After a short period of time, the teacher left and Mark told the therapist that he was mad at himself but was never reading again. The therapist told Mark that he would have another chance next week when the therapist would return to the school to help him once again. Mark, after much initial refusal, agreed that he would try again next week.

Prior to the therapist's return to the school, the therapist worked with Mark to practice the story, explore his fears, support his previous verbal accomplishments, and discuss the fact that this time when the therapist went to the school, Mark and he would not leave the school until Mark had read for his teacher. Mark was angry about this plan and told the therapist so repeatedly. At times he told the therapist he would never talk to him again and he would never read again. However, using a combination of humor, support, encouragement, and firm limit setting, the therapist was successful in getting Mark to agree to attempt to read in front of his teacher once again. The therapist returned to the school the next week. After receiving help reading the first word of the preselected story, Mark began reading quietly for the teacher. As Mark read, the therapist slowly repositioned the book so Mark was reading directly to the teacher. Once Mark completed his reading, the teacher asked him some preselected questions about colors, and Mark was able to answer her directly. Mark was reinforced verbally by the therapist and received his previously promised special toy surprise. This was a small stuffed animal with a watch attached (a watchdog). This had been carefully selected based on Mark's use of stuffed animals in therapy to express his feelings. Further, his teacher greatly praised his accomplishment. The therapist then left the school and the teacher brought Mark back to his class.

Mark read out loud to one additional child each day until he had read for the entire class. Mark then was required to increase his verbal behaviors by slowly beginning to answer attendance call and then answering preselected questions in front of the class.

When the therapist attempted to begin family therapy, the therapist was told by the family that Mr. Wilson often would not be able to attend sessions because of work. Further, he would not actively take part in the treatment or treatment suggestions. Efforts were made to engage Mr. Wilson in the therapeutic work by scheduling an evening appointment with Mr. Wilson and Mark approximately once per month. Through these appointments, Mr. Wilson became more involved and expressed feelings that in the past he had felt "left out" of the family.

In family sessions it was discovered that each family member would talk for Mark if he was in an uncomfortable situation. Mark might whisper his needs into a family member's ear in a public place and the family member would then respond, allowing Mark to avoid verbal interactions with nonfamily members. The Wilsons recognized this maladaptive response and began to set appropriate limits in this regard. They informed Mark that if he wanted something he needed to ask. This seems to be a simple, logical intervention; however, it was very difficult for the Wilsons to carry out and they were able to do so only after the family's dynamics and their facilitation of Mark's silence were worked through in family therapy sessions.

> Therapist: Mark is now speaking fairly easily in sessions and in school, and I wanted to make sure Mark received much of the credit for this because, as you know, it was not always this easy for him. But Mark couldn't have done it without you, because your support and attention mean everything to him, as you are the most important people in his life.
>
> Mother: We are very proud of Mark speaking, but he still has a hard time talking when we go out.
>
> Father: Just the other day we went to the mall and then stopped to get some lunch and Mark wouldn't talk.
>
> Therapist: Really? Mark, what happened?
>
> Mark: I just didn't want to talk.
>
> Therapist: What made it so hard to do?
>
> Mark: I don't know.
>
> Therapist: Mr. and Mrs. Wilson, what did you do when Mark didn't talk.
>
> Mother: Nothing. We just ignored him.
>
> Therapist: Okay, but what happened then? Can you go over what occured in a step-by-step manner?
>
> Mother: Well, we finished shopping and we were all getting hungry so we decided to go get some lunch. Mark wanted to go to Burger King so we went there but he wouldn't talk.
>
> Therapist: So, who ordered the food?
>
> Mother: Well, when we got to the head of the line, Mark whispered in his brother's ear and his brother ordered.
>
> Therapist: Oh. Huh. How did that happen?

Mother: Well, I guess we've all just gotten used to Mark not talking and communicating his needs to others by whispering in our ears.

Therapist: I see. The whole family sort of talks for Mark when he doesn't want to.

Mother: Yes, I guess we do. But if Mark doesn't whisper to us, how will he get what he wants?

Therapist: By talking himself.

Mother: But if he doesn't, what will happen?

Therapist: Well, I guess in this case, Mark wouldn't get his lunch at Burger King, but I bet when both of you let Mark know by your words and actions that he needs to communicate for himself, otherwise he won't get the things he wants, he will start talking. Is everybody ready to help Mark get over this next hurdle?

Mother :You're sure this won't hurt Mark?

Therapist: Absolutely not. He'll do great. He might miss a meal here or there or not get an ice cream cone or a treat that he wants, but as soon as he gets the idea that you're serious, things will work themselves out. It is important, though, once you set a limit, you must stick with it, even if Mark tries to wear you down like he has in the past.

Father: I'm ready to try it.

Therapist: How about you, Mrs. Wilson?

Mother: I'll do anything to help Mark.

Therapist: Good. Let's set up a plan to help get this started. Mark, I know you love ice cream, so I am going to ask your parents to take you and your brother out for ice cream later on this week, but you'll need to order for yourself if you want ice cream. Okay?

Mark: No, I won't.

Therapist: Okay. Then I guess you really didn't want that ice cream as much as I thought. Mr. and Mrs. Wilson, why don't you try that and we'll talk about what happened at the next appointment. Any questions?

Mother: No, I think I know what we have to do and I think we can do it.

Therapist: Good. Remember, what you're doing is going to really help Mark to get his mutism under control. Mark, I know this might be hard for you, but remember at first talking with me was very hard and then talking at school was very hard but you were able to do both of those things and look what's happened since then: you made a lot of new friends at school, you're having a lot more fun, and mom and dad are very proud of you. It might be hard at first, but I know you can do it. Mr. and Mrs. Wilson, Mark, I will plan on seeing you next week after you've gotten yourself that ice cream cone.

The Wilsons were further instructed to reward verbal behavior and ignore nonverbal behavior. At first, Mark protested, and did not ask for ice cream and thus did not receive any. He further attempted to test the Wilsons' resolve wherever he could but gradually he began being verbal in public places.

Additionally, six months into treatment, Mark's mother revealed that she would occasionally use silence when angry. Mark was described as paying attention but not appearing overly upset by it. This issue was then explored and worked through in the therapy.

Mark continued to talk about the bad guys and good guys in his head. The therapist introduced puppet play with Mark, creating a puppet character who refused to talk. The therapist asked Mark why the puppet wasn't talking and what could be done to help him. Mark slowly began talking about the puppet's fear of talking and having other people laugh at him and hate him. These fears were explored with Mark and he was given support and interpretations within the metaphor of the puppets.

During termination Mark's mother related, "He is a different child. The whole family has noticed. He seems happier and more confident and he hasn't had a temper tantrum in six months. He is still stubborn and hesitant around new people and new situations, but that is Mark."

Comments

Mark's case illustrates a particularly treatment-resistant child and family, but as such it illustrates some important points. Mark's ambivalence about his symptom became clear during the treatment as he was able, with the therapist and his family's help, to extricate himself from the cage his symptom had become. The mutism itself, as well as the control Mark was able to exercise over his family and teachers because of it, were seriously impairing Mark's development. It should also be noted that even in a child whose elective mutism was as family entrenched as Mark's, there was no symptom substitution or detrimental effect from treatment.

SUMMARY

A treatment approach for elective mutism developed at Hawthorn Center (Wright 1968) has been described and illustrated in this chapter. Underlying this approach is the realization that, despite the child's resistance, the child is very ambivalent about his symptoms. The child at some level realizes through this treatment approach that the therapist, unlike previous people in his life including parents, friends, teachers, and relatives, will not give in to his symptom. This is at some level comforting to the child, because it acknowledges the child's ambivalent feelings about not speaking while at the same time supporting his drive toward developmental progress and mastery. The child falls into being silent for many reasons. However, he has found that while it often provides tremendous secondary gains and a sense of power and control, he is frightened by having such power and control over significant adults. The child yearns to shout and scream, to play like other children, and to take part in social activities, but he finds he cannot extricate himself from his current situation. The firm approach the therapist takes in treatment is understood and at some level welcomed by the child. A positive relationship between therapist and child develops as treatment progresses. It is perhaps because of this that at Hawthorn Center, some elective mutes have returned to talk with their therapists years later when facing an unrelated difficult or traumatic situation. This illustrates the strength of the therapeutic alliance formed during the treatment of these children.

It is this therapeutic alliance that is the foundation of the Hawthorn Center approach. It allows these children to side with the healthy part of themselves that wants to play and speak as a normal child. When this has occurred, the feelings of needing to remain in control of themselves and their world through their mutism are no longer necessary.

REFERENCES

Black, B., and Uhde, T. W. (1992). Elective mutism as a variant of social phobia. *Journal of the American Academy of Child and Adolescent Psychiatry* 6:1090–1094.

Brown, J. B., and Lloyd, H. (1975). A controlled study of children not speaking at school. *Journal of Associated Workers of Maladjusted Children* 3:49–63.

Browne, E., Wilson, V., and Laybourne, P. C. (1963). Diagnosis and treatment of elective mutism in children. *Journal of the American Academy of Child Psychiatry* 2:605–617.

Diagnostic and Statistical Manual of Mental Disorders (1994). 4th ed. Washington, DC: American Psychiatric Association.

Fundudis, T., Kolvin, I., and Garside, R. (1979). *Speech Retarded and Deaf Children: Their Psychological Development*. London: Academic Press.

Hayden, T. L. (1980). Classification of elective mutism. *Journal of the American Academy of Child and Adolescent Psychiatry* 19:118–133.

Kolvin, I., and Fundudis, T. (1981). Elective mute children: psychological development and background factors. *Journal of Child Psychology and Psychiatry* 22:219–232.

Krohn, D., Weckstein, S., and Wright, H. (1992). A study of the effectiveness of a specific treatment for elective mutism. *Journal of the American Academy of Child and Adolescent Psychiatry* 31:711–718.

Kussmaul, A. (1877). *Die Storungen der Sprache*. Leipzig: F. C. W. Vogel.

Labbe, E. E., and Williamson, D. A. (1984). Behavioral treatment of elective mutism: a review of the literature. *Clinical Psychology Review* 4:273–294.

Parker, E. B., Elsen, T. F., and Throckmorton, M. C. (1960). Social casework with elementary school children who do not talk in school. *Social Work* 5:64–70.

Rutter, M. (1977). Delayed speech. In *Child Psychiatry: Modern Approaches*, eds. M. Rutter and L. Hersov. Oxford: Blackwell Scientific.

Sanok, R. L., and Ascione, F. R. (1979). Behavioral interventions for elective mutism: an evaluative review. *Child Behavior Therapy* 1:49–67.

Sanok, R. L., and Striefels, S. (1979). Elective mutism: generalization of verbal responding across people and settings. *Behavior Therapy* 10:357–371.

Tramer, M. (1934). Elektiver mutismus be: kindern. *Zeitschriftfur Kinder Psychiatrie* 1:30–35.

Wergeland, H. (1979). Elective mutism. *ACTA Psychiatrica Scandinavica* 59:218–228.

Wilkins, R. (1985). A comparison of elective mutism and emotional disorders in children. *British Journal of Psychiatry* 146:198–203.

Wright, H. L. (1968). A clinical study of children who refuse to talk in school. *Journal of the American Academy of Child Psychiatry* 7:603–617.

Wright, H. H., Miller, M. D., Cook, M. A., and Lihman, J. R. (1985). Early identification and intervention with children who refuse to speak. *Journal of the American Academy of Child Psychiatry* 24:739–746.

7

PHOBIC DISORDER

Alice G. Friedman
Donna B. Pincus
Edward P. Quinn

DESCRIPTION OF DISORDER

Fear is a normal response to a threat of harm, which can serve an adaptive function by facilitating avoidance of dangerous situations (Marks 1987). As genuine threats are plentiful during childhood, it is not surprising that fears are common in infancy and throughout childhood. When asked, most children will readily identify multiple fears (Ollendick 1983, Ollendick et al. 1989). Typically, such fears are mild and transient, and follow a predictable developmental sequence (Marks 1987). However, some children experience fears that persist, interfere with daily functioning, and are not age appropriate. When these fears are excessive, and not associated with an actual threat, they suggest a clinical level of fear, or a phobic disorder.

The characteristic feature of phobic disorders is the presence of excessive anxiety, which leads to avoidance of a feared object, event, or situation (phobic stimuli) and the experience of extreme levels of fear and anxiety when confronted with the perceived threat (*DSM-III-R*, American Psychiatric Association 1987). Phobic disorders are therefore classified as anxiety disorders in the recent *Diagnostic and Statistical Manuals of Mental Disorders* (*DSM-III-R*, American Psychiatric Association 1987, and *DSM-IV*, American Psychiatric Association 1994). Further, with only minor exceptions, the same criteria are used to classify phobic disorders in adults and children. The present chapter focuses exclusively on simple (or specific) phobias of childhood. While conceptually some instances of school refusal may reflect simple phobia of school, the topic is covered separately in this volume. Likewise, readers interested in social phobia and agoraphobia without history of panic disorder are directed to individual chapters devoted to those topics in the current text. Fears of medical procedures, though the focus of a substantial literature, are viewed as being conceptually different from phobias and therefore are not emphasized here.

Children can develop phobias to an endless array of situations, objects, and events. Recent studies have focused on children with fears of menstruation (Shaw 1990), telephones (Babbitt and Parrish 1991), water (Menzies and Clarke 1993), newspapers (Goldberg and Weisenberg 1992), and bowel movements (Eisen and Silverman 1991). In a survey of psychologists about types of fears and anxieties present in the children they treat, Silverman and Kearney (1992) reported that separation anxiety, school phobia, and fear of social situations represented over half of the cases of phobias. The next most prevalent included fears of tests and the dark. The remaining fears represented fewer than 4 percent of the referrals. The DSM-IV specifies five distinct types of phobias: animal type; natural environment type (e.g., heights and water); blood, injection, injury type; situational type (e.g., planes and elevators); and other type (those not otherwise classified). To date, there is little information about the prevalence of the specific phobia types in children.

Recent epidemiological surveys suggest that between 2 and 4 percent of children in the general population have clinical levels of fear that would qualify as a simple phobia (Anderson et al. 1987, Bird et al. 1988). Phobias are not a frequent reason for seeking psychological services as they account for fewer than 7 percent of the referrals for mental health services for children (Graziano and De Giovanni 1979, Silverman and Kearney 1992). Clinical levels of fear may actually be relatively rare or parents may view them as not sufficiently detrimental to a child's development to warrant treatment. In fact, the prognosis for children with simple phobias (without comorbidity) is excellent. Most phobias dissipate over time, even without treatment (Agras et al. 1972). It appears that those children who are brought to clinics for treatment often have additional anxiety-related disorders (Last, Strauss et al. 1987). These more severe problems, rather than the simple phobia, may prompt parents to seek treatment.

Concerns about the etiology of fears have fascinated researchers for decades. While there has been considerable debate about the origin of phobias (see Marks 1987), there is general consensus that phobias appear to be acquired and maintained by a complex interaction of classical, operant, or vicarious conditioning (Ollendick and King 1991). Exposure to phobic stimuli, or even anticipation of such an encounter, is accompanied by anxiety, resulting in avoidance of the fear-provoking cues and strengthening of the phobic response.

There has been surprisingly little systematic research on acquisition and treatment of childhood phobias. Most of what is known is based on case reports or studies using single subject design. There is now a fairly substantial literature on normal developmental fears, yet there is no reason to assume that these findings are pertinent to phobias. It is likely that phobias are acquired and maintained by different mechanisms than normal fears, and recent research supports this notion. For example, in a study of children with overanxious disorder, Strauss, Lease, and colleagues (1988) reported that more than 40 percent of their sample of children 12 years or older had a concurrent diagnosis of simple phobia. These children did not score higher than a normative sample on number and intensity of fears. Further, there is no evidence that children with multiple fears are more prone to phobias than those with fewer fears.

While normal fears and phobias may be attributable to different mechanisms, a child may be particularly vulnerable to certain phobias at certain ages. The onset of phobias may be temporally linked to the emergence of normal fears. Phobias that persist into adulthood appear to emerge at different times that may coincide with the normal emergence of the fear. For example, adults with animal phobias recall their emergence during the preschool years (Marks and Gelder 1966), while adults with blood or dental phobias recall their onset during mid-childhood or early adolescence (Ost 1987). Fear of animals typically emerges in children during the preschool years, while fear of bodily harm is not evident until later (Marks 1987).

DIFFERENTIAL DIAGNOSIS

There are a number of issues worth considering before a child is diagnosed with simple phobia. The first involves distinguishing among types of phobias. Simple or specific phobia refers to a circumscribed fear of a clearly delineated threat. Social phobia appears to be a more complex and disruptive disorder involving fears about being scrutinized, humiliated, or embarrassed by others. The onset of social phobia is usually during adolescence rather than earlier, as in the case of simple phobia (Strauss 1992). Fears related to social phobia may be quite specific, such as fearing embarrassment while giving a speech, or more global, such as fear of talking in front of other children. However, in each case the fear is rooted in concerns about the appraisal of others. The child is concerned about the negative judgments or scrutiny by others rather than fearing actual harm from others. As agoraphobia without history of panic disorder is virtually nonexistent in childhood it is less likely to present a problem for differential diagnosis. The essential feature of this disorder is fear of being unable to escape from a place or situation rather than fear of the place per se.

A second concern is distinguishing a simple phobia from other disorders where avoidance and anxiety may be important features but are symptoms of a more pervasive disorder. Excessive fears are frequent among children who meet criteria for a number of more serious disorders. Children with obsessive-compulsive disorder may appear to be phobic, since they may complain about a specific fear (such as fear of contamination). Such a child may engage in a ritual that may appear to be avoidance of phobic stimuli (such as ritualistically avoiding a contaminated area). However, this syndrome is characterized by repetitive behaviors and persistent intrusive thoughts, both of which are absent in children with simple phobias. Likewise, children with post-traumatic stress disorder may avoid a range of stimuli in an effort to avoid thoughts, feelings, or distress related to a past traumatic event. Generally a broad, rather than circumscribed, array of situations will elicit fear or anxiety. Further, an important feature of this syndrome is re-experiencing thoughts, feelings, or distress directly related to an event that is clearly out of the ordinary (such as rape, vehicle accident, fire). Children with specific phobias may recall a negative event associated with the fear (such as a dog bite) but it is rarely of a life-threatening magnitude.

A child with excessive anxiety related to separation from an attachment figure (usually a parent) would be diagnosed with separation anxiety disorder rather than simple or specific phobia. Children with pervasive anxiety that is generalized rather than focused on circumscribed stimuli would be diagnosed as generalized anxiety (or overanxious disorder of childhood according to DSM-IV). Reliable diagnosis is rendered more difficult by the high prevalence of comorbidity among children seeking treatment for anxiety related disorders (Strauss et al. 1988a, Strauss et al. 1988b).

Once the presence of more pervasive disorders has been ruled out, the next concern is distinguishing simple phobia from age-appropriate fears. In adults, distinguishing a fear from a phobia is relatively straightforward. An adult who is terrified by the thought of exposure to a dog clearly has a phobia. Such distinctions are more difficult in childhood because of the prevalence of fears among all children. Classifying a circumscribed fear as a phobia requires a consideration of the developmental progression of normal fears. Further, the term *phobia* typically implies that the fear is not only excessive but irrational and impervious to reason. Many age-appropriate childhood fears meet these criteria. A more relevant criterion to consider in decisions about whether a fear is sufficiently severe to warrant treatment is the extent to which a fear interferes with the life of the child and family. Parents are generally able to encourage their children to overcome fears by coaxing the child to approach feared objects, praising the child's efforts, and demonstrating that the fear is unwarranted. For most children these efforts are successful. When the fears persist despite such efforts and normal life is hampered by the child's fears, the family should probably consider treatment.

An additional concern involves the relationship between phobia and noncompliance. Sometimes a child's phobic behavior is actually not anxiety based. Rather, avoidant behaviors are maintained by environmental contingencies. In such cases, children may show very inconsistent patterns of avoidance behaviors. A child with long-standing disruptive nighttime behaviors may be fearless in the dark at times other than bedtime. Careful evaluation of the context within which fear is displayed, the response to phobic behavior by the family, and information about other instances of fear or noncompliance may provide clues to whether the behavior is anxiety based. However, fear responses across the three modalities (physiological, behavioral, subjective) are not necessarily correlated (Lang 1968). One can not infer lack of fear if the child exhibits avoidant behavior without reporting high levels of fear. Likewise, one can not infer lack of fear if the child reports high levels of fear but fails to show physiological or behavioral changes in the presence of the fearful stimuli. Therefore, in drawing conclusions about whether a child is fearful or noncompliant, one should consider information about the presence of noncompliance to other parental requests and in other contexts and determine whether the child can easily interact with or approach the phobic stimuli when the contingencies are slightly altered.

ASSESSMENT PROCEDURES

While a child may be brought to a clinic specifically for treatment of a phobia, it remains important to conduct a sufficiently thorough assessment to rule out the presence of other difficulties, as well as to provide enough information about the fear and its controlling variables to formulate a treatment plan (Ollendick and Francis 1988). Assessment of childhood simple phobias should include measures that evaluate the behavioral, subjective, and physiological aspects of fear and the context within which the fear is evident (Barrios and Hartmann 1988). Assessment of each of these response modalities can be accomplished directly by observing the child in feared situations or indirectly by relying on child and parent reports about the child. Most researchers advocate a multimethod approach to assessment including a combination of interviews, self-report instruments, parental report, and observational strategies (behavioral avoidance tests or direct observation) and home monitoring strategies. Because physiological measurement tends to be impractical in the clinic setting, information about the child's physiological response to exposure to phobic stimuli is usually gathered using indirect means, such as self or parental report. A crucial part of the assessment process is home monitoring, which should be initiated prior to treatment (to establish baseline levels of fear) and continued throughout treatment (to monitor treatment progress).

The selection of specific assessment strategies is dependent upon the age of the child. School-age children can complete questionnaires more easily and are generally able to verbalize their fears more effectively than younger children. Because younger children tend to be less accurate reporters and are less able to verbalize their fears, we rely more heavily upon parental report when conducting assessments of younger children.

We typically begin our assessment with an interview of the child and parents. We interview the parents first so that we have sufficient information to ask the child specific questions about his or her thoughts and behavior. Information gathered during the interview will serve as the foundation for the development of two critical assessment strategies (a behavioral avoidance test and home monitoring procedure) as well as a basis for decision making about treatment. While there are a number of standardized structured interviews designed to facilitate differential diagnosis of a broad range of childhood disorders, there is insufficient empirical evidence to suggest that they facilitate development of a treatment plan. Therefore, we rely primarily upon a standard behavioral interview.

The interview is structured to gather information about the circumstances surrounding acquisition of the fear, its duration, and which aspects of the fear are most problematic to the child and family. We gather very detailed information about the child's phobic behavior and its antecedents and consequences. To determine whether the child's fear is being inadvertently maintained by the family, we ask specific questions about how the family responds to the child while exhibiting fear and while being nonfearful, paying particular attention to aspects of the situation that may be inadvertently reinforcing the phobic behavior. To assess whether family members are modeling fearful behavior, we inquire about the current and past fears of other family members. It is also usually helpful to ask family members about their hypotheses about how the fear developed and what might be contributing to its maintenance. Likewise, it is informative to inquire about the child's and parents' previous attempts to alleviate the child's distress. The parents of an 8-year-old treated in our clinic for fear of being alone at night had actually given their child a machete to keep under the bed. They reasoned that arming him would help him feel capable of coping. Instead, it appeared to justify his fears, thereby increasing his terror.

A number of paper-and-pencil inventories may be useful for assessing the child's global level of anxiety, number and intensity of fears, and presence of additional problems. The Fear Survey Schedule for Children-Revised (FSSC-R, Ollendick 1983) may be helpful in assessing the child's perception of aspects of the environment that are fear evoking. This eighty-item fear survey, which covers a broad range of potentially threatening stimuli, yields scores for total fears as well as scores in each of five factors: fear of failure and criticism, fear of the unknown, fear of injury and small animals, fear of danger and death, and medical fears.

The Revised Children's Manifest Anxiety Scale (RCMAS, Reynolds and Richmond 1978) may also provide useful information about the nature and level of the child's anxiety. The RCMAS yields scores in three empirically derived subscales: physiological anxiety, worry/oversensitivity, and social concern/concentration. As these are self-report measures, there is always the possibility of response bias. A child who wants to appear brave may deny fears and anxieties. In that case, the lie scale of the RCMAS may be elevated. There are a number of additional self-report instruments designed to assess specific phobias (see Barrios and Hartmann 1988 for a comprehensive review). The child's subjective level of fear toward the specific phobic stimuli can be assessed using a Fear Thermometer (Walk 1956). The Fear Thermometer is a visual analogue scale that depicts a thermometer on which children rate their level of fear. Children are instructed to point to the height of the thermometer that corresponds to their level of fear when presented with phobic stimuli. This strategy circumvents language difficulties and appears to be readily understood by most children.

While the interview can assist in ruling out the presence of additional difficulties, it does not assist in a comparison of the target child with other children. We generally administer the Child Behavior Checklist (CBCL, Achenbach and Edelbrock 1986), a parental report of child behavior problems and social competency, to assist with such comparisons. The CBCL provides information about the presence of other problems and enables an informal assessment of concomitant changes in other areas following treatment. Additional difficulties revealed by the CBCL should be followed up with additional assessment strategies.

The instruments discussed thus far provide only indirect information about the child's motor response to fear. Behavioral avoidance tests (BATs) and observations of the child in the natural environment provide more direct means for assessing the child's behavior. The BAT is an analogue task designed to approximate the actual fear-evoking situation. The child is exposed to the phobic stimulus in a contrived, controllable setting and instructed to perform a series of graduated steps leading up to full confrontation with the fear-evoking stimulus. For children with fear of the dark, the BAT may be constructed so that the child remains in a room alone while the lights are gradually dimmed from full illumination to complete darkness in five steps. Variations of the BAT have been used to assess a wide range of phobias in children (Jersild and Holmes 1935, Friedman and Ollendick 1989). Potential problems with BATs include pragmatics of constructing a BAT in the clinic, presence of different demand characteristics associated with the BAT compared to the child's usual environment, and absence of the full stimuli configuration of the phobic object, rendering the BAT of questionable validity. Direct observation of the child, or construction of an observational rating scale to be used by the parents to rate their child, is often more practical and valid than the BAT. In both cases, a scale can be constructed using information from the interview to code the child's approach behaviors in graduated steps. The same information can be used to develop home monitoring forms to be used by the parents and child throughout treatment.

Home monitoring by the child and parent is an important component of assessment and treatment. Reactivity to home monitoring usually facilitates positive behavior change (Friedman and Ollendick 1989). The specific behaviors to be recorded should be clearly delineated. Selection of behaviors can be based on interview data and should reflect the agreed upon desired outcome. The forms should be easy to read, simple to complete, and devoid of any ambiguity about the criterion for recording a success.

ESTABLISHING TREATMENT GOALS

Once it is established that a child has a phobia, the first goal is to determine whether treatment is warranted. Phobias appear to dissipate even among children who have not been treated (Agras et al. 1972, Hampe et al. 1973). Hampe and colleagues (1973) compared improvement in children with phobias who received treatment to those assigned to a wait-list control group. Fourteen weeks later, significant reductions in fear were noted for all children, thereby challenging the assumption that change was attributable to the intervention rather than to developmental processes. Numerous studies have documented rapid improvement after very brief interventions (Friedman and Ollendick 1989, Menzies and Clarke 1993, Ollendick et al. 1991). In light of these findings, Graziano and colleagues (1979) suggest using a criteria of two years or extreme interference with the life of the child and family to establish the need for treatment. However, this seems like an excessive length of time. While fears may eventually dissipate without treatment, anxiety related to the fears may result in disruption of age-appropriate activities, increasing the risk of additional problems. We recommend considering extent of life interference rather than a specific time frame for deciding whether treatment is appropriate.

We typically will not treat children with age-appropriate fears unless they are causing extreme difficulties in the family. It is not unusual, for example, for parents of children below age 5 to request treatment in our Fear of the Dark Clinic. In many cases parents are unaware that certain fears are developmentally appropriate. In these instances, the treatment goal is to educate the parents and provide anticipatory guidance about what to expect as the child gets older. It is usually apparent that the parents actually know very little about child development and parenting practices, in which case we focus on educating the parents rather than changing the child's behavior.

The treatment goals for children with phobias are fairly straightforward. The overriding goal is to facilitate the child's competent interaction with the fear-evoking stimulus with concomitant decreases in subjective distress. In most cases, treatment should incorporate reducing the child's level of fear and should facilitate acquisition of new, more adaptive behaviors to reduce the probability of future problems (Evans 1989).

Assessment may reveal that the child and family have significant problems that are maintaining the fears, or may even appear unrelated to the fear, but that warrant more immediate attention. In this case, more extensive therapy is warranted. Here we stress the need to consider the child's difficulties in the context of other aspects of the child's life. Many children with medical problems, for example, develop extreme fear of invasive medical procedures. While the child may be resistant, disrupt the clinic, and even prolong the procedure, these are realistic fears rather than phobias. That is not to say that children should not be treated for these fears, as there are well-specified approaches to helping children cope effectively with medical procedures. However, the goal of treatment would be slightly different as treatment would generally acknowledge the realistic nature of the fear.

ROLE OF THE THERAPIST

In the treatment of phobias, the therapist takes an active role in educating the child and parent, encouraging the development of new skills, and facilitating exposure and coping with the feared object or situation. After the initial referral but before treatment, it is important for the therapist to outline to the family how therapy will proceed. Many families have little notion about the process of psychotherapy, particularly behavior therapy, except what they have garnered from television or similar sources.

Many parents have concerns about the hidden meaning of their child's fears. Part of the therapist's role is to educate families about the conceptualization of phobias. Conveying that the fears are understandable, treatable, and not indicative of deeper, more pervasive problems may help parents better understand the rationale underlying the treatment plan. The family can be reassured that treatment can be accomplished in a relatively brief period of time if the family cooperates and works together to solve the difficulties. The need for consistency and follow-through on all assignments should be stressed.

From the onset of treatment, it is important to establish the notion that the parents and child will have to take an even more active role in therapy than the therapist. Parents may expect that treatment will be conducted in the office during hourly sessions once a week. In fact, the family will actually be responsible for implementing and practicing strategies in the home environment. Therefore, during the initial session the therapist should establish the expectation that treatment may require changes in the family's routine and that the child and family may be asked to record behaviors and practice strategies between sessions.

TREATMENT STRATEGIES

The study of childhood phobia has served an important role in the development of behavior therapy. More than seventy years ago, Mary Cover Jones (Jones 1924) demonstrated the efficacy of desensitization techniques and modeling strategies to eliminate Peter's fear of rabbits (Barrios and Hartmann 1988). In 1935, Jersild and Holmes noted that childhood fears were successfully treated with graded exposure and use of activities and techniques that require "direct, active contact with or participation in the situation . . . " that is feared (p. 88). Little has changed about treatment recommendations in the subsequent sixty years: exposure, and activities that facilitate exposure, remain the most efficacious way to treat childhood phobias.

What has changed is the myriad of techniques that have been devised to facilitate exposure. Few of them have been subjected to adequately controlled study in children and many are simply downward extensions of approaches that have been successful with adults. Strategies that include explicit methods of exposure include imaginal and in vivo systematic desensitization (using relaxation or various forms of imagery), prolonged exposure (flooding, implosion, and reinforced practice), and modeling. Additional strategies focus on increasing the probability of exposure by altering existing contingencies (contingency management) or by altering the child's expectancies about the consequences of the feared object (cognitive strategies).

There continues to be little empirical data to facilitate making decisions about which of these particular approaches will be most effective for a given child. The few existing controlled studies of treatment efficacy continue to support the superiority of treatments that include in vivo exposure to those that rely on vicarious approaches (such as modeling) for treatment of phobia. In one recent study, Menzies and Clarke (1993) compared three fear-reduction strategies for treating children with water phobias. The study included forty-eight children living in Australia, where water-related activities are quite popular. Children received one of three interventions: (1) in vivo exposure where children were gradually exposed to water; (2) vicarious exposure where they observed a live model engage in water-related activities; or (3) in vivo exposure plus vicarious exposure. Children who received the in vivo exposure with or without vicarious exposure showed the greatest improvement. Those who received both approaches did no better than those who received only in vivo exposure.

In light of the paucity of empirical findings to guide selection of treatment strategies, most researchers and clinicians rely on a combination of strategies, integrated into a treatment package to maximize the potential for positive outcome. Typically these packages expose children to the feared object while teaching them cognitive strategies to cope more effectively with feared situations and help them adapt responses that are incompatible with phobic behavior. In addition, positive reward is used contingent upon approaching the feared object. Parents are taught specific skills to avoid inadvertently reinforcing phobic behavior. Finally, sometimes the child's environment is modified to enhance the likelihood that the child will successfully approach the phobic stimuli. We will briefly describe these interventions and then illustrate how they can be combined into an effective treatment.

The most common approach to treating phobias is systematic desensitization. In a study of acceptability of fear reduction procedures (King and Gullone 1990), professionals rated systematic desensitization as the most effective and most acceptable approach to treat childhood phobia. The basic tenet of this strategy is that the child's fear response (anxiety) can be inhibited by teaching an alternative behavior, such as imagery or relaxation strategies, that is incompatible with a fear response. The child is gradually exposed to phobic stimuli while practicing these new skills. The phobic stimuli may be presented via imagery or in actuality (in vivo). Systematic desensitization is generally conducted in three steps. First, relaxation (imagery and/or muscular) or cognitive strategies such as self-talk or other self-regulatory behaviors are introduced. The second step involves developing a fear hierarchy to be used during the actual desensitization sessions. The child and parents can assist in developing a hierarchy of situations from those evoking little anxiety to those associated with more extreme levels of fear. A hierarchy for a dog phobic child may begin with seeing a small caged dog while accompanied by an adult and proceed to being completely alone with a large dog. The third step involves using relaxation or cognitive strategies while faced with items from the fear hierarchy, presented in vivo or through imagery. Parents are instructed to coach their child to use the relaxation or cognitive exercises while faced with fear-evoking stimuli in the home.

A closely related strategy is emotive imagery. Emotive imagery (King et al. 1989, Lazarus and Abramovitz 1962) involves use of fear-inhibiting images associated with bravery, accomplishment, or success. The child imagines a hero assisting successful interaction with the phobic situation. The hero may be a cartoon character or a figure from television. The critical ingredient is the child's ability to imagine the hero during exposure to the phobic situation.

Strategies involving prolonged exposure are based on the assumption that fear will be attenuated when avoidance of the phobic stimuli is not possible. While differing in theoretical origins, flooding and implosion both involve prolonged exposure to vivid images of the fear-evoking stimuli. Since there is no compelling evidence to suggest the superiority of these approaches, we can see no reason to justify their use. Reinforced practice, on the other hand, is based on sound behavioral principles with empirical support. Reinforced practice uses a combination of prolonged exposure and contingency management to reduce phobic behavior. The strategy uses repeated graduated practice in approaching the fear-evoking stimuli along with reinforcement for small gains in performance, feedback about progress, and instructions designed to promote success (Leitenberg and Callahan 1973). Leitenberg and Callahan demonstrated the efficacy of this combination of procedures for increasing children's tolerance of the dark.

Contingency management, including reinforcement for approach behaviors and removal of positive consequences of fear-related behaviors, is included as an adjunctive approach in many treatment plans. Goldberg and Weisenberg (1992) reported successfully treating a child with an unusual phobia of newspapers with positive reinforcement (tokens exchangeable for rewards) for interacting with newspapers. Most of the support for contingency management is derived from single case studies (Babbitt and Parrish 1991) or studies that use contingency management as one aspect of treatment (e.g., Leitenberg and Callahan 1973, Friedman and Ollendick 1989). Successful contingency management is dependent upon accurately identifying the contingencies maintaining the avoidance and altering them to increase approach behaviors. For children with fear of the dark, parents often inadvertently reinforce the child's fear by sleeping with or comforting the child. Parents are taught how to deal more effectively with their child's behavior by setting clear expectations, using tokens (exchangeable for a tangible reward or extra time with parents), and praising to reward appropriate behaviors and ignoring phobic behaviors.

The fear reduction strategy that has been subjected to the most systematic study (e.g. Melamed and Siegel 1975) is modeling. Modeling involves teaching appropriate behaviors vicariously through observing someone safely interacting with phobic stimuli. Empirical support for modeling is derived primarily from studies of fear reduction in children with medical or dental fears. As noted above, such fears are not necessarily similar to simple phobias, since the fear of actual harm and pain is realistic (although sometimes out of proportion to actual pain). There continues to be little support for modeling alone as an effective fear-reduction strategy for phobias although it may be a useful intervention within a multicomponent treatment package.

Cognitive strategies are based on the premise that the child's expectations, images, beliefs, and thoughts mediate the child's response toward phobic stimuli. Cognitive strategies are designed to teach children to employ positive mediating strategies to control their behavior in problematic situations. Three prominent strategies include cognitive modeling, problem solving, and self-instruction (Hobbs et al. 1980). Cognitive modeling is similar to the strategy described above except that the model verbalizes the specific strategy used to demonstrate the desired behavior (approaching phobic stimuli). Problem-solving techniques involve teaching children specific strategies to generate solutions to problems. Self-instruction training involves teaching the child to self-verbalize appropriate coping behaviors. While there is limited support for use of cognitive strategies alone to treat childhood phobia, they are often used as part of multicomponent treatment programs.

Treatment packages typically use a combination of these strategies. While behavioral principles have guided the development of a broad array of techniques, the selection, sequencing, and timing of strategies to develop a coherent treatment plan have received less attention (Evans 1989). We typically administer a number of strategies concurrently in an effort to maximize the potential for change. However, this decision is not empirically derived. Rather, it is based on the premise (rather unscientific) that more is better. Further empirical study is necessary to test this hypothesis.

DEALING WITH COMMON OBSTACLES TO SUCCESSFUL TREATMENT

Most of the actual treatment for phobia takes place outside of the weekly therapy sessions. The family is given the primary responsibility for implementing strategies in the home environment and tracking the child's progress. The most common obstacle we have encountered is when families fail to follow through on treatment between sessions. This is evident when families forget to complete home monitoring, skip homework assignments, fill out all daily home monitoring forms immediately before the child's next session, or reschedule sessions on regular intervals. More problematic are situations where parents report that they completed assignments during the week while the child states clearly that this had not occurred.

Difficulties in completing assignments may be due to a number of factors. The family may have more extensive difficulties than were apparent during the assessment. In this case, it is possible that the behavior targeted for change is entirely inappropriate. For example, targeting reduction in a child's fear of the dark will not effect change if the function of the child's disruptive behaviors at night is to disrupt parental arguing. As parents may not recognize the functional component of their child's nighttime behavior and may not reveal marital problems to the therapist, the fact that the target for change is inappropriate may not be apparent until the treatment fails. When treatment does not appear to be working, or when initial gains are lost, the therapist should consider the possibility that the behavior targeted for change is inappropriate.

Noncompliance may be due to the nature of the tasks being assigned rather than a failure in choosing the correct targets for change. The assignments may simply be too difficult for the family to complete. Children may find the assignments involving exposure too fear provoking. Alternatively, some children treated in our clinic have lost interest in therapy, complaining that the assignments were too "Mickey Mouse." Parents may also have difficulty with assignments. Changing contingencies in the home requires a change in parental response to their child. It is reasonable to assume that parents have long-standing patterns of interacting with their child. Changing these patterns sometimes requires more effort and motivation than parents are willing to exert. Finally, parents may not fully understand the tasks assigned or the purpose of the assignments, and thus may not be motivated to comply with them on a regular basis. There are also many concrete obstacles that can contribute to parental noncompliance, including a chaotic home environment, lack of available time to spend with the child, or monetary problems precluding purchasing necessary supplies (such as tangible rewards for compliance).

In the course of setting up a home monitoring procedure and/or an operant component for parents and children, numerous obstacles may arise. It is often difficult to determine what will be a reasonable incentive for a child. The process of choosing an effective incentive appears to be largely dependent on the individual child, his or her age, interests, and preferences. The reinforcer must be salient enough to motivate the child without becoming mundane. Often parents are concerned that using a motivator is similar to a bribe, and thus may not follow through with using the reinforcer as directed. In some cases, the incentive chosen is not salient enough, and the child quickly becomes habituated to it. On a related note, naturally occurring reinforcers, in the form of praise and positive attention, are potent reinforcers for long-term behavior change. Parents who do not appreciate their child's efforts, or who minimize the distress their child experiences, may have difficulty recognizing positive behavior change.

Different treatment strategies appear to have differential acceptability with different aged children. Which children will respond to which components of a package is often unpredictable. For example, some younger children may have difficulty with being able to use imagery as a strategy, whereas older children could view certain imagery or relaxation scripts as being too childlike. Some children will rate relaxation exercise, for example, as being the most effective skill they use regularly in reducing their levels of fear, whereas other children will find cognitive self-statements to be more powerful.

Finally, a most troubling situation is when parents have historically used ridicule and humiliation to attempt to reduce their child's fears. In such families, the child may have difficulty accepting treatment and trusting the parents. Further, the child's feelings of self-competency are likely to be fairly low. In such instances, treatment must include bolstering the child's confidence prior to implementing specific fear-reduction strategies.

RELAPSE PREVENTION

Relapse prevention is less an issue with phobic disorder than with any of the other anxiety disorders. There is ample evidence to suggest that gains made during treatment are generally maintained (Graziano and Mooney 1982, Hampe et al. 1973). However, at the onset of treatment we discuss three issues pertinent to relapse prevention. The first focuses on the possibility that the child's behavior may appear to worsen before it improves. Depending upon the target for change, treatment often involves changing contingencies in the home. Children may react to the change with an increase in the undesirable behavior prior to improvement once the contingencies are clear.

The second issue focuses on the possibility that the child may experience temporary setbacks during treatment. These may be related to additional stressors experienced by the child or the family or lack of consistency on the part of the parents. Either way, the family should be prepared for the possibility of lapses and assured that the lapse will be temporary. When lapses occur, parents should be instructed to return to the last level of treatment that was successfully completed.

The third issue is planned generalization of treatment gains to other fear-provoking situations. Prior to termination, treatment should involve practice of strategies in fear-provoking situations that differ from the initial complaint. These may include situations that are reliably associated with fear and anxiety (e.g., getting an injection, giving a speech, taking a test) as well as those where fear is apparent but not anticipated. Parents can serve as therapist extenders by prompting the child to use fear-reduction strategies in a variety of situations. A concrete plan should be developed for dealing with the possibility of relapse following termination of treatment. Parents should be encouraged to first attempt to reinstate the treatment program on their own. If the child does not respond, the parents can return for booster sessions to strengthen their skills and, if necessary, learn additional strategies.

TERMINATION

The major goal of treatment is to facilitate the child's successful interaction with phobic stimuli along with decreased subjective distress during such exposure. Presuming that no additional problems arise during treatment, therapy should be discontinued once the child can approach phobic stimuli with confidence. Prior to termination, as noted above, the therapist should prepare the child and parents to continue to use the strategies following termination of treatment.

Effective treatment for phobic disorders of childhood can usually be accomplished fairly rapidly, and after this has been achieved, timely termination of therapy has a number of advantages. Families rarely become excessively dependent upon the therapist and perceive themselves as the agent of change. Treatment success can (and should) be attributed to the family's efforts rather than the skill of the therapist. We hope such a stance will increase the family's confidence in their own abilities to solve problems as they arise in the future. We advocate scheduling a booster session for one month following treatment. At that time, the therapist can evaluate maintenance of treatment gains and provide corrective feedback to the family.

CASE ILLUSTRATION (TYPICAL TREATMENT)

Description and History

Kevin was a 13-year-old white male referred by his parents for treatment of persistent, intense fear of the dark. His parents felt that his fear had become sufficiently intense that it was disrupting his daily functioning, including his ability to concentrate in school. Kevin refused to go to bed alone unless his radio was playing and room was fully illuminated. He typically woke his parents several times at night complaining of fears of intruders. The entire family was chronically fatigued and Kevin's teachers were beginning to complain about his frequent naps during class. In other ways, Kevin appeared to be a well-adjusted child. He had many friends, performed above average in school, and participated in several extracurricular activities.

Kevin's nighttime fears were problematic for him and his family in several ways. Despite having many friends, he refused to participate in any activity that would require him to spend the night away from home. He refused invitations to spend nights at the homes of friends because, as he reported, "I'm embarrassed to be scared of the dark." During the interview Kevin's parents revealed that an intruder had entered their home in the middle of the night when Kevin was 8 years old. Kevin was awakened by the sounds of the intruder and immediately called his parents, who were asleep. Kevin's parents reported that his fears appeared to have begun soon after this traumatic incident. Kevin could not remember the intruder incident.

The assessment session, consisting of interviews with Kevin and his parents, completion of the FSSC-R (Ollendick 1983), RCMAS (Reynolds and Richmond 1978), CBCL (Achenbach and Edelbrock 1983), and a BAT revealed that Kevin had several fears, all of which appeared to be related. He reported fear of being alone at home, fear of dying and of being killed, fear of being the only member of the household awake, and fear of being kidnapped. Results of the BAT suggested he could remain in a darkened room without anxiety but the situation was not really similar to the situation that evoked his fear. Results of the CBCL were within the normal range.

Kevin attended therapy willingly. He complained of being tired most of the time and wanting to feel like a "normal kid like the rest of [my] friends." His previous attempts to alleviate his fears included listening to music in bed, telling himself not to be scared, and reading before bedtime to distract himself. None of these strategies were very effective.

Kevin's fears clearly met the criteria for simple phobia. His fears were disruptive, persistent, out of proportion to an actual threat, and unrealistic. The goal of treatment was to (a) increase Kevin's tolerance to being alone at night, (b) teach him alternative strategies to cope with the dark, and (c) teach his parents more effective methods to encourage Kevin to tolerate the dark. This was accomplished using a combination of relaxation training, cognitive self-instruction, reinforcement for brave behaviors at night, and reinforced practice.

Synopsis of Therapy Sessions

Session 1

1. Review home monitoring completed by parents and child, discuss difficulties, problems, and progress (repeat each session). Provide home monitoring forms for the following week.
2. Meet with the child and review conceptualization of phobia (as a learned response to a potential threat) and treatment plan. Explain rationale behind relaxation training and cognitive self-instruction.
3. Begin relaxation training using the exact procedure the child will practice at home, in the presence of the fear-provoking stimuli. Inquire about the effectiveness of the exercise and give feedback and recommendations for improvement.
4. Explain the rationale behind cognitive self-talk. Have the child generate statements to use at night to assist feeling brave. Select three brief statements and rehearse them with child.

Example:

Therapist: What are things you can say to yourself as a reminder that there is really nothing to fear?

Client: Well, I know that it is totally ridiculous to be scared. I am too old for this. We have new locks on the doors and a high tech alarm system. There is really no reason to be scared.

Therapist: So at night can you remind yourself that you are safe?

Client: I guess I can remind myself that the house is safe and I am not chicken.

Therapist: How about the statements: "The house is safe and I am brave. I can take care of myself. I am brave and everything is all right."

5. Discuss need for regular practice in the presence of phobic stimuli.

6. Construct a fear hierarchy of realistic situations involving fear-provoking stimuli, from situations that are associated with mild discomfort to extreme levels of fear. Select the mildest situation to be practiced during the week with parents. Administer a Fear Thermometer (Walk 1956) to assess the child's level of fear associated with approaching the hierarchy situation (if high, construct a less aversive situation).

7. Meet with parents and review basic behavioral principles. Have parents generate possible ways they may have inadvertently reinforced their child's fears in the past. Develop concrete methods for more effectively handling the child's usual phobic behavior including a plan to explicitly reward approach behaviors. Delineate criteria for tangible reinforcers. Review the importance of consistency, praise, encouragement, and ignoring low-level distress behaviors.

8. Teach parents relaxation and cognitive self-instruction so that they may serve as coaches between sessions. Give parents a relaxation training script and jot down the child's self-instruction statements.

9. Design specific procedures for an vivo exposure situation, based on the hierarchy discussed above, for the child to complete at home between sessions. Anticipate potential obstacles to completing assignments; generate practical solutions for overcoming the obstacles.

Session 2

1. Review with the child the homework assignment and home monitoring from the previous week. Elicit explicit details about

the child's behavior during the exposure sessions, praising any signs of improvement while minimizing the importance of difficulties. Generate solutions to overcome apparent obstacles.

2. Repeat the Fear Thermometer (weekly) to assess the child's level of fear during exposure to the fear stimuli the previous week.

3. Transcribe information from home monitoring to a chart to graphically display the child's progress.

4. Observe the child complete relaxation and cognitive self-instruction and provide corrective feedback and praise. Modify statements as appropriate.

5. Discuss the next level of fear hierarchy and review potential obstacles to completion.

6. Meet with parents. Review parents' home monitoring from previous week and compare it to that of the child. Examine the graphic display of the home monitoring with the parents. Discuss apparent problems or inconsistencies across raters and provide corrective feedback if necessary.

7. Inquire about any difficulties parents may have encountered while attempting contingency management.

8. Discuss implementing the next level of the fear hierarchy. Identify additional obstacles that may arise.

Sessions 3–6

1. Generally repeat procedures from sessions 1 and 2. Continue to review home monitoring with parents and child.

2. Proceed to fear situations associated with increasing levels of distress. Deal with setbacks by repeating a homework assignment that was successfully accomplished prior to continuing with a more difficult one.

3. Continue to reinforce family's efforts. Chart progress weekly to evaluate treatment efficacy. Make adjustments in the treatment plan when difficulties become apparent.

Comments

This protocol outlines a program that was successful for treating Kevin's long-standing fear of the dark in four weeks. The program is based on a treatment package developed by Graziano and his colleagues (Graziano, Mooney et al. 1979). Previous studies (Friedman and Ollendick 1989, Graziano and Mooney 1980, Ollendick et al. 1991) have supported the efficacy of this approach for treating children with severe fears of the dark and disruptive nighttime behaviors.

Kevin and his parents were excited about the program and were diligent about completing assignments. His parents had relatively good parenting skills and needed only corrective feedback to make the necessary changes to encourage Kevin to cope more effectively with the dark. It might have been necessary to modify the program if the parents had been less competent. We typically begin with an extended initial session (two hours) with subsequent sessions being briefer. If assessment revealed additional problems, the timing of the interventions would be altered. Younger children and families with coexisting difficulties benefit from learning the strategies more gradually across sessions.

Assessment revealed that Kevin's fears were being maintained by parental response to his distress. It is possible that the self-control training was an unnecessary treatment component and that contingency management alone may have been effective. In one study (Campbell and Friedman 1994), similar levels of improvement were noted for dark-phobic children treated with exposure plus either operant or cognitive strategies. Future studies are warranted to determine whether certain strategies are more effective for different types of fears or for different children.

CASE ILLUSTRATION (OVERCOMING OBSTACLES)

Description and History

Anna was a 9-year-old Caucasian female who was referred for psychological intervention by her physician after her parents reported that she was experiencing fears of being alone at night. Her parents viewed these fears as interfering significantly with the family's routine. She frequently insisted on sleeping with her brother or sisters, and she often remained awake until the early hours of the morning. She was usually difficult to awaken the next morning and had difficulty concentrating in school. Her younger sister and brother had begun to mimic Anna's behavior by refusing to sleep in their own beds or even enter a dark room by themselves. Anna's parents had concerns about the impact of Anna's fears on the entire family.

Although the complaints related to nighttime were quite typical of children with nighttime fears, Anna's history and circumstances surrounding the fears were quite different. Anna was born with muscular dystrophy and was hospitalized for months at a time. Due to pulmonary complications she slept with a ventilator. At the time of the referral, she relied on a wheelchair and was frequently fatigued. Anna's parents were particularly concerned about how her lack of sleep would affect her health.

The family traced Anna's fears to an episode that occurred a year earlier when she had been hospitalized for diagnostic procedures. Shortly after her parents had left for the night she began to feel her heart beating faster until she felt it pounding. She stretched to press the hospital intercom, which was slightly beyond her reach. Ultimately, she was able to summon help, but she recalled the event as "traumatic." From that point on, she recalled being scared of being alone, and being scared of dark places.

During the initial interview, Anna was articulate and cooperative. She appeared to have a good understanding of the purpose of the session and conveyed that she had talked with a psychologist during a previous hospitalization. She readily discussed her fears, her medical condition, and the impact of both on her life at home and school. In terms of school, she noted that the wheelchair impeded her mobility, making it difficult for her to participate in as many activities as she would like.

Anna spoke of her fears in vivid detail. Her fears focused on fear of cardiac arrest and being "trapped in bed with a skeleton." She reported that during the night she started thinking about being left all alone and then being killed by the skeleton. She added that these ideas seemed unrealistic to her during the day but were very vivid at night. She described images of a skeleton (which resembled her brother) lying next to her bed. She also feared not being able to get out of the bed. Her efforts to cope with her fears included pulling the covers over her head to protect herself and calling out for her parents. She had not tried any other fear-reduction methods.

Anna's parents shared her concerns about her health. They responded immediately to her calls at night and often spent the night with her. They also believed that families should communicate their fears and concerns openly. Parental arguments, concerns about finances, and conflicts with extended family members were discussed with Anna, who often rendered her opinion about potential solutions. Anna's mother often confided with Anna that she was also frightened by Anna's medical difficulties. Anna often reassured her mother that things would work out well. Anna frequently spent much of the night talking with her mother.

Synopsis of Therapy Sessions

In this case, Anna's fears may have met criteria for simple phobia but there were obvious differences between her fears and those of Kevin (discussed above). Anna's fears were understandable within the context of her severe medical difficulties. It was apparent that the focus of her fears (skeleton in the bed) was unrealistic but that her fear of harm was justifiable. A related concern was the parents' inclusion of Anna in discussions about difficulties that were clearly the responsibility of the parents. Anna's parents did not recognize the negative impact their behavior had on Anna. Further, expression of fear appeared to be the most reliable way for Anna to get attention from her parents, who attended only to negative behaviors and who were preoccupied with their own problems.

Session 1

1. As Anna's fears were related to inability to summon help when needed, the initial session included Anna and her parents and focused on making concrete changes in the home environment to increase consistency of the family's routine and reassure Anna that she was safe. Plans included:

   a. Environmental changes to ensure ability to contact parents in an emergency. These included placing next to the bed an intercom to communicate with her parents and a fog horn to use in the event of an emergency.

   b. Structuring a regular nighttime routine to increase predictability. Parents were instructed to establish a regular bedtime with prompts at ten- and five-minute intervals prior to the deadline. Anna was instructed to call her parents on the intercom once a night to assure her of its functioning. Her parents would come in and help her with her exercises.

2. Initiate home monitoring to be completed by Anna each morning. Anna was instructed to record (a) level of fear the night before (using a Likert scale), (b) whether she utilized the intercom system or fog horn, and (c) whether she used any strategy to attempt to cope with the fear.

3. Construct a fear hierarchy of fear-evoking situations that include internal cues and environmental cues. Identify a prompt she can use to alert her parents when she is beginning to experience fear.

4. Establish criteria for concrete reinforcement that takes the potentially realistic nature of her fears into account. Criteria for reward include (a) going to bed on time, (b) sleeping in own bed throughout night, and (c) using the intercom only once a night (unless warranted by medical difficulties).

Session 2

1. Review home monitoring and chart progress with Anna.
2. Teach Anna emotive imagery skills. Identify a hero that she can imagine helps her during fear-evoking situations. Practice a scene by discussing how she believes her hero would help her reduce her fear. Begin with a scene on the low end of the fear hierarchy. After the scene, administer a fear thermometer to assess level of fear.
3. Delineate steps for problem solving using emotive imagery at bedtime. Anna decided she could turn on the overhead light and check the bed for reassurance and then use emotive imagery to facilitate feeling brave.
4. Homework assignment to use problem solving and emotive imagery each night. Continue home monitoring.
5. Meet with parents. Instruct parents in how their own fears impact on Anna's. Review age-appropriate methods of communication and problem solving. Parents were instructed not to discuss their own fears in front of Anna. Rather, their approach should be positive and hopeful, conveying a sense that they are confident rather than fearful.
6. Discuss need to distinguish realistic threats from irrational fears. Help parents plan method for differentially responding to the two sources of fear.
7. Instruct parents on use of emotive imagery. Parents were instructed to prompt Anna to use emotive imagery at the first signs of fear.
8. Encourage parents to continue home monitoring.

Session 3

1. Review home monitoring and progress during the week.
2. Continue discussions about contingency management and effective communication with parents.
3. Since the function of Anna's fear behavior appeared to be related to attention provided by the parents, it was reasonable to assume that her parents were not reinforcing more appropriate behavior. Teach parents better behavior management

skills to reduce the need for Anna to seek attention in maladaptive ways. Increase praise and attention contingent on adaptive functioning.

4. Parents were referred for marital therapy to help improve their method of solving problems and communicating with each other.

Sessions 4+

Continue monitoring and review Anna's progress. Continue with emotive imagery and progress through higher levels of the fear hierarchy in sessions. Alter the criteria for tangible reward to reflect Anna's increasing ability to cope effectively at night. Introduce the concept of generalization of strategies to other fear-evoking situations, including her fears about impending surgery.

Comments

In light of the more complex nature of the case, simply focusing on Anna's response at nighttime would have been ineffective. The parents had no understanding of concepts related to age-appropriate roles and methods of communication. Further, the function of the parents' inclusion of Anna in adult discussion warranted exploration. Treatment goals included (a) distinguishing real from imaginary threats; (b) altering the environment to minimize the potential for genuine harm; (c) teaching Anna self-control strategies to help her cope with her fears, whether realistic or phobic; and (d) instructing parents in developmental principles and effective communication. Last, exploration of the parents' method of communicating revealed significant marital problems warranting more extensive intervention.

Anna was able to learn the strategies fairly rapidly despite her parents' continued marital discord. However, unlike Kevin, treatment was not terminated once she was able to cope with being alone in bed at night. She had significant difficulties in other spheres, including peer relations and depression. Thus, the target for treatment changed once she successfully mastered the strategies described above.

SUMMARY

Selection of assessment and intervention strategies for childhood phobia remains more an art than a science. Behavior therapy has contributed to the development of numerous techniques, many of which appear to be effective. However, aside from exposure, there is little empirical information to guide the clinician and researcher in selection of specific strategies for particular children. As noted earlier, our approach has been to combine techniques that have some empirical support in the hopes that multiple components will ensure the inclusion of at least one approach that will be effective for a given child. The same dilemma is associated with choice of assessment strategies. While it is customary to advise use of a multimodal, multichannel approach to assessment, we typically rely primarily upon direct observation and information gathered during the behavioral interview. The incremental advantage of including multiple measures for the development of a treatment plan remains uncertain.

Interest in children's phobias has increased markedly during the past decade. A number of researchers are now conducting more systematic study of issues related to diagnosis, assessment, and treatment of childhood phobia. We hope these efforts will result in more definitive suggestions about which treatments are most effective for which children.

REFERENCES

Achenbach, T. H., and Edelbrock, C. (1983). *Manual for the Child Behavior Checklist and Revised Child Behavior Profile.* Burlington, VT: University of Vermont, Department of Psychiatry.

Agras, W. S., Chapin, H. H., and Oliveau, D. C. (1972). The natural history of phobia. *Archives of General Psychiatry* 26:315-317.

Anderson, J. C., Williams, S., McGee, R., and Silva, P. (1987). DSM-III disorders in preadolescent children. *Archives of General Psychiatry* 44:69-76.

Babbitt, R. L., and Parrish, J. M. (1991). Phone phobia, phact or phantasy?: an operant approach to child's disruptive behavior induced by telephone usage. *Journal of Behavior Therapy and Experimental Psychiatry* 22:123-129.

Barrios, B. A., and Hartmann, D. P. (1988). Fears and anxieties. In *Behavioral Assessment of Childhood Disorders,* ed. E. J. Mash and L. G. Terdal, 2nd ed., pp. 196-262. New York: Guilford.

Bird, H. R., Canino, G., Rubio-Stipec, M., et al. (1988). Estimates of the prevalence of childhood maladjustment in a community survey in Puerto Rico. *Archives of General Psychiatry* 45:1120-1126.

Campbell, T. A., and Friedman, A. G. (1994). *Effects of cognitive and operant therapy on decreasing children's nighttime fears.* Manuscript submitted for publication.

Diagnostic and Statistical Manual of Mental Disorders (1987). 3rd ed. rev. Washington, DC: American Psychiatric Association.

Diagnostic and Statistical Manual of Mental Disorders (1994). 4th ed. Washington, DC.: American Psychiatric Association.

Eisen, A. R., and Silverman, W. K. (1991). Treatment of an adolescent with bowel movement phobia using self-control therapy. *Journal of Behavior Therapy and Experimental Psychiatry* 22:45-51.

Evans, I. M. (1989). A multi-dimensional model for conceptualizing the design of child behavior therapy. *Behavioural Psychotherapy* 17:237–251.

Friedman, A. G., and Ollendick, T. H. (1989). Treatment programs for severe nighttime fears: a methodological note. *Journal of Behavior Therapy and Experimental Psychiatry* 20:171–178.

Goldberg, J., and Weisenberg, M. (1992). The case of newspaper phobia in a 9-year-old child. *Journal of Behaviour Therapy and Experimental Psychiatry* 23:125–131.

Graziano, A. M., and De Giovanni, I. S. (1979). The clinical significance of childhood phobias: a note on the proportion of child-clinical referrals for the treatment of children's fears. *Behaviour Research and Therapy* 17:161–162.

Graziano, A. M., DeGiovanni, I. S., and Garcia, K. A. (1979). Behavioral treatment of children's fears: a review. *Psychological Bulletin* 86:804–830.

Graziano, A. M., and Mooney, K. C. (1980). Family self-control instructions for children's nighttime fear reduction. *Journal of Consulting and Clinical Psychology* 48:206–213.

Graziano, A. M., and Mooney, K. C. (1982). Behavioral treatment of "night fears" in children: maintenance of improvement at 2 1/2- to 3-year follow-up. *Journal of Clinical and Child Psychology* 50:598–599.

Graziano, A. M., Mooney, K. C., Huber, C., and Ignaziak, D. (1979). Self-control instructions for children's fear reductions. *Journal of Behavior Therapy and Experimental Psychiatry* 10:221–227.

Hampe, E., Noble, H., Miller, L. C., and Barrett, C. L. (1973). Phobic children 1 and 2 years posttreatment. *Journal of Abnormal Psychology* 82:446–453.

Hobbs, S. A., Moguin, L. E., Tyroler, M., and Lahey, B. (1980). Cognitive behavior therapy with children: has clinical utility been demonstrated? *Psychological Bulletin* 87:147–165.

Jersild, A. T., and Holmes, F. B. (1935). Methods of overcoming children's fears. *Journal of Psychology* 1:75–104.

Jones, M. C. (1924). A laboratory study of fear: the case of Peter. *Journal of Genetic Psychology* 31:308–315.

King, N., Cranstoun, F., and Josephs, A. (1989). Emotive imagery and children's night-time fears: a multiple baseline design evaluation. *Journal of Behavior Therapy and Experimental Psychiatry* 20:125–135.

King, N., and Gullone, E. (1990). Acceptability of fear reduction procedures with children. *Journal of Behavior Therapy and Experimental Psychiatry* 21:1–8.

Lang, P. J. (1968). Fear reduction and fear behavior: problems in treating a construct. In *Research in Psychotherapy*, vol. 3, ed. J. M Shlier. Washington, DC: American Psychological Association.

Last, C. G., Strauss, C. C., and Francis, G. (1987). Comorbidity among childhood anxiety disorders. *Journal of Nervous and Mental Disease* 175:726–730.

Lazarus, A. A., and Abramovitz, A. (1962). The use of emotive imagery in the treatment of children's phobias. *Journal of Mental Science* 108:191–195.

Leitenberg, H., and Callahan, E. J. (1973). Reinforced practice and reduction of different kinds of fears in adults and children. *Behaviour Research and Therapy* 11:19–30.

Marks, E. (1987). The development of normal fear: a review. *Journal of Child Psychology* 28:667–697.

Marks, I. M., and Gelder, M. G. (1966). Different ages of onset in varieties of phobia. *American Journal of Psychiatry* 123:218–221.

Melamed, B. G., and Siegel, L. J. (1975). Reduction of anxiety in children facing hospitalization and surgery by use of filmed modeling. *Journal of Consulting and Clinical Psychology* 43:411–521.

Menzies, R. G., and Clarke, J. C. (1993). A comparison of in vivo and vicarious exposure in the treatment of childhood water phobia. *Behaviour Research and Therapy* 31:9–15.

Ollendick, T. H. (1983). Reliability and validity of the Revised Fear Survey Schedule for Children. *Behaviour Research and Therapy* 21:685–692.

Ollendick, T. H., and Francis, G. (1988). Behavioral assessment and treatment of childhood phobias. *Behavior Modification* 12:165–204.

Ollendick, T. H., Hagopian, L. P., and Huntzinger, R. M. (1991). Cognitive-behavior therapy with nighttime fearful children. *Journal of Behavior Therapy and Experimental Psychiatry* 22:113–121.

Ollendick, T. H., and King, N.J . (1991). Origins of childhood fears: an evaluation of Rachman's theory of fear acquisition. *Behaviour Research and Therapy* 29:117–123.

Ollendick, T. H., King, N. J., and Frary, R. B. (1989). Fears in children and adolescents: reliability and generalizability across gender, age, and nationality. *Behavior Research and Therapy* 27:19–26.

Ost, L. G. (1987). Age of onset in different phobias. *Journal of Abnormal Psychology*. 96:223–229.

Reynolds, C. R., and Richmond, B. O. (1978). What I think and feel: a revised measure of children's manifest anxiety. *Journal of Abnormal Child Psychology* 6:271–280.

Shaw, J. (1990). Menstruation phobia treated by cognitive correction: a case report. *Journal of Behavior Therapy and Experimental Psychiatry* 21:49–51.

Silverman, W. K., and Kearney, C. A. (1992). Listening to our clinical partners: informing researchers about children's fears and phobias. *Journal of Behavior Therapy and Experimental Psychiatry* 23:71–76.

Strauss, C. C. (1992). Developmental differences in expression of anxiety disorders in children and adolescents. In *Anxiety across the Lifespan: A Developmental Perspective*, ed C. G. Last, pp. 63–77. New York: Springer.

Strauss, C. C., Last, C. G., Hersen, M., and Kazdin, A. E. (1988a). Association between anxiety and depression in children and adolescents with anxiety disorders. *Journal of Abnormal Child Psychology* 16:57–68.

Strauss, C. C., Lease, C. A., Last, C. G., and Francis, G. (1988b). Overanxious disorder: an examination of developmental differences. *Journal of Abnormal Child Psychology* 16:433–443.

Walk, R.D. (1956). Self ratings of fear in a fear invoking situation. *Journal of Abnormal and Social Psychology* 52:171–178.

8

CHRONIC ANXIETY

Andrew R. Eisen
Linda B. Engler

DESCRIPTION OF DISORDER

The definition of chronic anxiety in children is continually evolving and is inextricably connected to the diagnostic nomenclature. In 1962, chronic anxiety, then referred to as "overanxious reaction," became a formal diagnostic category in the *Diagnostic and Statistical Manual of Mental Disorders* (*DSM*, American Psychiatric Association 1962). Characteristic features included persistent anxiety, fears, self-consciousness, and somatic concerns (Jenkins 1968). Nevertheless, this category stimulated little research. With the advent of *DSM-III* and *DSM-III-R* (American Psychiatric Association 1980, 1987), chronic anxiety was referred to as overanxious disorder (OAD) and included similar but increasingly precise diagnostic criteria. Despite the refinements of the revised *DSM* systems, however, little research has been conducted to date on OAD.

According to *DSM-III-R* (American Psychiatric Association 1987), the essential feature of OAD was excessive or unrealistic worry that was not circumscribed in nature. Characteristic features also included excessive performance concerns, marked self-consciousness, and strong reassurance needs. Additionally, somatic complaints, including headaches, stomachaches, muscle tension, sweating, and shakiness, were common (Eisen and Silverman 1993, Kendall et al. 1991, Last 1991, Silverman and Eisen 1993).

DSM-III-R criteria for OAD have been criticized on a variety of grounds. First, an absence of impairment guidelines may have led to an overdiagnosis of the disorder (Silverman and Eisen 1993). Second, OAD lacked diagnostic distinctness because of its vague content (Klein and Last 1989; Silverman and Eisen 1993) and symptom overlap with other anxiety disorders (Beidel 1991). Due to these problems, the diagnostic category for chronic anxiety in children was changed in *DSM-IV* (American Psychiatric

Association 1994). In this system, OAD is subsumed under the revised category of generalized anxiety disorder (GAD). The central feature of GAD continues to be excessive and unrealistic worry; however, associated physical tension symptoms have considerably diminished in number (i.e., from eighteen to six symptoms) and include "restlessness, easily fatigued, difficulty concentrating, irritability, muscle tension, and sleep disturbance" (p. 436). Throughout the chapter we will use the terms *chronic anxiety*, *OAD*, and *GAD* interchangeably.

Although numerous investigators have examined prevalence rates of child/parent reports of childhood fears, worries, and general tension, prevalence data for specific *DSM-III/DSM-III-R* child anxiety disorders is just beginning to emerge. For example, Last and colleagues (1987a) and Mattison and colleagues (1988) indicated that 23–29 percent of children evaluated at specialty clinics for anxiety disorders were diagnosed with OAD. However, these percentages reflected general, not primary, diagnoses of OAD. With respect to primary diagnosis, Silverman and colleagues (Silverman and Eisen 1992, Silverman and Nelles 1988) found the prevalence of OAD to be 8–14 percent in clinical samples. Prevalence data from community samples indicated rates of OAD at 2.8–3.6 percent (Anderson et al. 1987, Bowen et al. 1990).

DIFFERENTIAL DIAGNOSIS

Recent evidence has indicated that children with OAD experience additional problems including separation anxiety disorder (SAD), simple phobia (SP), panic disorder (PD), social phobia (SOP), affective disorders and test anxiety (e.g., Beidel and Turner 1988, Last et al. 1987a, Strauss et al. 1988). For example, Last and colleagues (1987a) indicated that the most common additional diagnoses for overanxious children are SAD (30 percent), SP (27 percent), and PD (15 percent). The coexistence of OAD and PD is similar to Barlow and colleagues' (1986) finding that one-third of adults diagnosed with GAD also met the criteria for PD.

Social phobia also appears to be a frequent comorbid diagnosis with OAD. Last and colleagues (1987b) indicated that 36 percent of overanxious children met *DSM-III* criteria for SOP. Other investigators have confirmed this finding (Bernstein and Garfinkel 1986, Kashani and Orvaschel 1988). Overanxious children frequently presented with affective disorders as well (e.g., Last et al. 1987a, Strauss et al. 1988). In Last and colleagues' (1987a) sample, 34 percent of youngsters with OAD were diagnosed with major depression. This finding was similar to research indicating adult comorbidity of anxiety and affective disorders (e.g., Barlow 1988). Finally, Beidel and Turner (1988) found 60 percent of elementary school children with significant test anxiety had concomitant diagnoses of child anxiety disorders, including 24 percent with OAD. Thus, test anxiety appeared to be an important characteristic of OAD.

In *DSM-III-R*, differential diagnosis of OAD was relatively clear for most of the anxiety disorder categories. For example, excessive worry was not focused on major attachment figures (SAD), unfamiliar people (avoidant disorder), circumscribed stimuli (SP), panic attacks (PD), perceived inability to escape or get help in a certain place (agoraphobia), and was not bizarre and disturbing in nature (OCD). On the other hand, differential diagnosis became more precarious when comorbid social anxiety emerged. For example, in *DSM-III-R*, social phobic (e.g., fear of being embarrassed, humiliated) and overanxious features (e.g., performance concerns, self-consciousness) often overlapped. Because of the frequent commonalities of worries and social anxieties, Klein and Last (1989) suggested that diagnoses of both OAD and SOP were frequently warranted in youngsters. Perhaps in *DSM-IV*, the categories of GAD (which contains no social evaluative features) and social anxiety disorder will become more diagnostically distinct.

ASSESSMENT PROCEDURES

While an extensive literature exists regarding the assessment of general childhood anxiety via cognitive, behavioral, and physiological measures (Barrios and Hartmann 1988, Silverman and Kearney 1993), the literature is sparse with respect to OAD. This section will discuss current efforts to assess chronic anxiety in youngsters.

The clinical interview has become one of the most prominent and widely used assessment instruments in this area (e.g., Edelbrock and Costello 1984, Silverman and Kearney 1993). Several investigators have developed structured interviews to assess for a wide range of psychopathology in children and adolescents. The coverage and utility of the interview schedules with respect to the *DSM-III/III-R* childhood anxiety disorder categories vary considerably.

Several structured clinical interviews have been employed with overanxious children. These include the Diagnostic Interview Schedule for Children (DISC, Costello et al. 1985), Child Assessment Schedule (CAS, Hodges et al. 1982), Interview Schedule for Children (ISC, Kovacs 1985),

Schedule for Affective Disorders and Schizophrenia for School-Age Children (K-SADS, Puig-Antich and Chambers 1978), and Anxiety Disorders Interview Schedule for Children (ADIS-C and ADIS-P, Silverman and Eisen 1992, Silverman and Nelles 1988). For the most part, these interview schedules have yielded adequate reliabilities for diagnosing anxiety disorders (see Silverman 1991, in press, for reviews).

The ADIS-C (child version) and ADIS-P (parent version) are used at the Child Anxiety Disorders Clinic (CADC) at Fairleigh Dickinson University because of their greater coverage of the *DSM-III-R* childhood anxiety disorder categories compared to the other interview schedules. Recent data (Silverman and Eisen 1992) indicate that the ADIS-C (kappa = .85) and ADIS-P (kappa = .64) can be used to reliably diagnose OAD using a test-retest paradigm.

A wide variety of self-report measures have also been used in the assessment of anxiety disorders in children, and several of these measures have particular relevance in identifying salient characteristics of overanxious children. Three self-report measures that are particularly useful in assessing anxiety proneness or chronic anxiety are the Revised Children's Manifest Anxiety Scale (RCMAS, Reynolds and Richman 1978), the State-Trait Anxiety Inventory for Children (STAIC, Spielberger 1973), and the Child Anxiety Sensitivity Index (CASI, Silverman et al. 1991). Each of these scales is composed of both cognitive and somatic factors. For example, the RCMAS contains physiological, concentration, and worry/oversensitivity indices, of which the latter possesses the greatest utility for assessing OAD (Mattison et al. 1985, Mattison and Bagnatto 1987, Mattison et al. 1988).

Two self-report measures that are useful in assessing the cognitive component of OAD are the Negative Affectivity Self-Statement Questionnaire (NASSQ, Ronan et al. in press) and the Children's Negative Cognitive Error Questionnaire (CNCEQ, Leitenberg et al. 1986). The NASSQ and CNCEQ are useful for identifying self-defeating thought patterns that are associated with anxiety and depression.

Two measures that are useful in assessing the performance and social evaluative features of OAD are the Test Anxiety Scale for Children (TASC, Sarason et al. 1958) and the Social Anxiety Scale for Children-Revised (SASC-R, La Greca and Stone 1993). Other child self-report measures that we find useful at the CADC include the Piers-Harris Self-Concept Scale (PHSCS, Piers 1984), the Fear Survey Schedule for Children-Revised (FSSC-R, Ollendick 1983), the Daily Life Stressors Scale (Kearney et al. 1993), and the Children's Depression Inventory (CDI, Kovacs 1983).

In addition to the aforementioned child self-report measures, we administer several parent-completed measures at the CADC to achieve a multisource assessment. These measures assess parental ratings of child behavior, for example, Child Behavior Checklist (CBCL, Achenbach 1991), and parental psychopathology, for example, Fear Questionnaire (FQ, Marks and Mathews 1979), Beck Depression Inventory (BDI, Beck et al. 1961), Dyadic Adjustment Scale (DAS, Spanier 1976), and Parental Expectancies Scale (PES, Eisen et al. 1994). The PES measures parental expectancies concerning children's school performance, extracurricular activities, popularity, household responsibilities, and potential success in life.

In keeping with the tripartite assessment approach, it is important to assess the motoric and physiological channels of anxiety. Unfortunately, the literature is slim with respect to these two areas. While investigators have developed rating scales to observe children's anxiety in various settings, such as preschools (Glennon and Weisz 1978) and hospitals (e.g., Melamed and Siegel 1975, Melamed et al. 1975), and during peer interactions (O'Connor 1969), these scales have not been employed to observe overanxious children. The primary problem with OAD is that its pervasive nature may make it difficult to identify circumscribed anxiety elicitors (Silverman and Eisen 1993). When employing behavioral observation procedures in OAD, it is important to look for stimuli that evoke anxiety in specific situations such as tests and social interactions (Eisen and Silverman 1994, Strauss 1988). The role of behavioral observations in OAD awaits future research.

A modest amount of research has been conducted on the psychophysiological assessment of child anxiety (e.g., Beidel and Turner 1988, Melamed and Siegel 1975, Melamed et al. 1978, Van Hasselt et al. 1979). This literature indicates that heart rate (HR) and sweat gland activity are the most useful measures in assessing changes associated with stress and relaxation (Silverman and Kearney 1993). However, psychophysiological assessment with overanxious children is just beginning to be explored (Beidel and Turner 1988; Eisen and Silverman 1994). In our work with overanxious youth, we assess HR via a Computer Instruments Corporation (CIC) UNIQ Heart Watch (model 8799). With this instrument it is possible to assess HR during behavioral observations. Preliminary data indicate that the CIC HR watch yields reliable test-retest results in phobic children (Chapinoff 1992).

ESTABLISHING TREATMENT GOALS

In the case of chronic anxiety, it may be difficult to pinpoint specific problem areas due to a lack of circumscribed anxiety elicitors; therefore, accompanying elements of anxious apprehension such as somatic complaints and/or cognitive distortions need to be addressed. Because chronic anxiety is pervasive in nature, however, some triggering events may be present. Such events include performance (e.g., tests, sports), social (e.g., oral presentations, parties), and family (e.g., illness) situations.

The goals of an anxiety management program for chronically anxious youngsters should aim to (1) reduce generalized anxiety, (2) target somatic complaints and cognitive distortions, (3) attenuate avoidance behavior, and (4) address problematic comorbid disorders. This can be accomplished via relaxation and breathing exercises, cognitive restructuring, a graduated sequence of exposure-based homework assignments, and parent training techniques. It is important for clinicians to identify variables that are *maintaining* a child's anxious apprehension. These variables (e.g., specific situations, somatic complaints, cognitive distortions, parental attention for anxious behaviors) will determine the treatment procedure(s) that are implemented.

ROLE OF THE THERAPIST

Kendall (1991) described the therapeutic posture of the cognitive-behavioral child therapist as containing three essential elements. They are the therapist as consultant, the therapist as diagnostician, and the therapist as educator. First, the therapist as consultant promotes the development of independent, problem-solving skills. The therapist does not necessarily prescribe the single best solution to the child's anxiety but must convince the client that there are a variety of potentially successful strategies that can be evaluated in terms of their utility for the child and family.

The therapist as diagnostician goes beyond the client's verbal description of the problem and integrates information from a variety of sources in order to establish diagnoses and prescribe particular treatments associated with the anxiety-related symptoms. Finally, the therapist as educator teaches the child to engage in independent thought processes and increased behavioral control. The therapist further assists the child to develop areas of strength and minimize areas of weakness.

TREATMENT STRATEGIES

Currently, there exists an extensive literature on the cognitive-behavioral treatment of specific childhood fears and phobias such as test anxiety and nighttime fears (see Silverman and Eisen 1993, Silverman and Rabian 1993 for reviews), but few investigations have examined the treatment of diffuse anxiety characteristic of OAD. Only recently have investigators applied cognitive-behavioral treatment strategies with overanxious children (Eisen and Silverman 1993, Eisen and Silverman 1994, Kane and Kendall 1989, Kendall 1994).

Kane and Kendall (1989) employed a treatment package (sixteen to twenty sessions) with four overanxious children, 9 to 13 years of age, using a multiple baseline design. This integrated treatment program (see Kendall et al. 1992 for full explication) included a variety of cognitive-behavioral components. Cognitive strategies included self-control elements (self-monitoring, self-evaluation, and self-reinforcement) that formed a cognitive coping plan. Behavioral components included imaginal and in vivo exposures, relaxation training, modeling, role-plays, and contingency management procedures. Additionally, homework assignments were given each week to help reinforce and generalize the skills taught during therapy sessions.

The results indicated that all children experienced improvement on parent (CBCL), clinician (modified Hamilton scale), and child self-report (STAIC-T) measures. Although treatment gains were generally maintained at posttreatment and follow-up, two children continued to experience some difficulties in the clinical range (i.e., somatic complaints and total internalizing factor on CBCL).

Recently, Kendall (1994) compared his integrated treatment protocol to a wait-list control group in the first randomized clinical trial with anxious youth. Sixty-four percent of these children, aged 9 to 13, received *DSM-III-R* diagnoses of OAD. Multimethod assessment included child (e.g., RCMAS, STAIC, FSSC-R, CDI), parent (CBCL), and teacher (Teacher Report Form, TRF, Achenbach and Edelbrock 1983) reports as well as behavioral observations (Glennon and Weisz 1978).

The results indicated significant improvements for the treated children as compared to the wait-list controls on child and parent measures. In fact, 64 percent of the treated youngsters (compared to 5 percent of the controls) did not receive an anxiety diagnosis at posttreatment. Treatment gains were generally maintained at one-year follow-up. Although the results of this randomized trial are impressive, the specific ingredients responsible for behavior change were impossible to determine due to the combination of treatment procedures employed.

Eisen and Silverman (1993) examined the specific contributions of relaxation training/exposure (RT) and cognitive therapy/exposure (CT) with four overanxious children, 6 to 15 years of age, using a multiple baseline design. Each subject received both RT and CT (counterbalanced), followed by combined treatment. Subjects were administered eighteen biweekly sessions with each condition lasting three weeks.

The CT intervention was similar to the cognitive component of Kendall and colleagues (Kane and Kendall 1989, Kendall et al. 1992) and emphasized self-control elements in the form of a cognitive coping plan. The major components of the RT intervention included an awareness of somatic symptoms when scared and a progressive muscle relaxation exercise for eleven body parts (Ollendick and Cerny 1981). Both interventions included a graduated sequence of imaginal and in vivo exposures to relevant fear/anxiety-provoking situations associated with the child's distressing thoughts/physical symptoms (based on hierarchy), homework assignments, and relapse prevention exercises. The combined intervention incorporated all elements of the two previous treatments.

The results indicated that all interventions were associated with diminished anxiety based on child (RCMAS, STAIC-T, CDI), parent (CBCL, parent rating of severity), and clinician ratings (ADIS-C) and were generally maintained at posttreatment and follow-up. Like the Kane and Kendall study, two subjects continued to experience some difficulties in the clinical range (e.g., CBCL scales: somatic complaints, anxious/obsessive). In both investigations, these subjects experienced extensive diagnostic comorbidity. The most interesting finding, however, was that interventions were most effective when they appeared "matched" to a subject's problematic response class. In other words, children benefitted most from CT, RT, and their combination if they experienced primarily cognitive symptoms, primarily somatic complaints, or both cognitive and somatic symptoms, respectively.

This finding coupled with adult anxiety investigations (Ost et al. 1981, Ost et al. 1982) suggesting the efficacy of matched or prescriptive treatments prompted Eisen and Silverman (1994) to examine the effectiveness of matched and mismatched treatments with overanxious children. Eisen and Silverman (1994) matched and mismatched cognitive-behavioral interventions with four overanxious children, 8 to 12 years of age, using a multiple baseline design. Assessment data were used to identify children with either a cognitive (i.e., CNCEQ, RCMAS, daily diaries) or somatic (CBCL, CASI, heart rate in an in vivo behavioral observation) problematic response class. Treatments consisted of CT and RT, and both interventions contained an exposure component.

The first two subjects were identified as having somatic and cognitive problematic response classes respectively, and received matched treatment.

Subject 1 (somatic) received RT whereas subject 2 (cognitive) received CT. Each treatment protocol consisted of ten biweekly sessions. The third and fourth subjects both initially received ten sessions of mismatched treatment (i.e., CT for somatic and RT for cognitive), followed by ten sessions of matched treatment.

The results indicated that matched treatments were superior to mismatched treatments. Three of four subjects receiving matched treatments scored within normal limits on self-report (child and parent) measures, behavioral observations, and physiological data. In fact, these subjects did not receive a *DSM-III-R* diagnosis of OAD at posttreatment based on independent clinician ratings (e.g., ADIS-C). These findings were generally maintained at six-month follow-up. Although subject 2 (matched CT) markedly improved, he was still experiencing some difficulties (CNCEQ, CBCL) at posttreatment and follow-up. Interestingly, this subject was experiencing several severe comorbid disorders. This finding is consistent with other OAD investigations (Eisen and Silverman 1993, Kane and Kendall 1989, Kendall 1994). Subjects receiving mismatched treatments experienced uneven improvements and failed to satisfy positive end-state functioning. This investigation lends preliminary support to the efficacy of prescriptive treatments in OAD.

DEALING WITH COMMON OBSTACLES TO SUCCESSFUL TREATMENT

Eisen and Kearney (1995) discuss a number of factors that can interfere with optimal treatment success when working with anxious youth. These factors differ in the degree to which they can interfere with treatment progress and in the degree to which they can be overcome.

The first obstacle is a lack of motivation on the part of the parent and/or child. A parent may lack the required motivation to exert the degree of energy needed to change patterns of behavior that have become habitual. For example, this can occur if parents accomodate their anxious child by allowing her to sleep in their bedroom. In this case, parents will need to make a commitment to taking the child back to her bedroom each time she comes into theirs and handling the increase in demanding behavior that can result from this new pattern of parental response.

A child can also demonstrate a lack of motivation to fully invest herself in the treatment program. This can result from lack of information about the beginning phase of treatment and from feeling little control regarding the decision to engage in the treatment. These obstacles can be overcome by focusing on building rapport and setting an expectation for success in terms of how the treatment will help the child to do something she would like to do but is currently unable to do (e.g., sleep at a friend's house).

Another obstacle that may relate to lack of motivation is noncompliance in the form of poor attendance and failure to complete homework assignments (e.g., diaries, exposures). Parents may be uncomfortable with the treatment procedures (e.g., placing the child in anxiety-provoking situations). Explanations of the need to shape behavior and habituate to anxiety, and the effects of parental accomodation can be helpful in alleviating some noncompliance. It is more likely, however, that the child will evidence directly noncompliant behavior with regard to the treatment process. Children may find exposures to anxiety-producing stimuli to be unpleasant, may not wish to commit themselves to the task of completing daily diaries, and may find aspects of the treatment sessions somewhat uncomfortable. In addition, a pattern of noncompliant behavior at home may have arisen through the "criticism trap" (Silverman 1989) where the parent learns that yelling terminates noncompliant behavior and children learn to engage in noncompliant behavior to gain attention. It is helpful to increase the attractiveness of completing the treatment program and work with the parents to reduce negative interactions with the child at home.

Another factor that can interfere with optimal treatment progress is parental modeling of fearful coping behavior for their children. Instead of learning to confront and cope effectively with anxiety-provoking situations, children may continue to learn to be fearful by observing their parents' responses during exposures. If this occurs, parents can be taught to serve as a coping rather than an anxious model by maintaining a calm posture during exposures (e.g., Kendall 1991).

Parental overprotection can provide an additional obstacle to successful treatment, especially when parents do not permit their children to be exposed to potentially fearful situations. The key to addressing this resistance is to alleviate parental anxiety. This can be accomplished by designing a graduated sequence of exposure-based homework assignments for the child and emphasizing shaping procedures with parents (Silverman 1989).

Unrealistic parental expectancies, like parental overprotection, may be the product of good intentions but result in increased anxiety for a child. High parental expectations can result in increased achievement when goals are appropriate for a child's level of ability and/or interest. However, unrealistic parental expectations that exceed a child's ability can produce increased anxiety, avoidance, and oppositional behavior.

In some of the cases we treat at the CADC, parental psychopathology is present and can interfere with treatment outcome. Not only can parents be overprotective and have unrealistic expectations, but parents of anxious children sometimes experience severe psychological disorders, such as depression, panic disorder, or alcoholism. Generally, we find that parental psychopathology need not interfere with treatment. In rare instances, however, we do encounter parents whose psychopathology interferes with their ability to participate in and/or complete the treatment program (e.g., inconsistent parenting, emotional/physical abuse). In such cases, we find it is best to recommend an appropriate treatment referral for the parent. Individual parent treatment may be a necessary precursor for the parent and child to focus on the anxiety treatment program. In other cases, however, concurrent parental treatment is sufficient for the family to be able to comply with the treatment program.

Last, successful treatment can be hampered when an anxious child is experiencing other comorbid disorders (see Perrin and Last, this volume) such as depression, attention deficit hyperactivity disorder, or oppositional defiant disorder. The severity of comorbid disorders will determine the necessity for treatment modifications or referral to other sources.

RELAPSE PREVENTION

Kendall and colleagues (Kendall 1991, Kendall and Treadwell 1993) noted that the assumption that therapy cures anxiety can be unfortunate and deceiving. Therapists and clients must be aware that the possibility of relapse exists and needs to be addressed. Kendall and Treadwell (1993) suggested several guidelines for relapse prevention at the conclusion of treatment. First, children should be encouraged to develop "effort attributions" (p. 169) regarding their newly gained control of anxiety symptoms. Children who believe that their own hard work is responsible for improvement during treatment will be more likely to continue self-reinforcement of their own efforts for partial successes after treatment. Children should also be encouraged to attribute increased anxiety symptoms after treatment as "lapses in effort" (p. 169) rather than relapses. Children who expect lapses and partial successes will be less likely to attribute them to personal ineptitude. Children need to be taught to recognize lapses as temporary and a signal for them to return to active problem-solving efforts (Kendall and Treadwell 1993, Silverman 1989).

Silverman and Eisen (1993) stated that relapse prevention must be "explicitly programmed and structured" (p. 189) in the treatment program for maintenance of progress. They devote an entire session to relapse prevention (Silverman 1989) and review the major ideas again in a subsequent session. Relapse prevention begins by reviewing a child's progress in therapy and helping her develop an expectation that progress will be maintained and continued, especially if newly gained coping skills continue to be utilized. Children are cautioned that slips will occur, but this is openly discussed in terms of how to handle such an event. This discussion is supplemented by a handout that specifies a plan for steps to take if a slip should occur. Educating parents on the likelihood of and suggested plan for resolution of slips is seen as an essential component of relapse prevention.

Kendall and Treadwell (1993) also suggested that continued therapeutic contact (phone or booster sessions) can be helpful in reassuring the child that progress is not lost and that the child is capable of returning to her problem-solving plan. Preventive booster sessions can help the child cope with anticipated anxiety-provoking events in a more proactive, independent manner.

TERMINATION

The end of the therapy program is a time where the child may experience a variety of conflicting feelings. Silverman and Eisen (1993) suggested using this time to review a child's progress in therapy and discuss the child's feelings about termination. Feelings may range from sadness about leaving therapy and difficulty separating from the therapist to excitement at having become more independent and effective at confronting fears. Children should be encouraged to develop feelings of confidence in their ability to continue using the skills they have learned and that they will continue to improve in their anxiety management abilities. Carefully programmed relapse prevention activities can help promote a positive outlook toward posttreatment functioning.

CASE ILLUSTRATION (TYPICAL TREATMENT)

Description and History

Kevin is a 12-year-old white male referred to the CADC for evaluation of chronic general fearfulness and an inability to relax. His primary complaints included multiple somatic symptoms (stomachaches, headaches, tension, nausea, body pains, and constipation) that were associated with taking tests, schoolwork, waking up at night, and new situations. During the interview, Kevin exhibited a fidgety restlessness and had difficulty relaxing. His eye contact and affect were appropriate and he was fully cooperative in answering the examiner's questions. Based on the ADIS-C, Kevin received a primary diagnosis of OAD (moderate severity) and mild social and specific phobias (e.g., traveling by plane). Self-report data (e.g., FSSC-R, TASC, CASI, and the SASC-R) were consistent with the diagnostic impressions. Due to Kevin's extreme test anxiety, he was asked to complete the Block Design subtest of the WISC-III with concurrent assessment of fear and HR. The latter measure was substantially elevated (i.e., 20 beats per minute above baseline) during the performance phase of the exposure and was seen to be in need of modification.

During the parent interview, Kevin's mother described her son as "anxiety prone" and indicated that he had had difficulty relaxing since he was a toddler. Additionally, she indicated that Kevin worried a great deal about "performance" concerns (e.g., taking tests, sports). Although Kevin's school performance was satisfactory, his mother felt that he wasn't fulfilling his potential. Based on the ADIS-P, Kevin received diagnoses of OAD (moderate severity) and mild social and specific phobias. Parent-completed questionnaires indicated that Kevin was experiencing excessive somatic complaints (e.g., CBCL) and that his mother was placing undue pressure on him to succeed in school and in general (e.g., PES). Finally, Kevin's mother was experiencing multiple fears (e.g., FQ), was not depressed (e.g., BDI), and her marital relationship was intact (e.g., DAS).

Synopsis of Therapy Sessions

After an initial evaluation (interview and questionnaires), families are asked to attend a consultation in which specific feedback is given regarding the nature of the youngster's anxious apprehension and maintaining variables. Following family consent for treatment, children are trained in self-monitoring (i.e., daily diaries) and asked to keep track of relevant situational variables, fearful thoughts, avoidance behavior, and daily ratings of anxiety for a baseline period of one to two weeks (Silverman 1989). Although primary responsibility for completing the diaries rests with the child, factors such as age, maturity, cognitive level, and motivation will determine whether or not this task becomes a family endeavor. In addition, during the consultation we often design a simulated exposure and concurrently assess fear ratings and HR.

At the CADC, therapy sessions are divided into separate child and parent segments with the last portion of the therapy session devoted to the entire family. The child session is conducted first because the focus of the program is directed at targeting and alleviating the child's anxious apprehension. The parent session is provided to educate family members regarding the therapeutic ingredients of the program and to facilitate maintenance and generalization of treatment effects. In Kevin's case, because he was experiencing primarily somatic complaints, we opted for a prescriptive approach that emphasized progressive relaxation training (Ollendick and Cerny 1981) coupled with imaginal and in vivo exposures. In the following section, we briefly outline such a protocol on a session-by-session basis (Kendall et al. 1992, Silverman 1989).

Session 1

1. Establish rapport, review baseline diaries, and address any motivational or compliance difficulties.
2. Present somatic conceptualization of anxious apprehension. Identify physical sensations associated with fear and avoidance and replace with controlled breathing and relaxation exercises.
3. Construct a fear hierarchy (both child and parent sessions). The idea is to identify six to ten scenarios that can serve as exposures. It is helpful to highlight at least two situations each of mild (e.g., anxious apprehension without avoidance), moderate (e.g., considerable anxious apprehension with a nagging reluctance to participate), and extreme (heightened anxious apprehension with or without strong avoidance behavior) severities. At the CADC, we use a 0–8 scale to rank order the severity of situations. With younger children, we use a Fear Thermometer (Melamed et al. 1978), which differentiates fear levels by increasingly hot colors. In the case of chronic anxiety, it may be difficult to identify circumscribed anxiety elicitors. Thus, it is important to identify situations that trigger anxious apprehension. In Kevin's case, his hierarchy was composed primarily of performance-based (e.g., tests, schoolwork, competitive sports) and novel (e.g., parties) situations.
4. Assign homework assignments (HW): daily diaries and list of problematic physical sensations experienced.

Session 2

1. Review diaries and HW (emphasize role of somatic sensations).
2. Finalize hierarchy.
3. Review rationale about muscle tensing and controlled breathing to relax.
4. Introduce first half of progressive muscle relaxation script (Ollendick and Cerny 1981) that emphasizes tensing and relaxing the hands and arms, arms and shoulders, shoulders and neck, and jaw. (Make audiotape for child.)
5. Practice relaxation exercises (model/role-play).
6. Assign HW: daily diaries, practice relaxation exercises twice daily (with and without tape).

Session 3

1. Review diaries and HW. Assess compliance about practicing relaxation exercises.
2. Introduce the second portion of the relaxation script, which emphasizes tensing the jaw, face and nose, stomach, and legs and feet (record for child on the same audiotape).
3. Practice relaxation exercises (model/role-play).
4. Introduce diaphragmatic breathing exercises (King 1980). Imagery is used in the form of a hot air balloon ride. A child is encouraged to take a journey to a far-off and exciting place. As a child describes her expedition (with therapist assistance), she breathes in and breathes out, making a SSSSSS sound. It is explained to a child that her breathing fuels the hot air balloon. To facilitate this imagery, we have a picture of a hot air balloon in the therapy room.
5. Practice breathing exercises (model/role-play).
6. Explain how relaxation can be used as a coping strategy and model using an anxiety-provoking situation not relevant to the child.
7. Conduct an imaginal exposure using the lowest item on the child's hierarchy.

Example:

Therapist: Kevin, what happens when you do your homework at night?
Client: I start to get very tense [biting lips].

Therapist: Can you be more specific?

Client: My stomach gets tight . . . I have trouble thinking.

Therapist: Kevin, I would like you to sit back in your chair and close your eyes [dim lghts]. Try to relax all the muscles in your body. I want you to imagine that you are doing your last math assignment. . . . Where are you now?

Client: I'm in my room sitting on my bed.

Therapist: Can you describe what you see?

Client: I'm looking at my desk . . . it's a mess. I'm thinking that I don't want to do my homework.

Therapist: What physical sensations are you experiencing?

Client: Well . . . my stomach is tight, my hands are sweating . . . and my head is starting to hurt.

Therapist: How tense are you on that zero to four scale?

Client: Maybe a two . . .

Therapist: Kevin, I want you to practice your breathing exercises. Where will you be going today?

Client: How about Maine?

Therapist: Sounds good. . . . Okay, start your breathing exercises to fuel the hot air balloon.

Kevin breathes in through his nose and breathes out through his mouth, making a SSSSSS sound. This process should continue until a child is breathing in a slowed, rhythmic fashion.

Therapist: Kevin where are you now?

Client: I'm floating over the ocean.

Therapist: What do you see?

Client: I see beaches . . . people . . . many rocks.

Therapist: What does the breeze feel like?

Client: Oh . . . it's great! Nice and cool.

Therapist: What is your rating on that zero to four scale?

Client: Still a two.

Therapist: Check your fuel.

Client: It's low . . . [Kevin begins breathing exercises].

Therapist: Kevin, could you go back to your homework?

Client: No . . . I'm distracted.

Therapist: What are you thinking about?

Client: What if my mom and teacher doesn't think it's good enough?

Therapist: Has that ever happened?

Client: Not really. . . .

Therapist: How tense are you right now on that zero to four scale?

Client: Still a two . . . maybe a little more.

Therapist: Which relaxation exercises will you perform now to reduce your anxiety?

Client: I will clench my fists . . . stretch my arms and shoulders, clench my teeth . . . wrinkle up my forehead [Kevin performs each exercise].

Therapist: Great! How do you feel?

Client: Pretty relaxed.

Therapist: How is your homework coming along?

Client: I'm almost finished . . . I think I did a pretty good job.

8. Assign HW: daily diaries, practice relaxation and breathing exercises, first in vivo exposure during the week (same as imaginal in this session).

Sessions 4 +

1. Continue to conduct imaginal (in session) and in vivo exposures (out of session) to increasingly anxiety-provoking items on the hierarchy using the relaxation and breathing techniques as a coping strategy.
2. Continue to assign the daily diaries, relaxation and breathing exercises (practice twice daily).
3. Teach family members to replace ineffective strategies (e.g., overprotection, criticism) to address their child's anxious apprehension with encouragement to use the relaxation and breathing exercises.
4. Discuss relapse prevention and termination issues.
5. Make arrangements for periodic follow-up visits.

Comments

This protocol is recommended for anxious youth experiencing primarily somatic complaints and heightened physiological arousal (Eisen and Kearney 1995, Eisen and Silverman 1994). In Kevin's case, other adjunctive treatment strategies such as cognitive therapy and contingency contracting were unnecessary because cognitive distortions and compliance issues were not problematic. In fact, preliminary data (Eisen and Silverman 1994) suggest that a prescriptive relaxation training/exposure protocol is effective in alleviating negative self-statements without any specific cognition targeting.

At the conclusion of the ten-week program, Kevin scored within normal limits on somatic measures (CASI, CBCL, and HR) and treatment gains were maintained for over one year. Although this approach appears promising, overanxious children often experience a combination of cognitive and somatic symptoms as well as extensive comorbidity. For this reason, assessment data should determine the type of intervention strategies employed and comprehensiveness of the treatment program. In this way, children and their families will receive the most effective and economical treatment program possible.

CASE ILLUSTRATION (OVERCOMING OBSTACLES)

Description and History

Jennifer was a 13-year-old white female referred to the CADC for an evaluation of chronic worry and sadness. Her primary complaints were multiple worries regarding family, personal harm, being teased, and hospitals. During the interview her eye contact was marginal and her affect was restricted. The majority of her answers to the examiner's questions were short, terse responses. She fidgeted throughout the interview and asked to be excused to the restroom on several occasions. Jennifer did speak freely, however, about her parents' relatively recent divorce (two years ago). Within minutes she began to cry and continued to do so sporadically throughout the interview. Based on the ADIS-C, Jennifer received a primary diagnosis of OAD (severe) and several comorbid diagnoses that included dysthymia (moderate-severe), social phobia (moderate), and several specific phobias that were of mild to moderate severity (e.g., blood, hospitals). Self-report data were consistent with diagnostic impressions and indicated heightened levels of negative affectivity (NASSQ, CNCEQ), worry (RCMAS), multiple fears (FSSC-R), and borderline levels of clinical depression (CDI).

Based on the parent interview, Jennifer's mother indicated that her daughter was always "high strung" and an avid worrier, yet a pleasant and sociable individual. Her mother also indicated that Jennifer had lost some interest in her friends and had become increasingly withdrawn since the time of the divorce. Based on the ADIS-P, Jennifer received a primary diagnosis of OAD (severe) with moderate to severe comorbid diagnoses of dysthymia and social phobia. Parent-completed questionnaires indicated that Jennifer was withdrawn and anxious/depressed (CBCL) and that her mother had elevated expectancies concerning her schoolwork (PES). Last, Jennifer's mother was experiencing multiple fears (FQ) and borderline levels of clinical depression (BDI).

Synopsis of Therapy Sessions

Following consent for treatment and training in self-monitoring (i.e., daily diaries), we opted for a prescriptive approach emphasizing cognitive self-control procedures (e.g., Kendall et al. 1992, Silverman 1989) because Jennifer was experiencing primarily anxious and depressogenic cognitions. We describe such an approach on a session-by-session basis.

Sessions 1–3

1. Establish rapport, review baseline diaries, address motivational or compliance difficulties.

Overcoming Obstacles:

Review of Jennifer's baseline diaries indicated sporadic performance. She indicated that she was just "too tired" to keep track of her thoughts all the time. In addition, her mother's "nagging" attempts at fostering compliance proved futile. For this reason, a contingency contracting component was added to the program. Contingent reinforcers (e.g., movie rentals, new clothes) not only enhanced her compliance with the daily diaries but also renewed her enthusiasm for the program.

2. Create a supportive atmosphere to foster a therapeutic alliance. In Jennifer's case, the first few sessions were largely devoted to discussions of nonthreatening topics. This was necessary to help establish trust and build momentum so that Jennifer could marshal enough energy to fully participate in the treatment program.
3. HW: daily diaries, list of frequently experienced negative self-statements (anxious and depressive).

Session 4

1. Review diaries and HW (emphasize cognitive distortions).
2. Present cognitive conceptualization of negative affectivity. Identify cognitive distortions that help maintain anxiety, depression, and avoidance and employ cognitive restructuring techniques to combat negativistic thinking.

3. Construct exposure hierarchy. Jennifer's hierarchy consisted primarily of family (ambivalent relationship with her father, household responsibilities) and social issues (e.g., being teased at school). Despite her love for her father, Jennifer avoided him due to strong feelings of guilt and anxious apprehension. One goal of the program was to teach Jennifer to confront her father and realistically appraise her associated negativistic thoughts and feelings.
4. Introduce cognitive techniques (e.g., Beck and Emery 1985, Kendall et al. 1992, Silverman 1989).
5. Practice cognitive techniques (model/role-play).

Example:

Client: I didn't go to school today [frowning].

Therapist: Why not?

Client: Everyone would have made fun of me. They would think my clothes looked ridiculous. It's just that . . . well . . . we don't have much money and mom is working so hard. . . . It's just not fair!

Therapist: Jennifer, who is *everyone*?

Client: Two girls in my social studies class . . .they just don't like me.

Therapist: What do they do?

Client: They laugh at me when I walk past them in the hallway.

Therapist: How often does that happen?

Client: Well . . . maybe once a week.

Therapist: Are these two girls your friends?

Client: No way! No one likes them.

Therapist: Does anyone else make fun of your clothes?

Client: Not really.

Therapist: So what you're saying is that maybe once a week, two girls, who no one cares for, might laugh at you because they don't like your clothes?

Client: Yes . . .

Therapist: Do you like your clothes?

Client: Well yes . . . I think they're pretty neat.

Therapist: So what is the worst thing that could happen if you went to school today?

Client: The worst thing?. . .Well . . . those two girls might laugh at me but I would just ignore them because no one likes them anyway.

Therapist: Great! Will you go to school tommorow?

Client: Definitely!

6. HW: daily diaries, practice cognitive techniques in relevant situations during the week.

Session 5

1. Review diaries and compliance in practicing cognitive techniques.
2. Finalize hierarchy.
3. Review therapy rationale: Employ cognitive restructuring techniques to replace negativistic thinking.
4. Introduce self-control acronym. In our work with anxious youth, we use the **STOP** acronym (Silverman 1989), which stands for the following:
   S: Scared? (recognize anxiousness)
   T: Thoughts? (fearful in nature, worries)
   O: Other thoughts? (coping in nature)
   P: Praise? (positive self-evaluations)
   The idea is for youngsters to **STOP their anxiety.** We find the concrete nature of this acronym to be extremely useful in helping children successfully apply self-control strategies.
5. Practice (model/role-play) using the STOP acronym in several anxiety-provoking situations.
6. Conduct imaginal exposure using lowest item on the hierarchy.

Example:

Therapist: Jennifer, I want you to imagine visiting your father this weekend. Can you describe what you see?
Client: I'm sitting in my room alone, crying and feeling very nervous.
Therapist: Why are you Scared?
Client: My mom is calling me and telling me to get ready.
Therapist: Thoughts?
Client: My dad will spend all his time with his wife and my stepbrother. He doesn't love me. . . . I'll do something to upset him.
Therapist: Other thoughts?
Client: Well . . .
Therapist: How much time does your dad spend with you over the weekend? Can you give me a percentage?
Client: Maybe 40 percent of the time. . . . He spends a lot of time with my stepbrother.
Therapist: How old is he?

Client: One.

Therapist: Do you spend time with your stepbrother?

Client: Yes! I'm with him all the time. He's so cute!

Therapist: So if you and your dad are always with your stepbrother how much time do you actually spend with your dad?

Client: I guess I'm with him most of the time, but he doesn't spend much time talking to me.

Therapist: So what can you do?

Client: I can try to talk to him more.

Therapist: Great! Jennifer, do you think your dad doesn't love you?

Client: Well . . . not really. . . . It's just that he is very preoccupied with his new life. It's hard for him to find time for me. I'm not sure where I fit in, and I don't get to see him very often.

Therapist: Is that why you're nervous about making mistakes and upsetting him?

Client: Yes . . . I mean if I upset him, he won't want to spend any time with me at all?

Therapist: How do you upset him?

Client: You know . . . like if I spill my drink or stain my shirt during dinner.

Therapist: How often does that happen?

Client: A few times. . . .

Therapist: What does your dad do?

Client: He calls me clumsy. . . .

Therapist: Has he ever said that you can't come visit him?

Client: No.

Therapist: Can you come up with some coping thoughts?

Client: Well . . . if I make a mistake, my dad might call me clumsy but I know he loves me and he always seems to enjoy my visits.

Therapist: Jennifer, can you Praise yourself?

Client: I'm proud of myself. I didn't want to go visit my dad and was very nervous and the visit turned out well.

Therapist: Great!

   7. HW: Daily diaries, first in vivo exposure during the week (same as imaginal in this session).

Sessions 6 +

   1. Continue to conduct imaginal (in session) and in vivo exposures (out of session) to increasingly anxiety-provoking items on the hierarchy using cognitive self-control techniques.

2. Continue to assign daily diaries.
3. Teach family members to replace ineffective coping strategies (e.g., overprotection, criticism) to address their child's anxious apprehension with encouragement to use the STOP acronym.

Overcoming Obstacles:

Due to her own anxiety, Jennifer's mother overprotected her daughter in two ways. First, she provided Jennifer with incessant reassurance to allay her worries, which served to maintain Jennifer's anxiety. Second, she viewed the exposures as too anxiety provoking and was resistant in helping to carry them out. This, in turn, offset Jennifer's motivation and enthusiasm. For this reason, Jennifer's mother was instructed to systematically shape her daughter's behavior. She was asked to provide support for coping behaviors and encourage her daughter to use the STOP acronym whenever she displayed fearful behaviors. The combination of Jennifer's diminished reassurance seeking (because her mother no longer gave her extended attention) and successful early exposures (in this case, conducted in an extremely gradual manner) enhanced her mother's confidence in the program and marshaled her support so that Jennifer could successfully complete all of the exposures.

4. Discuss relapse prevention and termination issues.
5. Make arrangements for periodic follow-up visits.

Comments

This protocol is recommended for anxious youth experiencing primarily cognitive symptoms (Eisen and Kearney 1995, Eisen and Silverman 1994). In Jennifer's case, because her motivation and enthusiasm were lacking at times (i.e., depressed affect, parental overprotection), a contingency contracting program was implemented. However, a relaxation protocol was unnecessary because Jennifer did not experience excessive somatic complaints.

At the conclusion of the fourteen-week program, Jennifer scored within normal limits on several self-report measures (NASSQ, CNCEQ, and CDI) but was still experiencing moderate degrees of worry (RCMAS) and anxious apprehension (CBCL). During follow-up visits (i.e., every three months), Jennifer continued to demonstrate improvements. This correlated with her mother's increasingly realistic expectancies of her behaviors (PES).

SUMMARY

The category of chronic anxiety is continuing to change. With OAD now subsumed under GAD in *DSM-IV*, researchers and mental health professionals will need to identify developmental differences in GAD across the lifespan. With respect to children and adolescents, special attention will need to be devoted to child variables such as the nature of symptoms (worry, somatic complaints), developmental status, and motivational and compliance issues. Parent (nature of symptoms, expectancies), family (dyadic adjustment), and diagnostic variables (comorbidity) also need to be addressed. The two OAD cases provided in this chapter illustrated the variability associated with chronic anxiety with regard to symptomatology, treatment, course, and outcome; hence, a prescriptive treatment approach is suggested (e.g., Eisen and Kearney 1995, Eisen and Silverman 1994, Kearney and Silverman 1990). Perhaps, with a coordinated research effort involving children, adolescents, and adults, chronic anxiety will become more fully understood and increasingly treatable.

REFERENCES

Achenbach, T. M. (1991). *Manual for the Child Behavior Checklist/4-18 and 1991 Profile*. Burlington: University of Vermont Department of Psychiatry.

Achenbach, T. M., and Edelbrock, C. (1983). *Manual for the Teacher's Report Form and Teacher Version of the Child Behavior Profile*. Burlington, VT: University of Vermont Department of Psychiatry.

Anderson, J. C., Williams, S., McGee, R., and Silva, P. A. (1987). DSM-III disorders in pre-adolescent children: prevalence in a large sample from the general population. *Archives of General Psychiatry* 44:69–76.

Barlow, D. H. (1988). *Anxiety and its Disorders: The Nature and Treatment of Anxiety and Panic*. New York: Guilford.

Barlow, D. H., DiNardo, P. A., Vermilyea, B. B., et al. (1986). Co-morbidity and depression among the anxiety disorders: issues in diagnosis and classification. *Journal of Nervous and Mental Disease* 174:63–72.

Barrios, B. A., and Hartmann, D. P. (1988). Fears and anxieties in children. In *Behavioral Assessment of Childhood Disorders*, ed. E. J. Mash and L. G. Terdal, 2nd ed., pp. 196–262. New York: Guilford.

Beck, A. T., and Emery, G. (1985). *Anxiety Disorders and Phobias: a Cognitive Perspective*. New York: Basic Books.

Beck, A. T., Ward, C. H., Mendelson, M., et al. (1961). An inventory for measuring depression. *Archives of General Psychiatry* 41:561–571.

Beidel, D. C. (1991). Social phobia and overanxious disorder in school age children. *Journal of the American Academy of Child and Adolescent Psychiatry* 30:545–552.

Beidel, D. C., and Turner, S. M. (1988). Comorbidity of test anxiety and other anxiety disorders in children. *Journal of Abnormal Child Psychology* 16:275-287.

Bernstein, G. A., and Garfinkel, B. D. (1986). School phobia: the overlap of affective and anxiety disorders. *Journal of the American Academy of Child and Adolescent Psychiatry* 20:235-241.

Bowen, R. C., Offord, D. R., and Boyle, M. H. (1990). The prevalence of overanxious disorder and separation anxiety disorder: results from the Ontario Child Health Study. *Journal of the American Academy of Child and Adolescent Psychiatry* 29:753-758.

Chapinoff, A. (1992). *Test-retest reliability of heart response in children with phobic disorder.* Unpublished master's thesis, Florida International University, Miami FL.

Costello, E. J., Edelbrock, C. S., and Costello, A. J. (1985). Validity of the NIMH diagnostic interview schedule for children: a comparison between psychiatric and pediatric referrals. *Journal of Abnormal Child Psychology* 13:579-595.

Diagnostic and Statistical Manual of Mental Disorders (1962). 2nd ed. Washington, DC: American Psychiatric Association.

Diagnostic and Statistical Manual of Mental Disorders (1980). 3rd ed. Washington, DC: American Psychiatric Association.

Diagnostic and Statistical Manual of Mental Disorders (1987). 3rd ed. revised. Washington, DC: American Psychiatric Association.

Diagnostic and Statistical Manual of Mental Disorders (1994). 4th ed. Washington, DC: American Psychiatric Association.

Edelbrock, C., and Costello, A. J. (1984). Structured psychiatric interviews for children and adolescents. In *Handbook of Psychological Assessment*, ed. G. Goldstein and M. Hersen, pp. 276-290. New York: Pergamon.

Eisen, A. R., and Kearney, C. A. (1995). *Practitioner's Guide to Treating Fear and Anxiety in Children and Adolescents: A Cognitive-Behavioral Approach.* Northvale, NJ: Jason Aronson.

Eisen, A. R., and Silverman, W. K. (1993). Should I relax or change my thoughts? A preliminary examination of cognitive therapy, relaxation training, and their combination with overanxious children. *Journal of Cognitive Psychotherapy: An International Quarterly* 7:265-279.

Eisen, A. R., and Silverman, W. K. (1994). *A preliminary examination of matched and mismatched cognitive-behavioral interventions for overanxious disorder.* Manuscript in preparation.

Eisen, A. R., Spasaro, S., Kearney, C. A., et al. (1994). *Reliability and validity of the parental expectancies scale (PES).* Manuscript in preparation.

Glennon, B., and Weisz, J. R. (1978). An observational approach to the assessment of anxiety in young children. *Journal of Consulting and Clinical Psychology* 46:1246-1257.

Hodges, K., Kline, J., Stern, L., et al. (1982). The development of a child interview for research and clinical use. *Journal of Abnormal Child Psychology* 10:173-189.

Jenkins, R. L. (1968). Classification of behavior problems of children. *American Journal of Psychiatry* 125:1032–1039.

Kane, M. T., and Kendall, P. C. (1989). Anxiety disorders in children: a multiple baseline evaluation of a cognitive-behavioral treatment. *Behavior Therapy* 20:499–508.

Kashani, J. H., and Orvaschel, H. (1988). Anxiety disorders in mid-adolescence: a community sample. *American Journal of Psychiatry* 145:960–964.

Kearney, C. A., Drabman, R. S., and Beasley, J. F. (1993). The trials of childhood: the development, reliability, and validity of the daily life stressors scale. *Journal of Child and Family Studies* 2:371–388.

Kearney, C. A., and Silverman, W. K. (1990). A preliminary analysis of a functional model of assessment and treatment for school refusal behavior. *Behavior Modification* 14:340–366.

Kendall, P. C. (1991). Guiding theory for therapy with children and adolescents. In *Child and Adolescent Therapy: Cognitive-Behavioral Procedures*, ed. P. C. Kendall, pp. 3–22. New York: Guilford.

Kendall, P. C. (1994). Treating anxiety disorders in youth: results of a randomized clinical trial. *Journal of Consulting and Clinical Psychology* 62:100–110.

Kendall, P. C., Chansky, T. E., Friedman, M., et al. (1991). Treating anxiety disorders in children and adolescents. In *Child and Adolescent Therapy: Cognitive-Behavioral Procedures*, ed. P. C. Kendall, pp. 131–167. New York: Guilford.

Kendall, P. C., Chansky, T. E., Kane, M. T., et al. (1992). *Anxiety Disorders in Youth: Cognitive-Behavioral Interventions*. Needham, MA: Allyn and Bacon.

Kendall, P. C., and Treadwell, K. (1993). Overanxious disorder. In *Handbook of Prescriptive Treatments for Children and Adolescents*, ed. R. T. Ammerman, C. G. Last, and M. Hersen, pp. 159–177. Needham, MA: Allyn and Bacon.

King, N. J. (1980). The therapeutic utility of abbreviated progressive relaxation: a critical review with implications for clinical practice. In *Progress in Behavior Modification*, eds. M. Hersen, R. E. Eisler, and P. Miller, vol. 10. New York: Academic Press.

Klein, R. G., and Last, C. G. (1989). Anxiety disorders in children. *Developmental Clinical Psychology and Psychiatry* 20:1–140. New York: Sage.

Kovacs, M. (1983). *The children's depression inventory: A self-rated depression scale for school-aged youngsters.* Unpublished manuscript, University of Pittsburgh.

——— (1985). The Interview Schedule for Children (ISC). *Psychopharmacology Bulletin* 21:991–994.

La Greca, A. M., and Stone, W. L. (1993). Social anxiety scale for children-revised: factor structure and concurrent validity. *Journal of Clinical Child Psychology* 22:17–27.

Last, C. G. (1991). Somatic complaints in anxiety disordered children. *Journal of Anxiety Disorders* 5:125–138.

Last, C. G., Hersen, M., Kazdin, A. E., et al. (1987a). Comparison of DSM-III separation anxiety and overanxious disorders: demographic characteristics and patterns of comorbidity. *Journal of the American Academy of Child and Adolescent Psychiatry* 26:527–531.

Last, C. G., Strauss, C. C., and Francis, G. (1987b). Comorbidity among childhood anxiety disorders. *Journal of Nervous and Mental Disease* 175:726–730.

Leitenberg, H., Yost, L. W., and Carroll-Wilson, M. (1986). Negative cognitive errors in children: questionnaire development, normative data, and comparisons between children with and without self reported symptoms of depression, low self-esteem, and evaluation anxiety. *Journal of Consulting and Clinical Psychology* 54:528–536.

Marks, I. M., and Mathews, A. M. (1979). Brief standard self-rating for phobic patients. *Behaviour Research and Therapy* 17:263–267.

Mattison, R. E., and Bagnatto, S. J. (1987). Empirical measurement of overanxious disorder in boys 8 to 12 years old. *Journal of the American Academy of Child and Adolescent Psychiatry* 26:536–540.

Mattison, R. E., Bagnatto, S. J., and Brubaker, B. H. (1988). Diagnostic utility of the revised Children's Manifest Anxiety Scale in children with *DSM-III* anxiety disorders. *Journal of Anxiety Disorders* 2:147–155.

Mattison, R. E., Bagnatto, S. J., Brubaker, B. H., and Humphrey, F. J. (1985). *Discriminant validity of the revised children's manifest anxiety scale with DSM-III anxiety disorders.* Unpublished manuscript.

Melamed, B. G., and Siegel, L. J. (1975). Reduction of anxiety in children facing hospitalization and surgery by use of filmed modeling. *Journal of Consulting and Clinical Psychology* 43:511–521.

Melamed, B., Weinstein, D., Hawes, R., and Katin-Borland, M. (1975). Reduction of fear related dental management problems using filmed modeling. *Journal of the American Dental Association* 90:822–826.

Melamed, B., Yurcherson, R., Fleece, E. L., et al. (1978). Effects of filmed modeling on the reduction of anxiety-related behaviors in individuals varying in level of previous experience in the stress situation. *Journal of Consulting and Clinical Psychology* 46:1357–1367.

O'Connor, R. D. (1969). Modification of social withdrawal through symbolic modeling. *Journal of Applied Behavior Analysis* 2:15–22.

Ollendick, T. H. (1983). Reliability and validity of the revised fear survey schedule for children (FSSC-R). *Behaviour Research and Therapy* 21:685–692.

Ollendick, T. H., and Cerny, J. A. (1981). *Clinical Behavior Therapy with Children.* New York: Plenum.

Ost, L. G., Jerremalm, A., and Johansson, J. (1981). Individual response patterns and the effects of different behavioral methods in the treatment of social phobia. *Behaviour Research and Therapy* 19:1–16.

Ost, L. G., Johansson, J., and Jerremalm, A. (1982). Individual response patterns and the effects of different behavioral methods in the treatment of claustrophobia. *Behaviour Research and Therapy* 20:445–460.

Piers, E. V. (1984). *Piers-Harris Children's Self-Concept Scale: Revised Manual.* Los Angeles: Western Psychological Services.

Puig-Antich, J., and Chambers, W. J. (1978). *Schedule for Affective Disorders and Schizophrenia for School-age Children (K-SADS).* Unpublished manuscript.

Reynolds, C. R., and Richman, B. O. (1978). What I think and feel: a revised measure of children's manifest anxiety. *Journal of Abnormal Child Psychology* 6:271–280.

Ronan, K. R., Kendall, P. C., and Rowe, M. (in press). Negative affectivity in children: development and validation of a self-statement questionnaire. *Cognitive Therapy and Research*.

Sarason, S. B., Davidson, K. S., Lighthall, F. F., and Waite, R. R. (1958). A test anxiety scale for children. *Child Development* 29:105–113.

Silverman, W. K. (1989). *Self-control manual for phobic children*. Unpublished treatment protocol. Florida International University, University Park, Miami, FL.

_____ (1991). Diagnostic reliability of anxiety disorders in children using structured interviews. *Journal of Anxiety Disorders* 5:105–124.

_____ (in press). Structured diagnostic interviews. In *Handbook of Phobic and Anxiety Disorders in Children*, ed. T. H. Ollendick, N. J. King, and W. Yule. New York: Plenum.

Silverman, W. K., and Eisen, A. R. (1992). Age differences in the reliability of parent and child reports of child anxious symptomatology using a structured interview. *Journal of the American Academy of Child and Adolescent Psychiatry* 31:117–124.

_____ (1993). Overanxious disorder in children. In *Handbook of Behavior Therapy with Children and Adults: A Developmental and Longitudinal Perspective*, ed. R. T. Ammerman and M. Hersen, pp. 189–201. Needham, MA: Allyn and Bacon.

Silverman, W. K., Fleisig, W., Rabian, B., and Peterson, R. A. (1991). The Child Anxiety Sensitivity Index. *Journal of Clinical Child Psychology* 20:162–168.

Silverman, W. K., and Kearney, C. A. (1993). Behavioral treatment of childhood anxiety. In *Handbook of Behavior Therapy and Pharmacotherapy for Children: A Comparative Analysis*, ed. V. B. Van Hasselt and M. Hersen, pp. 33–53. Needham, MA: Allyn and Bacon.

Silverman, W. K., and Nelles, W. B. (1988). The anxiety disorders interview schedule for children. *Journal of the American Academy of Child and Adolescent Psychiatry* 27:772–778.

Silverman, W. K., and Rabian, B. (1993). Simple phobias. *Child and Adolescent Psychiatric Clinics of North America* 2:603–622.

Spanier, G. B. (1976). Measuring dyadic adjustment: new scales for assessing the quality of marriage and similar dyads. *Journal of Marriage and the Family* 38:15–28.

Spielberger, C. D. (1973). *Manual for the State-Trait Anxiety Inventory for Children*. Palo Alto, CA: Consulting Psychologists Press.

Strauss, C. C. (1988). Behavioral assessment and treatment of overanxious disorder in children and adolescents. *Behavior Modification* 12:234–251.

Strauss, C. C., Lease, C. A., Last, C. G., and Francis, G. (1988). Overanxious disorder: an examination of developmental differences. *Journal of Abnormal Child Psychology* 16:57–68.

Van Hasselt, V. B., Hersen, M., Bellack, A. S., et al. (1979). Tripartite assessment of the effects of systematic desensitization in a multi-phobic child. *Journal of Behavior Therapy and Experimental Psychiatry* 10:51–55.

9

PANIC DISORDER WITH OR WITHOUT AGORAPHOBIA

Christopher A. Kearney
Wesley D. Allan

DESCRIPTION OF DISORDER

Panic disorder with or without agoraphobia in youngsters represents a fascinating but highly controversial syndrome. Such fascination is derived primarily from the diversity of symptomatology characteristic of this population. According to the *Diagnostic and Statistical Manual of Mental Disorders* (*DSM-IV*; American Psychiatric Association 1994), panic disorder subsumes continuing panic attacks or "discrete period(s) of intense fear or discomfort" (p. 395) that usually develop quickly and peak in intensity within ten minutes. In addition, significant behavior change (e.g., driving only small distances) and ongoing concerns about future attacks (e.g., where they may occur) and what might happen in the event of an attack (e.g., blocked escape) for at least one month are required for the diagnosis.

A panic attack consists of four of the following somatic and cognitive symptoms: heart palpitations, sweating, trembling, feeling short of breath or smothered, feeling of choking, chest pain, nausea, dizziness, derealization or depersonalization, fears of uncontrollability or losing one's mind, fear of dying, numbness or tingling, and chills or hot flushes (American Psychiatric Association 1994, p. 395). Symptoms with an asterisk are displayed by over two-thirds of youngsters with panic disorder (Kearney and Silverman 1992). Persons may also experience frequent "limited symptom attacks" involving fewer than four symptoms (Barlow 1988), or infrequent panic attacks (i.e., "nonclinical panic," Norton et al. 1992).

Panic attacks are typically unexpected or uncued in nature, initially occurring without warning and terrifying the recipient. Panic attacks that are situationally bound or cued in nature are more representative of syndromes such as specific or social phobia, but also occur in persons with advanced panic disorder. For example, one may experience an uncued panic attack following an accident, an experience with new peers, or a school event. Subsequent attacks may be uncued and/or triggered by environmental stimuli that remind the person of the original, highly aversive attack (e.g., risk of physical danger, evaluative situations, sexual arousal, sporting activities; Warren and Zgourides 1988).

In addition to symptoms characteristic of panic attacks, persons with panic disorder may display agoraphobia, or "anxiety about being in places or situations from which escape might be difficult (or embarrassing) or in which help may not be available in the event of having an unexpected or situationally predisposed panic attack" (American Psychiatric Association 1994, p. 396). As a result, one may avoid potentially unpleasant situations such as shopping malls or school, or require the presence of a safety person who must accompany one and provide comfort in case of an attack. One may also have agoraphobia without a history of panic disorder, but this is unusual. Therefore, this chapter will focus primarily on persons with panic disorder with agoraphobia.

The fascination with panic disorder is tempered, however, by ongoing controversy about the applicability of the diagnosis to youngsters. Investigators of panic disorder in adolescents, for example, often rely on assessment procedures that lack reliability, multiple informants, composite diagnoses, and considerations of cued-uncued panic and developmental factors (Kearney and Silverman 1992). In addition, the existence of panic in those under age 12 years has been disputed because their level of cognitive development often hampers their interpretation of aversive somatic symptoms (Griegel et al. 1991, Nelles and Barlow 1988). For example, many children experience hyperventilation but do not attribute its cause to harmful internal factors such as heart problems.

As a result, the epidemiology of panic disorder in youngsters remains unclear. The prevalence of panic disorder in high school students is about 1 percent (Lewinsohn et al. 1993, Whitaker et al. 1990), which is slightly less than that for adults (Brown and Deagle 1992; Myers et al. 1984, Norton et al. 1985, Von Korff et al. 1985). However, the prevalence of panic disorder in clinical samples is reportedly as high as 15 percent (Alessi et al. 1987), and the prevalence of panic attacks in the general adolescent population may be even higher (King et al. 1993, Macaulay and Kleinknecht 1989, Ollendick et al. 1994, Warren and Zgourides 1988). In addition, panic disorder seems to be more common in females than males, and peak age of onset is between 15 and 19 years (Last and Strauss 1989, Von Korff et al. 1985). Because of the controversy surrounding the diagnosis of panic disorder in youngsters, this chapter will focus on both children with somatic complaints that resemble panic attacks (e.g., hyperventilation) and adolescents with panic attacks and disorder.

DIFFERENTIAL DIAGNOSIS

Panic disorder appears to be comorbid with a variety of other anxiety, affective, personality, eating, and externalizing syndromes, although the most common is separation anxiety disorder (Kearney and Silverman 1992). A relationship between separation anxiety and panic has been discussed at length because of tantalizing data from several adult- and child-based studies. For example, many adults with panic disorder report childhood histories of separation anxiety (Perugi et al. 1988, Raskin et al. 1982). With respect to youngsters, Weissman and colleagues (1984) found that children of adults with depression and panic/agoraphobia exhibited more separation anxiety than children of adults with depression and/or generalized anxiety disorder. In addition, Hayward and colleagues (1989) revealed that adolescents with panic attacks were more likely to have separated or divorced parents than those without panic attacks. The authors suggested that "early loss, or sensitivity to separation" (p. 1062) may predispose one to develop later panic attacks.

Among samples of psychiatrically hospitalized children, the comorbidity of separation anxiety and panic has been reported to be 59 percent (based on ten of seventeen cases from Alessi and Magen 1988 and Alessi et al. 1987). Among outpatient samples, comorbidity has been reported to be 38 percent (based on nineteen of fifty cases from Bradley and Hood 1993, Last and Strauss 1989, and Vitiello et al. 1990). In addition, Biederman and colleagues (1993) found that 75 percent of children with separation anxiety disorder displayed agoraphobia at a three-year follow-up compared to 7 percent of those without separation anxiety disorder. Finally, several studies indicate that the treatment of both separation anxiety and panic disorder in youngsters can be accomplished via imipramine (e.g., Gittelman-Klein and Klein 1980). These data have led some authors to hypothesize that separation anxiety is either a precursor to, or a childhood version of, adult panic (e.g., Abelson and Alessi 1992, Alessi and Magen 1988). However, other authors conclude that a direct relationship between separation anxiety and panic/agoraphobia does not exist and that additional research is required (e.g., Thyer 1993).

Other problems common to persons with panic disorder include depression, anger, and general behavioral inhibition. Depression in youngsters with panic is comorbid in approximately 44 percent of cases (based on twenty-four of fifty-four cases from Alessi et al. 1987, Bradley and Hood 1993, and Last and Strauss 1989). With respect to anger, Schreier (1992) noted several child clinical cases where anger may have been a variant of panic. Such cases have been found in adults as well (Fava et al. 1990). Finally, several authors have noted a relationship between adolescent panic disorder, general fearfulness and avoidance in new situations, and oppositional behavior (e.g., Biederman et al. 1993, Bradley and Hood 1993).

These comorbidity data may reveal how some children with specific anxiety disorders or other problems are predisposed toward panic disorder in adolescence or adulthood. Because many symptoms of the disorders discussed here resemble panic disorder, some investigators (e.g., Biederman et al. 1993) propose that an "anxiety diathesis" may exist whereby milder anxiety disorders lead to panic disorder. Several factors that may contribute to this process include (1) modeling avoidance and fearful reactions to certain situations, (2) being rewarded for seeking reassurance and physical proximity to others, and/or (3) obtaining attention via externalizing behaviors (e.g., Biederman et al. 1993, Bowlby 1973, Perugi et al. 1988). Clinicians are thus encouraged to be sensitive to these behaviors when assessing and treating youngsters with initial anxiety disorders as well as later panic disorder.

ASSESSMENT PROCEDURES

Given the diversity of cognitive, behavioral, and somatic symptoms of panic attacks and diagnoses comorbid with panic disorder, an eclectic and in-depth assessment procedure that focuses on each is recommended. We strongly suggest, however, that a full medical evaluation precede or parallel a psychological one (although youngsters with uncomplicated panic disorder or primarily somatic complaints often present to pediatric clinics first; Garland and Smith 1990). Clinicians should consider the possibility of an organic basis for severe somatic symptoms like nausea/vomiting, dizziness, and heart palpitations. With respect to the latter, therapists should be particularly aware of the relationship between panic attacks and mitral valve prolapse (MVP), a cardiac condition characterized by abnormal systolic displacement of the mitral leaflets into the left atrium (Perloff and Child 1987). Several researchers have noted that MVP is common in adults (Gorman et al. 1988) and possibly youngsters (Kearney et al. 1992) with panic attacks and disorder.

With respect to a psychological evaluation, priority should be given to obtaining information on (1) severity and frequency of panic attacks and related symptomatology, (2) cognitive distortions and level of anticipatory anxiety, and (3) extent of avoidant behavior. Common procedures for obtaining this information include the interview, child self-report instruments, parent and teacher checklists, and physiological measurement. Unfortunately, many assessment techniques for adolescent panic disorder are based on adult versions of anxiety measures (Last 1993; e.g., the Structured Clinical Interview for *DSM-III-R*, Spitzer et al. 1986) that may lack substantial psychometric quality when used for youngsters.

A notable exception is the Anxiety Disorders Interview Schedule for Children (ADIS-C, Silverman and Nelles 1988), which was designed to assess for a variety of disorders in youngsters but particularly those related to anxiety. Child and parent versions of the interview have been developed and each displays adequate reliability and validity (Silverman and Eisen 1992). With respect to panic disorder, the interview assesses for feeling "scared for no reason at all," frequency of panic, settings in which panic occurs, and potentially concurrent agoraphobia. Child and parent reports are integrated by the clinician, who derives a composite diagnosis if applicable. Because the interview is semistructured, information on the antecedents and consequences of a particular client's panic episode may also be solicited. Interrater agreement for panic disorder and agoraphobia from child and parents ADIS reports has been reported to be over .90 (Silverman and Nelles 1988).

Following the interview, clinicians may wish to utilize self-report data to obtain more detailed information. Although few assessment devices are available specifically for youngsters with panic disorder, King and colleagues (1993) devised a panic attack questionnaire for adolescents based on earlier measures (e.g., Norton et al. 1985). On this new measure, panic attacks are defined prior to questions concerning "time to maximum onset, duration, symptomatology, life interference, and avoidance" (p. 113), among others. Although no psychometric data were presented, the authors found that almost 43 percent of their sample reportedly experienced a panic attack. The reliability and validity of self-report data in this area has not been well established, however, so the clinician is encouraged to cautiously employ a variety of such measures to evaluate the major themes discussed at the beginning of this section.

Other self-report measures applicable to youngsters with panic and/or agoraphobia include the (1) Fear Survey Schedule for Children-Revised (Ollendick 1983), which contains several items pertaining to medical fears (e.g., "not being able to breathe"); (2) Children's Manifest Anxiety Scale-Revised (Reynolds and Paget 1983), which incorporates three factors relevant to panic (i.e., physiological anxiety, worry/oversensitivity, concentration); (3) trait scale of the State-Trait Anxiety Inventory for Children (Spielberger 1973), which evaluates somatic and cognitive complaints resembling those of panic (e.g., "I worry too much, I notice my heart beats fast"); (4) Children's Anxiety Sensitivity Index (CASI, Silverman et al. 1991), a measure of the extent to which one believes his/her anxiety symptoms will produce aversive consequences (the reader is cautioned that the CASI may be more useful for adolescents than children; Chorpita et al. 1994); (5) Social Anxiety Scale for Children–Revised (La Greca and Stone 1993), which may assist in the assessment of social avoidance; and (6) Children's Depression Inventory (Kovacs and Beck 1977), which may be used to assess for concurrent depressive symptoms. In many cases, particularly for children or young adolescents, the use of such questionnaires will help solicit additional and potentially critical information that was not volunteered during an interview.

Clinicians should also attempt to assess parent and teacher reports of panic symptomatology and avoidance in their clients as well as familial problems that may contribute to the disorder. With respect to the former, for example, the Child Behavior Checklist (CBCL, Achenbach 1991a) may be used to assess internalizing symptoms like worrying, fear, anxiety, nervousness, obsessions, and self-consciousness as well as somatic complaints like dizziness, nausea, and fatigue. Externalizing symptoms potentially related to the disorder (e.g., running away) may also be examined. The Teacher's Report Form (TRF, Achenbach 1991b) may be used to solicit pertinent teacher reports on social avoidance and the effects of panic symptomatology on academic functioning.

With respect to familial problems, clinicians should evaluate distal factors that could maintain or exacerbate a youngster's panic symptoms. These factors include dysfunctional family environment (e.g., enmeshment), marital conflict, and ongoing family stressors. Finally, a continual assessment of physiological symptoms is recommended. Suggested procedures are discussed in more detail elsewhere (see Beidel and Stanley 1993), but particular attention should be paid to heart and respiratory rates and sweat gland activity (Silverman and Kearney 1993). In addition, between-session records of panic attacks and their duration, severity, symptomatology, and antecedents and consequences should be kept by parents and youngsters. This will ensure minimal reliance on retrospective analysis and an ongoing barometer of treatment progress.

ESTABLISHING TREATMENT GOALS

Because panic attacks are the key symptom of panic disorder, cause significant distress, and produce avoidance, their remediation is usually the first step in therapeutic protocols. Indeed, most treatment outcome studies of youngsters with panic disorder were designed primarily to reduce panic attacks and related avoidant behavior (e.g., Ballenger et al. 1989). To initially enhance this process, the clinician must pay close attention to developing trust and rapport, organizing intervention sessions with the client, and easing anticipatory anxiety about therapy attendance. Subsequently, one should concentrate on restructuring the client's cognitive distortions and diminishing fearfulness associated with somatic symptoms. Finally, a therapist will need to focus on the most intransigent symptom of behavioral avoidance, which in many cases has been well-rewarded and is resistant to change. The reader is encouraged to consult other avoidant behavior-related chapters in this handbook, particularly school refusal behavior, social anxiety, and sleep disorders.

The focus of treatment for panic disorder is typically the youngster who displays panic attacks and comorbid problems such as depression. However, panic is often inadvertently or deliberately reinforced by others in a youngster's environment. For example, parents may provide substantial attention to somatic complaints such as hyperventilation (particularly if they experience paniclike symptoms themselves), or teachers may provide escape from schoolwork by sending a student with panic to the nurse's office. Proximal reinforcers such as these should be ascertained and addressed at length. Finally, because separation anxiety and panic may be closely intertwined, the parent–child relationship may be an important focus of treatment as well.

ROLE OF THE THERAPIST

The primary roles of the therapist who treats panic disorder in youngsters will include clinician, educator, supporter, and mediator. With respect to the clinical role, therapists will need, of course, to institute specific procedures (e.g., restructuring, relaxation training, in vivo exposure) that directly ameliorate the cognitive, somatic, and behavioral symptoms of panic attacks. However, clinicians will need to spend almost as much if not more time educating their clients about the phenomenology of panic. Specifically, youngsters should be informed about (1) what constitutes panic disorder, (2) the symptomatology of panic attacks, including the interrelationship of cognitive, somatic, and behavioral responses, and (3) the fact that panic disorder is not uncommon and one is not "crazy" or "weird" for experiencing the problem (Craske and Barlow 1990). In addition, clients should be well informed about the expectations and structure of the proposed treatment program. Such an education process should be ongoing during therapy.

In cases where extensive behavioral avoidance is present, the therapist will also need to provide considerable encouragement and support when engaging the client in exposure to feared internal and external stimuli. This is particularly true when addressing stimuli (e.g., cars, bedrooms, classrooms, shopping malls) associated with the original and other severe panic attacks. In addition, the therapist must reduce any anticipatory anxiety potentially associated with therapeutic attendance. A consistent process of increasing the client's sense of self-efficacy via extensive recordkeeping, for example, may enhance motivation and response to treatment. Finally, the clinician may have to assume the role of mediator in cases where familial variables substantially impinge upon the disorder. Examples include separation anxiety regarding a safety person, parent–child conflict over avoided situations, and marital disputes. Also, the therapist may need to provide direct or referral services for parents who display psychopathologies (e.g., anxiety states) that provide a model for a youngster's panic and/or impede therapeutic progress.

TREATMENT STRATEGIES

Few treatment outcome studies are available for youngsters with panic disorder. Several researchers have, however, investigated the efficacy of pharmacotherapy with this population. For example, Biederman (1987) examined three children with paniclike symptoms including somatic complaints characteristic of panic attacks. Moderate doses of the benzodiazepine clonazepam were successful in reducing phobic and avoidant behaviors over several months. Ballenger and colleagues (1989) treated three youngsters with panic disorder and agoraphobia with the antidepressant imipramine and/or the anxiolytic alprazolam for at least one year. This treatment, combined with unspecified psychotherapy, produced abated "panic attacks, separation anxiety, and fear and avoidance of crowds and public places" (p. 922).

Finally, Black and Robbins (1990) treated four adolescents with panic disorder with the antidepressants imipramine or desipramine. Three were successfully treated for phobic avoidance and related problems such as somatic complaints over several weeks to months. Although these investigators concluded that childhood panic disorder does exist and may be treated pharmacologically, they also acknowledged the need for well-controlled, placebo-comparative designs to fully evaluate the efficacy of this treatment. In many severe cases where other interventions have failed, however, drug treatment may be an effective and preferable method.

With respect to psychological interventions, no systematic evaluations of their utility in youngsters are available. However, the construction of a psychological approach to ameliorate panic in this population may be made from those fashioned for adults (Acierno et al. 1993) and youngsters with other anxiety disorders. Again, such an approach would likely be more applicable to adolescents than children because an adolescent's cognitive developmental level more closely approximates that of an adult. However, interventions designed specifically for the remediation of somatic complaints could be employed with children who display precursory panic symptoms such as hyperventilation, dizziness, or muscle tension.

The construction of a psychological treatment for panic in youngsters may be derived from Craske and Barlow's (1990) Mastery of Your Anxiety and Panic (MAP) program for adults and Kendall and colleagues' (1992) FEAR program for children and adolescents with other fear/anxiety disorders. The two methods have similar components, and include the identification of cues that trigger panic, cognitive therapy and coping skills, somatic control exercises, interoceptive and in vivo exposure, and evaluation and reward. Specifically, clients are taught to manage and control negative cognitive distortions, dysfunctional breathing patterns and other visceral problems, and avoidance. Craske and Barlow's (1990) treatment protocol is designed to reduce panic attacks, anticipatory anxiety, and avoidance over fifteen sessions. Outcome data indicate these procedures to be effective for these behaviors in over 85 percent of adults with panic disorder (e.g., Barlow et al. 1989, Klosko et al. 1990).

In conjunction with procedures mentioned earlier to establish initial treatment goals and focus, clients should be taught and required to self-monitor the precipitants (e.g., behavior, emotions) of panic. Self-monitoring should help the client identify cue patterns that trigger panic attacks and achieve subsequent control of these attacks. Physiological symptoms of panic may then be addressed via rebreathing and relaxation training. For example, clients may be taught to concentrate on breathing through the nose only, maintaining a regular inhalation rate, and practicing diaphragmatic respiration (Wolpe and Rowan 1988). In addition, a progressive muscle relaxation procedure could be introduced whereby one systematically tenses and releases various muscle groups (e.g., hands, Jacobsen 1938). These somatic control exercises provide skills to control the aversiveness of panic and potentially limit the perceived need for avoidance.

Subsequent cognitive restructuring involves a careful examination of the client's self-statements and inaccurate perceptions of surrounding events. For example, one may misinterpret panic symptoms as a heart attack or believe that everyone in a classroom will laugh during his/her panic attack. Cognitive restructuring procedures such as decentering, decatastrophization, palliative techniques, and hypothesis testing may be used (e.g., Foreyt and McGavin 1989). With respect to the latter, for example, a therapist could ask a client to identify the perceived probability of a specific event (e.g., laughter from others) and then test this hypothesis via empirical evidence derived from real-life occurrences. In many cases, clients are shown that they grossly overestimate the probability of negative events. For children and young adolescents, an emphasis on coping skills may be most appropriate (Grace et al. 1993).

Finally, an emphasis should be placed on exposure to internal and external cues that trigger panic attacks and subsequent avoidance. Clients may be gradually exposed to situations (e.g., hyperventilation, exercise, driving) that produce potentially aversive internal reactions (e.g., dizziness). Eventually, the client should habituate to the situation and experience less fear and avoidance. Subsequently, clients could be asked to recall and possibly revisit stimuli associated with their first or most aversive panic attack. Treatment may then focus on other avoided situations, withdrawal of safety persons, and the elimination of medication if appropriate. Evaluation of and systematic rewards for successful progress should also pervade the treatment process.

Clinicians may also need to implement treatment techniques that address familial variables contributing to a youngster's panic (e.g., attention). Such tactics include contingency management, in which case parents or others may be instructed to reward youngsters for appropriate nonpanic behavior (e.g., brave self-statements) and downplay or ignore inappropriate illness behaviors (e.g., somatic exaggerations, school refusal behavior). Problem-solving and communication skills training are also recommended if high levels of conflict are present. In addition, family therapy may be needed to modify enmeshed parent–child relationships that foster dependent panic behaviors and social avoidance. Finally, marital therapy could be necessary in cases where parents cannot maintain a uniform strategy for addressing a youngster with panic disorder.

Given the diagnostic comorbidity evident in this population, treatment strategies must also be flexible enough to account for concurrent depression, other anxiety disorders, and externalizing problems. For example, one par-ticular condition that often requires inpatient treatment is primary depres-sion with secondary panic disorder (Jacob and Lilienfeld 1991). With respect to externalizing problems, clinicians should pay special attention to sub-stance abuse or the self-medication of one's anxiety (Warren and Zgourides 1988). Finally, given that panic disorder in youngsters is more likely to occur in adolescents than children, clinicians should be particularly aware of normal, pubescent developmental variables that could affect treatment length or structure. For example, many teenagers experience "imaginary audiences" (Elkind 1976), or the misperception that others are specifically concentrating on a unique aspect of their body. An exacerbation of this phenomenon may require more in-depth cognitive restructuring during therapy than that needed only for panic.

DEALING WITH COMMON OBSTACLES TO SUCCESSFUL TREATMENT

Common obstacles to successfully treating panic disorder in youngsters will be divided here into three categories: problems that occur before treatment, problems with pharmacological treatment, and problems with psychological treatment. With respect to problems before treatment, the most prevalent are (1) excessive anticipatory anxiety that prevents therapeutic attendance, and (2) addressing the incorrect primary diagnosis. In the former case, clinicians should be prepared to conduct extensive telephone discussions or schedule a home visit to initiate therapy if necessary. In the latter case, symptoms of adolescent panic often appear to be the youngster's most serious complaints when actually they are secondary to anger, depression, another anxiety disorder, or relationship difficulties. In addition, youngsters are often referred for panic disorder when only severe anticipatory anxiety is present. Manifes-tations of the latter include school refusal behavior or externalizing problems such as aggression or inattention (Garland and Smith 1990). Clinicians are thus encouraged to make a full determination of which problems produce the most interference in their client's life.

In addition, many panic symptoms are the result of drug or medical conditions that should be addressed first. Examples of common drugs that simulate acute anxiety reactions include bronchodilators, caffeine, and other stimulants such as cocaine. Examples of medical conditions that simulate panic reactions include cardiovascular (e.g., arrythmias), metabolic (e.g., hypoglycemia), neurologic (e.g., epilepsy), and pulmonary (e.g., pneumothorax) disorders (Fontaine 1991). In cases where a clinician suspects the possibility of any of these, an initial referral to a physician is recommended. Should any of these conditions not be addressed when in fact they primarily contribute to "panic," then treatment efficacy will suffer considerably.

General obstacles to successful pharmacological treatment include parental proscription, reluctance on the youngster's part to ingest drugs, subtherapeutic or inappropriate doses, too limited a drug trial, potential drug dependency especially in cases of past alcohol or other drug abuse, questions of safety during pregnancy, withdrawal problems, possible ineffectiveness in long-term outcome, relapse, and side effects that precipitate dropout or other problems (Sheehan and Raj 1991, Walker et al. 1991). Typical drugs for panic disorder in youngsters include the anxiolytics clonazepam and alprazolam and the antidepressants imipramine and desipramine.

Common side effects of alprazolam and clonazepam include lethargic or hyperactive behavior, aggression, ataxia, hypotonia, irritability, and memory and cognitive impairment (Carpenter and Vining 1993, Werry and Aman 1993). With respect to imipramine and desipramine, common side effects include sedation or potential stimulant-like effects and a variety of physiological symptoms that often simulate panic (e.g., dizziness, tremors, nausea, palpitations, chest pain, and sweating, Viesselman et al. 1993). Should an adolescent referred for panic disorder begin to experience such symptoms following the intake of medication, the likelihood of dropout or resistance to other procedures is substantial. Clinicians are thus urged to carefully consider the ramifications of pharmacologic treatment and educate their clients about such procedures in a detailed fashion.

Obstacles are also common to the psychological treatment of panic disorder in youngsters. For example, panic attacks or anticipatory anxiety may increase significantly at the onset of treatment when a youngster realizes that a serious attempt is now being made to alleviate the condition. In these cases, clinicians are encouraged to extend and intensify the educational elements that compose part of the psychological intervention for this population. In addition, important competing conditions that affect treatment direction (e.g., pregnancy, substance abuse, personality disorder, extreme social anxiety, poor accessibility to services, Sheehan and Raj 1991, Walker et al. 1991) may be present and should be addressed prior to and during the therapeutic process.

Other important obstacles to psychological intervention can be divided into those affecting the cognitive, somatic, and behavioral treatment of panic. For example, clinicians should be aware that a client's cognitive development may be insufficient for the purpose of restructuring maladaptive thoughts. In addition, a youngster may have difficulty comprehending that the presence of only cued or limited-symptom panic attacks represents an improvement from previously spontaneous, uncued attacks. With respect to somatic treatment, clinicians should carefully monitor the possibility that youngsters will misuse procedures such as rebreathing training and inadvertently increase their anxiety. With respect to behavioral treatment, particularly of avoidance, clinicians must be continually vigilant for sudden cessations in exposure to feared stimuli. Especially in cases of severe avoidance, one should monitor on a daily basis the client's levels of activity and exposure to new situations.

Other problems that can occur anytime during the therapeutic process include (1) lack of client compliance and motivation, (2) incongruent amelioration of panic symptoms (e.g., somatic but not behavioral), and (3) emergence of new situations after the remission of panic that create difficulties in adjustment (e.g., entering a new classroom, Sheehan and Raj 1991). With respect to the first problem, clinicians should provide as much education as possible during assessment and early treatment about upcoming therapeutic components, organize therapy sessions in detail with the client, and monitor compliance to medical regimens. In addition, daily logbooks of panic attacks and related symptomatology should be required to assess for sudden decreases in adherence to the treatment protocol.

Youngsters with panic may also encounter situations in which some aspects of the disorder remit while others continue to be problematic. A common example is the remission of panic attacks but maintenance of anticipatory anxiety and avoidant behavior (Fyer et al. 1991). In these cases, clinicians may suggest a low-dose benzodiazepine to ease anxiety about exposure to feared situations like those associated with the original panic attack. Extensive relaxation training, encouragement from the therapist and family members, and daily records of even very slight improvements should also take place.

Finally, a youngster may experience new situations during recovery from panic that were previously unexpected but now cause substantial obstacles to future progress. Examples include (1) new family dynamics such as loss of support or attention with reduced panic symptoms, (2) increased familial conflict, (3) worsening of other, previously less severe disorders such as depression or phobia, and (4) exposure to new school and social situations. In these cases, clinicians may need to schedule additional treatment sessions during the week to address alternative issues. Intensive family therapy with contingency management procedures, communication and problem-solving training, and revisions of the panic treatment components already utilized with the client (e.g., cognitive restructuring, in vivo exposure) are recommended.

Overall, the treatment of panic disorder in youngsters is potentially replete with diversions and stumbling blocks, but these obstacles can be overcome by relying on the consistent implementation of a few, key procedures. These include education about the disorder and subsequent treatment practices, development of rapport, family intervention, and a focus on compliance. In many cases, the remediation of obstacles will be as important to the amelioration of panic as the active treatment procedures themselves.

RELAPSE PREVENTION

Relapse prevention of panic disorder is defined broadly along a continuum between the recurrence of any cued or uncued panic attack and the reintroduction of panic attacks sufficient to result in severe avoidant behavior (Zitrin et al. 1983). Many investigators prefer a middle-of-the-road approach, however, and define relapse as a "recurrence of spontaneous panic attacks leading to interference with functioning" (Fontaine 1991, p. 365). For youngsters, interference with functioning could involve disruptions in peer and familial relationships, school attendance and academic performance, recreational activities, and/or driving and maintaining a job. Approximately one-third of persons successfully treated for panic disorder will relapse within two years of treatment termination (Fontaine 1991).

The prevention of relapse for this population may be best accomplished via periodic monitoring of pharmacological interventions in addition to cognitive therapy, problem-solving skills, and specialized psychoanalysis. Doses of medication should be frequently checked for decreases in effectiveness and increases in side effects. Cognitive therapy is effective for reducing long-term problems related to disorders marked by thought distortions (e.g., depression) and possibly panic (e.g., Emmelkamp et al. 1986). Problem-solving training could focus on teaching the youngster to identify new social or academic problems that may induce future panic as well as coping and other skills to alleviate their aversiveness (e.g., Kleiner et al. 1987). Specialized psychoanalysis or supportive psychotherapy may be useful for those with concurrent personality disorders or difficulties with exposure to new situations. Whatever method is used, however, the clinician is encouraged to maintain contact with a youngster with panic disorder for at least two years after therapy termination (Fontaine 1991).

TERMINATION

A recommended criterion for ending treatment for a youngster with panic disorder and/or agoraphobia is the remission of panic attacks, anticipatory anxiety, and avoidance of key areas in the person's life (e.g., social functions). As part of (1) the initial educational process about panic disorder and (2) the design and implementation of a structured treatment protocol (e.g., Craske and Barlow 1990), procedures for determining treatment termination should be communicated to the client. As a result, he or she should not be surprised or distressed when the issue arises later.

Emmelkamp and Bouman (1991) indicated that terminating treatment for this population will occasionally be more difficult for clients who are dependent or perceive any panic symptom as relapse. In these cases, the authors recommend the use of (1) symptom prescription, or asking clients to "produce and confront their feared or avoided situations in real life" (p. 425), (2) encouraging self-efficacy in the client and emphasizing the increasingly minimized therapist role, and (3) reframing "relapses" as opportunities to practice cognitive, somatic, and behavioral exercises learned during therapy. In addition, clients should be encouraged to respond to hypothetical situations devised by the therapist. Inappropriate or incomplete responses should be addressed at length. Appropriate family intervention should also be considered for excessively dependent parent–child relationships.

At the conclusion of therapy, the clinician may wish to re-administer pretreatment assessment measures to confirm areas of progress. Both the youngster and family members should be instructed to contact the therapist if any debilitating panic attacks or significant avoidance recur. In addition, referral to other agencies specializing in behaviors related to panic disorder (e.g., substance abuse, depression, suicidal ideation) may be necessary.

CASE ILLUSTRATION (TYPICAL TREATMENT)

Description and History

Amanda was a 15-year-old white female referred by her parents and school nurse for acute and recurring panic attacks. Approximately six months before, Amanda experienced initial panic at a local library one evening while completing a difficult homework assignment in geometry. According to her report, Amanda felt "stressed" and "exhausted" when faced with several problems she had difficulty comprehending. She then experienced several sudden physiological changes, including sweaty palms, dizziness, difficulty breathing, and a "racing heart." Amanda reportedly felt quite anxious and confused about the experience, thinking she was "losing her mind." After two or three minutes, she snatched up her belongings and ran from the library to the cooler air outside. Her anxiety reaction subsided quickly, and she proceeded home without incident.

Amanda reported that this initial experience, while highly unpleasant, was not repeated for several weeks. During this time, however, she avoided the library and preferred to work at a "safer" environment at home. Approximately seven weeks after her initial anxiety reaction, Amanda experienced a full-blown panic attack during her geometry class at school. In addition to the somatic complaints experienced earlier, Amanda felt nauseous and ran from the room without permission to the nurse's office, where she asked for an ambulance to take her to the hospital. The nurse, noting that the symptoms were subsiding, instead asked Amanda to lie down and rest. After thirty minutes, Amanda's initial panic had dissipated but she insisted on going home. She was allowed to do so.

Over the course of the next five weeks, Amanda experienced five similar panic attacks. Each occurred in geometry class between 12:30 and 1:15 P.M. and caused Amanda a substantial amount of embarrassment. Interestingly, these attacks always came immediately before, during, or after an examination or request that Amanda provide a theoretical proof on the blackboard. After this five-week period, Amanda refused to go to school after 12:30 P.M. to avoid potential panic attacks. She became increasingly noncompliant with parent and teacher requests, and was therefore referred for treatment.

During the interview, Amanda was highly cooperative and verbal, discussing at length her cognitive and somatic complaints. In fact, she provided detailed information about her heart and respiration rates during panic and nonpanic states. She seemed particularly interested in whether she was experiencing initial symptoms of schizophrenia, which she had read about in health class. Amanda reported severe anticipatory anxiety about her afternoon classes and discussed her adamant refusal to return. When asked about the library, she reported not having returned there since the initial panic episode. Amanda's parents and school nurse confirmed these accounts and revealed Amanda to be a generally normal adolescent who was academically talented but also somewhat dependent. Questionnaire data indicated that Amanda was particularly fearful of aversive social or evaluative situations. In addition, she appeared to place an inordinate amount of self-worth on her academic performance. She was diagnosed with panic disorder with mild to moderate agoraphobia.

After extensive discussions with Amanda and her parents, teachers, and school nurse, an initial treatment plan was developed. This consisted of cognitive restructuring, relaxation and rebreathing training, and in vivo exposure to avoided situations. Amanda and her parents were asked to complete daily logbooks about Amanda's anxiety and panic symptomatology. Consultation with school officials was maintained to facilitate Amanda's reintegration into afternoon classes and minimize social ostracization.

Synopsis of Therapy Sessions

Before any specific therapeutic procedures are employed to treat panic disorder in youngsters, a complete education should be provided about the disorder and its prevalence, symptomatology, course, and prognosis. The youngster should also be made aware of the effectiveness of cognitive-behavioral treatments for panic disorder. Motivation and compliance with the treatment procedures should be stressed. In addition, the youngster should understand the relationship between cognitions, somatic reactions, and overt behaviors.

The subsequent treatment of panic disorder in youngsters often involves the separate targeting of various cognitive, somatic, and behavioral symptoms. In addition, many clinicians prefer to target cognitive and somatic symptoms first to reduce the aversiveness of panic attacks before discussing avoidance. In some cases, however, the clinician may prefer to address all symptom types in each session. As a result, a treatment protocol is outlined here in sections that separately pinpoint cognitive, somatic, and behavioral symptoms as well as one that addresses all components and other issues.

Section 1 (Cognitive)

1. Review the completed baseline child and parent logbooks, discussing compliance, problems, or questions (repeated each session).
2. Outline the expected course of therapy with the youngster. Explain the concepts of cognitive distortion, cognitive restructuring, and what specific techniques (e.g., hypothesis testing)

will be used. Introduce how and when the techniques will be used for that particular youngster.

3. Review specific cognitions that precede, coincide with, and follow a typical panic attack for the youngster. Concentrate on those that tend to aggravate the aversive reaction (e.g., thoughts of dire physical harm and death, others closely watching and making judgments, loss of control, going crazy).

4. Encourage the youngster to review negative self-statements and disabuse false notions and catastrophizations. Example:

Client: When I have those heart and breathing feelings, I just have to get away.

Therapist: Away? What is it that you think will happen if you stay?

Client: I'm not sure, but I think everyone around me will feel sorry for me or be scared and want to stay away from me. I'd be totally embarrassed.

Therapist: What if you did feel that way? What is the worst that could happen?

Client: I don't know, maybe I would feel weirder . . . although I don't know how.

Therapist: So, the physical symptoms are the worst part about it all?

Client: Yes, but they're pretty bad.

Therapist: Yes, I know the physical symptoms are uncomfortable, but I wonder if they seem worse when you think others are judging you?

Client: Maybe . . . I know if less people are around, it's not so bad. Maybe I do blow it out of proportion sometimes.

Therapist: Maybe that's what's so bad, and makes you run away.

Section 2 (Somatic)

1. Explain in detail to the youngster the somatic exercises of relaxation and rebreathing training. Emphasize the importance of regular practice and utilization during and after a panic episode.

2. Begin relaxation training by asking the youngster to systematically tense and release various muscle groups (e.g., hands, face, stomach, Jacobsen 1938). Audiotape the procedure and instruct the youngster to practice twice daily and during any panic-related symptoms. In addition, instruct the youngster to

identify particularly tense muscle groups during a panic episode and concentrate on those areas.

3. Begin rebreathing training by asking the youngster to maintain a regular respiratory rate and breathe "from the dia-
phragm." Instruct the youngster to engage in this practice
during a panic episode to reduce overbreathing and increased
arousal (Craske and Barlow 1990).

4. Ask family members to monitor these somatic exercises to
ensure their regular practice and efficiency.

Section 3 (Behavioral)

1. Explain in detail to the youngster the concept of in vivo
exposure. Explain that the lessening of panic attacks and/or
their severity should allow him/her to better approach certain
feared stimuli.

2. Design a hierarchy of avoided situations from those that are
least to most anxiety provoking. Choose five to ten severely
problematic areas.

3. Pair relaxation training with each item on the hierarchy and
instruct the youngster to gradually increase his/her approach
to each object or situation. Be sure to include stimuli particular to the youngster's initial and/or subsequent panic attacks.

4. If applicable and necessary, begin to expose the youngster to
stimuli (e.g., exercise) that increase arousal related to panic.
Instruct the youngster to engage in the relaxation training
procedures.

Section 4 (Overall and termination)

1. During each session, review current progress, education about
the disorder, and cognitive, somatic, and/or behavioral techniques. If possible, integrate such techniques (e.g., relaxation
with imaginal exposure).

2. Maintain contact with school officials and others who may be
instrumental in helping to reduce the client's avoidance.
Encourage the youngster to continue regular social activities.

3. Intermittently discuss issues of treatment structure and eventual termination when appropriate.

4. Engage family members in contingency management procedures if applicable and/or recommend pharmacotherapy if
necessary.
5. Following termination of therapy, schedule follow-up telephone conversations and booster sessions if necessary. Encourage the youngster to contact the therapist should any
future problems arise.
6. Provide a referral for any related problems (e.g., substance
abuse).

Following six weeks of intensive therapy, Amanda reported that
her overbreathing and muscle tension had subsided to a moderate
extent and that her ability to control her catastrophic cognitions had
dramatically improved. As a result, Amanda was able to resume school
attendance in the afternoon. Further therapy was geared toward
interoceptive exposure (Craske and Barlow 1990) of remaining physical
symptoms (e.g., dizziness) and tutoring to reduce academic stress.
Amanda's parents reported that their daughter seemed more confident
in social situations, although dependent behavior was sometimes displayed. At six-month follow-up, Amanda reported occasionally mild
paniclike symptoms but no full-blown panic attacks.

Comments

The treatment of panic disorder in youngsters will likely require an integrative effort using several prescriptive techniques. However, clinicians may
sometimes find that reliance on one set of techniques more than another is
mandated. For example, a client may display distressful thoughts without
avoidance or undue avoidance without aversive somatic complaints. In
addition, the use of somatic exercises to control hyperventilation or related
physical symptoms may be necessary and sufficient for children and young
adolescents. Conversely, a combination of cognitive and somatic treatment
techniques for older adolescents is advised, and behavioral techniques to
reduce agoraphobic avoidance are appropriate and can be employed with
most youngsters with panic. In addition, all clients should be given detailed
information about their symptoms and actively participate in the development of a treatment plan.

Finally, we urge clinicians to note that many of the procedures described here have been shown to be quite useful for adults but not as yet for
children and adolescents with panic disorder. We note that cognitive ther-

apy, systematic desensitization and relaxation training, and in vivo exposure have been successfully used by therapists to treat several anxiety-related disorders in this population. However, their efficacy for the complicated and not yet fully understood syndrome of panic disorder with agoraphobia remains highly speculative. Clinicians are thus encouraged to consider the developmental status of their client's intellectual, social, and physical abilities before implementing any psychological and/or pharmacological treatment procedure.

CASE ILLUSTRATION (OVERCOMING OBSTACLES)

Description and History

Theresa was a 16-year-old white female referred by her parents and cardiologist for moderate, recurring panic attacks and other problems. During an initial interview, Theresa reported experiencing several limited-symptom panic attacks during the past two years. The initial attack, which occurred when she was at a day party with friends, consisted primarily of heart palpitations and sweating. Because Theresa was consuming alcohol at the time, she attributed these sensations to her drinking. Over the next two years, however, Theresa intermittently experienced similar sensations when with her friends in public places (e.g., shopping malls, restaurants). Her anxiety about these sensations was moderate and usually subsided if she excused herself to use the restroom.

Theresa also reported that, during the past year, her parents had become increasingly combative about recent financial difficulties and methods of disciplining Theresa for status offenses (e.g., breaking curfew, purchasing liquor). Theresa, who was not performing well academically, felt depressed and steadily began to withdraw from her family. She increasingly spent time with her friends but noticed that her intermittent episodes of somatic complaints were worsening. Approximately twice per month, Theresa experienced now severe symptoms of heart palpitations, sweating, dizziness, and tremors when with her friends or when her parents were arguing. She occasionally missed school because of these sensations and sometimes purchased alcohol to relieve the symptoms.

Approximately four weeks ago, Theresa experienced her most severe panic episode in the cafeteria at school. Her symptoms resembled those of earlier episodes but were apparently of significantly longer duration this time. Theresa went to the nurse's office where she was instructed to rest and was later sent home. Theresa subsequently confided to her mother her symptom patterns and history. Theresa's mother, who had occasionally experienced similar but mild symptoms over the past few years, scheduled an appointment with a cardiologist. The cardiologist found a very slight heart murmur that did not appear to account for the psychological symptoms that Theresa was experiencing. As a result, Theresa and her parents were referred for treatment.

Theresa's mother and father generally confirmed these recent events but emphasized Theresa's externalizing problems as particularly nettlesome. They were especially concerned with her recent school refusal behavior and alcohol use. Questionnaire data indicated that Theresa was not highly fearful of particular objects or situations but did show some moderate negative affectivity (anxiety and depression) about large group settings. In addition, she displayed considerable discomfort about her paniclike somatic symptoms. Family assessment measures revealed a vacillation between detachedness and conflict. Theresa was diagnosed with limited-symptom panic attacks with mild to moderate agoraphobia. Secondary symptoms included those related to depression and substance abuse.

After consultation with the nurse and principal from Theresa's school, an initial treatment plan was devised for Theresa and her family. Although the primary focus was Theresa's paniclike symptoms, secondary targets included family disagreements and Theresa's response to peer pressure. Also, in response to requests from Theresa's parents and with Theresa's approval, treatment was to focus on the youngster's school refusal behavior, depression, and alcohol use. Both Theresa and her parents were instructed to complete daily logbooks of anxiety, depression, panic symptomatology and frequency, and related externalizing problems.

Synopsis of Therapy Sessions

Theresa's case represents one with numerous obstacles, including the presence of limited-symptom panic attacks, familial difficulties, and comorbid depression, substance abuse, and school refusal behavior. The lengthy history of these problems also represents a potential drawback for treatment. As a result, treatment should serve to reduce the aversiveness of somatic symptoms, target absenteeism and related behaviors, and coordinate a familial response. Therefore, a synopsis of treatment sessions is provided along sections that separately address each of these problem sets.

Section 1 (Panic attacks)

1. Review the completed baseline child and parent logbooks, discussing compliance, problems, or questions (repeated each session).
2. Explain to the youngster the expected course of therapy, including procedures to address panic attacks. Implement treatment techniques discussed earlier to ameliorate the frequency and severity of panic attacks.
3. Given this youngster's primarily somatic complaints with respect to panic attacks, concentrate on somatic control exercises such as rebreathing and relaxation training. The client should practice these exercises extensively and employ them as a substitute for self-medication via alcohol use.
4. Address the cognitive aspects of the client's panic attacks, providing education about cognitive distortions and engaging in restructuring techniques (e.g., hypothesis testing, decatastrophization). Utilize these to target symptoms of depression as well.

Section 2 (School refusal behavior and social avoidance)

1. Integrate procedures for reducing panic attacks with those for reducing related social avoidance and school refusal behavior. Assessing the function of school refusal behavior (see Kearney, this volume) is recommended. Be sure to explain upcoming procedures to the client.
2. Role-play specific situations that are most problematic for the client, especially those related to aversive panic attacks and subsequent escape. For example, if the client often displays the somatic symptoms of a panic attack in social situations where she knows few people, have the client practice appropriate cognitive, somatic, and behavioral responses in analogue settings that resemble such situations. Model appropriate responses for the client if necessary and provide detailed feedback.
3. Establish a schedule for resuming full-time school attendance with the client, parents, and school officials. If possible, instruct the client to attend classes that are not highly aversive.

Gradually reintroduce more difficult-to-attend classes as treatment of agoraphobic avoidance progresses.

4. Begin reducing agoraphobic avoidance as much as possible. Instruct the client to practice appropriate cognitive, somatic, and behavioral responses in real-life situations. Review progress extensively. Example:

Therapist: Even though you seemed to have overcome many of your panic symptoms, you've mentioned that eating lunch with your friends remains one of the toughest situations to practice your [cognitive and somatic] exercises. What happens to make this the case?

Client: I start to feel upset and worry that I'll lose everything and go back to square one. I also have other feelings that I don't have in other places, like floating in the air. I bet that sounds weird.

Therapist: No, I kind of expect that you'll feel anxious sometimes, but remember that the more you practice your exercises, the easier it gets. Remember when this happened with other situations in which you had problems adjusting? Also, you have some new skills now that should help even when you experience a different symptom. Let's go ahead and review them.

Section 3 (Familial conflict and secondary variables)

1. Conduct family therapy sessions to address issues of conflict between parents and between parents and the youngster. Explain in detail the reciprocal relationship between the youngster's panic/avoidance, substance use, withdrawal, and familial infighting.

2. Utilize contingency contracting to address school refusal behavior and alcohol use. Institute a system of rewards and punishers for appropriate and inappropriate behavior. Be sure that all family members agree to the contract before signing and implementing the contract.

3. Conduct parent training sessions to help the parents present a unified front in addressing their youngster's panic and related externalizing problems. If necessary, provide services or a referral for marital therapy.

Section 4 (Other issues)

1. Address issues of termination and relapse prevention intermittently throughout the therapeutic process. Have the client

present solutions to new, hypothetical familial and extrafamilial situations that may precipitate paniclike symptoms.

2. Continue to maintain contact with school officials to monitor and review reintegration into regular classroom settings.

3. Following termination, schedule intermittent booster sessions to address new problematic situations or antecedents to panic and/or avoidance. Maintain periodic telephone or written contact with the youngster and parents for at least two years following termination.

4. Provide referral services for specific problems that may require additional attention.

Following three months of therapy, Theresa reported that her physiological symptoms had diminished considerably and that alcohol use to reduce their severity was no longer needed. Her externalizing behaviors (e.g., breaking curfew) were lessened to a moderate degree but continued to be problematic. Theresa's parents confirmed this report and indicated their desire to focus therapy on other family issues. With everyone's consent, structural and strategic family therapy continued for the next several months to address areas of conflict. With respect to Theresa's panic symptoms, however, their absence was maintained at six-month follow-up.

Comments

The treatment of limited-symptom panic attacks with comorbid psychopathology represents a significant challenge to therapists who address this population. Instead of prescribing a package treatment to specifically address symptoms of panic, the therapist will have to decide on a unique combination of interventions to address concurrent internalizing and externalizing problems. In addition, when avoidance involves school refusal behavior or other key areas of the youngster's life, a crisis management approach may need to be adopted. Treatment duration in these cases is likely to be longer than in a case of circumscribed panic.

A client's use of alcohol or other drugs to self-medicate panic symptomatology is also a significant obstacle to treatment. Approximately 13 percent of adolescents with panic attacks ingest drugs to relieve social anxiety and physical symptoms related to the disorder (Warren and Zgourides 1988). Unlike adults, however, who often have adequate knowledge regarding the effects of alcohol and other drugs, youngsters may quickly develop abusive patterns with serious mental, physical, legal, and financial ramifications. Hence, the treatment of substance abuse and panic disorder must sometimes coexist. In such cases, though, clinicians are urged to exercise extreme caution when considering the use of pharmacotherapy to ease panic.

SUMMARY

Although the classification, assessment, and treatment of panic disorder and agoraphobia in adults has received a substantial amount of research attention in recent years, the same cannot yet be said for youngsters with the disorder. As a result, this chapter has focused on the extant literature and an extrapolation from knowledge about adult panic disorder. Future research must concentrate on whether the clinical picture of panic disorder is qualitatively different across childhood, adolescence, and adulthood. In addition, course, prognosis, and specific assessment and treatment strategies for this population must be investigated further. Although panic disorder and agoraphobia represent fascinating aspects of psychopathology in youngsters, the syndromes remain largely mysterious. Given that most persons with panic disorder experience their initial symptoms in childhood or adolescence, however, the study of panic in youngsters should receive a greater priority among clinical researchers.

REFERENCES

Abelson, J. L., and Alessi, N. E. (1992). Discussion of "Child panic revisited" (letter). *Journal of the American Academy of Child and Adolescent Psychiatry* 31:114–116.

Achenbach, T. M. (1991a). *Manual for the Child Behavior Checklist/4-18 and 1991 Profile*. Burlington: University of Vermont Department of Psychiatry.

———— (1991b). *Manual for the Teacher's Report Form and 1991 Profile*. Burlington: University of Vermont Department of Psychiatry.

Acierno, R. E., Hersen, M., and Van Hasselt, V. B. (1993). Interventions for panic disorder: a critical review of the literature. *Clinical Psychology Review* 13:561–578.

Alessi, N. E., and Magen, J. (1988). Panic disorder in psychiatrically hospitalized children. *American Journal of Psychiatry* 145:1450–1452.

Alessi, N. E., Robbins, D. R., and Dilsaver, S. C. (1987). Panic and depressive disorders among psychiatrically hospitalized adolescents. *Psychiatry Research* 20:275–283.

Ballenger, J. C., Carek, D. J., Steele, J. J., and Cornish-McTighe, D. (1989). Three cases of panic disorder with agoraphobia in children. *American Journal of Psychiatry* 146:922–924.

Barlow, D. H. (1988). *Anxiety and Its Disorders: The Nature and Treatment of Panic and Anxiety.* New York: Guilford.

Barlow, D. H., Craske, M. G., Cerny, J. A., and Klosko, J. S. (1989). Behavioral treatment of panic disorder. *Behavior Therapy* 20:261–282.

Beidel, D. C., and Stanley, M. A. (1993). Developmental issues in measurement of anxiety. In *Anxiety Across the Lifespan: A Developmental Perspective,* ed. C. G. Last, pp. 167–203. New York: Springer.

Biederman, J. (1987). Clonazepam in the treatment of prepubertal children with panic-like symptoms. *Journal of Clinical Psychiatry* 48:38–41.

Biederman, J., Rosenbaum, J. F., Bolduc-Murphy, E. A., et al. (1993). A 3-year follow-up of children with and without behavioral inhibition. *Journal of the American Academy of Child and Adolescent Psychiatry* 32:814–821.

Black, B., and Robbins, D. R. (1990). Panic disorder in children and adolescents. *Journal of the American Academy of Child and Adolescent Psychiatry* 29:36–44.

Bowlby, J. (1973). *Attachment and Loss: Vol. II. Separation, Anxiety, and Anger.* New York: Basic Books.

Bradley, S. J., and Hood, J. (1993). Psychiatrically referred adolescents with panic attacks: presenting symptoms, stressors, and comorbidity. *Journal of the American Academy of Child and Adolescent Psychiatry* 32:826–829.

Brown, T. A., and Deagle, E. A. (1992). Structured interview assessment of nonclinical panic. *Behavior Therapy* 23:75–85.

Carpenter, R. O., and Vining, E. P. G. (1993). Antiepileptics (anticonvulsants). In *Practitioner's Guide to Psychoactive Drugs for Children and Adolescents,* eds. J. S. Werry and M. G. Aman, pp. 321–346. New York: Plenum.

Chorpita, B. F., Albano, A. M., and Barlow, D. H. (1994). *The Childhood Anxiety Sensitivity Index: considerations for children with anxiety disorders.* Unpublished manuscript.

Craske, M. G., and Barlow, D. H. (1990). *Therapist's Guide for the Mastery of Your Anxiety and Panic (MAP) Program.* Albany, NY: Graywind.

Diagnostic and Statistical Manual of Mental Disorders (1994). 4th ed. Washington, DC: American Psychiatric Association.

Elkind, D. (1976). *Child Development and Education.* New York: Oxford.

Emmelkamp, P. M. G., and Bouman, T. K. (1991). Psychological approaches to the difficult patient. In *Panic Disorder and Agoraphobia: A Comprehensive Guide for the Practitioner,* eds. J. R. Walker, G. R. Norton, and C. A. Ross, pp. 398–429. Pacific Grove, CA: Brooks/Cole.

Emmelkamp, P. M. G., Brilman, E., Kuiper, H., and Mersch, P. P. (1986). The treatment of agoraphobia: a comparison of self-instructional training, rational emotive therapy, and exposure in vivo. *Behavior Modification* 10:37–53.

Fava, M., Anderson, K., and Rosenbaum, J. F. (1990). "Anger attacks": possible variants of panic and major depressive disorders. *American Journal of Psychiatry* 147:867–870.

Fontaine, R. (1991). The role of the primary care physician in the treatment of panic disorder. In *Panic Disorder and Agoraphobia: A Comprehensive Guide for the*

Practitioner, eds. J. R. Walker, G. R. Norton, and C. A. Ross, pp. 352–367. Pacific Grove, CA: Brooks/Cole.

Foreyt, J. P., and McGavin, J. K. (1989). Anorexia nervosa and bulimia nervosa. In *Treatment of Childhood Disorders*, eds. E. J. Mash and R. A. Barkley, pp. 529–558. New York: Guilford.

Fyer, A. J., Sandberg, D., and Klein, D. F. (1991). The pharmacologic treatment of panic disorder and agoraphobia. In *Panic Disorder and Agoraphobia: A Comprehensive Guide for the Practitioner*, eds. J. R. Walker, G. R. Norton, and C. A. Ross, pp. 211–251. Pacific Grove, CA: Brooks/Cole.

Garland, E. J., and Smith, D. H. (1990). Panic disorder on a child psychiatric consultation service. *Journal of the American Academy of Child and Adolescent Psychiatry* 29:785–788.

Gittelman-Klein, R., and Klein, D. (1980). Separation anxiety in school refusal and its treatment with drugs. In *Out of School*, eds. L. Hersov and I. Berg, pp. 321–341. New York: Wiley.

Gorman, J. M., Goetz, R. R., Fyer, M., et al. (1988). The mitral valve prolapse–panic disorder connection. *Psychosomatic Medicine* 50:114–122.

Grace, N., Spirito, A., Finch, A. J., Jr., and Ott, E. S. (1993). Coping skills for anxiety control in children. In *Cognitive-Behavioral Procedures for Children and Adolescents: A Practical Guide*, eds. A. J. Finch, Jr., W. M. Nelson III, and E. S. Ott, pp. 257–288. Boston: Allyn & Bacon.

Griegel, L. E., Albano, A. M., and Barlow, D. H. (1991). *"Do children panic?" revisited: Yes they do!* Paper presented at the meeting of the Association for the Advancement of Behavior Therapy, New York, NY, November.

Hayward, C., Killen, J. D., and Taylor, C. B. (1989). Panic attacks in young adolescents. *American Journal of Psychiatry* 146:1061–1062.

Jacob, R. G., and Lilienfeld, S. O. (1991). Panic disorder: diagnosis, medical assessment, and psychological assessment. In *Panic Disorder and Agoraphobia: A Comprehensive Guide for the Practitioner*, eds. J. R. Walker, G. R. Norton, and C. A. Ross, pp. 16–102. Pacific Grove, CA: Brooks/Cole.

Jacobsen, E. (1938). *Progressive Relaxation*. Chicago: University of Chicago Press.

Kearney, C. A., and Silverman, W. K. (1992). Let's not push the "panic" button: a critical analysis of panic and panic disorder in adolescents. *Clinical Psychology Review* 12:293–305.

Kearney, C. A., Williams de Coronado, M., and Cheeseman, P. (1992). *Mitral valve prolapse and negative affectivity in adolescents*. Paper presented at the meeting of the Western Psychological Association, Portland, OR, May.

Kendall, P. C., Chansky, T. E., Kane, M. T., et al. (1992). *Anxiety Disorders in Youth: Cognitive-Behavioral Interventions*. Boston: Allyn & Bacon.

King, N. J., Gullone, E., Tonge, B. J., and Ollendick, T. H. (1993). Self-reports of panic attacks and manifest anxiety in adolescents. *Behaviour Research and Therapy* 31:111–116.

Kleiner, L., Marshall, W. L., and Spevack, M. (1987). Training in problem-solving and exposure treatment for agoraphobics with panic attacks. *Journal of Anxiety Disorders* 1:219–238.

Klosko, J. S., Barlow, D. H., Tassinari, R., and Cerny, J. A. (1990). A comparison of alprazolam and behavior therapy in treatment of panic disorder. *Journal of Consulting and Clinical Psychology* 58:77–84.

Kovacs, M., and Beck, A. T. (1977). An empirical-clinical approach toward a definition of childhood depression. In *Depression in Childhood: Diagnosis, Treatment, and Conceptual Models*, eds. J. G. Schulterbrandt and A. Raskin, pp. 1–25. New York: Raven.

La Greca, A. M., and Stone, W. L. (1993). Social Anxiety Scale for Children-Revised: factor structure and concurrent validity. *Journal of Clinical Child Psychology* 22:17–27.

Last, C. G. (1993). Introduction. In *Anxiety across the Lifespan: A Developmental Perspective*, ed. C. G. Last, pp. 1–6. New York: Springer.

Last, C. G., and Strauss, C. C. (1989). Panic disorder in children and adolescents. *Journal of Anxiety Disorders* 3:87–95.

Lewinsohn, P. M., Hops, H., Roberts, R. E., et al. (1993). Adolescent psychopathology: I. Prevalence and incidence of depression and other *DSM-III-R* disorders in high school students. *Journal of Abnormal Psychology* 102:133–144.

Macaulay, J. L., and Kleinknecht, R. A. (1989). Panic and panic attacks in adolescents. *Journal of Anxiety Disorders* 3:221–241.

Myers, J. K., Weissman, M. M., Tischler, G. L., et al. (1984). Six-month prevalence of psychiatric disorders in three communities. *Archives of General Psychiatry* 41:959–967.

Nelles, W. B., and Barlow, D. H. (1988). Do children panic? *Clinical Psychology Review* 8:359–372.

Norton, G. R., Cox, B. J., and Malan, J. (1992). Nonclinical panickers: a critical review. *Clinical Psychology Review* 12:121–139.

Norton, G. R., Harrison, B., Hauch, J., and Rhodes, L. (1985). Characteristics of people with infrequent panic attacks. *Journal of Abnormal Psychology* 94:216–221.

Ollendick, T. H. (1983). Reliability and validity of the Revised Fear Survey Schedule for Children (FSSC-R). *Behaviour Research and Therapy* 21:685–692.

Ollendick, T. H., Mattis, S. G., and King, N. J. (1994). Panic in children and adolescents: a review. *Journal of Child Psychology and Psychiatry* 35:113–134.

Perloff, J. K., and Child, J. S. (1987). Clinical and epidemiologic issues in mitral valve prolapse: overview and perspective. *American Heart Journal* 113:1324–1332.

Perugi, G., Deltito, J., Soriani, A., et al. (1988). Relationship between panic disorder and separation anxiety with school phobia. *Comprehensive Psychiatry* 29:98–107.

Raskin, M., Peeke, H. V. S., Dickman, W., and Pinsker, H. (1982). Panic and generalized anxiety disorders: developmental antecedents and precipitants. *Archives of General Psychiatry* 39:687–689.

Reynolds, C. R., and Paget, K. D. (1983). National normative and reliability data for the Revised Children's Manifest Anxiety Scale. *School Psychology Review* 12:324–336.

Schreier, H. A. (1992). Panic disorder and anger attacks (letter). *Journal of the American Academy of Child and Adolescent Psychiatry* 31:369.

Sheehan, D. V., and Raj, B. A. (1991). Treatment of the difficult case with panic disorder. In *Panic Disorder and Agoraphobia: A Comprehensive Guide for the Practitioner*, eds. J. R. Walker, G. R. Norton, and C. A. Ross, pp. 368–397. Pacific Grove, CA: Brooks/Cole.

Silverman, W. K., and Eisen, A. R. (1992). Age differences in the reliability of parent and child reports of child anxious symptomatology using a structured interview. *Journal of the American Academy of Child and Adolescent Psychiatry* 31:117–124.

Silverman, W. K., Fleisig, W., Rabian, B., and Peterson, R. A. (1991). Childhood Anxiety Sensitivity Index. *Journal of Clinical Child Psychology* 20:162–168.

Silverman, W. K., and Kearney, C. A. (1993). Behavioral treatment of childhood anxiety. In *Handbook of Behavior Therapy and Pharmacotherapy for Children: A Comparative Analysis*, eds. V. B. Van Hasselt and M. Hersen, pp. 33–53. Boston: Allyn & Bacon.

Silverman, W. K., and Nelles, W. B. (1988). The Anxiety Disorders Interview Schedule for Children. *Journal of the American Academy of Child and Adolescent Psychiatry* 27:772–778.

Spielberger, C. D. (1973). *Manual for the State-Trait Anxiety Inventory for Children*. Palo Alto, CA: Consulting Psychologists Press.

Spitzer, R. L., Williams, J. B. W., and Gibbon, M. (1986). *Structured Clinical Interview for DSM-III-R (SCID)*. Unpublished manuscript.

Thyer, B. A. (1993). Childhood separation anxiety disorder and adult-onset agoraphobia: review of evidence. In *Anxiety across the Lifespan: A Developmental Perspective*, ed. C. G. Last, pp. 128–147. New York: Springer.

Viesselman, J. O., Yaylayan, S., Weller, E. B., and Weller, R. A. (1993). Antidysthymic drugs (antidepressants and antimanics). In *Practitioner's Guide to Psychoactive Drugs for Children and Adolescents*, eds. J. S. Werry and M. G. Aman, pp. 239–268. New York: Plenum.

Vitiello, B., Behar, D., Wolfson, S., and McLeer, S. V. (1990). Diagnosis of panic disorder in prepubertal children. *Journal of the American Academy of Child and Adolescent Psychiatry* 29:782–784.

Von Korff, M. R., Eaton, W. W., and Keyl, P. M. (1985). The epidemiology of panic attacks and panic disorder: results of three community surveys. *American Journal of Epidemiology* 122:970–981.

Walker, J. R., Ross, C. A., and Norton, G. R. (1991). A final word: pragmatic considerations for the practitioner. In *Panic Disorder and Agoraphobia: A Comprehensive Guide for the Practitioner*, eds. J. R. Walker, G. R. Norton, and C. A. Ross, pp. 504–519. Pacific Grove, CA: Brooks/Cole.

Warren, R., and Zgourides, G. (1988). Panic attacks in high school students: implications for prevention and intervention. *Phobia Practice and Research Journal* 1:97–113.

Weissman, M. M., Leckman, J. F., Merikangas, K. R., et al. (1984). Depression and anxiety disorders in parents and children. *Archives of General Psychiatry* 41:845–852.

Werry, J. S., and Aman, M. G. (1993). Anxiolytics, sedatives, and miscellaneous drugs. In *Practitioner's Guide to Psychoactive Drugs for Children and Adolescents*, eds. J. S. Werry and M. G. Aman, pp. 391–415. New York: Plenum.

Whitaker, A., Johnson, J., Shaffer, D., et al. (1990). Uncommon troubles in young people: prevalence estimates of selected psychiatric disorders in a nonreferred adolescent population. *Archives of General Psychiatry* 47:487–496.

Wolpe, J., and Rowan, V. C. (1988). Panic disorder: a product of classical conditioning. *Behaviour Research and Therapy* 26:441–450.

Zitrin, C. M., Klein, D. F., Woerner, M. G., and Ross, D. C. (1983). Treatment of phobias: I. Comparison of imipramine hydrochloride and placebo. *Archives of General Psychiatry* 40:125–138.

10

OBSESSIVE-COMPULSIVE DISORDER

Anne Marie Albano
Lenna S. Knox
David H. Barlow

INTRODUCTION

The chronic and debilitating course of obsessive-compulsive disorder (OCD) has been well documented in the literature (e.g., Flament et al. 1990, Karno et al. 1988; Rapoport 1988, Riggs and Foa 1993). Tragically, this disorder has gone underreported and undertreated in children. Although epidemiological and pharmacological research on childhood OCD has burgeoned in the past decade, the development and evaluation of effective psychosocial interventions are lacking. In this chapter we first describe the phenomenology of OCD in children and adolescents. We then review current diagnostic and assessment procedures and describe a new behavioral treatment program for OCD in children and adolescents. The remainder of the chapter is focused on actual case descriptions of two patients, a relatively typical OCD child and a clinically challenging case.

DESCRIPTION OF THE DISORDER

Recent epidemiological studies of OCD in children and adolescents have identified the mean age of onset ranging from 9.0 years to 12.8 years (Flament et al. 1988, Last and Strauss 1989, Riddle et al. 1990), with one study reporting onset as low as 2 years of age (Swedo et al. 1989). Onset appears to occur earlier in boys than girls, yielding a predominance of males in younger samples and equal male to female ratios in older samples. The early onset of the disorder has also been confirmed by the retrospective reports of adult

OCD patients. In one study, Lo (1967) found that 22 percent of eighty-eight adult OCD patients endorsed onset before age 15.

The symptoms of OCD in children and adolescents are strikingly similar to those found in adults. Common are obsessions involving contamination, sexual themes, religiosity, or aggressive/violent images. At the Child and Adolescent Program of the Center for Stress and Anxiety Disorders, we have observed children with OCD complain of an inability to stop "hearing" intrusive and recurrent songs or rhymes, fears of catching a life-threatening illness such as cancer or AIDS, and seeing images of their parents in coffins. Compulsions involving washing, checking, ordering, and arranging have been noted in child cases as well (Flament et al. 1988, Last and Strauss 1989, Riddle et al. 1990). In one case at our clinic, a young boy was overcome with anxiety while at Disney World, and feared some terrible disaster would befall his family unless he touched all the lines in the parking lot. In children, obsessions without compulsions are relatively rare, as is also true for adults. Interestingly, the literature reveals that in 90 percent of child OCD cases the symptom patterns change over time (Swedo et al. 1989). For example, parents will report their child having started with checking locks and cupboards, but having replaced such behaviors by counting or arranging rituals.

Investigators have noted that as many as 50–60 percent of children receiving diagnoses of OCD experience severe impairment in global functioning (Berg et al. 1989, Last and Strauss 1989, Whitaker et al. 1990). Such impairment reflects the interference of the disorder in the child's personal, social, and academic life. Children and adolescents with nighttime rituals find themselves unable to invite friends to sleepovers and embarrassed by their repeated refusal to accept such invitations. Ordering and arranging rituals become difficult to hide from schoolmates as the rituals become more elaborate and time consuming. Frequently, homework becomes an overwhelming daily struggle, as the child may spend hours with repeated checking and erasing. A straightforward multiple-choice test may trigger continuous checking rituals, with the child failing to complete the test within the allotted time. Although adolescence is generally a time to foster independence from the family and accept personal responsibility for one's own behavior, the adolescent with OCD will find such tasks extremely difficult and anxiety producing. Rituals may keep the adolescent from engaging in usual teenage activities, such as dating or driving. Moreover, leaving home for college will be particularly challenging, due to the impact of leaving the family system that has evolved around the OCD and the potential for being discovered by college peers.

Perhaps the most glaring finding reported in the recent literature is the evidence supporting the chronicity and intractability of this disorder. As in adults, OCD appears to follow a chronic but fluctuating course (Swedo et al. 1989). In a two-year follow-up study of the National Institute of Mental Health adolescent epidemiological project, 31 percent of those adolescents who had received an initial current or lifetime diagnosis of OCD received a current diagnosis at follow-up, and 25 percent received a diagnosis of subclinical OCD. Of those who had received an initial current or lifetime subclinical OCD diagnosis, 10 percent received a current diagnosis of OCD and 40 percent received a diagnosis of subclinical OCD (Berg et al. 1989). More recently, Leonard et al. (1993) reported the results of their prospective two- to seven-year follow-up study of fifty-four pediatric OCD patients who had participated in controlled treatment trials with clomipramine followed by a variety of interim treatments. On follow-up, twenty-three (43 percent) of the subjects still met diagnostic criteria for OCD, and only three (6 percent) were considered in full remission. Thirty-eight subjects (70 percent) were taking psychoactive medication at follow-up. Overall, the group as a whole was considered improved despite continued OCD symptomatology, as only ten subjects (19 percent) were rated unchanged or worse. This study illustrates the chronicity of the disorder, in that despite multiple interventions and potent psychopharmacological treatment, the symptoms of OCD persist for a significant subgroup of patients.

DIFFERENTIAL DIAGNOSIS

Comorbid psychiatric disorders occur in 62–74 percent of OCD children and adolescents, with anxiety disorders most prevalent, and with mood disorders less than reported in adults (Flament et al. 1988, Last and Strauss 1989, Riddle et al. 1990, Swedo et al. 1989). Additionally, high rates of tics and Tourette's disorder are associated with this population (Grad et al. 1987, Leonard et al. 1992, Pauls et al. 1986). Consequently, differential diagnosis of OCD in children is rarely straightforward.

The relatively common co-occurrence of other anxiety disorders and anxiety symptoms among children with OCD makes differential diagnosis complex. For example, children with OCD will frequently display phobic avoidance of objects or situations that trigger their obsessions. A child who fears contamination by germs may avoid using public restrooms or refuse to use classroom supplies shared by other students. Touching an animal, even the beloved family dog or cat, may evoke extreme fear of germs such that the child begins to avoid the animal. Such behavior may resemble the avoidance of a specific phobic. In severe cases, fears of contamination may result in school refusal behavior, giving the appearance of agoraphobia. Thus, the nature of the child's fear must be carefully delineated for accurate diagnosis. For specific phobics, the child typically fears a circumscribed object or event (e.g., being bitten by a dog, getting lost at school), and escape or avoidance of the stimulus reduces the child's distress. A friend can lock the dog in the basement, resulting in a phobic child feeling safe and relieved. However, for the OCD child, the animal has already spread germs throughout the house, and as such the contamination fears persist in the dog's absence. Additionally, the OCD child will be compelled to ritualize (e.g., wash hands) to neutralize his or her anxiety. Such ritualistic behavior is not observed in specific phobics.

Generalized anxiety disorder (GAD) is characterized by excessive worry about a number of life circumstances and may be accompanied by somatic complaints in children and adolescents. GAD worry may be distinguished from obsessions in that worry typically represents excessive concern over real-life situations, such as academic reports, popularity and friendships, or athletic competition. Conversely, obsessive ruminations are more likely to focus on unrealistic or extremely unlikely events. Riggs and Foa (1993) note that in some cases the content of an obsessional fear may reflect events that can realistically occur, such as illness befalling a family member. However, in such cases, the individual greatly exaggerates the realistic probability of such occurrences. In addition, compulsions are not evidenced in GAD behavior.

Compulsive rituals may take the form of repetitive motor behaviors similar to those observed in Tourette's disorder and tic disorders. In OCD, the behaviors are purposeful and goal directed, aimed at neutralizing the distress triggered by obsessive thoughts. Conversely, stereotyped motor behaviors of Tourette's or tic disorders are usually involuntary and unintentional. Similarly, the stereotypic behavior of autism or pervasive developmental disorder can be differentiated from OCD. In the former, the behavior is performed in the absence of any identifiable anxiogenic trigger. However, in OCD a cognitive or overt behavioral trigger can usually be identified. The presence of language delays or effective nonverbal communication skills may complicate diagnosis in these cases.

Riggs and Foa (1993) provide a number of additional guidelines for the differential diagnosis of OCD. First, OCD may present with nonbizarre obsessions of delusional intensity. OCD can best be differentiated from delusional disorder on the basis of the presence of associated compulsions. Second, although some patients may manifest thoughts with clearly bizarre content, OCD may be differentiated from schizophrenia on the basis of a lack of positive schizophrenic symptoms (e.g., loose associations, hallucinations, thought insertion or broadcasting, inappropriate affect). At times, however, an individual may present with sufficient symptoms for a dual diagnosis of OCD and thought disorder. Finally, although depressive disorders are thus far less often identified in OCD children than adults, the two disorders may co-occur. Riggs and Foa point out that depressives may present with ruminations about unpleasant life events, but these patients typically do not try to suppress or avoid such thoughts. Moreover, ruminations are typically common in depressives and congruent with depressed mood.

ASSESSMENT PROCEDURES

In our clinic, children and adolescents undergo a comprehensive assessment battery designed to examine the triple response system of anxiety (cognitive, physiological, and behavioral). Additionally, information is gathered from multiple sources, including the child, parents, and clinician. At times, teacher ratings or behavioral observations are obtained. Such assessment allows the clinician to identify and quantify specific symptoms and rate symptom severity, and thus provides a basis for evaluating clinical change. Moreover, the comprehensive nature of the assessment provides a framework for understanding the impact of the disorder on multiple areas of the child's functioning (social, familial, academic). In addition to assisting the therapist in identifying targets for treatment, a functional analysis of the problems aids our understanding of the developmental and phenomenological parameters of these disorders in children. The choice of assessment measures within each response system is guided by the child's presenting diagnosis. Below we describe our battery for evaluating obsessive-compulsive symptomatology in children.

Diagnostic Interview

A structured diagnostic interview is highly recommended for reliable differential diagnosis of OCD. Although several such interviews are available (see Silverman 1991 for a review), the Anxiety Disorders Interview Schedule for Children and Parents (ADIS-C/P, Silverman and Nelles 1988) was developed specifically to provide accurate differential diagnosis among the anxiety disorders, affective disorders, and externalizing disorders of childhood. In addition, the ADIS-C/P interviews provide screening questions for psychotic symptomatology. When conducting the ADIS-C/P the child is seen first, followed by an independent interview of the parents. Information obtained from the child interview is not openly used during the parent interview. Diagnoses from each interview are then combined to form a composite diagnosis following specific guidelines (Silverman 1991). For each diagnosis identified, a clinical severity rating is assigned ranging from 0 to 8, with adverb qualifiers defining selected points of severity (e.g., 0 = absent symptomatology – no disruption in functioning, 4 = moderate symptomatology – definitely disturbing/disabling, and 8 = severe symptomatology – very severely disturbing/disabling). Consequently, the ADIS-C/P provides an efficient mechanism for tracking overall treatment progress and patterns of symptom remission through follow-up assessments. In addition, the ADIS-C/P provides questions for assessing the triple response system of anxiety for each individual diagnosis. The clinician is able to access information regarding the child's beliefs and interpretation of the problem, rate the child's physiological reactivity and assess for panic symptomatology, and gain an understanding of the behavioral mechanisms involved in escape/avoidance or other methods of coping with the anxiety. Silverman (1991) reports good Kappa coefficients of .84 and .83 for the ADIS-C and ADIS-P, respectively, and .78 for the composite OCD diagnosis. The ADIS-C/P is currently being revised to be consistent with *DSM-IV* (Silverman et al. 1994).

Following the diagnostic evaluation, the therapist should conduct a pretreatment assessment to collect data on the client's specific OCD symptomatology. Such data will serve as a basis for evaluating the progress and rate of treatment, and for identifying targets for specific behavioral interventions. Basic assessment consists of the administration of a standardized inventory for obsessive-compulsive symptomatology and the construction of an individualized hierarchy of external and internal fear cues and corresponding Subjective Units of Distress (SUDS) ratings. In addition, the client is also given instruction in the use of a continuous self-monitoring diary to complete during a pretreatment baseline and for the duration of treatment.

Child Self-Report Measures

Initially, the child is administered the Leyton Obsessional Inventory–Child Version (LOI-CV; Berg et al. 1986), a forty-four-item downward extension of the adult version of this instrument. The individual items of the LOI-CV test for the presence of persistent thoughts, checking, fears of dirt and/or dangerous objects, cleanliness, order, repetition, and indecision. The forty-four items are presented to the child on 3 × 5 index cards, and first sorted into "Yes" or "No" slots of an answer box. "Yes" responses are then re-sorted for perceived resistance, and again for degree of interference. The LOI-CV provides a total item subscale ("Yes" score) and two ratings of subjective distress. The resistance subscale quantifies the child's struggle to fight intrusive thoughts or images and resist performing compulsive rituals; the interference subscale provides a rating of subjective distress and perceived disruption in functioning.

Using information obtained during the ADIS-C/P interviews and the LOI-CV, the therapist then assists the child in constructing a ten-item Obsessive-Compulsive Hierarchy (OCH) of fear cues, focused on external and internal cues and their associated consequences, avoidance, and rituals. Using a visual thermometer, the therapist assists the child in anchoring ratings of perceived distress due to each OCD symptom on a 0–8 subjective units of distress (SUDS) scale. The thermometer assists the child in more accurately expressing his or her level of distress and avoidance of OCD triggers by providing a visual stimulus. Parent input is solicited to validate the parameters of each hierarchy item. These "Top Ten" items will then become the targets of intervention in treatment.

Children are also instructed in the use of a daily diary, in which they record the occurrence and frequency of the ten hierarchy items, along with any other OCD symptoms they may experience. In the diary, the child notes the date, time, place, and people present for each OCD episode. They then record what they were thinking, what they felt physically, and what they did. Finally, an overall SUDS rating, resistance rating, and interference rating are assigned on the same 0–8 scale for each episode. The diary provides the therapist with an ongoing evaluation of the course of the disorder and feedback on how the child is progressing through treatment.

In addition to the aforementioned self-report measures, we often obtain measures of related symptomatology from the child. Measures of trait anxiety, generalized anxiety, fearfulness, and depression may be easily accessed through paper and pencil methods. Such evaluation will allow the therapist to assess the impact of treatment on comorbid conditions and to evaluate the child's overall coping ability and response.

Behavioral Observation

Unfortunately, behavioral observation in the natural setting may be costly and time consuming, and at present there are no published coding scales for rating the behavioral expression of childhood OCD. However, we are currently evaluating the validity and reliability of a standardized behavioral avoidance task (BAT) for OCD. The goal of the BAT is to obtain both a self-report of anxiety and a behavioral measure of resistance, that is, the amount of time spent resisting the compulsion until habituation to the anxiety occurs. In the BAT, the child is imaginally exposed to two situations from his or her hierarchy, items three and eight, representing relatively low and moderate anxiety, respectively. For each situation, the child is told to imagine as vividly as possible the scene described in the item and the ensuing consequence (e.g., "imagine swallowing contaminated saliva, think about how it will taste, what will happen, etc."). To prevent the possibility of covert compulsions, the child is asked to describe the scene verbally as it progresses, with prompts from the therapist. At the same time, no directions are given pertaining to compulsions. Each task lasts eight minutes or until the occurrence of a compulsion is noted, or the child asks to stop. SUDS ratings (from 0–100) are taken every minute during the task. In addition to SUDS ratings, the therapist records the duration of the exposure, time of escape, and presence of compulsions. The BAT provides important clinical information about the behavioral limits of the child's tolerance for anxious symptomatology and serves as an objective measure of clinical change.

Parent-Report Measures

In our clinical work with children and adolescents, we have noted that parents often describe critical incidents that have occurred, such as observing their child repeating songs or phrases, touching objects in a certain manner or number of times, and showing excessive slowness in dressing and grooming. To enhance the accuracy of reporting and to gain important information about the antecedents, consequences, and parameters of these situations, we ask parents to complete a parent diary form for each episode of obsessive and/or compulsive behavior that they observe or may receive information about secondhand (e.g., teacher report of OCD incidents). Similar to the children's diary, the parent form requests information about the date, time, situation, and people present. The parents are asked to provide a short narrative about what they observed, how they responded to the incident, and how their child responded. Parents also give an overall 0–8 interference rating for each episode. This method of assessment provides important cross-informant information and a quantifiable rating of critical anxiety-producing incidents that parents are privy to during the course of treatment.

Future Directions

The complex nature of anxiety and the pervasive disruption across all aspects of the child's life experiences calls for the development of measures that will maximize our understanding of the disorder and facilitate appropriate treat-ment planning. Currently, we are evaluating several additional assessment modalities for anxiety disorders in youth. For example, few studies of the psychophysiological responding of anxious children exist (Beidel 1988, 1989), and no studies have evaluated the responding of obsessive-compulsive youth. In our clinic, we are currently collecting data on the physiological responding of OCD children during the BAT tasks, to understand the parameters of physiological responding in children in general and anxious children in particular.

In addition, assessment of family communication patterns in response to anxiety-provoking situations can be quantified to examine the differential effects of treatment on the parent–child relationship. A "Family BAT" methodology has been developed at our clinic, where the child and parents are presented with an anxious scenario corresponding to their child's pre-senting complaint. For example, in a case of obsessional slowness, the family is asked to discuss this situation: "Your family has dinner reservations with friends in one-half hour, yet your son/daughter is not ready to go. This has been a problem, causing you to be late for many engagements. Discuss this with your son/daughter." The discussion is taped and then coded for communication style, level and type of affective expression, and method of resolution. Similar methods can be easily adapted in clinical practice and provide invaluable information about the impact of the disorder and subse-quent treatment response on the family.

ESTABLISHING TREATMENT GOALS

Information gained from a thorough pretreatment assessment will provide the targets for intervention, through the examination of the functional relationships between fear cues and the avoidance or ritualistic behaviors maintaining the disorder.

External and Internal Fear Cues

According to Riggs and Foa (1993), fear cues may be either tangible objects in the environment or thoughts and images that the person experiences. We have observed that fear cues are experienced as specific and idiosyncratic for each individual child. For example, although it is not uncommon for OCD children to fear contamination, one child may fear contracting a disease by shaking hands with strangers but consider his or her own family members safe. However, another child may fear touching any other person, including his or her parents and siblings.

It is of paramount importance that the therapist uncover fear cues both external (objects, persons, situations) and internal (thoughts, images, impulses) for each individual child during the pretreatment assessment. Internal fear cues may be triggered by external situations. For example, one adolescent feared his parents had suddenly died whenever he saw or heard emergency service vehicles. Such cues were experienced both in his everyday real life and when watching television programs, prompting him to picture his parents dead and resulting in frantic searches to locate their whereabouts.

Fear cues should be identified and described in full detail. Such descriptions may involve elaborate and fairly distressing scenes; however, it is essential for effective treatment that the therapist uncover all aspects of the cue in the child's imagination. For each identified fear cue, a SUDS rating should be taken and recorded. The goal of treatment will be to effect a decrease in SUDS ratings through habituation, accomplished via continued and prolonged exposure to both imaginal and in vivo fear cues.

Feared Consequences

Similar to adult OCD patients, many child and adolescent patients fear that something terrible may happen if they fail to perform their ritualistic behaviors. Although Riggs and Foa (1993) caution that it is important to uncover the specific details of the patient's feared consequences, due to cognitive-developmental limitations it is sometimes difficult for the child to identify a specific fear. Young children (roughly up to age 8) will report "something bad will happen," but may not be able to elaborate on what the consequence might be. Adolescents will sometimes minimize their self-reported feared consequences, although behavioral avoidance measures and parental report may reveal higher levels of anxiety. Specific and elaborate details of the child's feared consequences are necessary to plan effective exposure sessions. The use of drawings, puppets, or story-telling tasks may facilitate the uncovering of feared consequences.

Avoidance Behavior and Rituals

Children may be secretive about their compulsions, and therefore a comprehensive assessment is necessary to uncover complete information about all methods of passive avoidance and rituals. Once again, information from parents may be helpful to supplement the child's report. For example, parents are more likely to notice obsessive slowness, elaborate eating or grooming behaviors, and checking or arranging rituals that the child may not consider as compulsive. It is important to inquire (of the child and parents) what will happen if the child is interrupted during a ritual or prevented from performing the ritual. If refraining from performing a ritual evokes distress, or if interruption results in repeating the ritual and/or distress, then the action should be targeted for intervention. The treatment goal is for the child to confront the fear cue without performing a neutralizing ritual.

Rituals may be passive, such as in avoiding specific objects or situations that evoke obsessive thoughts; or active, as in the case of repeated hand washing, checking, arranging, or counting. As previously noted, it is not uncommon for children to change the ritual during the course of the disorder, and during the course of treatment. Parents often report a change in ritualistic behavior, with more elaborate and interfering rituals resulting in their seeking intervention. During the response prevention component of treatment, when the child is instructed not to engage in the ritual, we sometimes observe a new behavior emerging. Riggs and Foa (1993) caution that therapists must be vigilant to such shifts in ritualistic behaviors and apply the treatment to any new symptoms.

In summary, the goals of treatment are focused on the extinction of fear in response to specific internal and external cues, and the cessation of the ritualistic behaviors or passive avoidance previously utilized in an attempt to neutralize the fear or prevent some catastrophic consequence. Although the obsessive-compulsive hierarchy (OCH) will serve as the targets for intervention, the OCH should be used as a guide and all aspects of the child's symptomatology should be subjected to intervention.

ROLE OF THE THERAPIST

The method employed in the psychosocial treatment of OCD, exposure and response prevention (ERP), is a demanding treatment and high levels of anxiety may be provoked during exposure exercises. Considerable courage and trust is asked of the child in enduring this anxiety without resorting to compulsions to ward off feared consequences and reduce the anxiety. Children with OCD have become practiced in using avoidance as their primary method of coping with their fears, and it may be difficult for them to learn to simply tolerate distress. They may attempt to abort the exposure, or may use such techniques as distraction or overt or covert compulsions to deal with the anxiety provoked by the exposure. Such avoidance behaviors may be extremely subtle, as when the child engages in fragmented compulsions such as an extra push while closing a door, rather than the full compulsion of reopening and closing the door. The therapist must be alert to such behaviors and ask the child to desist, as compulsions or distraction will negate the full effect of the exposure and actually act to maintain the child's anxiety.

The therapist must balance between firm adherence to exposure and response prevention rules and coercion. At the same time, the therapist gives the child encouragement to persist despite high anxiety, while denying the child reassurance regarding their fears. Tact and sensitivity are needed in walking these boundaries. Most children respond well to empathy for their distress coupled with a firm adherence to response prevention rules. The therapist can facilitate this process by carefully explaining the procedures for each exposure, including a detailed description of response prevention rules and what the child can expect during the exposure. If the therapist remains calm in the face of the child's anxiety, the child is more likely to believe that things are proceeding normally toward a good outcome.

In addition, tact and sensitivity are needed in working with the parents to change those behaviors that reinforce and maintain the OC symptoms. In working to change parental responses, the therapist must be careful not to imply that the parents have caused the OCD. Instead, parental responses to the compulsions can be described to the parents as their best attempt using commonsense parenting to help alleviate their child's distress. They can be told that, unfortunately, commonsense approaches that work well with other child behaviors backfire with OCD, and specialized techniques must be used, such as those presented in treatment.

TREATMENT STRATEGIES

The chronic course of childhood OCD, its resultant impairment in functioning, and its persistence into adulthood accentuate the importance of early intervention. Although investigators at the National Institute of Mental Health (NIMH) have examined the efficacy of pharmacological treatments for childhood OCD (e.g., Flament et al. 1985, 1987, Leonard et al. 1989, 1991, 1993), research examining the behavioral treatments for this population has lagged far behind the adult treatment research and child psychopharmacology research. Exposure and response prevention (ERP) is the most commonly employed and efficacious method examined in the adult psychosocial literature (see Riggs and Foa 1993, and Steketee 1991), yet controlled studies systematically evaluating its effectiveness with children and adolescents are lacking.

The behavioral conceptualization of obsessions as anxiety-increasing thoughts, images, or behaviors, and compulsions as anxiety-reducing behaviors or cognitions, has led to the development of very successful treatments for adult OCD (Steketee and Tynes 1991). Prolonged exposure to fear cues, combined with blocking of ritualistic responses, has proven to be highly effective in upwards of 75 percent of cases reported (Steketee and Tynes 1991). Moreover, maintenance of therapeutic gains and the generalizability of treatment effects have been well documented in this literature. Several studies have employed variations of response prevention in the treatment of childhood OCD (e.g., Apter et al. 1984, Francis 1988, Kearney and Silverman 1990, Mills et al. 1973). Of the child and adolescent patients reported in these studies as treated with response prevention, at posttreatment 33 percent were symptom free, 36 percent improved or much improved, and 31 percent experienced no change. It should be noted that these patients were treated with response prevention in combination with other therapies, and the only controlled studies evaluating response prevention alone were by Mills and colleagues (1973) and Francis (1988). As indicated in the adult literature, if the key to the treatment of OCD is to block compulsions while facilitating habituation to anxiogenic obsessive thoughts, then direct exposure to anxiety-provoking cues combined with response prevention should produce therapeutic effectiveness. Several uncontrolled case studies combined exposure and response prevention in the treatment of childhood OCD (Bolton and Turner 1984, Lindley et al. 1977, Ong and Leng 1979, Zikis 1983). Again, the ERP component was part of an overall treatment package, and not systematically applied nor evaluated, yet follow-up data suggest that overall the patients were much improved and maintained treatment gains up to one year.

Inclusion of Parents

Research has suggested that children are initially secretive about their OCD symptoms (Swedo et al. 1989), and that family members may become drawn into the compulsive rituals over time (Honjo et al. 1989, Riddle et al. 1990). Involvement in the child's rituals may be passive or active. Parents who tell their child that dinner is at six, when in fact dinner is at eight, may have learned to accept the child's obsessive slowness. Similarly, when family members avoid touching or moving certain objects in the home because the child becomes upset, they too have become passive participants in the ritual.

Active participation occurs when the family assists the child in completing the rituals, such as checking the closets, washing furniture or clothes repeatedly, or reciting songs. Such participation typically occurs as the parents attempt to allay the child's distress and anxiety, without realizing the nature of the disorder. In either case, involving parents in the active treatment process appears to be a necessary component of effective treatment.

Although most cognitive-behavioral therapists endorse the importance of parental involvement in treatment, most often parents are involved in some manner of contingency management, observation, or differential reinforcement. In the treatment of childhood OCD, only a limited number of studies actively incorporated the parents in some way into the exposure and response prevention protocol (e.g., Apter et al. 1984, Mills et al. 1973, Zikis 1983). No definitive statements can be made about parent involvement in this treatment, as involvement of parents has not been applied systematically, replicated, or evaluated. Given that parents and family members often become inadvertently involved in compulsive rituals, it seems reasonable to address this involvement directly by making the parents agents of change, as opposed to passive participants or contingency managers. Moreover, the extant literature on treatment of adult anxiety disorders has demonstrated the inclusion of a family member to enhance significantly the effects of treatment, and to address the sometimes severe interpersonal problems accompanying anxiety disorders as well (Barlow et al. 1984, Cerny et al. 1987). Several preliminary studies at our clinic have supported inclusion of parents in the active treatment component (e.g., Barlow and Siedner 1983). Recently we concluded a preliminary study evaluating the relative impact of parent involvement as compared to no involvement in the treatment of socially phobic teens (Albano, Marten, et al. 1994). We are presently evaluating the impact of training parents in the delivery of home-based ERP for childhood OCD patients (Albano, Knox, and Barlow 1994). A preliminary study conducted at our clinic has yielded promising results (Knox et al. 1993), and future controlled trials will focus on the impact of variables such as the child's age, comorbid psychiatric conditions, and the presence of parental psychopathology on treatment outcome.

Exposure and Response Prevention with Parent Participation

Recently, we developed an OCD treatment program for children and adolescents based largely upon the successful psychosocial methods employed by Edna Foa and colleagues (e.g., Foa et al. 1984, 1985, Riggs and Foa 1993), and incorporating parents in the home-based delivery of treatment (Knox et al.

1991). In the treatment of OCD, it is optimal to schedule several intensive and prolonged sessions per week. Such treatment is necessary to promote habituation to the anxiety and generalization of treatment effects across sessions. In our treatment program, patients are seen for approximately eighteen sessions scheduled over a three-month period. Initially, the child is seen three times weekly until session 12; sessions 13–16 are weekly, followed by two biweekly sessions for termination.

During the pretreatment assessment, the child and parent are trained in the accurate monitoring of OC symptoms (cognitive and overt behaviors). The initial phase of the program involves in-session exposure and response prevention, while training the parents and child in procedures for conducting exposure and response prevention homework. Imaginal and in vivo exposure to fear cues, both in the office and the child's home, and response prevention of rituals are initiated in session 1 and continue throughout the first phase of treatment.

During each session, the child is seen initially for individual time with the therapist. An imaginal exposure is conducted and taped for use in homework exposures. The therapist begins with a relatively low hierarchy item. Specific response prevention rules are discussed with the child for each exposure. For example, if the child's first item is "washing hands after touching doorknobs," then the rule would be that under no circumstances can he wash after touching a doorknob or any other common object that he believes may be contaminated. This includes using damp towels or wipes, rubbing hands on clothing or furniture, or any other method to cleanse the hands. The child is seated comfortably in a chair, while the therapist describes *in great detail* the particular item. Subjective ratings of anxiety (0–8), augmented by the use of a fear thermometer, are taken from the child at five-minute intervals. The objective is for the anxiety to peak at its maximal levels, and for the child to maintain focus on the anxiety until it naturally dissipates, without giving in to compulsions. If SUDS are then graphed, the therapist should observe an inverted U exposure curve. Following the imaginal exposure, an in vivo exposure is immediately conducted. Such exposures will involve the use of actual external fear cues (e.g., leaving a door unlocked, making mistakes on homework papers). Most in vivo exposures can be contrived in the office setting; however, sessions in the child's home are encouraged. Length of exposure will depend upon the child and the particular item, but it is not unusual for an imaginal exposure to last upwards of thirty minutes, and in vivo exposures thirty to sixty minutes. The therapist should conduct two exposures before bringing the parent(s) into the session for feedback. During the final phase of treatment, sessions 13–18, greater responsibility for conducting any continuing exposures is placed on the child, utilizing within-session time to provide feedback and evaluate homework. Details on devising and conducting both imaginal and in vivo exposures, and outlines of response prevention rules for children, may be found in Knox et al. (1991).

We have varied the point that parents are introduced into the active treatment process, and are currently evaluating the optimal time and amount of parent involvement. The case studies described at the end of this chapter illustrate involving parents after several individual sessions with the child. The therapist will spend some time alone with the parents explaining the behavioral model of anxiety and treatment rationale. The therapist then describes exposure and response prevention, and illustrates the technique by describing the child's previous exposures. Role-playing, with their child, is then utilized to begin training the parents in the ERP technique. The parents and child role-play an exposure, with the child purposefully violating response prevention rules. Parents are given corrective information and feedback. The child and parents are then given instruction in conducting both imaginal and in vivo exposures at home. Typically, both an imaginal and an in vivo exposure are conducted once daily between sessions, with the parents instructed to participate in both of these exposures. The child and parents are also given instruction in responding to particularly strong urges or compulsions that the child finds difficult to control. Gentle prompting of the child is suggested, with systematic ignoring of OCD behavior and reinforcing response prevention as an alternative behavior.

DEALING WITH COMMON OBSTACLES TO SUCCESSFUL TREATMENT

Due to the nature of this anxiety disorder, children and adolescents will want to avoid conducting exposures or may try to prematurely terminate an exposure. The therapist must pay careful attention to such behavior and use encouragement and a firm but understanding manner in explaining the rationale to the child. It is important to fully debrief the child after each exposure, and we have found that using visual cues, such as drawing the child's habituation curve for his/her inspection, helps the child in understanding the treatment process.

Comorbid conditions may also obstruct successful treatment. It is imperative that the most disabling condition be treated first, so as not to confound and dilute treatment effectiveness. Serious family dysfunction, major depression, and externalizing disorders of significant severity may interfere with the progress of this protocol. Similarly, if a child is referred on any type of psychotropic medication, we suggest that the dosage be stabilized prior to the initiation of the behavioral treatment and maintained throughout the treatment program. Following a period of symptom remission, medication discontinuation may be initiated with the coordinated efforts of the child's physician and therapist.

Parents may have become participants in their child's compulsive rituals and may become anxious themselves as their child experiences anxiety. They may be reluctant to conduct exposures without providing reassurance or other responses aimed at anxiety reduction. The therapist must be alert to any reluctance on the part of the parents and must emphasize that their child must confront fears to conquer them. The role-plays conducted during the parent sessions help to clarify desired parental responses to child behaviors during exposure.

RELAPSE PREVENTION AND TERMINATION

Because OCD follows a chronic course, relapse prevention may be crucial to the long-term maintenance of treatment gains. The final six sessions of our treatment focus on relapse prevention. Our first step in maintaining treatment gains is to teach the child the functional relationship between OC symptoms. Using examples from the child's own symptomatology, we step through the OCD cycle in the following order: the external trigger, the obsessive fears, the rise in anxiety, the compulsion, and the temporary decrease in anxiety. An example might go as follows: the child comes in contact with a contaminating object, experiences obsessive fears of illness to self or family, becomes anxious, washes his or her hands several times with strong soap to neutralize the contamination and obsessive fears, and anxiety temporarily subsides. The illustration of the OCD cycle is stepped through several times with the child, showing that the rise in anxiety reaches new heights with each repetition. The child learns explicitly what he or she has known all along: compulsions work temporarily to alleviate distress, but function in the long term to increase anxiety.

The child is then taught the treatment rationale in detail using the child's own treatment experiences to illustrate that anxiety decreases and obsessive fears remit without resorting to compulsions. This information is then applied to hypothetical future new symptoms and to the return of old symptoms. The child is instructed to wait it out or to stop and focus on obsessive fears and external triggers without compulsions until anxiety subsides. In addition, the child is encouraged to utilize anxiety as a prompt to conduct frequent mini-exposures to any triggers prompting residual anxiety. As the child learns treatment concepts, any overly strict response prevention rules are relaxed to more normal limits, while the child is praised for the use of coping skills.

Borrowing from the work of Kendall (1990), during the final session the child makes a video that incorporates the information learned in treatment and emphasizes coping skills for use in any future problems. The videotape is given to the child at the close of the session to take home. The child and parents are encouraged to view the videotape together if they have any problems and are unsure how to proceed.

In our experience in working with anxious children, it is more often the parents than the child who panic at the first sign of the child's anxiety. Parents commonly respond to normal anxiety or to small and most likely temporary upsurges in symptoms by abandoning treatment skills, returning to former symptom-reinforcing strategies, and complaining that their children have "returned to square one." Therefore it is extremely important to work with the parents as well as the child in ensuring the maintenance of treatment gains. Although the apparent focus of the maintenance sessions is on the child, parents are present at the close of each session while the child reviews for them the principles covered in each session. Parents are thus given an opportunity to hear the child voice common patient concerns and their solutions. Parents are also given the opportunity to voice their fears and to devise coping strategies for future use. We stress to the parents that fears of their child relapsing are a signal to continue or increase their use of the treatment skills rather than surrender to despair.

CASE ILLUSTRATION (TYPICAL TREATMENT)

Description and History

Casey was an 8-year-old Caucasian female with a three-year history of bedtime rituals. Obsessions included intrusive songs and fear of monsters, of spiders, of inability to sleep, and of swallowing at night. Compulsions included closing and checking the closet and cupboard doors, pushing toys and clothes out of sight, smoothing and "cuffing" the bedclothes, checking for cracks in the walls, holding saliva in her mouth, and repeating a song perfectly from beginning to end. Her rituals took approximately three hours each evening and were repeated after lights out for several hours. In addition, her parents were helping her perform the rituals to expedite the process. However, they reported that rather than decrease Casey's anxiety, the rituals became more elaborate and took longer. Nearly every night they would awaken to hear her repeating the rituals into the early hours of the morning. Although her symptoms were confined to mainly her own home, the severe disruption in sleep patterns began to interfere with her academic performance. At the time of intake, Casey was extremely distressed and, in fact, had begged her parents to take her to a doctor for help.

On the basis of the ADIS-C/P interviews, Casey received a principal composite diagnosis of OCD, and an additional diagnosis of overanxious disorder. Casey was not taking any psychotropic medication upon intake or during treatment. Although only 8 years of age, she was quite verbal and expressed her high motivation to "beat these feelings." She readily identified her obsessions and compulsions, and was able to anchor the duration of these symptoms by identifying the grade in which they had started. Not surprisingly, her parents were not aware that many of her habits were driven by frightening thoughts. For example, Casey described having to skip around a cul-de-sac at her grandmother's house whenever they visited. For Casey, this behavior prevented her family from dying. Her parents had no idea that the behavior was motivated by fear. Moreover, Casey's obsessions reflected developmentally expected fears. At night, she was afraid of monsters and other typical 8-year-old concerns. However, the magnitude of her fears, interference in her normal functioning, and unrelenting persistence warranted intervention. For Casey, her parents' reassurances were insufficient to calm her, and so she developed rituals in a desperate attempt to ward off these "monsters."

Casey was an only child in an intact dual-career family. Neither parent reported any current history of obsessive-compulsive disorder, anxiety disorder, or other psychopathology. Her father, however, reported having rituals as a child, which he "outgrew" by adulthood. Casey and her parents were explained the treatment rationale and course of therapy, and they agreed to participate. Due to his profession, Casey's father traveled often during the week, and hence it was decided that her mother would assist Casey in therapy. Her father attended parent conferences when available.

Pretreatment Assessment

In one pretreatment session, Casey was administered our standard assessment battery, described previously. On the Leyton Obsessional

Inventory, Casey identified a clinically significant number of symptoms, and moderate to severe levels of resistance and interference. An individual OC hierarchy was constructed, with associated subjective units of distress (Table 10–1). Casey and her therapist discussed each hierarchy item and devised scripts with elaborate scenes for treatment. In addition, Casey and her mother were instructed in the use of the diary forms and assigned a monitoring period of one full week. At the time of Casey's involvement at the clinic, we had not yet initiated the BAT portion of the assessment.

Synopsis of Therapy Sessions

Sessions 1–7

Casey appeared to understand from the onset of treatment that her compulsions were not reducing her anxiety and that, in fact, they probably were not preventing bad things from happening. Nevertheless, she felt powerless to control herself and gave in to her fearful thoughts. In session 1, Casey was imaginally exposed to a relatively low hierarchy item. First, response prevention rules were outlined. Casey was instructed that she had to listen to the script and could not think other thoughts or touch herself in any special ways to make the anxiety go away. The therapist then described the following scenario to Casey, while taking SUDS ratings at five-minute intervals throughout the forty-minute exposure:

Table 10-1. Casey's Obsessive-Compulsive Hierarchy

Hierarchy Item*	SUDS†
1. Breathe through nose and swallow saliva.	6
2. Song in head that keeps going and won't stop.	5
3. Not skipping around the circle at Nana's house.	5
4. Leave toys and clothes in sight of bed at night.	4
5. Hang clothes on door in bedroom and leave clothes hanging out of drawers when going to bed.	4
6. Leave bathroom cupboards open at bedtime.	4
7. Don't smooth bed down or cuff it at bedtime.	4
8. Leave tape off the crack in the wall and don't check the crack for spiders.	3
9. Leave closet door in bedroom open at bedtime.	3
10. Leave self damp after bath.	2

*Exposures begin with lower SUDS items.
†SUDS ratings on 0–8 scale.

Therapist: It is nighttime. Your parents have tucked you in and have gone to bed themselves. You reach over to shut the light off on the nightstand, and you notice that your bedroom door is open. The door is cracked just a bit, just enough for something to crawl out and into your room. It's dark in that corner, and you think you see something. You close the light and lie down. You hear a strange, scratching noise coming from the closet. It sounds like something is moving. What's your SUDS rating?

Client: [Points to thermometer] It's a seven.

Therapist: Stay with it. Tell me about what happens next.

Client: The closet door creaks open a bit more, and now I know that something is there. It can come get me. It's a monster.

Therapist: You begin to sweat. You want so badly to go and shut that door, but you stay in bed. You close your eyes, but the sound doesn't stop. It seems to be getting closer. You look over, and see a horrible face, with red eyes staring at you. You want to scream, but you know you can't. What's your SUDS rating now?

Client: Eight. This is the worst part.

Therapist: Okay, good, stay with the image. Tell me what happens next.

The exposure was taped and continued until Casey's SUDS ratings dropped to 25 percent of their initial level and she reported feeling minimal anxiety. She was instructed to play this tape at home, in her room, twice daily for homework. Also, a response-prevention rule was initiated, that she must leave her closet door open at night and had to look at the open door.

During the first seven sessions, Casey's mother was told that there might be an initial rise in anxiety, and that Casey should be practicing her homework on her own. The parents were not to prompt her to do the homework, but were to place responsibility on the child. Treatment progressed to involve in vivo exposures. The therapist made several home visits to conduct sessions in Casey's bedroom and bathroom, exposing her to opening closets, leaving clothes and toys around, and preventing her from neutralizing such anxiogenic cues.

Sessions 7–13

Casey continued to engage in at least two exposures with her therapist, with the length of each exposure lessening considerably. At session 7, Mrs. L. was seen individually and given instruction in conducting the exposures. Initially, Mrs. L. was surprised at the scary content of the imaginal scenes. However, it was explained to her that these were the images and thoughts that Casey was experiencing, and that Casey had embellished the scenes for the exposures. Role-plays were enacted to rehearse conducting the exposures.

> Therapist: Okay, I'll be Casey. Mom, can't we do this later?
>
> Mother: No, let's not put it off anymore. Okay, I'll start the tape. What is your, um, SUDS rating?
>
> Therapist: It's a three.
>
> Mother: Okay, we're ready to leave Nana's house, and you think that you won't see Nana again. Oh, my. She looks very sick to you. But you know if you skip around the circle, then she'll be okay. But you . . .
>
> Therapist: It's okay mom, I'm not feeling that scared anymore.
>
> Mother: Let's keep going anyway. Just listen. You can't get to skip the circle because we have to leave. You're feeling really scared about Nana, and you also start to think me and dad will be sick. You picture us in the hospital and you can't help us. If only you had skipped the circle. Um, what is your SUDS now?
>
> Therapist: Very good. Don't let her dissuade you from continuing with the script.
>
> Mother: This is really scary stuff. How could she think this?
>
> Therapist: Well, she has a vivid imagination, and the anxiety works like on autopilot to keep these kinds of thoughts coming. Let's do the scene again, this time, stop every now and then and ask Casey to tell you about the scene. That way, you know for sure that she's paying attention and it gives you more images to work with. Okay?

Mrs. L. was also given instruction in how to ignore Casey's OC behavior, but not Casey. The principle of differential reinforcement was explained, and examples from Casey and her mom's interactions were utilized. Next, the therapist observed Mrs. L. conducting an exposure with Casey, giving corrective feedback when indicated.

Sessions 14–18

Casey quickly progressed through her hierarchy and continued to engage in home-based exposures both with and without her mother's assistance. Interestingly, her motivation was so high that she requested the therapist expose her "to everything at once." And so, in an extended session Casey listened to tapes for all of her hierarchy items.

By session 14, Casey was no longer evidencing compulsive behaviors or reporting any distress or interference from obsessive thoughts. The remaining sessions were focused on relapse prevention and termination. Casey made a videotape, with her mother and therapist as assistants, in which she reported to other children how to "beat OCD."

At posttreatment assessment, conducted by an independent evaluator, there was no evidence of obsessive-compulsive symptomatology, and interestingly, although the overanxious disorder was not targeted in treatment, this condition also remitted. Results were maintained at three-month and one-year follow-up. Additionally, scores on the Leyton decreased to within normal limits.

Comments

Casey's successful treatment may be attributed to several factors. First, this child was highly motivated and easily engaged, and participated fully in the therapeutic regime. On pretreatment assessment her OCD was judged to be in the moderate range and was not yet interfering with social or academic functioning. Second, her parents, especially her mother, adhered to the treatment protocol and presented her for sessions without cancelling. Last, the family appeared to be relatively healthy and cohesive. Although this case represents a near model patient, the relative efficacy of the protocol was demonstrated by significant improvement and maintenance of gains.

CASE ILLUSTRATION (OVERCOMING OBSTACLES)

Description and History

Ernie was an 11-year, 2-month-old, Caucasian male referred for the assessment and treatment of severe compulsive rituals that included repeating, touching, and stepping rituals. During the diagnostic interview he initially denied obsessive fears in connection with these rituals, but upon further inquiry admitted that the compulsions were prompted by fears that harm would befall family members and pets. Ernie had been performing compulsions since the age of 10 years. At the time of the referral, he was engaging in compulsions for up to forty-five minutes at a time. His mother could not specify the total amount of time spent on compulsions per day, but declared that they occurred almost continually. He expressed little embarrassment about others observing the rituals and engaged in them freely at school.

Ernie's clinical picture was complicated by numerous additional diagnoses. He was under the care of a local psychiatrist for Tourette's disorder and was taking Clonidine at 100 mcg., 1/2 tablet three times daily. The tics had begun two years before his referral and included vocalizations, grunts, and head jerks. Ernie was able to distinguish readily between the tics and the compulsions. He also received additional diagnoses of overanxious disorder, separation anxiety disorder, dysthymia, enuresis, and simple phobia. Ernie attended fifth grade in a public elementary school. He was in primarily mainstream classes but attended some contained classes, and was accompanied to classes and assisted in his schoolwork by a classroom aide.

Ernie was attentive and cooperative during the first thirty minutes of the ninety-minute diagnostic interview. As the interview opened, he freely identified compulsions and tics as problems for which he needed help. He appeared bright and engaging although immature, and was initially open and talkative. However, he became increasingly distracted and less cooperative as the interview progressed. He appeared restless and distracted during the discussion of his OCD symptoms, and denied or minimized the symptoms of additional disorders. No compulsions or tics were observed during the interview, but Ernie was observed in the waiting room stepping in a ritualized pattern.

Ernie was from a working class family and lived with his mother, father, and 16-year-old brother. He had close contact with extended family members. The mother–son relationship appeared very enmeshed, and Mrs. C. described Ernie as almost completely disabled by the compulsions. The school reported that Mrs. C. frequently contacted them and requested that fewer demands be placed on Ernie. Ernie's father appeared more distant and did not attend the diagnostic interview or treatment sessions. According to Mrs. C.'s report, her husband was often impatient with Ernie and believed that Ernie's compulsions were primarily motivated by a desire for attention.

Although Ernie presented with a complicated clinical picture, it was judged that the greatest degree of distress and interference resulted from the obsessive-compulsive symptoms. Treatment for OCD was recommended. Further treatment recommendations to address additional concerns could be made if necessary following posttreatment assessment.

Pretreatment Assessment

Ernie participated in our standard assessment battery, which includes the Leyton Obsessional Inventory; the acquisition of a detailed description of the functional relationship between external cues, obsessive fears, and compulsive rituals; and hierarchy construction (Table 10-2). He was agitated and distractible during discussions of obsessive-compulsive symptoms, and his attention span was limited. Four sessions were necessary to obtain the complete information needed to plan exposure sessions. The assessment phase was used as a four-week medication washout period in addition, as Mrs. C. and their psychiatrist decided to discontinue the Clonidine due to insufficient response. Diary records indicated no change in the frequency of the compulsions during the assessment phase.

Ernie demonstrated little awareness of the connection between compulsive rituals and their external cues, and often substantial questioning was necessary before a clear functional relationship was obtained.

Therapist: You've told me that you feel like you have to do things like the footsteps and bouncing up and down. I'd like to get a list now of all the things you have to do when you feel like you

Table 10-2. Ernie's Obsessive-Compulsive Hierarchy

Hierarchy Item*	SUDS†
1. Sitting down or getting up without bouncing or repeating.	7
2. Walking without footstep or dance.	7
3. Getting dressed without repeating articles of clothing.	6
4. Touching walls and other objects just once.	6
5. Playing Nintendo or Game Boy without moving men back and forth, turning on and off, or picking up cord.	5
6. Going to bed without touching pillow, checking under bed, or moving blanket over and back.	5
7. Turning off lights, TV, turning sound up or down without repeating.	4
8. Eating without repeated touches to food and cup.	3
9. Doing homework without erasing and rewriting, flipping pages, or tapping pencil.	1
10. Shutting or locking windows, doors, drawers without repeating.	1

*Exposures begin with lower SUDS items.
†SUDS ratings on 0–8 scale.

have to do them, so we'll know what we want to work on together. Tell me about the things you feel that you have to do.

Ernie: Well, I have to do these footsteps when I'm walking sometimes. [demonstrates]

Therapist: Okay, when do you feel like you have to do them?

Ernie: When I'm walking on rock.

Therapist: What kind of rock?

Ernie: Like rock floors, like in our house.

Therapist: Are there other times that you have to do the footsteps?

Ernie: Well, it could be any floor. I do them outside, too.

Therapist: So it could be anything that you're walking on. What happens that makes you feel like you need to do the footsteps?

Ernie: Like if I'm walking someplace, like the hall between the long room to the kitchen, then I have to do them.

Therapist: Does it happen every time that you're walking to go someplace?

Ernie: Well, almost every time. Sometimes I'm thinking about something and I don't notice.

Therapist: What if I asked you to walk all around inside the clinic?

Ernie: Yeah, it would happen a lot then.

Therapist: Okay, so we know that you do the footsteps when you are walking to go someplace. I'd like you to watch this week and see if you can tell anything else about when they happen. Let's talk about some of the other things you feel like you have to do. What are they?

Ernie's report was compared to diary records and to his mother's report to ensure that a complete list was obtained. Ernie was then asked about obsessive fears related to his compulsions. He was reluctant to discuss these fears, but with coaxing eventually admitted fears of harm to family members or pets.

Therapist: We've talked about all the things that you feel like you have to do, and the times that you feel like you have to do them, like doing the footsteps when you're walking to go somewhere. What makes you feel like you have to do the footsteps . . . for instance, what would happen if you didn't do them?

Ernie: I don't know. I just have to do them. [Ernie became very restless at this point, and was squirming, tapping the arm of his chair, bouncing up and down, and becoming absorbed in the toy shelf.]

Therapist: Lots of people feel like something bad might happen if they don't do something like the footsteps to stop it. They feel like these thoughts are silly because they really know that they won't happen, or someone told them that they won't happen, but . . .

Ernie: Yeah, I think that something bad will happen to my mom or dad. Then I do the footsteps.

Therapist: Okay, that's a thought that lots of people with OCD have. What do you think might happen to your mom or dad if you didn't do the footsteps?

Synopsis of Therapy Sessions

Sessions 1–7

Child sessions consisted of homework review, imaginal and in vivo exposure, and homework assignment. Several sessions were conducted at Ernie's home, as the exposure content could not be easily contrived in the clinic setting. The majority of the sessions took place at the clinic. As in the assessment sessions, Ernie engaged in frequent interruptions, questioning, and fidgeting. These behaviors were conceptualized as serving the functions of attention seeking and distraction from anxiety, and were ignored except when they interfered with effective exposure exercises. During initial sessions, Ernie interrupted exposures frequently to ask how long exposures would last. The therapist responded to his first question by stating, "I know that you are really nervous right now, but I can't tell you when we will stop because this won't work if I do. It's very important that you sit quietly and listen to the tape without interrupting or thinking about anything but what's on the tape. In fact, it's so important that I will ignore any questions that you ask, and just keep on with the tape." Ernie indicated a willingness to continue under this rule, and the therapist ignored all further requests for information on how long exposures would continue.

When his questions were ignored, he fidgeted and muttered vocalizations like "shut up; no that wouldn't happen" during imaginal exposures, complained of dizziness, reeled and leaned against the walls, and engaged in subtle compulsions such as extra pushes or rattling door knobs when closing doors. During the first three sessions, Ernie continued avoidance behaviors despite requests that exposures be performed without compulsions or distractions. During each exposure, the therapist pointed out the first occurrence and subsequently ignored all further occurrences of avoidance behavior. The exposure was continued until all distracting, compulsive, and behavioral signs of anxiety ceased. If this could not be accomplished in the allotted session time, Ernie was informed that the exposure would be repeated in the next session.

In session 4, the exposure was halted after frequent complaints and avoidance attempts, and Ernie was given the choice of stopping the exposure or continuing without avoidance. He became tearful but continued without further complaints or compulsions. SUDS decreased and he appeared relaxed at the end of the procedure. He was praised for his compliance, and the connection between compliance and decrease in SUDS was pointed out.

> Therapist: What happened to your nervousness?
> Ernie: It went down.
> Therapist: Yes, it did. Why do you think it went down?
> Ernie: Because my writing wasn't as messy as I thought it would be. It got better the more I wrote.
> Therapist: Other times when we've done this, you stayed nervous— it didn't go down. What was different this time? Did you do anything different?
> Ernie: Well, I kept on writing, and I stopped arguing.
> Therapist: So when you did the writing without stopping or erasing and let yourself feel nervous, you saw that nothing bad happened and the nervousness went down?
> Ernie: Yeah, it goes down if I keep going.

In future sessions avoidance steadily declined, and Ernie responded instantly to requests to cease avoidance. By session 8, overt distraction, fidgeting, and compulsions were no longer observed, and SUDS declined rapidly during each exposure.

Through repeated exposures the child learns that anxiety decreases and feared consequences do not occur despite the absence of compulsions. A potential problem in treatment is when an event seems to confirm the client's fears regarding the consequences of refraining from rituals. Ernie reported such an event but coped with it well, using the experiences he had undergone in treatment.

> Ernie: My brother was in a car accident—but he's okay.
> Therapist: That's what we imagined last time, isn't it, that he would be in an accident?

Ernie: Yeah, but I know it didn't happen because of that or because I didn't do the OCD.

Therapist: How do you know that?

Ernie: Because I haven't been doing them all this time, and nothing happened before this. Besides, it was really snowy out, and he just learned how to drive. Other people had accidents too that night.

Sessions 7–13

Beginning with session 7, each child session was followed by a parent session. During these sessions Mrs. C. was given instruction in conducting home-based exposures and in the application of differential reinforcement to assist her in discontinuing behaviors that reinforce the compulsions.

As Ernie began to tolerate anxiety with less distress, Mrs. C. began to ignore the compulsions before this was suggested by the therapist. She reported that she was beginning to conclude that the compulsions were reinforced by attention as well as anxiety reduction, and that Ernie need not be completely disabled by his anxiety. Nevertheless, her responses were inconsistent, and she frequently returned to former patterns of encouragement or nagging in response to compulsions, particularly in response to new behaviors. Her encouragement was reframed as attention-giving reinforcement, and she agreed to return to the use of ignoring and positive reinforcement.

Mother: Ernie started a new thing. He's really trying, but sometimes he forgets and does a compulsion. Then he says, "Oops, I wasn't supposed to do that!"

Therapist: Hm, and what do you do then?

Mother: I think he's trying, but he forgets, so I tell him to remember what he learned here and to do what he's supposed to do.

Therapist: Sometimes behaviors that look new are the same old thing, just dressed in new clothes. Let's look at some of the compulsions we've dealt with successfully, and how we succeeded. In the past, Ernie used to touch his cup and plate over and over. What did you do in response?

Mother: I used to try to calm him down, and his father used to yell at him. Neither one worked—he just kept doing it. Then I started to think that maybe even when the nervousness made him do it, that he did it too for the attention. So I started to ignore it, and that worked.

Therapist: Okay, how does your response then compare with your response now?

Mother: You're saying that he's doing it for attention, and I should just ignore it again.

Therapist: It worked before. Do you think it might work again?

Mother: Maybe. And I should go back to praising him when he's doing a good job?

Therapist: That sounds like a good idea. Why don't we try ignoring the "oopses" and rewarding Ernie for coping, and see what happens. Let's act it out now, so we're all sure what we've agreed to do.

As Mrs. C.'s responses became more consistent, compulsions decreased. In addition, mother–son interactions in session were increasingly positive, with decreased attention-seeking behavior on Ernie's part, and decreased nagging and increased affectionate behavior on Mrs. C.'s part.

Session 14–19

At session 14, compulsions had decreased substantially but had not fully remitted. The remaining sessions focused on maintenance of gains, relapse prevention, and termination issues. Some difficulty was encountered when Ernie failed to use the steps generated in treatment for dealing with urges to ritualize "because they were too much work and I thought I could just stop on my own." Mrs. C. responded to Ernie's failure to use coping steps by again reminding him after each observed compulsion to use his steps. Further exposures to hierarchy items were discussed with Ernie and his mother, but it was decided that before resorting to exposures, Ernie should be allowed a chance to practice coping steps while Mrs. C. returned to ignoring the compulsions. Compulsions remitted almost completely, and this gain was maintained through the end of treatment.

Because Ernie displayed a strong attachment to the therapist, a substantial portion of each session was devoted to termination issues. Ernie was able to verbalize two main concerns regarding termination: fears of a relapse and sadness regarding the impending separation from the therapist. Relapse fears were addressed through emphasizing the skills-building nature of the treatment program and discussing methods of applying treatment techniques to vanquish hypothetical new symptoms or a resurgence of past symptoms. Sadness regarding the impending separation was addressed by utilizing similar past separations, for example with teachers, to normalize and restructure his fears regarding the separation.

Comments

This case presented several obstacles that are common to the treatment of childhood OCD. Ernie was initially secretive regarding the content of his obsessive fears. As with most children, he responded well when he was assured that most children with OCD experience unrealistic or excessive fears. Other children may make so immediate a compulsive response to anxiety that they may have difficulty identifying their obsessions. Repeated and in-depth questioning coupled with understanding of their difficulty may help them to arrive at a report of their fears.

Children may have difficulty giving a straightforward account of the external triggers for their compulsions. Instead they may focus on one isolated event, as when Ernie reported that walking on rock floors triggered his stepping compulsion. In some cases, the therapist must generate a list of detailed triggers for each compulsion before deriving an overreaching category. Parental report and diary records can assist in this process.

Many children engage in overt, covert, or fragmented compulsions or distraction during exposures. The therapist may confront the child during the exposure and ask that the avoidance behaviors cease. However, if the behaviors continue at a high level, the therapist must consider whether the instructions to cease are serving to reinforce the behavior. In such cases, the best strategy is to ignore the compulsions while continuing the exposure. Obvious attention-seeking behaviors such as complaints of dizziness and reeling into walls are more rare and can be ignored. Decisions as to when to confront the child regarding avoidance and when to ignore can be difficult, and the therapist may have to feel the way to the best solution. Regardless of the strategy chosen, the therapist should continue the exposure until all detectable avoidance behaviors have ceased, even if SUDS ratings decline before this point. If this is not possible in the available session time, the exposure should be repeated in the next session. In addition, we typically do not tell the child that the exposure will end when their SUDS have declined, as this encourages children to give low SUDS ratings to prematurely terminate the exposure. However, the child may be told that the exposure will continue and be repeated until avoidance ceases.

Another common obstacle in treatment is inconsistency in parental responses to compulsions. Rather than ignore the compulsions, Mrs. C.

responded with encouragement to utilize treatment skills. A reversion to this response was particularly likely when she saw a behavior as a new one. This can be conceptualized as a failure in generalization. The "new" behavior can be compared to old behaviors, and their similarity in function and thus in optimal parental response can be emphasized. In addition, the effects of intermittent reinforcement in strengthening child behaviors cannot be over-emphasized to parents. Praise for positive coping and "fun times together" were recommended to Mrs. C. as a way of giving Ernie the encouragement and attention he sought.

This case was complicated by a complex clinical presentation and an enmeshed mother–son relationship. These factors played out in treatment as attention-seeking and avoidance behaviors on Ernie's part, and hyperalertness to Ernie's behavior on Mrs. C.'s part. Despite these factors, treatment was carried out as specified in our manual, and a positive outcome was achieved. At a posttreatment assessment conducted by an independent interviewer, a diagnosis of anxiety disorder NOS was assigned to reflect residual overanxious concerns. Some compulsions remained at low levels, but Mrs. C. reported that the compulsions did not occur every day, took less than a minute when they did occur, and did not interfere with normal routine. Scores on the Leyton Obsessional Inventory were within normal range. It was judged that a continuing diagnosis of obsessive compulsive disorder was unwarranted. Nevertheless, the school reported that Ernie still required extensive behavioral management in class, and Mrs. C. was reluctant to have more academic demands placed on Ernie despite the remission of compulsions in the school setting. The mother–son relationship remained very enmeshed, with the father distant. While school officials expressed satisfaction with the remission of OC symptoms, they requested that referrals for further treatment be given to assist with the above problems. Referrals for family counseling were given. At a three-month follow-up assessment, obsessive-compulsive symptoms remained at posttreatment levels, and no clinical diagnoses were assigned. Mrs. C. reported that the family was in therapy.

SUMMARY

Despite the chronic and debilitating course of childhood OCD, only recently has attention turned to developing effective psychosocial methods of intervention. The treatment program described in this chapter shows promising results, yet empirical validation of the protocol is just under way. Moreover, the application of such an intense protocol in clinical practice may not be feasible, due to therapist time constraints and the limits of the parent's mental health care benefits. For that reason, the training of parents in conducting home-based exposures may facilitate treatment and clearly deserves further attention.

REFERENCES

Albano, A. M., Knox, L. S., and Barlow, D. H. (1994). *Training parents in the delivery of exposure and response prevention: a multiple baseline evaluation of a new treatment protocol.* Work in progress.

Albano, A. M., Marten, P. A., Holt, C. S., et al. (1994). *Cognitive-behavioral group treatment for social phobia in adolescents: a preliminary study.* Manuscript submitted for publication.

Apter, A., Bernhout, E. and Tyano, S. (1984). Severe obsessive compulsive disorder in adolescence: a report of eight cases. *Journal of Adolescence* 7:349–358.

Barlow, D. H., O'Brien, G. T., and Last, C. G. (1984). Couples treatment of agoraphobia. *Behavior Therapy* 15:41–58.

Barlow, D. H., and Seidner, A. L. (1983). Treatment of adolescent agoraphobics: effects on parent-adolescent relations. *Behaviour Research and Therapy* 21(5):519–526.

Beidel, D. C. (1988). Physiological assessment of anxious emotional states in children. *Journal of Abnormal Psychology* 97:80–82.

_____ (1989). Assessing anxious emotion: a review of psychophysiological assessment in children. *Clinical Psychology Review* 9:717–736.

Berg, C. J., Rapoport, J. L., and Flament, M. (1986). The Leyton Obsessional Inventory-Child Version. *Journal of the American Academy of Child Psychiatry* 31:84–91.

Berg, C. B., Rapoport, J. L., Whitaker, A., et al. (1989). Childhood obsessive-compulsive disorder: a two-year prospective follow-up of a community sample. *Journal of the American Academy of Child and Adolescent Psychiatry* 28:528–533.

Bolton, D., and Turner, T. (1984). Obsessive-compulsive neurosis with conduct disorder in adolescence: a report of two cases. *Journal of Child Psychology and Psychiatry and Allied Disciplines* 25:133–139.

Cerny, J. A., Barlow, D. H., Craske, M. G., and Himadi, W. G. (1987). Couples treatment of agoraphobia: a two-year follow-up. *Behavior Therapy* 18:401–415.

Flament, M. F., Koby, E., Rapoport, J. L., et al. (1990). Childhood obsessive-compulsive disorder: a prospective follow-up study. *Journal of Child Psychology and Psychiatry* 31:363–380.

Flament, M. F., Rapoport, J. L., Berg, C. J., et al. (1985). Clomipramine treatment of childhood obsessive-compulsive disorder. *Archives of General Psychiatry* 42:977–983.

Flament, M. F., Rapoport, J. L., and Murphy, D. L. (1987). Biochemical changes during clomipramine treatment of childhood obsessive-compulsive disorder. *Archives of General Psychiatry* 44:219–225.

Flament, M. F., Whitaker, A., Rapoport, J. L., et al. (1988). Obsessive compulsive disorder in adolescence: an epidemiological study. *Journal of the American Academy of Child and Adolescent Psychiatry* 27:764–771.

Foa, E. B., Steketee, G. S., Grayson, J. B., et al. (1984). Deliberate exposure and blocking of obsessive-compulsive rituals: immediate and long-term effects. *Behavior Therapy* 15:450–472.

Foa, E. B., Steketee, G. S., and Ozarow, B. (1985). Behavior therapy with obsessive-compulsives: from theory to treatment. In *Obsessive-Compulsive Disorder: Psychological and Pharmacological Treatment*, ed. M. Mavisskalian. New York: Plenum.

Francis, G. (1988). Childhood obsessive-compulsive disorder: extinction of compulsive reassurance-seeking. *Journal of Anxiety Disorders* 2:361–366.

Grad, L., Pelcovitz, D., Olsen, M., et al. (1987). Obsessive-compulsive symptomatology in children with Tourette's Disorder. *Journal of the American Academy of Child and Adolescent Psychiatry* 26:69–73.

Honjo, S., Hirano, C., Murase, S., et al. (1989). Obsessive-compulsive symptoms in childhood and adolescence. *Acta Psychiatrica Scandinavica* 80:83–91.

Karno, M., Golding, J. M., Sorenson, S. B., and Burnam, M. A. (1988). The epidemiology of obsessive-compulsive disorder in five U.S. communities. *Archives of General Psychiatry* 45:1094–1099.

Kearney, C. A., and Silverman, W. K. (1990). Treatment of an adolescent with obsessive-compulsive disorder by alternating response prevention and cognitive therapy: an empirical analysis. *Journal of Behavior Therapy and Experimental Psychiatry* 21:39–47.

Kendall, P. C. (1990). *The coping cap manual.* Unpublished manuscript. Philadelphia, PA: Temple University.

Knox, L. S., Albano, A. M., and Barlow, D. H. (1991). *Treatment of OCD in children: exposure and response prevention and parent training manual.* Unpublished manuscript: Albany: State University of New York.

———— (1993). *Parent involvement in the treatment of childhood OCD.* Paper presented at the 13th National Conference of the Anxiety Disorders Association of America, Charleston, SC.

Last, C. G., and Strauss, C. C. (1989). Obsessive-compulsive disorder in childhood. *Journal of Anxiety Disorders* 3:295–302.

Leonard, H. L., Lenane, M. C., Swedo S. E., et al. (1992). Tics and Tourette's disorder: a 2-to-7-year follow-up of 54 obsessive-compulsive children. *American Journal of Psychiatry* 149:1244–1251.

Leonard, H. L., Swedo, E., Lenane, M. C., et al. (1993). A 2-to-7-year follow-up study of 54 obsessive-compulsive children and adolescents. *Archives of General Psychiatry* 50:429–439.

Leonard, H. L., Swedo, S., and Rapoport, J. L. (1989). Treatment of obsessive compulsive disorder with clomipramine and desipramine in children and adolescents: a double blind crossover comparison. *Archives of General Psychiatry* 46:1088–1092.

_____ (1991). Diagnosis and treatment of obsessive-compulsive disorder in children and adolescents. In *Current Treatments of Obsessive-Compulsive Disorder*, ed. M. T. Pato and J. Zahor. Washington, DC: American Psychiatric Press.

Lindley, P., Marks, I., Philpott, R., and Snowden, J. (1977). Treatment of obsessive-compulsive neurosis with history of childhood autism. *British Journal of Psychiatry* 130:592–597.

Lo, W. H. (1967). A follow-up study of obsessional neurotics in Hong Kong Chinese. *British Journal of Psychiatry* 113:823–832.

Mills, H. L., Agras, W. S., Barlow, D. H., and Mills, J. R. (1973). Compulsive rituals treated by response prevention. *Archives of General Psychiatry* 28:524–529.

Ong, S. B. Y., and Leng, Y. K. (1979). The treatment of an obsessive-compulsive girl in the context of Malaysian Chinese culture. *Australian and New Zealand Journal of Psychiatry* 13:255–259.

Pauls, D., Leckman, J., Towbin, K., et al. (1986). Tourett's syndrome and obsessive compulsive disorder. *Archives of General Psychiatry* 43:1180–1182.

Rapoport, J. L. (1988). *The Boy Who Couldn't Stop Washing*. New York: Dutton.

Riddle, M. A., Scahill, L., King, R., et al. (1990). Obsessive compulsive disorder in children and adolescents: phenomenology and family history. *Journal of the American Academy of Child and Adolescent Psychiatry* 29:766–772.

Riggs, D. S., and Foa, E. B. (1993). Obsessive compulsive disorder. In *Clinical Handbook of Psychological Disorders*, ed. D. H. Barlow. New York: Guilford.

Silverman, W. K. (1991). Diagnostic reliability of anxiety disorders in children using structured interviews. *Journal of Anxiety Disorders* 5:105–124.

Silverman, W. K., Albano, A. M., and Barlow, D. H. (1994). *The Anxiety Disorders Interview Schedule for Children and Parents–DSM-IV version*. In preparation.

Silverman, W. K., and Nelles, W. B. (1988). The anxiety disorders interview schedule for children. *Journal of American Academy of Child and Adolescent Psychiatry* 27:772–778.

Steketee, G. S. (1991). When time is short, is there effective treatment for OCD? *The Behavior Therapist* 14:79.

Steketee, G. S., and Tynes, L. L. (1991). Behavioral treatment of obsessive-compulsive disorder. In *Current Treatments of Obsessive-Compulsive Disorder*, ed. M. T. Pato and J. Zahor. Washington, DC: American Psychiatric Press.

Swedo, S. E., Rapoport, J. L., Leonard, H., et al. (1989). Obsessive-compulsive disorder in children and adolescents. *Archives of General Psychiatry* 46:335–341.

Whitaker, A., Johnson, J., Shaffer, D., et al. (1990). Uncommon troubles in young people: prevalence estimates for selected psychiatric disorders in a non-referred adolescent population. *Archives of General Psychiatry* 47:487–496.

Zikis, P. (1983). Treatment of an 11-year-old obsessive-compulsive ritualizer and tiqueur girl with in vivo exposure and response prevention. *Behavioural Psychotherapy* 11:75–81.

11

POSTTRAUMATIC STRESS DISORDER

David P. Ribbe
Julie A. Lipovsky
John R. Freedy

DESCRIPTION OF DISORDER

The effects of trauma on children have been studied systematically only recently (Eth and Pynoos 1985, Lyons 1987, McNally 1991, Pynoos 1990, Sugar 1989, Terr 1985). Most posttraumatic stress disorder (PTSD) research to date has been focused on etiology, prevalence, and treatment of PTSD in adults. However, recent studies of children's psychological reactions to traumatic events suggest that children who are exposed to trauma may develop symptoms associated with PTSD, as well (McNally 1993). Types of stressors that have been examined for PTSD as an outcome among child populations include natural disasters (Jones and Ribbe 1991, Jones et al. 1994, Lonigan et al. 1991, McFarlane 1987a), sexual assault (Kiser et al. 1988, McLeer et al. 1988, Wolfe et al. 1989), warfare (Arroyo and Eth 1985), violent crime (Malmquist 1986, Pynoos et al. 1987), and accidents (Ribbe and Jones 1993, Yule and Williams 1990). Some children who are exposed to traumatic events develop PTSD, whereas others do not develop the disorder at all or develop a partial or subclinical PTSD. Still others show acute symptoms with a decline in symptoms over several days or weeks after the trauma (Keppel-Benson and Ollendick 1993).

PTSD is diagnosed when a child has experienced a traumatic event that would be perceived as markedly distressing to anyone, and then develops symptoms in each of three groups that persist for one month or more (see *DSM-III-R* criteria, American Psychiatric Association 1987). The first group of symptoms are those that involve a subjective reexperiencing of the traumatic event. In children, only one re-experiencing symptom is required to meet the diagnostic criterion. Re-experiencing symptoms include recurrent and intrusive thoughts about the trauma, trauma-related dreams, flashbacks of the trauma, repetitive play with trauma-related themes, and intense distress when exposed to reminders of the trauma. Children may suddenly act or feel as if the trauma is recurring.

Avoidance symptoms compose the second group of PTSD symptoms. Avoidance symptoms include avoiding thoughts or feelings associated with the trauma, avoiding reminders of the trauma, inability to recall some aspects of the event (amnesia), decreased interest in previously significant activities (or, in younger children, loss of previously acquired developmental skills such as bowel and bladder training, communication skills), feeling detached from others, restricted affective expression, and sense of a foreshortened future. Three symptoms from this group are required to meet the avoidance criterion.

The third group of symptoms is characterized by increased arousal. This arousal is manifested in sleep difficulties (trouble falling asleep, frequent waking, early waking, etc.), irritability, difficulty concentrating, hypervigilance, and physiological reactivity when exposed to stimuli associated with the trauma. To meet the increased arousal criterion, two symptoms from this group must be present.

PTSD in DSM-IV

While researchers are still attempting to define which PTSD symptoms are considered core symptoms and which are less central to the diagnosis (Vogel and Vernberg 1993), the *DSM-IV* criteria (American Psychiatric Association 1994) reflect several modifications in the symptoms and criteria considered essential for diagnosing PTSD under *DSM-III-R*. The first criterion (A) requires that the individual be exposed to a traumatic event in which he or she "has experienced, witnessed, or been confronted with an event or events that involve actual or threatened death or serious injury, or a threat to the physical integrity of oneself or others" (p. 427), in addition to having a response that involves intense fear, helplessness, or horror. For children, the response may be characterized by disorganized or agitated behavior.

The *DSM-IV* moves physiological reactivity to reminders of the trauma from the increased arousal criterion (D) to the re-experiencing criterion (B). In addition, the duration of the disturbance must be more than one month under *DSM-IV*. Finally, the *DSM-IV* includes a sixth criterion that was not in *DSM-III-R*. The F criterion specifies that the disturbance must cause "clinically significant distress or impairment in social, occupational, or other important areas of functioning." In children, impairment of functioning in school is an area in which posttraumatic responses are often observed. Under *DSM-IV*, PTSD will be classified as acute if the symptoms last less than three months; chronic if three months or more. If symptoms begin at least six months after the stressor, then PTSD with delayed onset is specified.

As in *DSM-III-R*, *DSM-IV* includes re-experiencing items that represent PTSD in children (e.g., repetitive play in which themes or aspects of the trauma are expressed, frightening dreams without recognizable content, trauma-specific re-enactment). However, the loss of previously acquired developmental skills among traumatized children is no longer elaborated as a potential avoidance symptom for children. The effect this change will have on case identification among children is uncertain at this time. The interested reader should see Schwarz and Kowalski (1991) for an early discussion of symptom threshold selection for PTSD in children.

Short- and Long-Term Reactions to Trauma

Short-term reactions to traumatic events are defined as those that are evident within the first three months following trauma (Vernberg and Vogel 1993). This period allows for most initial adaptation to daily routines and resuming social roles to take place (Rothbaum and Foa 1993). The most common psychological and behavioral symptoms manifested in children across all traumatic events in the short term are sleep disorders (bad dreams), persistent thoughts of the trauma, belief that another trauma will occur, conduct disturbances, hyperalertness, and avoidance of symbolic situations or stimuli reminiscent of the traumatic event (Frederick 1985).

Some short-term symptoms may continue into long-term symptoms. Fearful reactions, sleep difficulties including nightmares, psychophysiological reactions, and avoidance of symbolic situations or stimuli reminiscent of the traumatic event are some of the many chronic trauma-related symptoms reported in the literature (Frederick 1985, see also Vogel and Vernberg 1993). In response to most disasters, children's symptoms generally decrease substantially within months to a year, with nearly complete recovery between sixteen months and three years (Vogel and Vernberg 1993). Recovery from more chronic types of trauma, such as sexual assault, may be much longer, although the effects can be mitigated by early intervention (Lipovsky 1991a).

The symptom picture varies with factors specific to individual children and stressors (Kendall-Tackett et al. 1993). As mentioned above, not all children develop PTSD when exposed to potentially traumatic events. The most likely outcome of exposure to trauma among children is not necessarily the development of psychopathology (e.g., PTSD), but moderate to minimal levels of behavioral disruption and psychological distress. This may be due, in part, to individual differences such as the developmental level and capabilities of the child, gender, premorbid functioning, previous exposure to trauma, resources, coping style, and other individual factors. It may also be that children develop subclinical levels of PTSD, demonstrating a number of symptoms in one or two symptom groups but not in all three required to make a PTSD diagnosis. In addition, the *DSM* requires a minimum duration of one month for symptoms to warrant the diagnosis. Some children may exhibit PTSD symptoms for a few days or weeks following a trauma, but not long enough to meet the time criterion.

Situational or stressor factors also may play a part in the development of PTSD in children (Milgram et al. 1988, Lonigan et al. 1991, 1994, Pynoos et al. 1987). Children who are victims of violently intrusive events are particularly prone to experience PTSD with long-term psychological effects (Frederick 1985).

To distinguish between stressor types and their associated consequences, Terr (1991) has described two types of trauma. Type I traumas, such as exposure to a natural disaster, are typically one-time events characterized by a sudden and unpredictable onset. Type II traumas, such as childhood sexual or physical assault, are repeated, long-standing, or chronic traumas, which are often expected. Terr (1991) suggested that children exposed to Type I traumas are more likely to evidence classic PTSD symptoms such as repetition, avoidance, and hyperalertness. They are also more likely to have intact recollections of the trauma without amnesia. In contrast, children exposed to Type II traumas are more likely to demonstrate long-standing characterological problems. In addition, they may evidence increased detachment from others, sadness, restricted range of affect, dissociation, pervasive use of defenses, denial, and rage. Memories of Type II traumas are typically less vivid, as the repeated events blur over time.

Although there is no empirical evidence that the distinction between Type I and Type II traumas is valid, clinical experience suggests that there is utility in making the distinction for understanding the way in which symptoms develop and how they're expressed in children. This chapter focuses specifically on posttraumatic outcomes of two general types of traumatic stressors that affect children, natural disaster and sexual assault. These stressors reflect some of the qualitative differences in symptom expression associated with Type I and Type II traumas.

Natural Disaster

Natural disasters can be characterized as Type I traumas. In a review of the literature on traumatic stressors that produce PTSD in children, McNally (1993) concluded that few studies of the psychological consequences of disaster among children used *DSM-III* or *DSM-III-R* criteria to assess PTSD. Of the few studies of the psychological consequences of natural disasters that involved standardized assessment of PTSD, cases of PTSD have been rare (cf. Earls et al. 1988, Handford et al. 1986, Jones and Ribbe 1991, Jones et al. 1994). These findings are consistent with the adult disaster literature. In a review of the psychological consequences of disaster among adult populations, Rubonis and Bickman (1991) reported a 17 percent increase in clinically significant distress among adults. Few adults evidencing clinical levels of distress, however, met criteria for PTSD.

Earls and co-authors (1988) investigated the mental health effects of two disasters (flood and exposure to dioxin) on children aged 6 to 17, one year after the event. Using a structured psychiatric, diagnostic interview, they found that 10 percent of the children experienced symptoms severe enough to warrant a diagnosis of adjustment disorder following the flood. No children met the full criteria for a diagnosis of PTSD, but many children in the sample reported some PTSD symptoms. Chronic re-experiencing symptoms, particularly nightmares and "feeling as though it was happening again" were endorsed by 25 percent of the children one year after the offset of the disasters.

Handford and colleagues (1986) reported some findings that appear to contradict those of other studies of the long-term effects of a nuclear disaster on children. In a sample of thirty-five children ages 6 to 19 years, Handford found only moderate residual levels of anxiety and no evidence of abnormally high levels of behavioral or emotional problems. The authors speculated that it was because of the "silent," nonconcrete nature of the radioactivity hazard that determined the low levels of psychopathology among children. Similarly, Jones and Ribbe (1991) and Jones and co-authors (1994) found relatively low levels of PTSD symptoms among child and adolescent survivors of residential fires and wildfire disaster, perhaps owing to the less than sudden onset of many of the fires, or mediating effects of parents.

In the largest study completed to date that examined the effects of natural disaster (hurricane) on children, Lonigan and colleagues (1991, 1994) also found relatively low levels of PTSD. This finding may be due to lack of direct exposure to aspects of the disaster that would produce high levels of fear and anxiety or a sense of threat to life. However, an association was found between level of exposure and degree of PTSD symptomatology reported in this sample.

McNally (1993) concluded that there is little evidence that disasters produce PTSD in children, unless specific events that can occur during a natural disaster lead to PTSD, such as witnessing the injury or death of another person, or being directly exposed to life-threatening elements of the disaster. Similarly, Vogel and Vernberg (1993) concluded that there is evidence that severity and pattern of responses among children (including PTSD) are influenced by characteristics of the disaster (e.g., degree of life threat, injury, and loss), characteristics of the child (e.g., gender and age), and characteristics of the social context (e.g., family and community). However, the studies above and other studies show that children do evidence increases in behavioral and emotional distress following natural disasters. This distress does not usually reach clinical levels, but perhaps reflects the degree of disruption to children's daily routines (Lipovsky 1991a).

Despite relatively low levels of PTSD symptoms in children following disaster, symptoms and behaviors observed in children following a disaster do include some elements of the PTSD syndrome, which often warrant clinical attention. Lystad (1989) and Farberow and Gordon (1986) have documented some common behavioral difficulties that preschoolers, elementary school age children, and adolescents experience following a disaster (see Table 11-1).

Sexual Assault

Estimates of new child sexual assault (CSA) cases in the United States range from 150,000 to 200,000 each year (Finkelhor et al. 1984). The literature addressing mental health consequences is broad in focus and growing at an exponential rate. Based on a review of studies, Browne and Finkelhor (1986) concluded that between 46 percent and 66 percent of children who had been sexually assaulted show significant psychological impairment. Symptoms of depression and anxiety were common among child CSA survivors. PTSD as a consequence was not addressed within their review. Other short-term symptoms exhibited by child CSA survivors include sexualized behaviors, nightmares, social withdrawal or isolation, sleep difficulties, anger, acting out, somatic difficulties, and school difficulties (Beitchman et al. 1991, Kendall-Tackett et al. 1993).

While there are many potential psychological effects of CSA, PTSD has begun to receive increased attention in recent years. Different approaches to assessing symptomatology within different types of samples of abused chil-

Table 11-1. Age-Specific Reactions of Children to Disasters

Preschoolers	Elementary School Age	Pre-adolescents and Adolescents
Depression, sadness	Depression, sadness	Depression, sadness, suicidal ideation
	Withdrawal from peers	Withdrawal and isolation
Confusion	Confusion	Confusion
Irritability	Irritability	Irritability
Sleep problems:	Sleep problems	Sleep problems:
–night terrors	–night terrors	–night terrors
–nightmares	–nightmares	–nightmares
–interrupted sleep	–interrupted sleep	–sleeplessness
–bedwetting	–bedwetting	–withdrawal into
–need for night light	–need for night light	heavy sleep
General and specific fears:	General and specific fears:	Antisocial behaviors:
–fear of being left alone	–irrational fears: safety of	–stealing
–fear of strangers	buildings, lights in sky	–aggressive behavior
–weather fears (rain,	–weather fears	–acting out
lightning, high winds)	–safety fears	
–fears of darkness	–fears of darkness	
–fears of animals	–fears of animals	
–fear of sleeping alone	–fear of sleeping alone	
Eating problems	Headaches, nausea,	Physical complaints:
	physical complaints	headaches, stomach pain
Marked sensitivity	Visual or hearing	
to loud noises	problems	
Regressive behaviors:	School problems:	School problems:
–excessive clinging	–school refusal	–avoidance
–whining	–behavior problems	–disruptive behavior
–loss of bowel and/or	–poor performance	–academic failures
bladder control	–poor concentration	–poor performance
–asking to be dressed/fed	–distractibility	
–thumb sucking	–fighting	
–speech difficulties	–withdrawal from	
–immobility	interests, playgroups	
	–disobedience	

Adapted from Lystad (1989), and Farberow and Gordon (1986). Used by permission.

dren report rates of PTSD ranging from 21 percent to 48 percent among child victims of sexual assault (see Deblinger et al. 1989, Famularo et al. 1990, McLeer et al. 1988, 1992).

Early studies of the psychiatric morbidity among child survivors of sexual assault did not systematically assess PTSD (Burgess et al. 1984, Gomes-Schwartz et al. 1985). Deblinger and colleagues (1989) used a retrospective chart review of psychiatric inpatients to determine prevalence of

PTSD associated with sexual abuse and physical abuse. Overall, 20.7 percent of the sexually assaulted children appeared to meet the diagnostic criteria for PTSD. Group comparisons were made on the number of symptoms in each of the three PTSD categories, re-experiencing or repetitive phenomena, avoidant behaviors, and symptoms of autonomic hyperarousal. Sexually assaulted children evidenced more re-experiencing PTSD symptoms than did either physically assaulted or nonassaulted children. Both sexually assaulted and physically assaulted children showed tendencies to exhibit more symptoms in the avoidance/dissociative subcategory of PTSD than did nonassaulted patients. The sexually and physically assaulted children exhibited significantly more hyperarousal symptoms than the physically assaulted children. Despite the limitations of the retrospective methodology, this finding suggests that children who are exposed to multiple sources of trauma are more likely to evince increased arousal symptoms.

McLeer and colleagues (1988) directly assessed PTSD in samples of children presenting to an outpatient clinic. They found that 48 percent of the sample met *DSM-III-R* criteria for PTSD. Many children in the sample who did not meet full PTSD criteria exhibited partial PTSD symptoms. They also found that children with PTSD exhibited more externalizing and internalizing behaviors than children who did not have PTSD.

Despite methodological weaknesses and failure of many researchers to assess PTSD symptomatology specifically, results of these studies consistently demonstrate that a proportion of CSA survivors develop symptoms related to PTSD. These findings imply that child CSA survivors are at risk for developing PTSD. Therefore, children who are referred for behavioral or emotional problems should be screened routinely for CSA and PTSD (Lipovsky 1992).

DIFFERENTIAL DIAGNOSIS

As mentioned above, traumatized children frequently demonstrate symptoms of disorders other than PTSD. Conversely, children with other disorders may have PTSD as a comorbid diagnosis (Famularo et al. 1990). Often, children exhibit PTSD symptoms secondary to trauma that overlap with other symptom groups. For example, as part of the response to trauma, children may evidence affective constriction, which may overlap with depressive anhedonia (March and Amaya-Jackson 1993).

Traumatized children report more trauma-related fears than nontraumatized children (Dollinger et al. 1984). Saigh (1989) reported increased levels of anxiety, depression, and conduct problems among children with PTSD. Behavioral disturbances are more common among traumatized children than among nontraumatized children (Cohen and Mannarino 1988).

Livingston (1987) found significant psychiatric comorbidity among sexually assaulted children. The most common diagnoses in the sample were major depression with psychotic features (77 percent), attention deficit disorder (69 percent), overanxious disorder (62 percent), separation anxiety disorder (54 percent), and oppositional disorder (62 percent). Sirles and colleagues (1989) found Axis I disorders among 38 percent of sexually assaulted children in an outpatient clinic. Specifically, the most common conditions were adjustment disorders with depressed mood (28 percent) and conduct disorder (5 percent).

ASSESSMENT PROCEDURES

Various studies that have assessed PTSD in children and adolescents yield mixed findings. Some, such as Yule and Williams (1990), have found considerable support for the presence of PTSD in child and adolescent trauma victims, whereas others, such as Green and colleagues (1991) and Quarantelli (1985) have found contradicting evidence, both for and against PTSD in child and adolescent trauma victims. The inconsistency among studies may be due to a variety of methodological issues, including assessment procedures. Thus, an issue to keep in mind when assessing the traumatized child is that the uncertainty of PTSD diagnosis in children and adolescents may be due to the inadequacy of the instruments used to assess the presence or severity of the disorder in children and adolescents.

One safeguard against making invalid or unreliable diagnoses of PTSD in children is to employ a multimethod assessment strategy. The adult PTSD literature has consistently called for a multimethod assessment strategy, using the following five methods: (1) structured clinical interview; (2) determination of pre-trauma history and functioning; (3) psychometric assessment; (4) collection of behavioral and physiological response data; and (5) review of archival information (Lyons 1987, Solomon 1989).

Most of the instruments used to assess stress symptomatology in children have been structured interviews (e.g., Diagnostic Interview for Children and Adolescents-Revised, DICA-R, Reich and Welner 1990), self-report measures of depression and anxiety such as the Revised Children's Manifest Anxiety Scale (R-CMAS, Reynolds and Richmond 1978, Saigh 1989), the Children's Depression Inventory (CDI, Kovacs 1981; see Saigh

1989), the State-Trait Anxiety Inventory for Children (STAIC, Spielberger et al. 1970) or self-report instruments developed and validated with adult populations, such as the Impact of Event Scale (IES, Horowitz et al. 1979, Jones and Ribbe 1991, Malmquist 1986, Yule and Williams 1990). The IES has been used as a screening instrument for intrusion and avoidance symptoms, but it does not assess hyperarousal symptoms. The Children's Impact of Traumatic Events Scale (CITES, Wolfe et al. 1991), a measure of children's post-sexual abuse PTSD symptoms, includes a scale that assesses intrusive thoughts about the abuse, as well as about other PTSD symptoms. High scores on the CITES, however, do not necessarily confirm a diagnosis of PTSD (Lipovsky 1991b).

Structured and semistructured clinical interviews such as the DICA-R are considered to be the gold standard by which PTSD is diagnosed in children. However, reliability and validity data on many of these instruments are lacking, as many of these instruments have included PTSD sections only recently (March and Amaya-Jackson 1993). The Reaction Index (RI, Frederick 1988), for example, has been shown to be a valuable screening tool for the assessment of PTSD symptoms in children. It is limited, however, in that it does not provide a PTSD diagnosis.

Self-report measures such as the CDI and the RCMAS can be used to assess internalizing comorbid psychopathology. Although parents and teachers often underreport children's internal responses to trauma (e.g., intrusive imagery, efforts to avoid thoughts about the trauma) (cf. Handford et al. 1986, McFarlane 1987b), their assessment of children's behavioral responses to trauma can be useful. Parent and teacher reports on the Child Behavior Checklist (CBCL, Achenbach and Edelbrock 1983) and Conners Teacher Rating Scale (CTRS, Conners 1969) are useful for determining externalizing symptoms in children. Some studies, however, have found that children's scores on measures of depression and anxiety do not differ between traumatized groups and normative samples (Cohen and Mannarino 1988, Jones and Ribbe 1991, Wolfe et al. 1989). Such findings suggest that general measures of psychopathology may not detect PTSD among children (Keppel-Benson and Ollendick 1993). Another interpretation is that children are resilient and do not develop PTSD or PTSD-related symptoms. Despite relatively poor agreement between parent and child reports of distress, it is important to gather information from the parent or guardian regarding the child's behavior.

In a study of disaster effects among children, Earls and co-authors (1988) cautioned that structured interviews used with children may obtain a high prevalence rate of disorders identified through children's reports of psychiatric symptoms, because children tend to overreport subjective symptoms. They asserted that there is a tendency for the structured interview method to yield more children with multiple psychiatric diagnoses than is usually produced in a clinical examination. In addition, Pynoos and Nader (1988) argued that another problem with the reliability of children's self-report of symptoms is that they may not make general statements about their emotional state. It may be difficult, therefore, to estimate the prevalence or severity of certain PTSD symptoms. These conclusions underscore the need for more objective and reliable indicators of the impact of trauma, especially in the diagnosis of PTSD in children and adolescents.

In a comprehensive review of the literature of children's responses to disaster, Vogel and Vernberg (1993) highlighted the importance of directly asking children about their reactions to trauma rather than relying on parent or teacher reports exclusively. In general, children report more severe reactions to disaster than parents or teachers. This is especially true for internalizing symptoms, including PTSD symptoms.

ESTABLISHING TREATMENT GOALS

As described above, Type I and Type II traumas are likely to lead to different patterns of symptom expression in children. Therefore, when establishing treatment goals for a child who has been traumatized, the clinician must take into account the chronicity of the trauma, the level of exposure, and the characteristics of the individual child (developmental level, gender, social support systems, etc.) when formulating a treatment strategy. In addition, posttraumatic responses tend to be multifaceted. Thus, treatment goals should address multiple channels, including behavioral, affective, and cognitive aspects of the disorder. Because these three channels often are intertwined, the therapist must be sensitive to issues in each of these areas.

Traumatized children react to situations that remind them of the trauma with a fear response that is both classically and operantly conditioned. The fear response is manifested on three levels: physical, cognitive, and behavioral (Lang 1979). Physical reactions such as increases in heart rate, blood pressure, respiration rate, and muscle tension are automatic. Such reactions are considered an adaptive part of the fight or flight response when an inidividual perceives threat or danger. However, in the traumatized child victim, these responses recur repeatedly when the child is exposed to reminders of the trauma. The physical fear response may become maladaptive when it interferes with the child's ability to function in day-to-day activities when no threat is present.

The fear response is also reflected in cognitions, triggered by the child's thoughts. Following a traumatic event, children may experience unwanted images or thoughts about the trauma. These images or thoughts may persist despite the child's efforts to stop them. The intrusive nature of these cognitions may cause concentration difficulties and lead the child to feel that he or she has little control. Sometimes, intrusive cognitions take the form of nightmares about the accident or night terrors that leave the child awake in a state of fear with no recall of the content of the dream.

After a trauma, children also respond to the physical and cognitive fear response on a behavioral level. They may attempt to control further exposure to situations that evoke fear-producing physical reactions and cognitions by behaviorally avoiding situations that remind them of the trauma. Children may go to great lengths to avoid people, places, things, or situations that are associated with the trauma.

Sometimes the physical, cognitive, and behavioral fear responses occur separately. Most frequently, however, the three levels of fear response occur simultaneously or interact with one another. For example, having thoughts about the trauma may trigger physical reactions, which, in turn, may lead to avoidance behaviors that limit further exposure to fear-producing situations.

Effective treatment focuses on each of the three levels of the fear response. While specific treatment goals may be determined by the particular symptomatology of the child, general treatment goals are incorporated into the process. First, treatment is designed to help the child to understand the nature of the trauma as well as the effects of the trauma. Second, treatment approaches should facilitate the child's ability to talk and think about the trauma without embarrassment, significant anxiety, or other debilitating levels of negative affect. Third, intervention addresses presenting symptoms in order to reduce the intensity and frequency of intrusive, avoidant, and hyperarousal symptoms. Finally, distorted, faulty, or unhealthy cognitions, such as those related to issues of self-blame, personal power/control, safety, and interpersonal relationships are examined and modified to promote more adaptive ways of thinking about the trauma, self, and relationships.

Treatment focuses on the multiple consequences of trauma. The most immediate are those acute reactions to the trauma—crying, increased cling-ing, nightmares, bed-wetting, fears, phobias, avoidant behaviors, increased irritability, and so on. Following closely on the heels of the acute reactions are the grief/trauma responses, such as impaired social functioning, withdrawal, grief, anger, anxiety, decreased school performance, decreased self-esteem, behavioral disturbance, and so forth. Thus, these symptoms are appropriate targets for treatment, as well as the PTSD symptoms.

ROLE OF THE THERAPIST

When a traumatized child is referred to a clinician, the therapist takes on a multidimensional task that requires fortitude and courage. First, the therapist takes the role of witness, both to the trauma and to the healing process (see Lifton 1993). To assess the impact of the trauma and begin the healing process, the child must tell his or her story. Whether the child is able to articulate the story verbally, through art, or through play, the therapist becomes a witness to the child's inner experience. In the same moment, the therapist becomes a witness to the efforts of the child to make sense out of the events and his or her first steps toward dealing with the trauma.

Second, the therapist becomes a symbolic representation of that trauma. In re-enacting and re-exposing the child to the elements of the trauma, certain features of the trauma accrue to the therapist. The therapist must be prepared and willing to assume some of the negative valence associated with the trauma. The process of re-exposure therapy, whether it be through play or imaginal exposure or systematic desensitization, requires that the therapist be an empathetic yet firm guide.

At times, the child will be resistant to come to therapy. He or she will have difficulty approaching the therapist or telling the story again. At this point, the therapist needs to communicate understanding and empathy, acknowledging the conflict that the child experiences when he or she enters the office. Thus, in providing a supportive environment in which the child can safely confront the elements of the trauma, the therapist also accrues positive associations. For a period of time, the therapist may function as a danger signal to the child, indicating that he or she is about to re-experience unpleasant thoughts or feelings. However, as a child's distress begins to abate through repeated exposure to the memories of the trauma in the therapist's presence, the therapist's signal value becomes one of safety.

When a child has experienced a severe trauma, clinicians may experience countertransference reactions. According to Aptekar and Boore (1990), clinicians may have several of the following reactions to the traumatized child, all of which are countertherapeutic. First, the clinician may deny the child's problem and avoid talking about the untalkable. The clinician may feel personally overwhelmed by the traumatic story and the affect expressed by the child and his or her parents (see also Pollak and Levy 1989). In an attempt to minimize his or her own anxiety, the clinician may minimize the child's problems and dismiss them as transient. Avoidance of emotionally charged issues on the part of the therapist may interact with the avoidant behaviors of the child and his or her parents. This interaction may lead to more and more frequently missed appointments, or failure to see improvement in symptoms. Thus, the therapist may fail to allow the child time to help himself or herself gain a sense of self-efficacy and mastery over the situations and cues that contribute to his or her distress.

Another form of countertransference is overidentification with the child's trauma. This is particularly likely if the therapist has experienced a trauma similar to the child's, or if the therapist has a child of the same age or gender as the client. In such cases, the therapist may begin to experience symptoms similar to those of the child. He or she may become consumed with intrusive thoughts about the child's trauma, both during the day and at night. The therapist may experience dreams or nightmares about the child's trauma and develop fears and phobias related to the child's experience (Aptekar and Boore 1990).

Although this type of reaction to a child's trauma is probably rare among professional mental health providers, it nevertheless can be disruptive to the therapeutic process when it does occur, and steps should be taken to minimize its effect on the treatment process. In both cases, the therapist can combat the ill effects of countertransference by means of routine supervision or counseling from professional peers. This type of peer support can help the therapist to gain a more objective view on the impact of the child's trauma on his or her therapeutic interventions, as well as gain further insight into the impact of the trauma on the child him- or herself.

TREATMENT STRATEGIES

Little is known about the treatment of children with PTSD. Most of the literature about treatment contains case reports (e.g., McNeill and Todd 1986, Saigh 1986, 1987). Although no controlled studies of treatment of PTSD in traumatized children have been published to date, the literature does provide helpful information about the treatment of PTSD in children (Lipovsky 1992).

Ideally, treatment should begin relatively soon after the child is exposed to a traumatic event. With Type I traumas, the child is often able to discuss the event with some anxiety, and avoidance symptoms may not have set in if the child presents to treatment soon after the event (Terr 1991). Treatment in this type of situation should be very focused on the traumatic event and should include a strong psycho-educational focus on the normative course of recovery (Lipovsky 1991b; see also Pynoos and Nader 1990). In Type II traumas, with greater levels of avoidance, one generally is not seeing the child recently after the event. Therefore, it takes more time to establish rapport and to understand the child's coping styles.

As alluded to above, treatment of PTSD should include education about PTSD. Helping a child to understand natural responses to trauma and the symptoms of PTSD help reduce the child's fear of being "crazy." Such education may involve explaining how the symptoms developed from a learning perspective. This may help to normalize the process for children and assure them that their symptoms are understandable to the therapist and others. In addition, information about coping strategies can be helpful, particularly if coupled with rehearsal and feedback. Educational efforts should be directed at helping parents or guardians to understand the nature of the child's experience, his or her symptoms, and their own feelings. It is particularly helpful to assist the caretaker to learn appropriate responses to the child's distress.

Treatment strategies for dealing with PTSD symptoms among children include therapies often used with traumatized adults. Some of the most thoroughly researched interventions for PTSD in children are cognitive-behavioral therapies, such as systematic desensitization and imaginal exposure (Deblinger et al. 1990, Saigh 1992). Play therapy is another approach commonly used to treat young children who have been sexually assaulted. In each of these treatment modalities, the main goal is to re-expose the child to the elements of the trauma in a supportive and protective environment.

In most therapeutic interventions with traumatized children, the developmental level of the child needs to be considered in formulating a treatment approach. In general, younger children need more concrete instructions and examples of anxiety-reducing skills. For example, interventions that focus on clearing up cognitive distortions related to the trauma with younger children may incorporate techniques that are developmentally appropriate to the child, such as the use of coloring books, dolls, and toys to uncover beliefs, attitudes, and emotions related to the trauma. Similarly, interventions that focus on cue-controlled breathing should include concrete instructions, such as encouraging the child to pretend to blow up a balloon.

The cornerstone of treatment for traumatized children is the inclusion of direct focus on the traumatic experiences themselves (Berliner 1991). This focus provides opportunities to accomplish several therapeutic goals: (1) identify cues that may be associated with increased anxiety/distress and disconnect these negative associations; (2) identify maladaptive cognitions; and (3) promote emotional processing of the child's experiences. It is essential that the therapist attend carefully to the child's level of comfort within the treatment environment. Direct focus on trauma can evoke strong emotional reactions in children. Therefore, children and parents can become avoidant of a treatment process that moves quickly and does not take into account the child's level of distress.

Direct focus must be paced in such a way that the child feels that he or she has power and control within the therapeutic process. Focus on the traumatic events may proceed slowly, particularly in work with children exposed to chronically stressful events. Although direct focus on the trauma is essential, children with PTSD often have associated symptomatology that requires direct focus. For example, behavioral treatment strategies are helpful for addressing sexualized behaviors in sexually abused children or phobic behaviors in children who have survived a natural disaster.

Addressing the trauma directly can be facilitated by teaching the child anxiety-reduction strategies. Deep muscle relaxation techniques can produce a sense of calm and control that the child can employ when he or she begins to feel fearful or anxious. Ollendick and Cerny (1981) have provided detailed instructions about relaxation procedures with children. Essentially, the child is asked to sit comfortably, close his or her eyes, and, following the therapist's direction, focus attention on specific muscle groups. Deep muscle relaxation involves tensing, holding for ten seconds, and releasing those muscles in a progressive manner, usually moving from head to toes. This pattern is repeated two or three times for each muscle group.

In addition to tensing and releasing muscles, cue-controlled breathing can be incorporated into the procedure. This involves instructing the child to take a deep breath through the nose, hold for a count of three, then exhale while silently saying "relax" as the therapist says "relax." The sequence is repeated three times.

The calm that results from deep muscle relaxation and cue-controlled breathing techniques can become a conditioned response after several practice sessions. The child can begin to experience relief of fear and anxiety relatively quickly after learning the techniques, allowing him or her to be relaxed enough to think more clearly and feel some control over feelings. The child can practice these techniques in anxiety-producing situations outside of the therapy session.

Deep muscle relaxation can be used in a systematic desensitization manner as well. This technique requires that the child and therapist construct a hierarchy of fear-producing stimuli (images, thoughts, sounds, situations) that progresses from those that are slightly distressing to those that are highly distressing. While in a state of relaxation induced through progressive muscle tensing and releasing, the child is presented with stimuli at the less distressing end of the hierarchy. Over several sessions, stimuli of increasing distress value are presented. With time, the repeated pairing of the incompatible state of relaxation with distressing stimuli leads to a reduction in fear and anxiety in the presence of those stimuli. Thus, children can learn to engage the relaxation response as a coping mechanism when confronted with stimuli or situations that arouse fear or anxiety.

Distraction techniques are also helpful in reducing anxiety in children. The therapist helps the child construct a pleasant, imaginal scene, particularly one in which the child feels safe (i.e., a "safe place"). When the child feels overwhelmed with negative affect, he or she can imagine the safe place to reduce the anxiety. Another distraction approach is to engage in a board game with the child while discussing more difficult issues. Engaging in other activities helps to reduce negative feelings.

Children often develop distorted perceptions of the trauma and its consequences. They may develop complex belief systems about the conditions, real or imagined, that led to the event, complicated it, or led to a less desirable outcome. Such cognitions may compound the distress that the child experiences. It is possible that, when children begin to act on misinterpretations and distorted beliefs, they inadvertently create more difficulties in their physical and social environment that further impair functioning or intensify anxiety.

The goal of cognitive treatment techniques, then, is to correct or stop faulty thinking about the antecedents, behaviors, and consequences associated with the trauma, discover the source of faulty belief systems or misinterpretations, and substitute those cognitions with more appropriate and adaptive thoughts. Cognitive clarification with children can be accomplished through direct discussion of the trauma and the child's beliefs and experience of it. For younger children, play or drawings can be useful techniques for uncovering faulty beliefs.

Sometimes, a functional analysis of a child's distressing symptoms is called for (Lipovsky 1992). When symptoms occur in a defined setting with specifiable antecedents, behavioral responses, and reinforcing consequences, it may be helpful to assist the child to recognize patterns of situations and behaviors. Then, the child and the child's caregivers can be enabled to change the contingencies that maintain the patterns of re-exposure and distress.

Thought-stopping is a technique used to interrupt ruminative thinking associated with trauma. When utilizing this procedure, it is important to prepare the child for what is going to happen, in order not to frighten him or her. Essentially, the therapist instructs the child to think about the trauma for a brief period. Then the therapist loudly says "Stop!" The therapist should then ask the child if the thoughts are continuing. If so, the procedure is repeated until the thoughts stop. The child can then be trained to stop his or her own intrusive, distressing, or ruminative thoughts in this way, first overtly, then covertly.

Role-playing can be useful to help the child engage in behaviors that are more adaptive. Role-playing can uncover distorted cognitions or beliefs and reveal other dysfunctional responses. A valuable variation of this technique is role-reversal, where the therapist takes the role of the child and the child takes the role of other people in his or her sphere of functioning. Role-reversal may help the child confront his or her maladaptive beliefs about others' thoughts and feelings toward him or her. Role-playing can also be helpful in teaching children self-protective skills that may help school-aged children who are at risk for sexual abuse learn how to identify and avoid situations that may lead to traumatization (Wurtele et al. 1989).

Exposure therapy is, perhaps, the central element of successful treatment of traumatized children. Consistent re-exposure to reminders of the trauma allows the multifaceted fear response (physical arousal, intrusive cognitions, and behavioral avoidance) to extinguish in the absence of real danger. As the level of the fear response decreases, the child can begin to feel, think, talk, and approach situations without being overwhelmed. Exposure to fear-producing situations, thoughts, and feelings can be produced imaginally without need for direct exposure to the actual traumatic situation.

In therapy, exposure can be effected by encouraging the child to tell the story of the trauma. The child may attempt to tell the story quickly and in a matter-of-fact manner (without emotion). However, the therapist's task is to help the child focus on sensory details, thoughts, impressions, affective states, and physical sensations at each part of the trauma. The therapist should have the child tell the story slowly, in minute detail, reporting every aspect of his or her experience. The child should be encouraged to recall sights, sounds, smells, physical sensations, and thoughts related to the traumatic event(s).

This part of therapy may be the most difficult for the therapist because of the child's tendency to try to escape or avoid confronting the traumatic memories. For extinction of the fear response to occur, the therapist must encourage the child to stay with the fear-producing memories to the point that he or she reaches a level of emotional arousal similar to that experienced during the traumatic incident. Attempts by the child to escape or avoid this level of distress must be prevented until he or she begins to show signs of calming down. The most intense period of exposure may take several minutes, during which the therapist may become aware of his or her own level of discomfort. It is important for the therapist to be aware of his or her own tendency to avoid confronting the most distressing parts of the traumatic memory, because, in so doing, the client's avoidance is reinforced.

Exposure can be facilitated through a number of techniques, including retelling the trauma story over and over again in detail (as described above), artwork depicting the trauma and/or experiences subsequent to the trauma (Berliner 1991, Pynoos and Eth 1986), writing down accounts of the trauma and thoughts and feelings related to it, acting out the trauma, or expressing reactions to the trauma through movement. Many of these techniques can be employed outside the therapy session, as well as during therapy.

Treatment Following Natural Disaster

Vernberg and Vogel (1993) identified a number of intervention strategies for treating child victims of disaster in the short- and long-term adaptation phases after disaster. From a review of the disaster literature, they concluded that future adjustment to the impact of disaster is largely determined in the short-term postdisaster period (twenty-four hours to three months). Intervention during this time is important in influencing how children will adapt in the long term. Children's defenses are activated in this period, which may cloud the emotions more associated with the trauma itself (Gillis 1991, 1993, Pynoos and Nader 1988). Intervening before the defenses obscure or distort memory of the trauma may enhance children's coping (Yule 1993).

Whether treatment is provided in the context of classroom interventions, small groups, family therapy, or individual therapy, children who have survived disaster need to address several psychological issues (Vernberg and Vogel 1993): (1) accept the events; (2) identify, label, and express emotions; (3) regain a sense of mastery and control; and (4) resume age-appropriate roles and activities (see Klingman 1987, Pynoos and Nader 1988). Accomplishing these goals in any therapeutic context requires sensitivity to the child's developmental level. In general, younger children benefit more from concrete repetitions and clarification of the disaster's events (Pynoos and Nader 1989). To this end, coloring books that help children record their experiences specific to disaster, thoughts, and feelings have been developed. For example, a coloring book, "My Fire Story," was developed to help school-age children work through the Santa Barbara wildfire (Oklan 1990). This was distributed through schools, mental health agencies, and disaster relief organizations following the fire. Such materials can be used in the therapeutic context to help children talk about their experiences and fears.

Treatment Following Sexual Assault

Lipovsky (1992) outlined several general objectives for the treatment of child survivors of CSA. Within an individual approach to treatment, the first goal of therapy is to help children understand the nature of the trauma they have experienced, as well as to realize the effects that the trauma has had on their lives. Second, treatment should help children to talk and think about the abuse experience without embarrassment or significant anxiety. Third, PTSD symptoms should be reduced in intensity and frequency. Finally, distorted or faulty cognitions about the trauma and about the child him- or herself should be corrected.

DEALING WITH COMMON OBSTACLES TO SUCCESSFUL TREATMENT

There are many obstacles to treating traumatized children. Certain types of difficulties are encountered by clinicians rendering therapeutic services to children with PTSD resulting from natural disasters. Other difficulties are common when providing services to children who have been traumatized through sexual or physical assault.

Natural Disaster

One of the primary obstacles to treating psychological problems in children following disaster is obtaining access to children. Lindy (1986) described the presence of a "trauma membrane" that shields disaster victims from outside influences. Access to disaster victims is granted only to those people who are perceived as highly respected or helpful by the community affected by the disaster. Even then, access to victims of disaster may be granted only by the sanction of community leaders (Wilkenson and Vera 1989). Thus, assessing the degree of distress and treating postdisaster symptoms among children is often accomplished in a community context. Pynoos and Nader (1988, 1990) outlined community approaches to providing psychological first aid and treatment to children who have been exposed to large-scale trauma such as disaster or community violence (see also Blom et al. 1991). Essentially, community intevention may be administered through many channels, including through emergency room and other hospital personnel and through coordinated efforts of mental health professionals and school officials. In addition, educating the community about the psychological effects, course of adjustment, and coping skills via the media is an effective way of overcoming treatment obstacles following disaster (Freedy et al. 1992).

Sexual Assault

Although many factors may contribute to unsuccessful treatment with child CSA survivors, Lipovsky (1992) identified three obstacles that are particularly specific among this group of traumatized children. First, a child may avoid engaging in exposure techniques. At this point, the therapist must explore what causes avoidance and reluctance to deal with some aspect of the trauma, then help the child find ways of approaching the topic without experiencing overwhelming distress.

Addressing avoidance in treatment of traumatized children is probably the most essential part of treatment, but it is also the most challenging. Most children, particularly those who have experienced ongoing trauma, are reluctant if not actively opposed to talking about their experiences. This is part of the disorder. Avoidance can serve to limit children's exposure to situations, feelings, thoughts, and so forth that are a part of normal child development. Thus, the child may miss important experiences because he or she is unable to engage in them due to fear associated with the traumatic event.

Approaches to avoidance continue throughout the therapeutic process. The child may be taught anxiety reduction strategies, and distraction techniques such as talking while playing a game can help reduce anxiety that arises when a child approaches uncomfortable trauma-related materials. Additionally, distancing techniques, such as the use of therapeutic stories (e.g., Davis 1988), or using drawings to help the child express feelings or describe the trauma, can facilitate approaching the material.

Before talking about an uncomfortable topic with a child, it is often helpful to provide a rationale to the child about why it is important to talk about unpleasant experiences. It often helps to ask the child what would make it easier to talk about uncomfortable experiences. Then, a number of strategies to facilitate talking about the events can be employed, including those suggested by the child.

One approach that may help the child talk about an uncomfortable topic is to limit the amount of time spent on that topic in the therapy session. The time limit can be specified and controlled by the child by setting a timer. It is also possible to start out by discussing an uncomfortable event by talking about the least scary, uncomfortable, or unpleasant event, then chaining it to another, more upsetting event. Then the therapist and child can talk about the difference between the events. Sometimes suggesting that the child write the events in a story fashion helps.

A second impediment to treatment is the response of authorities to the child's disclosure of sexual abuse. Difficulties with the court system often include confusion about visitation privileges, concerns about the child giving testimony in court, and who will receive psychotherapy. Often, the legal process and the changes it brings in the child's life exacerbate distress in the child. In such situations, the therapist needs to be proactive in educating other professionals about the needs of the child and in making sure the child's best interests are protected (Lipovsky 1992).

The third obstacle to treatment is the therapist's own reaction to the child's trauma and sexual issues. In order to be competent to recognize and deal with therapist difficulties, therapists should be well trained in child development, child psychopathology, legal issues, and therapeutic techniques with sexual assault victims. Here, again, it is recommended that therapists maintain a network of other professionals who can provide objective and emotional support.

RELAPSE PREVENTION

As detailed above, the primary approach to reducing the PTSD-like symptoms in traumatized children is re-exposure to the stimuli associated with the trauma. Repeated exposure leads to extinction of the hyperarousal response and avoidance behaviors. As with any behavioral extinction strategy, however, conditioned fear and avoidance responses are likely to recur spontaneously from time to time. Efforts to reduce recurring PTSD symptoms may include equipping the child with various coping skills (e.g., relaxation, cue-controlled breathing, thought-stopping). In addition, it may be helpful to predict some degree of relapse following termination. Reviewing with the child and his or her caretakers the coping stategies that have been acquired and encouraging the child to use them as often as symptoms return may increase the likelihood that the child will use the skills.

TERMINATION

Positive indicators that therapy may be terminated appropriately include a decrease in the child's PTSD symptoms (i.e., intrusive, avoidant, and hyperarousal symptoms) to levels that no longer interfere with normal, day-to-day functioning (Lipovsky 1992). At the end of therapy, the child should be able to talk about his or her feelings without becoming too distressed. The child should feel a sense of mastery and control over encounters with situations, people, or objects that remind him or her about the trauma.

Termination following successful completion of therapy often includes a review of the process of therapy, retelling the traumatic story, and summarizing the skills, benefits, and resources gained in therapy. For younger children, it may be most helpful to review the gains of therapy with his or her caretakers. In addition, the therapist may predict the occurrence of situations that will be difficult for the child in the future as he or she encounters significant developmental milestones (e.g., puberty, intimate relationships) or situations reminiscent of the original trauma. The therapist should encourage the child and the parents to seek therapeutic assistance if such situations provoke a recurrence of symptoms.

CASE ILLUSTRATION (TYPICAL TREATMENT)

Description and History

Mary was a 9-year-old girl who had been molested by her stepfather over a two-year period. Her mother was quite distressed by the disclosure but was able to be supportive. Mary was experiencing nightmares, moderate anxiety, and moderate depressive symptoms. Mary was also having difficulty in school, displaying behavioral problems such as not attending to the teacher and not staying in her seat in class. She also was rather withdrawn from the other children.

Mary had talked with the police and the Department of Social Services (DSS) about the sexual abuse, providing sufficient detail to justify proceeding with the case. In therapy, Mary was initially reluctant to talk about the abuse experiences. She was able, however, to draw a picture of one event in which her stepfather had touched her genital area outside her clothes.

Synopsis of Therapy Sessions

Initial sessions with Mary were focused on assessing her current behavioral functioning and establishing rapport. The therapist explained that many children are touched in an uncomfortable way by their parents and that children have all sorts of different feelings about this. The therapist clarified that treatment sessions would help to figure out how Mary was feeling about what had happened to her, to see whether her feelings were having an effect on her behavior, and to make sure that she understood what had happened to her and who was at fault.

The therapist made use of drawings (e.g., kinetic family drawing as well as free drawings) to facilitate Mary's discussion of her current situation. Additionally, the therapist explored the frequency and occurrence of Mary's symptoms with both the child and her mother. In the third session, the therapist explained the diagnosis of PTSD to Mary and her mother, normalizing these symptoms as understandable reactions to the sexual assaults that Mary had experienced. A treatment plan, including the use of skill building (e.g., relaxation) and discussion of the abuse, was described to Mary and her mother. Mary was instructed in the use of cue-controlled deep breathing.

> Therapist: We're going to practice a little exercise that can help you feel calmer if you begin to feel anxious when we talk about uncomfortable things. I'd like you to sit back in your chair, and let all your muscles relax. Now, Mary, I want you to take a deep breath [child inhales], now hold your breath for a few seconds, now let your breath all the way out and tell yourself "relax . . . calm . . . relax." [child complies] Great! Let's try it again [repeats procedure]. Now, how are you feeling?
> Client: That was kind of fun. I feel pretty good!
> Therapist: Good. Now, Mary, you can use this breathing when you are feeling nervous or jumpy. I will remind you to use it when we are talking about things and you seem to be feeling nervous. I think you will find that it helps you to relax, even when you are thinking about what has happened to you.

Sessions 4 to 6 were focused on teaching Mary the full body relaxation response (see Ollendick and Cerny 1981 for a sample script for teaching children the relaxation response), explaining the relationship between thoughts, feelings, and behaviors in language appropriate to her developmental level, and contining work on building trust. Mary was able to discuss her experiences after disclosing (her experiences with DSS, fear that her mother would be angry with her, fear that others would know that she had been abused, etc.). The relaxation response was used to ensure that Mary did not become overly anxious in discussing these topics. Drawings and puppet play were the primary modes with which Mary communicated during her sessions.

> Client: [Sitting on the floor, playing with some girl dolls]
> Therapist: Do you play with other children at school?
> Client: The other kids don't like me. I don't want to play with them.

Therapist: Show me what the children at school do.

Client: [Placing one doll to the side and forming the others into a circle]

Therapist: [Pointing to the doll on the side] Who is this?

Client: Me. And those are kids in my class—they think they are better than I am.

Therapist: What do they do that makes you think that?

Client: They just do. They won't play with me. They say mean things to me. They don't want to play with me 'cause of what my stepfather did.

Therapist: What is it that they say that tells you they don't want to play with you because of what your stepfather did?

Client: Well, they say that my stepfather probably did this because I wanted him to and because I liked it.

Therapist: And what do you think?

Client: I did not like it.

Therapist: So the other kids really don't know what happened.

Client: I guess. But why would they say things then?

Therapist: What do you think?

Client: I don't know. [Role-play follows in which Mary expresses what she believes the other children think about her and her abuse experience. The therapist helps Mary recognize faulty assumptions about the meaning of other children's behavior toward her. She helps Mary remember that she did not want her stepfather to touch her and provides information about adults who abuse children. In particular, the therapist emphasizes that adults should know better and that their job is to protect children. The therapist does not automatically tell Mary that the abuse was not her fault, but helps Mary to recognize this by focusing on her stepfather's choice to ignore what was important to her. With the dolls as props, the therapist also helps Mary practice appropriate social and assertive skills around the issue of addressing her peers about their beliefs concerning the abuse.]

Sessions 7 to 10 began to focus more directly on the abuse experiences themselves. While Mary had been able to address postdisclosure experiences in previous sessions with only moderate anxiety, she became rather distressed when she was directed to think and communicate about the abuse itself. Cognitive techniques were employed, particularly addressing possible threats that her stepfather may have made. It was clear that Mary had been threatened and she was reassured by both the therapist and Mary's mother. Mary continued to resist the therapist's attempts to address the abuse directly. Mary displayed her avoidance by changing the subject, directing the therapist to a game in the office, and merely shutting down. When the therapist encouraged Mary to describe an incident in which her stepfather touched her under/inside her clothes, Mary stopped talking. She became unsettled and anxious.

Client: Why do we have to talk about this? It makes me feel bad.

Therapist: I understand that you feel bad when you are talking about this. We can use your deep breathing to help you feel less bad.

Client: I don't want to do that. I will still feel bad.

Therapist: What feels bad about talking about what your stepfather did?

Client: I get embarrassed.

Therapist: You know, most kids do feel embarrassed talking about what adults have done to them. I know it's hard to talk about these things. What I want to do is to help you talk about this stuff so you don't feel embarrassed any more. I think you will find that when we talk about it you will feel embarrassed at first but that the bad feelings will start to get smaller. Until we talk about it though, the bad feelings will stay inside – talking helps to get those feelings out. Let's talk about the time that your stepfather touched you *outside* your clothes first.

Client: Okay – that isn't so hard [interchange around this event – Mary described what happened, how she felt, what she was thinking].

Therapist: How was this time different from a time when your stepfather touched you *under* your clothes?

Client: Well, that seemed more scary.

Therapist: So you were more afraid. Did it seem more real to you?

Client: Well, I knew it wasn't an accident.

Therapist: What did your stepfather say to you about this? [dialogue continued about this more uncomfortable experience]

Sessions 11 to 15 involved continued work directly on Mary's abuse experiences. Through drawings and puppets she was able to describe what had happened to her, express feelings about the events, her stepfather, and her need to keep the abuse a secret. The relaxation response was used frequently during the early sessions of this phase of treatment, but as Mary became more comfortable with her position of control over the feelings she experienced, this coping strategy was not needed as much. There were many points during these sessions when Mary was reluctant to proceed. The therapist was always responsive to Mary's discomfort and always encouraged her to proceed. If Mary strongly resisted, the therapist redirected the focus to a less uncomfortable topic and revisited the distressing subject at a later time.

Client: I don't want to talk about this right now.

Therapist: What is uncomfortable today?

Client: I just don't want to and you can't make me.

Therapist: You're right, Mary, I can't make you, and I won't make you. Our sessions will not be like the abuse when a grown-up didn't pay attention to what you wanted. But, you know that I think it is very important to talk about what happened so your uncomfortable feelings about the sexual abuse can get smaller. How have you felt after talking about some of the abuse in other sessions?

Client: It wasn't so bad, but we probably have to talk about some of the really scary things next and I just don't want to.

Therapist: Let's do some deep breathing and help you feel better. [Deep breathing exercise] Now, how do you feel?

Client: I feel better, but I still don't want to talk about this.

Therapist: Can you draw your feelings? [Child draws a picture indicating that she feels scared.] I see that today is a touch day for you. Let's draw how you would like to feel. [Child draws a happy picture.] What would help you to feel this way?

Client: If the abuse never happened.

[Discussion then focuses on how Mary's life would be if the abuse had never occurred. The therapist provides support and reinforces Mary's ability to talk about her feelings and indicates that they will come back to the abuse itself some other time, but that right now, it is fine to focus on her feelings.]

Comments

Over the course of this relatively uncomplicated case, Mary became more relaxed both at home and in school. She learned that she did not have to tell other children of her experiences and that she displayed no tell-tale signs that she had been abused. Mary also learned that she could use her deep breathing or relaxation in situations in which she felt anxious. Her nightmares and behavioral problems decreased in frequency. Anxiety and depressive symptoms were reduced significantly and Mary's mother enrolled the child in a community recreation program. Mary's peer relationships improved greatly, as she became less fearful of others' responses toward her. The rapid improvement in this child was facilitated by her extremely supportive mother and by the child's willingness to approach uncomfortable topics. It should be kept in mind that many cases will require much more time, adjunctive interventions, and more restraint on the part of the therapist in helping the child to address frightening thoughts, feelings, and memories. This child's experiences were relatively mild in the sense that there was no sexual penetration and no actual physical violence. The child was, however, threatened with violence if she disclosed. Children whose experiences are more violent and threatening may be expected to be more avoidant of the therapeutic process designed to facilitate their recovery.

CASE ILLUSTRATION (OVERCOMING OBSTACLES)

Description and History

The following account describes a case that presented significant obstacles to providing treatment to a young girl who had been raped. Specifically, the mother's distress about the rape and its consequences was the most significant obstacle to making therapeutic progress with the child.

Kathee was a first grader who was referred to therapy by the County Sheriff's Department after she was raped by a 13-year-old boy in her neighborhood. One month after the rape, Kathee was accompanied to the intake interview by her mother, Mrs. W. According to Mrs. W., Kathee had difficulty sleeping at night, frequent nightmares, nighttime enuresis, difficulty concentrating in school, and increased aggression at school. Until the time of the rape, Kathee was making a good adjustment to school. She also avoided going near the woods where the rape occurred. In addition, Kathee had been indiscriminately telling everyone she met that she had been raped, causing concern for her mother and teacher.

Kathee was playing outside with her brother and some other neighborhood children in a play fort in the nearby woods when a 13-year-old boy, Thomas, told her to come with him to another part of the woods to "get something" for the fort. When they were away from the other children, he pushed Kathee on the ground and took her clothes off. Her back was scratched by branches on the ground as she fell. He then attempted to penetrate her vagina with his penis. Kathee reported that she was yelling at the time, while the assailant laughed. Her brother, Ronald, heard Kathee yelling and came to find her. When he reached the scene, Kathee was crying and putting on her clothes and Thomas was running away. Thomas came back to the scene and began pulling Kathee's arm, while Ronald took her other arm, trying to pull her away from Thomas. Thomas eventually let go and Kathee and Ronald ran home.

Ronald entered the house first and told his mother what had happened. Kathee initially did not say what had happened, but after being examined by her parents, told them about her experience. She was then taken to the emergency room, where a representative of a victim assistance group assisted them for a time. The family then waited for more than ten hours for Kathee to be examined, which made the experience extremely upsetting for Mrs. W. The medical examination found positive evidence of penetration.

By court order, the assailant was removed from his home and placed in a residential treatment center. Mrs. W. indicated that she was concerned that the Sheriff's Department would not be objective in gathering evidence and statements from her family because the assailant's father was a deputy sheriff with the county. Incidentally, Mrs. W. reported that she was the daughter of a police officer. This was important, because she believed that the assailant's father could "work the system" to make sure that his son was not prosecuted.

Synopsis of Therapy Sessions

The first session was spent gathering information about Kathee's rape experience from Kathee and her mother. In addition, information about how Kathee, her family, and community responded to the incident was obtained through interview and behavioral observation. In the initial session, Kathee presented as a somewhat overweight child who was dressed in boys' clothes. She spoke surprisingly openly and freely about the details of her rape experience. She showed appropriately sad affect when describing how she felt about what had happened. Kathee appeared to be calm and relaxed throughout the interview. Kathee patiently answered all the questions in the children's self-report assessment packet when they were read aloud to her. Although it appeared that she tended to positively endorse most items, she was able to give evidence of her thoughts and feelings to support many of her responses. She colored pictures of a boy and a girl and described their feelings and behaviors in detail.

> Therapist: Kathee, I wonder if you could draw me a picture of a girl who is your age.
>
> Client: Okay. [Draws girl with crayons]
>
> Therapist: Kathee, tell me about the picture.
>
> Client: [Pointing to girl's face] See, there are tears on her face. She's crying 'cause she's sad.
>
> Therapist: Why is she sad?
>
> Client: 'Cause a mean boy hurt her. [Holds her back] See, I got scratches there [lifts back of shirt to reveal scratches].
>
> Therapist: I see. Tell me how that happened.
>
> Client: Okay. [Tells story of the assault in detail]
>
> Therapist: Now draw me a picture of a boy.
>
> Client: Okay. [Draws boy figure] See, he's laughing, 'cause he gets all the Christmas presents he wants.
>
> Therapist: What's the boy's name?
>
> Client: [Uses name of assailant.] He lives near me. [Affect turns sad] I don't like to go near his house anymore. I stay in my house or in the yard when my mom is there.
>
> Therapist: Kathee, you look kinda sad . . . [Kathee nods]. You know, most kids do feel kinda sad when something scary happens to them. You and I are going to talk about what happened to you so that you won't feel so sad or scared. We will learn how to do some breathing and relaxation exercises to help you feel better when we talk about uncomfortable things.

In contrast, Mrs. W. appeared to be more distressed than Kathee. During the intake session (and throughout much of therapy), she spoke in angry tones and in a sarcastic manner about the way in which the case was handled by the police and the hospital. She appeared to be pessimistic about the outcome of the legal process and the treatment of the offender. She voiced many concerns about how she and her husband should act around Kathee and Ronald, admitting that they frequently displayed their anger about the rape and its consequences at home.

The second and third sessions focused on teaching Kathee the relaxation response and cue-controlled breathing, techniques that she mastered readily. Initially, therapy dealt directly with the traumatic experience, as well as some of the problems that were related to the disclosure of the incident. Kathee and the therapist drew pictures together as they talked about the rape incident. Kathee talked about how the other children at school were mean to her and tried to start fights with her. She talked about how the teacher made her go into time-out every day. Episodes of enuresis and nightmares declined notably after the onset of therapy.

In sessions 4 through 6, Kathee reported an increase in nightmares and fighting at school and with her brother. She had begun to wet the bed again, and had started to wet herself at school. In the time spent with Mrs. W. during these sessions, it became apparent that she was becoming more and more distressed about the legal processes related to the rape and about neighbors' and teachers' reactions to the incident. It appeared that the increase in Kathee's symptoms might be linked to Mrs. W.'s distress levels. At this point, the therapist began to use half the session to continue talking with Kathee and the other half to spend time teaching Mrs. W. the relaxation exercises, educating her about posttraumatic adjustment, and coaching her about positive ways to express feelings at home.

Therapist: How have things been going this week?

Mother: Kathee's been getting into more fights with her brother at home. She's also become much more "touchy." For instance, when she and her father and brother were playing rough the other day, she got very upset when someone touched her genital area.

Therapist: What happened then?

Mother: Kathee started screaming and crying. My husband got very upset and started yelling at her to "chill out." We all got pretty upset. We decided that they shouldn't play rough any more. [With angry tone] When is all this going to stop? This really makes me mad that this boy could do this to our family . . .

Therapist: It's going to take some time. Mrs. W., let's do the deep breathing exercises we learned last week. [Repeats exercise three times.] Now, how does that feel?

Mother: Better. I really need to relax more. I've been yelling a lot at home.

Therapist: It seems like you've been under quite a bit of stress lately. I know that your business is struggling financially, the assailant has returned to the neighborhood, there's been more tension at home, Kathee's symptoms have intensified, and so on.

Let's look at some ways to reduce some of the distress

everybody's feeling at home. First, it may be helpful to understand that Kathee's reaction to being touched in her private area, even inadvertently, may bring back some scary feelings for her. That's one of the things we talk about in therapy. It's normal for her to have an increase in symptoms when reminders of the event occur—even therapy can be a reminder. But, the goal of therapy is to help her talk about what happened, how it made her feel, and so on, until she feels more comfortable about talking and thinking about such things. It's important for you and your husband to understand how she's feeling, and to be supportive of her when she has a strong reaction like the one she had the other day. You and your husband can anticipate that such reactions will take place from time to time. You can plan to respond with gentle assurance that she is safe until she calms down. It's very important to control the level of your own reaction, so she does feel safe. You both can practice your relaxation exercises when these situations recur.

It's probably equally important to be aware of how you talk about family stresses in front of Kathee and her brother. A suggestion would be that you discuss problems with your husband when the children are not present. If you're feeling stressed by dealing with the authorities and with Kathee's teacher over this issue, talk privately with your husband or other adults about your concerns. I'm concerned that Kathee is picking up on the frustration and anger you and your husband feel, and that is creating stress for her, thus increasing her nightmares and fighting at school and so on. [Discussion continues about ways in which Mrs. and Mr. W. can cope more effectively with opposition from the authorities.]

Sessions 7 through 12 consistently focused on direct exposure to the rape trauma with Kathee through play with dolls, coloring, and retelling the rape experience. Cognitive distortions and faulty beliefs about the trauma and about people's reactions to the trauma were uncovered and addressed primarily through these media with Kathee. Mr. W. and brother Ronald were brought in for two family sessions in which the concerns of the family were addressed. Ronald was asked to draw pictures about the parts of the incident that he witnessed. He talked about his feelings as well.

During this time, Kathee's nightmares became less frequent. The daytime and nighttime wetting stopped. The family began to attend therapy more sporadically, canceling two sessions and missing one. When Kathee indiscriminately began telling everyone she met that she had been raped, Mrs. W. brought Kathee back to therapy under pressure from Kathee's teacher.

Therapist: Kathee, you've been doing real well in therapy. You can talk about what happened to you without feeling too uncomfortable. That's good. Let's talk for a few minutes about how to know *when* to talk about the time Thomas raped you.

Client: Okay.

Therapist: You know that it's okay to talk about what happened and how you feel about it here, with me. And it's okay to talk with your mom and dad about these things, too. Sometimes, it might

be okay to talk to your teacher, too, because she needs to know how to help you when you're feeling upset. Now let's talk about when you shouldn't talk about what happened. Most kids your age, Kathee, don't understand about what happened. It's probably not important for them to know what Thomas did. If you're in school, and you feel that you need to talk to somebody, tell your teacher that you want to talk. She can help you decide who to talk to. [Role-play using dolls followed, modeling appropriate disclosure. The therapist provided corrective feedback and reinforcement for appropriate responses.]

In the final sessions of therapy, the focus continued to be directly on Kathee's feelings and experiences. During this time, it became evident that Mrs. W. perceived that Kathee's teacher was selectively treating Kathee differently in class. She reported that the teacher was sending antagonistic messages home on Kathee's report card, accusing Mrs. W. of keeping Kathee up too late at night, not reading to her enough, and so forth. The time spent with Mrs. W. during the final sessions focused on reframing the teacher's behavior and comments as constructive suggestions rather than accusations. The therapist focused attention on how Mrs. W.'s defensive behavior around Kathee may have had the effect of causing the teacher and other authorities involved in the case to react negatively, thus creating more difficulties that had negative consequences for Kathee. In this instance, the therapist took a proactive approach as an advocate for Kathee. Specifically, he set up a meeting with Kathee's parents, the teacher, and himself as moderator to educate the teacher about the course of post-trauma adjustment and how to respond to Kathee's needs, and to facilitate productive communication between Kathee's parents and teacher.

The therapist also acted as Kathee's advocate through the legal process. He provided Kathee's parents with information about applying for victim assistance from the state, how to communicate their concerns to the county solicitor, and what to expect during the court process. He wrote a letter of support to the solicitor who was scheduled to try the case, which described the impact of the rape on Kathee and her family and their efforts and gains in therapy, and made an appeal for appropriate treatment and consequences for the assailant. These types of efforts were considered to be a valuable part of the therapeutic healing process in this case.

Although not all of Kathee's problems were resolved, she did evidence an overall reduction of symptoms by the time therapy ended. Her nightmares had declined significantly, and she was no longer wetting herself. She continued to be able to talk about the rape trauma comfortably and with appropriate affect. After several approximations, Kathee and her family were able to walk together through the section of the woods where the assault occurred. Some difficulties in her relationships with peers remained.

Comments

Kathee's case was rife with obstacles that could detract from the primary focus of dealing directly with the trauma. While the goals of therapy are to help the child understand what happened to him or her, to be able to talk about what happened without excessive anxiety, and to reduce symptoms, it may become necessary to do a broad assessment of factors outside the individual child that may interfere with attaining those goals. Such factors may include the reactions of parents, siblings, teachers, and peers, or the machinations of the legal system. Therapists can take an active role in reducing such impediments by educating individuals who influence the child's life about how to respond appropriately to the child, providing information about services that provide support to children and families who have been traumatized, and facilitating communication between those who are involved in the child's case.

SUMMARY

Many gaps exist in the knowledge and understanding of the etiology, prevalence, course, and treatment of PTSD in traumatized children. The technology for assessing PTSD in children is still underdeveloped. Much of what is known about the treatment of traumatized children is derived from clinical experience. In sum, the current status of the empirical foundation for understanding PTSD in children is limited, although it clearly is growing. The information we have regarding the epidemiology, course, and core symptoms of PTSD in children is largely based upon research conducted with small, often biased samples using measures of PTSD symptomatology that have not been validated. The challenges for future research are to specify the circumstances under which children develop PTSD following exposure to traumatic events, define the course of the disorder, and evaluate treatment effectiveness. A growing literature about PTSD in children coupled with greater efforts at standardizing assessment procedures and new initiatives to conduct controlled treatment outcome studies suggest that progress is being made in that direction.

REFERENCES

Achenbach, T. M., and Edelbrock, C. (1983). *Manual for the Child Behavior Checklist and Revised Child Behavior Profile.* Burlington, VT: University of Vermont, Department of Psychiatry.

Aptekar, L., and Boore, J. A. (1990). The emotional effects of disaster on children: a review of the literature. *International Journal of Mental Health* 19:77–90.

Arroyo, W., and Eth, S. (1985). Children traumatized by Central American warfare. In *Post-traumatic Stress Disorder in Children*, ed. S. Eth and R. S. Pynoos, pp. 103–120. Washington, DC: American Psychiatric Press.

Beitchman, J. H., Zucker, K. J., Hood, J. E., et al. (1991). A review of the short-term effects of child sexual abuse. *Child Abuse and Neglect* 15:537–556.

Berliner, L. (1991). Clinical work with sexually abused children. In *Clinical Approaches to Sex Offenders and Their Victims*, ed. C. R. Hollin and K. Howells, pp. 209–228. Chichester, England: Wiley.

Blom, G. E., Etkind, S. L. and Carr, W. J. (1991). Psychological interventions after child and adolescent disasters in the community. *Child Psychiatry and Human Development* 21:257–266.

Browne, A., and Finkelhor, D. (1986). Impact of child sexual abuse: a review of the research. *Psychological Bulletin* 99:66–77.

Burgess, A. W., Hartman, C. R., McCausland, M. P., and Powers, P. (1984). Response patterns in children and adolescents exploited through sex rings and pornography. *American Journal of Psychiatry* 141:656–662.

Cohen, J., and Mannarino, A. (1988). Psychological symptoms in sexually abused girls. *Child Abuse and Neglect* 12:571–577.

Conners, C. K. (1969). A teacher rating scale for use in drug studies with children. *American Journal of Psychiatry* 126:884–888.

Davis, N. (1988). *Therapeutic Stories to Heal Abused Children.* Author.

Deblinger, E., McLeer, S. V., Atkins, M., et al. (1989). Post-traumatic stress in sexually abused children, physically abused, and non-abused children. *Child Abuse and Neglect* 13:403–408.

Deblinger, E., McLeer, S. V., and Henry, D. (1990). Cognitive behavioral treatment for sexually abused children suffering post-traumatic stress: preliminary findings. *Journal of the American Academy of Child and Adolescent Psychiatry* 29:747–752.

Diagnostic and Statistical Manual of Mental Disorders (1987). 3rd ed., revised. Washington, DC: American Psychiatric Association.

Diagnostic and Statistical Manual of Mental Disorders (1994). 4th ed. Washington, DC: American Psychiatric Association.

Dollinger, S. J., O'Donnell, J. P., and Staley, A. A. (1984). Lightning-strike disaster: effects on children's fears and worries. *Journal of Consulting and Clinical Psychology* 52:1028–1038.

Earls, F., Smith, E., Reich, W., and Jung, K. G. (1988). Investigating psychopathological consequences of a disaster in children: a pilot study incorporating a structured diagnostic interview. *Journal of the American Academy of Child and Adolescent Psychiatry* 27:90–95.

Eth, S., and Pynoos, R. S., eds. (1985). *Post-traumatic Stress Disorder in Children.* Washington, DC: American Psychiatric Press.

Famularo, R., Kinscherff, R., and Fenton, T. (1990). Symptom differences in acute and chronic presentation of childhood post-traumatic stress disorder. *Child Abuse and Neglect* 14:439–444.

Farberow, N. L., and Gordon, N. S. (1986). *Manual for Child Health Workers in Major Disasters DHHS Publication #86-1070.* Washington, DC: U.S. Government Printing Office.

Finkelhor, D., Hotaling, G., Lewis, I. A., and Smith, C. (1984). Sexual abuse in a national survey of adult men and women: prevalence, characteristics, and risk factors. *Child Abuse and Neglect* 14:19–28.

Frederick, C. J. (1985). Children traumatized by catastrophic situations. In *Perspectives on Disaster Recovery,* ed. J. Laube and S. A. Murphy, pp. 110–130. Norwalk, CT: Appleton-Century-Crofts.

_____ (1988). *Reaction Index to Psychic Trauma Form C (Child).* (Available from C. J. Frederick, Ph.D., Psychological Services, 69/B116B, Veterans Affairs Medical Center, 1301 Wilshire Boulevard, Los Angeles, CA 90073.)

Freedy, J. R., Resnick, H. S., and Kilpatrick, D. G. (1992). Conceptual framework for evaluating disaster impact: implications for clinical intervention. In *Responding to Disaster: A Guide for Mental Health Professionals,* ed. L. S. Austin, pp. 3–23. Washington, DC: American Psychiatric Press.

Gillis, H. M. (1991). Assessment and treatment of post-traumatic stress disorder in childhood. In *Innovations in Clinical Practice: A Source Book, vol. 10,* ed. P. A. Keller and S. R. Heyman, pp. 245–257. Sarasota, FL: Professional Resource Exchange.

Gillis, H. M. (1993). Individual and small-group psychotherapy for children involved in trauma and disaster. In *Children and Disasters,* ed. C. F. Saylor, pp. 165–186. New York: Plenum.

Gomez-Schwartz, B., Horowitz, J. M., and Sauzier, M. (1985). Severity of emotional distress among sexually abused preschool, school-age, and adolescent children. *Hospital and Community Psychiatry* 36:503–508.

Green, B. L., Korol, M., Grace, M. C., et al. (1991). Children and disaster: age, gender, and parental effects on PTSD symptoms. *Journal of the American Academy of Child and Adolescent Psychiatry* 30:945–951.

Handford, H. A., Mayes, S. D., Mattison, R. E., et al. (1986). Child and parent reaction to the Three Mile Island nuclear accident. *Journal of the American Academy of Child Psychiatry* 25:346–356.

Horowitz, M., Wilner, N., and Alvarez, W. (1979). Impact of event scale: a measure of subjective stress. *Psychosomatic Medicine* 41:209–218.

Jones, R. T., and Ribbe, D. P. (1991). Child, adolescent, and adult victims of residential fire. *Behavior Modification* 15:560–580.

Jones, R. T., Ribbe, D. P., and Cunningham, P. (1994). Psychosocial correlates of fire disaster among children and adolescents. *Journal of Traumatic Stress* 7:117–122.

Kendall-Tackett, K. A.., Williams, L. M., and Finkelhor, D. (1993). Impact of sexual abuse on children: a review and synthesis of recent empirical studies. *Psychological Bulletin* 113:164–180.

Keppel-Benson, J. M., and Ollendick, T. H. (1993). Post-traumatic stress disorder in children and adolescents. In *Children and Disasters,* ed. C. F. Saylor, pp. 29–43. New York: Plenum.

Kiser, L. J., Ackerman, B. J., Brown, E., et al. (1988). Post-traumatic stress disorder in young children: a reaction to purported sexual abuse. *Journal of the American Academy of Child and Adolescent Psychiatry* 27:645–649.

Klingman, A. (1987). A school-based emergency crisis intervention in a mass school disaster. *Professional Psychology: Research and Practice* 18:604–612.

Kovacs, M. (1981). *The Children's Depression Inventory.* Pittsburgh, PA: University of Pittsburgh Press.

Lang, P. J. (1979) A bio-informational theory of emotional imagery. *Psychophysiology* 16:495–511.

Lifton, R. J. (1993). From Hiroshima to the Nazi doctors: the evolution of psychoformative approaches to understanding human stress syndromes. In *International Handbook of Traumatic Stress Syndromes,* ed. J. P. Wilson and B. Raphael, pp. 11–23. New York: Plenum.

Lindy, J. D. (1986). An outline for the psychoanalytic psychotherapy of post-traumatic stress disorder. In *Trauma and its Wake* (vol. 2), ed. C. R. Figley. New York: Brunner/Mazel.

Lipovsky, J. A. (1991a). Children's reaction to disaster: a discussion of recent research. *Advances in Behaviour Research and Therapy* 13:185–192.

_____ (1991b). Posttraumatic stress disorder in children. *Family and Community Health* 14:42–51.

_____ (1992). Assessment and treatment of post-traumatic stress disorder in child survivors of sexual assault. In *Treating PTSD: Cognitive-Behavioral Strategies*, ed. D. W. Foy, pp. 127–164. New York: Guilford.

Livingston, R. (1987). Sexually and physically abused children. *Journal of the American Academy of Child and Adolescent Psychiatry* 26:413–415.

Lonigan, C. J., Shannon, M. P., Finch, A. J., et al. (1991). Children's reactions to a natural disaster: symptom severity and degree of exposure. *Advances in Behaviour Research and Therapy* 13:135–154.

Lonigan, C. J., Shannon, M. P., Taylor, C. M., et al. (1994). Children exposed to disaster: II. Risk factors for the development of post-traumatic symptomatology. *Journal of the American Academy of Child and Adolescent Psychiatry* 33:94–105.

Lyons, J. A. (1987). Posttraumatic stress disorder in children and adolescents: a review of the literature. *Developmental and Behavioral Pediatrics* 8:349–356.

Lystad, M. (1989). Special programs for children. In *Innovations in Mental Health Services to Disaster Victims*, ed. M. Lystad, pp. 151–160. Washington, DC: National Institute of Mental Health.

Malmquist, C. P. (1986). Children who witness parental murder: post-traumatic aspects. *Journal of the American Academy of Child and Adolescent Psychiatry* 25:320–325.

March, J. S., and Amaya-Jackson, L. (1993). Posttraumatic stress disorder in children and adolescents. *PTSD Research Quarterly* 4:1–5.

McFarlane, A. C. (1987a). Posttraumatic phenomena in a longitudinal study of children following a natural disaster. *Journal of the American Academy of Child and Adolescent Psychiatry* 26:764–769.

_____ (1987b). Family functioning and overprotection following a natural disaster: the longitudinal effects of post-traumatic morbidity. *Australian and New Zealand Journal of Psychiatry* 21:210–218.

McLeer, S. V., Deblinger, E., Atkins, M. S., et al. (1988). Post-traumatic stress disorder in sexually abused children. *Journal of the American Academy of Child and Adolescent Psychiatry* 27:650–654.

McLeer, S. W., Deblinger, E., Delmina, H., and Orvaschel, H. (1992). Sexually abused children at high risk for posttraumatic stress disorder. *Journal of the American Academy of Child and Adolescent Psychiatry* 31:875–879.

McNally, R. J. (1991). Assessment of posttraumatic stress disorder in children. *Psychological Assessment: A Journal of Consulting and Clinical Psychology* 3:531–537.

_____ (1993). Stressors that produce posttraumatic stress disorder in children. In *Posttraumatic Stress Disorder: DSM-IV and Beyond*, ed. J. R. T. Davidson and E. B. Foa, pp. 57–74. Washington, DC: American Psychiatric Press.

McNeill, J. W., and Todd, F. J. (1986). The operant treatment of excessive verbal ruminations and negative emotional arousal in a case of child molestation. *Child and Family Behavior Therapy* 8:61–69.

Milgram, N. A., Toubiana, Y. H., Klingman, A., et al. (1988). Situational exposure and personal loss in children's acute and chronic stress reactions to a school bus disaster. *Journal of Traumatic Stress* 1:339–352.

Oklan, A. K. (1990). *My Fire Story: A Guided Activity Workbook for Children, Families, and Teachers*. Kentfield, CA: Psychological Trauma Center Press.

Ollendick, T. H., and Cerny, J. A. (1981). *Clinical Behavior Therapy with Children*. New York: Plenum.

Pollak, J., and Levy, S. (1989). Countertransference and failure to report child abuse and neglect. *Child Abuse and Neglect* 13:515–522.

Pynoos, R. S. (1990). Post-traumatic stress disorder in children and adolescents. In *Psychiatric Disorders in Children and Adolescents*, ed. B. D. Garfinkel, G. A. Carlson, and E. B. Weller, pp. 48–63. Philadelphia, PA: W. B. Saunders.

Pynoos, R. S., and Eth, S. (1986). Witness to violence: the child interview. *Journal of the American Academy of Child and Adolescent Psychiatry* 25:306–319.

Pynoos, R. S., and Nader, K. (1988). Psychological first aid and treatment approach to children exposed to community violence: research implications. *Journal of Traumatic Stress* 1:445–473.

—— (1989). Prevention of psychiatric morbidity in children after disaster. In *Prevention of Mental Disorders, Alcohol, and Other Drug Use in Children and Adolescents*, ed. I. D. Scheffe, I. Philips, and N. B. Enzor, pp. 225–271. Washington, DC: U. S. Government Printing Office.

—— (1990). Children's exposure to violence and traumatic death. *Psychiatric Annals* 20:334–344.

Pynoos, R. S., Frederick, C., Nader, K., et al. (1987). Life threat and posttraumatic stress in school-age children. *Archives of General Psychiatry* 44:1057–1063.

Quarantelli, E. L. (1985). An assessment of conflicting news on mental health: the consequences of traumatic events. In *Trauma and Its Wake*, ed. C. Figley, pp. 173–215. New York: Brunner/Mazel.

Reich, W., and Welner, Z. (1990). *Diagnostic Interview for Children and Adolescents-Revised*. Washington University.

Reynolds, C. R., and Richmond, B. O. (1978). What I think and feel: a revised measure of children's anxiety. *Journal of Abnormal Child Psychology* 6:271–280.

Ribbe, D. P., and Jones, R. T. (1993). *Chronic psychological and psychophysiological sequelae among adolescent bus crash survivors*. Paper presented at the meeting of the American Psychological Association, Toronto, Ontario, Canada, August.

Rothbaum, B. O., and Foa, E. D. (1993). Subtypes of posttraumatic stress disorder and duration of symptoms. In *Posttraumatic Stress Disorder: DSM-IV and Beyond*, ed. J. R. T. Davidson and E. B. Foa, pp. 23–35. Washington, DC: American Psychiatric Association.

Rubonis, A. V., and Bickman, L. (1991). Psychological impairment in the wake of disaster: the disaster-psychopathology relationship. *Psychological Bulletin* 109:384–399.

Saigh, P. A. (1986). *In vitro* flooding in the treatment of a 6-year-old boy's posttraumatic stress disorder. *Behaviour Research and Therapy* 24:685–688.

_____ (1987). *In vitro* flooding of an adolescent's posttraumatic stress disorder. *Journal of Clinical Child Psychology* 16:147–150.

_____ (1989). The validity of the *DSM-III* posttraumatic stress disorder classification as applied to children. *Journal of Abnormal Psychology* 98:189–192.

_____ (1992). The behavioral treatment of child and adolescent posttraumatic stress disorder. *Advances in Behaviour Research and Therapy* 14:247–275.

Schwarz, E. D., and Kowalski, J. M. (1991). Posttraumatic stress disorder after a school shooting: effects of symptom threshold selection and diagnosis by *DSM-III*, *DSM-III-R*, or proposed *DSM-IV*. *American Journal of Psychiatry* 148:592–597.

Sirles, E. A., Smith, J. A., and Kusama, H. (1989). Psychiatric status of intrafamilial child sexual abuse victims. *Journal of the American Academy of Child and Adolescent Psychiatry* 28:225–229.

Solomon, S. D. (1989). Research issues in assessing disaster's effects. In *Psychosocial Aspects of Disaster*, ed. R. M. Gist and B. Lubin, pp. 308–340. New York: Wiley.

Spielberger, C. D., Gorsuch, R. L., and Lushene, R. E. (1970). *Manual for the State-Trait Anxiety Inventory*. Palo Alto, CA: Consulting Psychologists Press.

Sugar, M. (1989). Children in a disaster: an overview. *Child Psychiatry and Human Development* 19:163–179.

Terr, L. C. (1985). Psychic trauma in children and adolescents. *Psychiatric Clinics of North America* 8:815–835.

_____ (1991). Childhood traumas: an outline and overview. *American Journal of Psychiatry* 148:10–20.

Vernberg, E. M., and Vogel, J. M. (1993). Task force report: Part 2: Interventions with children after disasters. *Journal of Clinical Child Psychology* 22:485–498.

Vogel, J. M., and Vernberg, E. M. (1993). Task force report: Part I: Children's psychological responses to disasters. *Journal of Clinical Child Psychology* 22:464–484.

Wilkenson, C. B., and Vera, E. (1989). Clinical responses to disaster. In *Psychosocial Aspects of Disaster*, eds. R. Gist and B. Lubin, pp. 229–267. New York: Wiley.

Wolfe, V. V., Gentile, C., and Wolfe, D. A. (1989). The impact of sexual abuse on children: a PTSD formulation. *Behavior Therapy* 20:215–228.

Wolfe, V. V., Gentile, C., Michienzi, T., et al. (1991). The Children's Impact of Traumatic Events Scale: a measure of post-sexual-abuse PTSD symptoms. *Behavioral Assessment* 13:359–383.

Wurtele, S. K., Kast, L. C., Miller-Perrin, C. L., and Kondrick, P. A. (1989). Comparison of programs for teaching personal safety skills to preschoolers. *Journal of Consulting and Clinical Psychology* 57:505–511.

Yule, W. (1993). Technology-related disasters. In *Children and Disasters*, ed. C. F. Saylor, pp. 105–122. New York: Plenum.

Yule, W., and Williams, R. M. (1990). Posttraumatic stress reactions in children. *Journal of Traumatic Stress* 3:279–295.

12

SLEEP DISORDERS

Jodi A. Mindell
Laurie Cashman

INTRODUCTION

Children experience a large number of sleep disorders (for a complete review see Mindell 1993). Only a few of these disorders will be reviewed in this chapter. Those will include sleep disorders that do have an anxiety component and those disorders that people often assume have an anxiety component but actually do not. It is important in evaluating and treating sleep problems that this distinction be clearly made and that myths and beliefs about sleep problems as they relate to anxiety are dispelled.

DESCRIPTION OF DISORDERS

Before discussing any of the sleep disorders it is important to just mention the classification system of these disorders, as this terminology will be referred to throughout this chapter. Sleep disorders are basically classified into two major categories, the dyssomnias and the parasomnias, as delineated by the International Classification of Sleep Disorders (ICSD, Diagnostic Classification Steering Committee 1990). The dyssomnias include those disorders that result in difficulty either initiating or maintaining sleep, or involve excessive daytime sleepiness. The parasomnias, on the other hand, are disorders that disrupt sleep after it has been initiated and are disorders of arousal, partial arousal, or sleep stage transitions. They are disorders that intrude into the sleep process but usually do not result in complaints of insomnia or excessive sleepiness. Note that these terms, as they are defined by the ICSD, differ slightly from their use in the American Psychiatric Association's *DSM-IV* (1994). *DSM-IV* defines dyssomnias as those sleep disorders in which the predominant disturbance is in the amount, quality, or timing of sleep and that can produce either insomnia or excessive sleepiness. The parasomnias are described as sleep disorders that involve an abnormal event occurring during sleep and the predominant complaint focuses on the disturbance, not on its impact on sleeping or wakefulness. Both methods of defining these terms, however, result in the same classification of disorders.

For the purposes of this chapter, sleep disorders will be discussed as they pertain to anxiety. As mentioned above, many believe that troubled sleep is a reflection of underlying emotional difficulties, primarily anxiety or stress. However, there is very little evidence for this assumption and little support for the belief that emotional state or presleep cognitions disrupt sleep (Dollinger et al. 1988). Although few sleep problems have a psychopathological basis, the discussion of the specific sleep disorders that follows is organized by those disorders that may have anxiety as a basis, followed by a selection of common sleep disorders seen in children and adolescents that are not related to anxiety.

Sleep Disorders that May Have an Anxiety Component

Adjustment Sleep Disorder

Some sleep disorders are environmentally related. Adjustment sleep disorder is a form of insomnia related to emotional arousal caused by acute stress, conflict, or an environmental change (ICSD 1990). It is often seen in children following a move or before the first day of school. The duration of such a sleep problem is often days.

Hospitalized children often experience an adjustment sleep disorder. Hospitals, and all that goes with being hospitalized, can be a major disrupter of sleep, and children who are hospitalized often develop sleep problems (Beardslee 1976, Prugh et al. 1953, White et al. 1988). Hospitalization also may exacerbate preexisting sleep difficulties (Anders and Weinstein 1972). Hagemann (1981) found that hospitalized children, ages 3 to 8, lose up to 25 percent of their normal sleep time because of difficulties falling asleep and delays in sleep onset. Studies have been done exploring means to reduce sleep difficulties in hospitalized children. Surprisingly, White and her colleagues (1990) found that children were more distressed and had longer latency to sleep onset when parents were present at bedtime or when children listened to a parent-recorded story compared to those children who listened to a stranger-recorded story at bedtime or had no intervention. They suggest that hospitalized children may have more difficulties falling asleep at night when reminders of home are present. These data are in contrast to popular opinion. A survey of 400 psychiatrists found that 44 percent believed that mothers should sleep in a hospitalized child's room whenever possible (Pietropinto 1985). Other suggestions to help hospitalized children sleep include instructing the nursing staff to institute more structured bedtimes for the children and to modify the hospital environment (e.g., dimmed lights, reduced noise, television off) to reduce interferences with sleep. Mild sedatives may also be used for hospitalized children experiencing sleep problems (Besana et al. 1984).

Not only do hospitalized children have difficulties with sleep, but so may children with chronic illnesses or acute medical disturbances (Dinges et al. 1990, Mindell et al. 1990, Miser et al. 1987). For example, children with severe burns often experience nightmares (Noyes et al. 1971, Tarnowski et al. 1987). One study (Roberts and Gordon 1979) successfully treated a 5-year-old child who was having nightmares secondary to burns over 30 percent of her body. Nightmares were eliminated within a two-week period through the use of response prevention and systematic desensitization. Unfortunately, few studies have targeted sleep problems related to other medical conditions and much more needs to be done.

In general, few studies have explored treatments for adjustment sleep disorders, other than those related to hospitalization, since these problems often resolve naturally over time. In some cases, though, often associated with ongoing stressors, this form of sleep disturbance may last as long as several months. If treatment is sought, psychological therapies typically focus on the disrupting events. With resolution of the precipitating event, the sleep problems typically dissipate with sleep returning to normal.

Nighttime Fears

Fear of the dark is common in children and frequently leads to sleep problems. This is a normal, developmental occurrence in young children. Many of these fears are learned through simple conditioning (Hewitt 1981). For example, the bedroom may be a source of anxiety for some children, especially if the bedroom is the place where the child is sent as punishment. Also, if the child has a nightmare or awakens distressed in the middle of the night, a parent typically comes into the room, turning on the light. Thus, a child may associate light with comfort and associate darkness with distress or nightmares.

A number of studies have successfully treated nighttime fears in children using cognitive-behavioral techniques. Several studies have incorporated relaxation training, self-monitoring of nighttime behavior, verbal self-control training, and positive reinforcement to decrease severe nighttime fears (Graziano and Mooney 1980, 1982, Graziano et al. 1979). Ollendick and colleagues (1991) found that reinforcement for engaging in appropriate nighttime behavior and self-control procedures was successful in reducing nighttime fears in two children. In their study, they found that the most important component of treatment was contingent reinforcement. In summary, fear of the dark, which is common in young children, is often a result of associative learning. Although most children will outgrow their fears, in severe cases cognitive-behavioral treatments are effective.

Nightmares

Nightmares occur in about 10–50 percent of all children between the ages of 3 and 6 years (ICSD 1990). Following a gradual onset, nightmares typically decrease in frequency over time. A small percentage of children will continue to have nightmares throughout adolescence, and even possibly into adulthood (ICSD 1990). Nightmares occur during periods of rapid eye movement (REM) sleep, in contrast to sleep terrors, which happen during slow-wave sleep earlier in the night. Table 12-1 delineates the unique characteristics of nightmares versus sleep terrors, which will be discussed later. Nightmares usually involve fears of attack, falling, or death (Kales et al. 1980). Although 50 percent of individuals with recurrent nightmares have no associated psychopathology, in some, especially adults, nightmares are associated with schizotypal personality, borderline personality disorder, and schizophrenia.

Stressful periods and traumatic events will exacerbate the occurrence of nightmares. For example, studies have found that distressing or frightening events such as automobile accidents or death of a relative are associated with increased nightmares (Erman 1987). In contrast, however, one study surpris-

Table 12-1. Characteristic Features of Sleep Terrors/Confusional Arousals and Nightmares

	Sleep Terrors/ Confusional Arousals	Nightmares
Time of night	first 1/3 of night	mid to last 1/3
Behavior	variable	very little motor behavior
Level of consciousness	unarousable or very confused if awakened	fully awake
Memory of event	amnesia	vivid recall
Family history	yes	no
Potential for injury	high	low
Frequency	common	very common
Stage of sleep	deep NREM	REM

ingly found that parents' most common causal attribution for nightmares was overtiredness, with stress not highly rated as a factor (Fisher and Wilson 1987). Others at risk for nightmares are those who have experienced significant physical or emotional distress. In addition, some medications are associated with nightmares. These include some beta blockers and antidepressants. Other medications produce nightmares as withdrawal symptoms including alcohol, barbiturates, and benzodiazepines. All in all, though, we know little about the causes of nightmares in children.

Treatment strategies for nightmares have focused on anxiety reduction techniques such as relaxation and imagery, often combined with other behavioral strategies such as systematic desensitization (Cavior and Deutsch 1975) or response prevention (Roberts and Gordon 1979). One 13-year-old girl was successfully treated for nightmares using reinforcement and anxiety management techniques (Kellerman 1980). Others have used cognitive-behavioral treatments, including dream reorganization (Palace and Johnston 1989). Dream reorganization involves both systematic desensitization with coping self-statements and guided rehearsal of mastery endings to dream content. However, for most families, reassurance that nightmares are part of normal child development is beneficial and all that is necessary, especially to decrease the likelihood that the child will be treated as though psychologically disturbed.

Sleep Bruxism

Sleep bruxism, which involves grinding or clenching the teeth during sleep, occurs in over 50 percent of infants, typically beginning at 10 months of age (ICSD 1990, Kravitz and Boehm 1971). Adult bruxism usually begins during adolescence. Although there is little evidence for an underlying psychological disorder, bruxism often increases during times of stress, for example, the night prior to a major test or during problems with friends (Funch and Gale 1980, Rugh and Solberg 1975). Bruxism may cause dental problems, such as abnormal wear of teeth or periodontal tissue damage, and may also be related to headaches or jaw pain. The research to date on bruxism is primarily with adult populations. Studies have found bruxism to be amenable to EMG-activated biofeedback (e.g., Casas et al. 1982, Kardachi et al. 1978, Kardachi and Clarke 1977, Piccione et al. 1982, Wagner 1981) and stress management approaches (Casas et al. 1982, Hartmann 1989). An excellent review of the use of biofeedback for bruxism in adults is provided by Cassisi and colleagues (1987). Unfortunately, few studies have researched the efficacy of treatment programs for bruxism in children.

Sleep Disorders without an Anxiety Component

Confusional Arousals and Sleep Terrors

Confusional arousals occur almost universally in children before the age of 5 years (Ferber 1985a), and are much less common in older children. Confusional arousals primarily occur in the first part of the night and are characterized by confusion during and following arousals from sleep (ICSD 1990). The child is often disoriented, has slowed speech, and is slow to respond to commands or questions. This confusional behavior may last from several minutes to hours. Typically, treatment is not recommended and children outgrow this sleep problem. Little research has been done in this area.

Sleep terrors occur in about 3–6 percent of all children and are more intense than confusional arousals (Broughton 1968, DiMario and Emery 1987, Soldatos and Lugaresi 1987). Sleep terrors, also known as night terrors or pavor nocturnus, begin suddenly with a piercing scream or cry and the child appears intensely fearful (ICSD 1990). Sleep terrors usually occur within 90–120 minutes of sleep onset and typically during the first period of slow wave sleep. The child is usually extremely agitated, often unresponsive to attempts at soothing, and may even become more agitated if held. If awakened, the child may be confused and disoriented.

Although sleep terrors and confusional arousals appear to be anxiety based, they are not. Parents often are worried that daytime concerns or worries are being manifested at night in the form of sleep terrors. This is not true. Sleep terrors are a developmental phenomenon, most common in children ages 4 to 12, and tend to resolve by adolescence (Kales et al. 1979, Kales et al. 1977). Night terrors have a genetic component, in that there is usually a family history (Kales, Soldatos, and Kales 1980) and they are considered a disorder of impaired arousal (Broughton 1968). One study that conducted a factor analysis on a multitude of sleep problems found that those items associated with night terrors were not in any way related to items associated with anxiety (Fisher and McGuire 1990). Unfortunately, many individuals unwittingly assume that night terrors are a form of child anxiety, which continues to perpetuate the myth (e.g., Auchter 1990, Taboada 1975).

As with many sleep disorders, little is known about treating these problems. Two case studies successfully utilizing behavioral methods have been reported in the literature (Kellerman 1979, 1980). Hypnosis also has been utilized as a treatment for night terrors (Koe 1989, Kramer 1989). Sometimes, pharmacological treatments have been successful. Studies have found diazepam (Valium) to be effective (Fisher et al. 1973, Glick et al. 1971), but relapse may occur when the drug is stopped. Other studies have reported successful treatment with a short-acting benzodiazepine, midazolam (Popo-viciu and Corfariu 1983), with alprazolam, a triazolobenzodiazepine (Cameron and Thyer 1985), and even low doses of a tricyclic antidepressant (Reite et al. 1990). The use of medications to treat sleep terrors is controversial, with some individuals (e.g., Weissbluth 1984) arguing strongly against their use. Other treatments have also been attempted. Agrell and Axelsson (1972) significantly reduced sleep terrors following adenoidectomy in a group of twenty-three children. Unfortunately, no further studies have replicated the benefits of adenoidectomy for children with sleep terrors.

Recently, studies have begun to look at the treatment of sleep terrors and confusional arousals with scheduled awakenings (Lask 1988). Scheduled awakenings involve the behavioral alteration of the child's sleep patterns. For example, in one case a 7-year-old boy experienced, on average, three to four sleep terrors per week for approximately four years. Following a two-week regimen of scheduled awakenings, no future sleep terrors occurred. It is unclear what exactly is the mechanism of change. It may be that scheduled awakenings give an individual practice in changing sleep stages, as parasomnias occur during sleep stage transitions. Or, it may be that scheduled awakenings simply interrupt sleep at the time of the night at which a parasomnia is likely to occur. However, no matter what the mechanism of change is, scheduled awakenings appear to be effective. The efficacy of this intervention is being further studied.

Sleepwalking

Another parasomnia common in children is sleepwalking. Chronic sleepwalking is experienced by approximately 1–6 percent of children, with as many as 15 percent of all children having at least one such episode (Anders 1982, Broughton 1968, ICSD 1990, Soldatos and Lugaresi 1987). When sleepwalking, the child is often difficult to awaken, and upon awakening appears confused. Sleepwalking is most prevalent in children between the ages of 4 and 8 years and usually disappears spontaneously after adolescence. The frequency of the behavior can vary from infrequently to several times a week. Sleepwalking can be exacerbated or induced by fever, sleep deprivation, environmental noises, and some medications, such as lithium, prolixin, and desipramine (Klackenberg 1982). Little is known about treatment for sleepwalking in children. Typically, parents are told to safety-proof the house; for example, to make sure all doors leading outside the house are locked and upstairs windows are secure. Otherwise, parents are reassured about their child's sleepwalking and informed that sleepwalking is usually a benign, self-limited maturational occurrence (Berlin and Qayyum 1986).

Rhythmic Movement Disorder

Many children fall asleep while rocking their body, rolling back and forth, or banging their head. Rhythmic movement disorder is characterized by stereotyped movements that occur at sleep onset or when awakening from sleep (ICSD 1990). Body rocking, head rolling, or head banging are very common in infants, with 60 percent of 9-month-olds doing one of these behaviors. Until 2 years of age, 22 percent of children continue to engage in one of these behaviors, and they are seen in approximately 5 percent of children after 2 years. Injuries are uncommon and typically treatment is not instituted, as this behavior is usually benign and self-limiting and thus dissipates on its own. These behaviors, again, are not a sign of anxiety or emotional disturbance; rather they have a neurophysiological basis (Horne 1992). The only major concern about this sleep disorder is that it can be disruptive to the family and can have psychosocial consequences in older children and adolescents.

Delayed Sleep Phase Disorder

A common event that occurs especially with adolescents is staying up late at night. Some adolescents completely shift their sleep-wake schedule. The end result is that they may have symptoms of sleep-onset insomnia and extreme difficulty awakening at a desired time in the morning (ICSD 1990). Many adolescents do not go to sleep until the early morning hours and are unable to awaken on weekdays for school. On weekends, the adolescents have no problems sleeping but do so on a delayed phase, often going to sleep at 2:00 AM and awakening anywhere from noon to 2:00 PM. These individuals have little success trying to advance their timing of sleep onset to a more appropriate schedule. Approximately 7 percent of adolescents are sleep phase delayed (Thorpy et al. 1988). The end result for many children and adolescents with this sleep disorder is difficulties in school, primarily because of chronic absenteeism and tardiness (Carskadon et al. 1988).

The primary mode of treatment for this disorder is chronotherapy (Czeisler et al. 1981). The first step in this program is stabilizing sleep at the phase delayed times, for example 3:00 AM to noon. For the next week to ten days, the sleeping period is delayed by three hours every day until the desired sleeping times occur. For example, on night 1 sleep is to occur from 6:00 AM to 3:00 PM and on night 2 from 9:00 AM until 6:00 PM. The imposed scheduling of sleep must be strictly followed for treatment to be effective. Once sleep is occurring at the appropriate times, the new schedule must be rigidly adhered to, given that it is easy for these individuals to return to a delayed sleep phase pattern. Some adolescents will be resistant to treatment. In those cases, psychological issues will need to be addressed.

Obstructive Sleep Apnea and Narcolepsy

No chapter on sleep disorders can be written without at least a mention of the two major sleep disorders, sleep apnea and narcolepsy. Obstructive sleep apnea is a breathing disorder that involves repetitive episodes of upper airway obstruction during sleep, often causing a reduction in blood oxygen saturation (Guilleminault et al. 1981, ICSD 1990). These apneic episodes cause frequent arousals and brief awakenings throughout the night. Most individuals with apnea are unaware of these occurrences. In comparison with adults, in which apneic episodes are often associated with snoring and are easy to identify, diagnosis in children is more difficult (Brouilette et al. 1982). Children with this disorder may be excessively sleepy during the day. During sleep, these children may snore or have agitated arousals. The mean age at diagnosis for children with sleep apnea is 7 years (Mauer et al. 1983), and it is more common in boys (Guilleminault and Anders 1976). Children who are morbidly obese (greater than 150 percent ideal body weight) are also at increased risk for sleep apnea (Mallory et al. 1989). In children with sleep apnea, the most common form of treatment involves surgery to remove the airway obstructions (e.g., Guilleminault and Dement 1988). Tonsillectomy and/or adenoidectomy relieves symptoms in about 70 percent of all child cases. Other treatments are also recommended, including weight loss (Roth et al. 1988) and nasal continuous positive airway pressure (CPAP, Guilleminault et al. 1985).

Narcolepsy is characterized by excessive sleepiness, often presenting itself as repeated episodes of naps or lapses into sleep of short duration throughout the day (Guilleminault 1986, ICSD 1990, Mitler et al. 1987). Another common symptom that is unique to narcolepsy is cataplexy, which involves the sudden loss of bilateral muscle tone following the occurrence of strong emotions (e.g., laughter, elation, anger). This loss of muscle tone can be as minor as a mild sensation of weakness involving facial sagging or slurred speech, or can be as severe as complete postural collapse. Cataplexy typically lasts from a few seconds to several minutes, with complete and immediate recovery. Narcolepsy occurs in a very small portion of the population, approximately 0.03–0.16 percent, with onset typically not occurring until adolescence. This disorder is rarely diagnosed in preteenaged children. There is no known cure for narcolepsy, so treatment focuses on the management of this disorder, typically with medications such as tricyclic antidepressants and

CNS stimulants, such as pemoline, methylphenidate, or dextroamphetamine (Wittig et al. 1983).

DIFFERENTIAL DIAGNOSIS

Often the presenting complaints for the above sleep disorders are similar, for example, insomnia, excessive daytime sleepiness, or unusual behaviors during the night. It is important to conduct a thorough evaluation to fully assess which specific sleep disorder the child is experiencing. Thus, differential diagnosis in the area of sleep disorders is essential.

Differentiation between a sleep disorder and other medical or psychological problems is also important. A child with what looks like night terrors may actually be having seizures during sleep. In other cases, difficulties at bedtime may be symptomatic of a more general problem with noncompliance. Nighttime fears may be just one aspect of a child with extensive fears.

Furthermore, delayed sleep phase syndrome should always be assessed before a diagnosis of school refusal is made. Some of the effects of sleep phase disorder, which results from interference with one's circadian rhythm, are evident in children and adolescents given a diagnosis of school refusal (for a complete discussion of school refusal see Chapter 2). Children and adolescents with delayed sleep phase syndrome are often irritable and moody during the daytime. In addition, sufferers of this sleep disturbance may appear anxious or even neurotic, especially after several months of the disorder (Horne 1992). These symptoms of sleep phase disorder may also be present in school refusal behavior, whether it is a result of separation anxiety, school phobia, social withdrawal, or depression (Burke and Silverman 1987). Given the similar characteristics of each disorder, it appears likely that sleep phase disorder may sometimes present as school refusal, especially among adolescents who constitute the majority of individuals with delayed sleep phase syndrome. A differential diagnosis of delayed sleep syndrome should be ruled out by evaluating the presence of delayed sleep onset and the presence of excessive daytime sleepiness.

ASSESSMENT PROCEDURES

A thorough evaluation of sleep disorders involves a number of steps. The first step is the completion of a sleep history. All aspects of the sleep-wake cycle need to be reviewed. Areas that need to be addressed include evening activities such as television watching, medications, intake of caffeinated beverages, bedtime, and bedtime routines. During the night, areas to be evaluated include latency to sleep onset, behaviors during the night, and the number and duration of nighttime awakenings. In the morning, the time of awakening, sleepiness, and initial behaviors upon arising should be evaluated. During the day, sleepiness, naps, meals, caffeine intake, medications, and feelings of anxiety and depression should be reviewed. Details about abnormal events such as night terrors, confusional arousals, respiratory disturbances, seizures, and enuresis should be collected. Medication intake should also be reviewed, as many medications can affect sleep. A review of psychological symptoms during the day is also important. Symptoms of anxiety and depression can be the result of lack of sleep. For example, feelings of fatigue, irritability, and sluggishness may simply be the result of sleep deprivation.

The second step in the evaluation of sleep problems is the keeping of sleep diaries. A typical sleep diary includes information on the time to bed, sleep latency, number and duration of nighttime awakenings, time of arising in the morning, total sleep time, and duration and time of naps. For the most useful information, two weeks of baseline sleep diaries should be kept. This way sleep patterns can clearly be evaluated.

In cases in which there is a concern about an underlying physiological problem, polysomnography (PSG) is an essential component of assessment. Even in some cases in which the client does not report any physiological symptoms it may be important to completely evaluate the person's sleep. Many clients are unaware of snore arousals or sleep apnea that may be interrupting their sleep and resulting in complaints of insomnia and daytime sleepiness. Polysomnography typically consists of an overnight sleep study in which recordings of oxygen saturation, nasal and oral airflow, thoracic and abdominal respiratory movements, limb muscle activity, and electroencephalogram (EEG) are taken. As an adjunct to a PSG, a multiple sleep latency test (MSLT) is often conducted. This test, which is performed in two-hour intervals throughout the day following the overnight study, evaluates the client's level of daytime sleepiness. The MSLT consists of four twenty-minute nap opportunities given at two-hour intervals. Measures of sleep latency are taken. If sleep occurs, the nap is terminated fifteen minutes after sleep onset.

Most PSGs and MSLTs are conducted at accredited sleep disorders centers. A typical patient seen at a sleep disorders center will undergo an initial evaluation that will include medical and sleep history and a physical examination. Following the initial evaluation a decision will be made as to whether polysomnographic testing is warranted. If so, the testing is scheduled for a later date and the patient will spend the night at the center. In the cases of children or adolescents, a parent or other adult is usually allowed to stay with the client. Following the collection of all information, a diagnosis is reached and a treatment plan would ensue. Often the sleep disorders center staff will send all information to the referring agent or, if appropriate, will institute treatment.

Another important aspect of assessment with sleep disorders that are related to anxiety is a thorough evaluation of other anxiety disorders (see additional chapters for a complete review). In relation to sleep problems, an evaluation for panic disorder is important, as some adolescents do experience nocturnal panic attacks. These panic attacks are more often seen in adults with a concomitant diagnosis of panic disorder, but it is worth evaluating. Nocturnal panic attack symptoms are typically similar to daytime symptomatology and rarely occur without the presence of daytime panic attacks.

Other life events that may be related to acute sleep problems are significant life stressors. Failure in school, death in the family, or a recent move can all contribute significantly to a sleep problem that resembles insomnia. A thorough evaluation should include questioning about school performance, social functioning, and family functioning. A recent change in a family's financial status can result in sleeping problems in children even if the parents do not believe that the child is aware of such problems. Often children, and especially adolescents, are much more aware of tensions in a family than parents are aware. Thus, it is important that a thorough evaluation of all aspects of sleep and daytime functioning be conducted.

ESTABLISHING TREATMENT GOALS

After a diagnosis is made, the treatability of the disorder must be established. As mentioned previously, some sleep disorders are not amenable to treatment. If the sleep difficulty is treatable, then the goal of treatment is to reduce the incidence or severity of the problem. However, if the presenting problem is not curable—for example, if it is developmentally based—then treatment should aim at prevention and coping with the problem.

The treatment of sleep disorders varies widely according to the particular diagnosis and unique individual and family influences, but some commonalities are evident. Education is an important component of treatment and should include an explanation and discussion of etiological factors, prevalence, defining characteristics, prognosis, and common treatments. The development and implementation of an individualized treatment strategy, with proper consideration of its effect on and receptivity by the family, is the next step. Interventions may focus on sleep hygiene, scheduled awakenings, or bright light therapy. Evaluation at specified time intervals is recommended to assess the efficacy of the prescribed treatment. These evaluations should also identify possible noncompliance issues. Finally, alternative treatments may be required, which may require further assessment and/or consultation with professionals in related disciplines.

ROLE OF THE THERAPIST

A therapist has multiple roles in cases of sleep disorders. First, therapists often have to evaluate for physiological aspects that may contribute to sleep disorders. A therapist must have a thorough grounding in sleep medicine before attempting to evaluate and treat children with sleep problems. Therapists must also be cognizant of when to refer for specialized services. It is often important to seek a complete sleep assessment, including an overnight polysomnogram and multiple sleep latency test. Most hospitals in major cities have an accredited sleep disorders center. You can also call the American Sleep Disorders Association at (507) 287-6006 to find the nearest sleep disorders center. Contact with a physician, especially one with knowledge about sleep and sleep disorders, may also be necessary. Often a complete medical examination is a key component to your evaluation and if medications are warranted a physician will be necessary.

Usually, the most important role that a therapist in sleep disorders undertakes is that of educator and reassurer. Parents will often look to you as their source of facts. Very often education about sleep problems is the essential component of treatment. Usually this education brings with it reassurance that what the child is experiencing is normal and benign. Many parents have lived with this problem for years and often have not told anyone about it. Hearing that other children or adolescents have similar experiences is often crucial to treatment. In addition, it is important to dispel myths about sleep that many individuals believe. It is often assumed that adolescents need less sleep than adults (not true; they actually need more sleep than adults) or that snoring is normal and means that the person is experiencing "good, deep sleep" (also not true, and in some cases snoring may be a sign of a more serious problem such as sleep apnea).

In other situations, such as with prolonged adjustment sleep disorder or nighttime fears, the therapist may need to institute treatment. Treatment may include, in these cases, cognitive-behavioral techniques such as verbal self-control, positive reinforcement, relaxation, and guided imagery. In other cases, the institution of a strict sleep schedule is crucial. Given that there are a multitude of sleep disorders, it is difficult to provide information on each specified treatment. However, someone who is treating sleep disorders in children and adolescents needs to be familiar with the different disorders and treatment modalities.

TREATMENT STRATEGIES

The treatment strategies delineated in each case will depend upon the specific sleep problem that is diagnosed. This section will discuss each sleep disorder discussed above that is possibly related to anxiety and provide recommendations on treatment strategies.

For children with an adjustment sleep disorder, the problem typically resolves with time. Once the stressor dissipates or the child acclimates to the environmental change, normal sleep usually resumes. If sleep problems persist, treatment usually should first focus on the disrupting events. For example, if sleep becomes disturbed following a death in the family, treatment would focus on issues related to the death. Once this problem is resolved, any sleep disturbances should also resolve. If the sleep problem does not improve significantly, treatment may need to focus on the new sleep issues, such as reestablishing previous sleep habits or education about proper sleep hygiene.

Nighttime fears are extremely common in young children, especially fear of the dark. In these instances, parents should reassure the child but set limits on their and their child's behavior so that the behavior does not become reinforced. For example, checking closets and leaving a low nightlight on is reasonable, but starting to sleep with the child every night is not. For persistent fears, a combination of cognitive-behavioral therapies is successful. A treatment package combining relaxation training, self-monitoring of nighttime behavior, and positive reinforcement is recommended.

Persistent nightmares, similar to adjustment sleep disorders, may be the result of an environmental stressor. In these cases, as discussed above, treatment should focus on the stressful events. For children for whom there is no identifiable precipitating event, efforts should be made to try to identify other factors that are exacerbating the occurrence of nightmares such as medications or sleep deprivation. In other cases, anxiety management strategies such as relaxation training and positive imagery can be successful. It is important to remember, however, that nightmares are common. Therefore, for many families reassurance that nightmares are a part of normal child development is all that is necessary.

Sleep bruxism can also be the result of stress. For these cases, like other sleep disorders associated with anxiety, stress management strategies can be effective. In severe cases, and in those cases in which there are already resulting dental problems, referral to a dentist or orthodontist for a night-guard is appropriate.

In addition to any sleep disorders present, many children have other problems that need to be recognized. Some children who are referred for a sleep problem have other difficulties including learning disabilities, attention deficit–hyperactivity disorder, family difficulties, and school problems. If you are a therapist who specializes in sleep disorders, you may choose to refer families for the appropriate specialized services. Otherwise, it is important in seeing a child or adolescent to conduct a thorough psychological evaluation and then prioritize your client's needs. In cases of bedtime struggles, it may be that the family has a more general problem with noncompliance that is affecting all aspects of the child's behavior, not just bedtime behavior. In other cases, family therapy may be the most appropriate treatment choice.

Another issue pertaining to childhood sleep disorders is that most clients are seen on a short-term basis. Contact with a child or adolescent may consist solely of one or two sessions with follow-up appointments made as necessary. Often a child is sent for an evaluation and all conclusions and treatment suggestions made are simply reported back to the referring agent. In other cases, treatment may be prolonged and evolve over a longer period of time, although rarely longer than months except in cases of sleep apnea or narcolepsy. However, even in these longer term cases, treatment is typically focused and goal-directed, oriented about sleep issues.

DEALING WITH COMMON OBSTACLES TO SUCCESSFUL TREATMENT

The most common obstacle to the treatment of sleep disorders in children and adolescents is that often there is no effective treatment. You can't get rid of some sleep disorders! Infrequent sleepwalking, sleeptalking, or night terrors are typically not treatable, nor should there be any need to treat these problems. These common parasomnias are often benign disorders that may dissipate with time or may continue throughout a lifetime. What is important in terms of these disorders, as discussed above, is simple reassurance and preventative methods. In some cases, prevention is the best treatment. Many sleep disorders are exacerbated by sleep deprivation. Sleep problems may also become worse with the use of alcohol and with other drug use. It is important to talk to parents and children about these possibilities and work with them to establish good sleep habits.

Another obstacle to treatment is that in some cases the child or adolescent is resistant to change. This resistance occurs especially with adolescents, whether they have delayed sleep phase disorder or other sleep disorders. Adolescents are often dealing with issues of individuation and independence. One area in which they are trying to achieve independence is with their sleep patterns. Often, a parent telling a teenager to go to bed at a specific time may backfire and the adolescent will simply stay up longer out of sheer will.

And, last, parents may also be invested in some children's sleep problems. At times a child's sleep problem may be beneficial to the parent. A parent who is required to sleep with his/her child during the night or whose child sleeps in the parents' bed may be avoiding marital problems or sexual difficulties. Often, there is resistance to changing these bad habits. In these cases, discussion of these issues would be appropriate, and individual or family therapy may be warranted.

RELAPSE PREVENTION

As mentioned previously, an important aspect of treatment of sleep disorders is the identification of factors that are likely to precipitate sleep difficulties, such as sleep deprivation and life stressors. It is essential that children, adolescents, and adults alike get enough sleep every night. In adolescents and adults, this requirement is eight hours a night. In children, it varies according to age. There are a number of publications available that provide information on the amount of sleep required by children at varying ages (e.g., Ferber 1985b). Other life events and stressors may also cause sleep problems to recur. Illness, death in the family, and moving may all lead to an increase in sleep problems. The period of time right before returning to school in the fall or prior to a stressful exam period also may cause sleep disturbances in some children and adolescents. Other things that can lead to a return of sleep problems are a change in where the person sleeps, for example at a friend's house or on a camping trip. With such a change, sleep disorders such as sleep terrors, sleepwalking, and sleeptalking are likely to occur. Thus, parents and children need to be informed about these potential problem areas so attempts at prevention can be made and so that the family knows that this is likely to be a temporary problem.

One of the toughest sleep problems to treat, and one that is likely to relapse, is delayed sleep phase disorder. The child or adolescent who becomes sleep phase delayed in the first place is likely to be an "owl." An owl, in comparison to a "lark," is someone who has a tendency to be an evening person. Larks, on the other hand, are morning types. Owls are likely to have an ongoing battle with the tendency to phase delay sleep. Their inclination is to go to bed late at night, or early in the morning hours, and sleep later in the day. People with this tendency who need to wake early in the morning, as children and adolescents do to attend school, will always need to be diligent about maintaining a regular sleep schedule and resist the urge to stay up late at night, especially on weekends.

TERMINATION

In cases of sleep disorders, treatment goals are typically well defined and termination occurs either when the sleep problem has resolved or when the question has been answered. Often sleep problems in children are treated in sleep disorders centers that utilize a medical model. That is, a client comes to the clinic with a specific complaint, requesting an evaluation and possible treatment. An evaluation is completed and a treatment plan is developed. Most times, treatment is conducted by the clinician at the center. However, in some cases the best treatment may be surgery, in which case the client is referred to the proper surgeon. In other cases, sleep is not the primary issue but it is more of a problem with compliance or anxiety. In these instances, the client and clinician work together to decide who is the most appropriate treatment agent, whether it be the staff at the sleep disorders center or another therapist who may be more accessible or appropriate. Across the board, though, therapy is focused and goal oriented, and thus termination occurs naturalistically. In some cases, though, the problem is ongoing, and follow-up appointments will need to be scheduled on an annual or semi-annual basis.

CASE ILLUSTRATION (TYPICAL TREATMENT)

Description and History

Melissa, a 9-year-old girl, was referred to the Sleep Disorders Center because she was sleepwalking, sleeptalking, and sitting up in bed asleep. Between the ages of 2 and 3 and again at age 6, Melissa had several episodes of sleepwalking. In the three months prior to her visit, Melissa had several more episodes. One episode was on a school trip when her teachers reported prolonged sleeptalking and sleepwalking. The first night of the trip Melissa also had a slight fever. Since her school trip, Melissa had three more events involving sleepwalking and sleeptalking. Melissa had no recollection of any of the episodes and did not remember any nighttime awakenings. Rather, she denied that these events occurred.

Melissa generally went to bed between 8:30 and 9:00 P.M., took fifteen to sixty minutes to fall asleep, and got up at 7:00 A.M. on school days, but usually slept later on weekends. Melissa always had to be awakened on school days. Melissa stated that she often worried about things prior to falling asleep and believed that she worries more than most girls her age. As an infant and young child she had a habit of rocking back and forth on her hands and knees while falling asleep. Later, and until age 5, she sucked on a blanket while falling asleep.

Melissa's physical examination was normal. She lived with her parents and fraternal twin sister. Melissa was doing well in school, but she had some increased stress recently because she had just started a new school. In addition, Melissa's mother reported that Melissa was often "spacey" at home and at school, and was "easily distracted." Melissa stated that these episodes were related to daydreaming and being bored.

Synopsis of Therapy Sessions

Our initial impressions were that Melissa was experiencing parasomnias including sleepwalking and sleeptalking. Because of the recent significant increase in frequency and severity of these behaviors and her history of daytime distractibility, the possibility of an underlying sleep disrupter or seizure disorder needed to be explored. Thus, an all-night polysomnogram was conducted. The results of the polysomnogram were consistent with normal sleep except for sudden arousals and behavior consistent with parasomnias. (It is difficult for individuals to sleepwalk during a PSG because of the electrodes.) She did not have any other other sleep disrupters and her EEG was normal.

During the follow-up session, the above results were discussed with Melissa and her mother. Since the initial intake, Melissa had not experienced any further episodes of sleepwalking or sleeptalking, at least as observed by her parents. The nature of parasomnias was discussed, including that this is a benign disorder that does not denote psychological difficulties. It was recommended that Melissa maintain a very regular sleep schedule and avoid sleep deprivation. In addition, home safety precautions should be taken. Her mother was asked to continue to observe Melissa's sleep behaviors and contact us in one month to report on her nighttime behaviors. In addition, if at any time in the future Melissa had a dramatic increase in her incidents of sleepwalking and sleeptalking, she was to return for additional evaluation and treatment.

Comments

The above case illustrates the importance of a thorough evaluation for all underlying physiological causes of sleep problems. In addition, the importance of understanding the nature of sleepwalking and sleeptalking and being able to convey this information to the family was essential. In this case, no treatment was warranted, although preventative techniques were discussed.

CASE ILLUSTRATION (OVERCOMING OBSTACLES)

Description and History

Raji, a 14-year-old boy, had a long-term history of anxiety at bedtime, nightmares, frequent nighttime awakenings, delayed sleep phase syndrome, and daytime sleepiness. On weekdays, Raji generally went to bed at 1:00 A.M., took up to a half hour to fall asleep, and woke at 7:00 A.M. On weekends and during the summer, Raji went to bed anytime between 2:00 and 4:00 A.M. and would rise between noon and 2:00 P.M. From the time he was young, Raji required one of his parents to be present at bedtime until he fell asleep because of his extensive fears. His fears were primarily of someone robbing the house, spiders, and noises. On weekends, when Raji went to sleep much later than his parents and thus they could not stay with him, he would leave all the lights on and have the television playing. He also locked all the doors and windows to his room and made sure his shutters were shut, whether his parents were present or not. He described having anxious thoughts and a racing pulse when trying to fall asleep. Once asleep, Raji would awaken several times during the night, typically because of bad dreams. After a bad dream he would usually go and awaken one of his parents to stay with him.

One area that became clear from his sleep history was that Raji had snored since he was a young child. He snored every night and throughout the night. He had never awakened himself with a snore but had infrequently awakened gasping and had been observed to have breathing pauses while he slept. In addition, Raji often had a morning headache. Last, Raji reported that he was often sleepy during the day. He had a history of falling asleep at school, but said this was only when he "chose to."

In terms of his personal history, Raji lived with his parents and 15-year-old sister. He was in the tenth grade with below-average performance in school, although he scored very high on standardized tests. It became clear throughout the interview that there was a tremendous amount of tension in the household with a great deal of arguing between Raji and his parents. Raji was extremely belligerent toward his parents and rebellious. He constantly talked back to his parents, especially his father. Raji's parents were extremely concerned about his behavior at home and at school.

On physical exam, it was clear that Raji was slightly overweight at 168 pounds and 5 feet, 6 inches. In addition, he had enlarged tonsils and a shallow hypopharynx. We decided to have Raji undergo a polysomnogram (PSG) and multiple sleep latency test (MSLT), given his history of snoring and breathing pauses that were suggestive of sleep apnea. Furthermore, Raji's schedule and mild daytime sleepiness were consistent with sleep deprivation, that is, inadequate total nighttime sleep. Thus, he was put on a strict sleep schedule with a bedtime of 10:30 P.M. and a wake time of 7:30 A.M.

Synopsis of Therapy Sessions

All physiological sleep disorders need to be assessed and treated first, as they may be the underlying cause of his problems with anxiety. Raji's PSG results were significant for loud snoring. He also had approximately 100 snore arousals during the night, meaning that 100 times he was awakened by his own snoring. In addition, Raji had a number of apneic events, on average four times per hour. The results of the PSG were clearly consistent with a breathing disorder that would significantly contribute to Raji's difficulties falling asleep at night, his nighttime awakenings, and his daytime sleepiness. His breathing disorder clearly was causing disruption of his sleep. This problem, in addition to his erratic sleep schedule, was likely to account for many of his sleep problems.

A number of recommendations were made to Raji and his parents at the next visit. First, it was recommended that Raji be evaluated by an ear/nose/throat specialist for a tonsillectomy and adenoidectomy for his significant snore-related arousals and his mild sleep apnea. Raji was quite resistant to the idea of surgery and insisted that the only way he would consider it is if it was scheduled when school was in session rather than during a holiday. Second, it was suggested that Raji maintain a strict sleep schedule as outlined above. Given that Raji was resistant to suggestions made by his parents, it was recommended that Raji take responsibility for his sleep schedule and that his parents were not to interfere, until at least several weeks after he had surgery. Raji appeared to take this suggestion seriously and stated that he would be compliant with the imposed sleep schedule. In addition, he was pleased that his parents would not interfere. Third, a recommendation was made for family therapy, as there was a great deal of tension in the household and the family had difficulty communicating. Raji was clearly going through a rebellious time and his parents were having difficulty managing him. In the meantime, Raji was asked to maintain a sleep log and an appointment was made for six weeks later, enough time for surgery and recovery to take place.

Raji returned for a follow-up session approximately nine weeks later, after several cancelled appointments. Raji did undergo surgery, but only an adenoidectomy was done. It is unclear why the surgeon decided not to do a tonsillectomy, which was clearly warranted in this case. Raji and his parents stated that Raji's snoring was much better, although he continued to experience mild snoring. Raji reported that the surgery was the "worst experience of his life" and he was never returning to the ENT specialist. Raji was still sleepy during the day, but his sleep schedule had not continued to improve. He was now going to bed during the week at 12:30 A.M. and maintaining his late-night weekend schedule. He was insistent that he did not want to miss specific shows on late-night television and there was no reason to get up at a reasonable hour on weekends because there was nothing to do and no good morning television programs. Given that Raji continued to snore and maintain a poor sleep schedule, it was difficult to ascertain what was accounting for his daytime sleepiness. To evaluate whether Raji still had a breathing disorder and a return for a tonsillectomy was warranted, a repeat polysomnogram was recommended. Until the issue of a breathing disorder was resolved, we could not begin to treat his anxiety problems, as much of it might resolve with treatment of the former. At this point, Raji became belligerent not only to his parents but also to the therapist, insisting that he was never returning for an overnight study, nor was he willing to undergo surgery again. Further-more, he was not willing to continue to work on his sleep schedule. As Raji's parents were not able to insist on Raji undergoing further testing, therapy came to a standstill. Strong recommendations were made for the family to seek family therapy, but his parents did not seem willing to pursue it given Raji's resistance to this idea, also.

Comments

The above case illustrates the difficulties in differentiating physiological bases for sleep problems and an anxiety disorder. The necessity of pursuing sleep assessment was instrumental in this case, as at least a major part of this client's problem was related to an underlying breathing disorder that needed to be treated. Furthermore, the above case delineates the difficulties often found when treating adolescents and when family issues are involved.

SUMMARY

Sleep disorders are a common problem found in children and adolescents. Sometimes these sleep disorders are anxiety related, but often they just appear to be so. Many people believe that, because a child looks anxious, especially during night terrors or following a nightmare, the primary contrib-uting factor for the sleep problem is psychological. In most cases, however, sleep problems are not the result of underlying psychopathology but are physiologically or behaviorally based.

In sum, given the prevalence of these problems in the child and adolescent population, it is important for all therapists to become knowledge-able about sleep and sleep disorders. This information is essential whether or not the therapist is going to treat the client directly or is going to refer for specialized services. We all spend about one-third of our lives sleeping, or trying to sleep; thus, we should understand as much as we can about it.

REFERENCES

Agrell, I. G., and Axelsson, A. (1972). The relationship between pavor nocturnus and adenoids. *Acta Paedopsychiatrica* 39:46–53.

Anders, T. F. (1982). Neurophysiological studies of sleep in infants and children. *Journal of Child Psychology and Psychiatry and Allied Disciplines* 23:75–83.

Anders, T. F., and Weinstein, P. (1972). Sleep and its disorders in infants and children: a review. *Journal of Pediatrics* 22:137–150.

Auchter, U. (1990). Anxiety in children: an investigation on various forms of anxiety. *Acta Paedopsychiatrica* 53:78–88.

Beardslee, C. (1976). The sleep wakefulness pattern of young hospitalized children during nap time. *Maternal-Child Nursing Journal* 5:15–24.

Berlin, R. M., and Qayyum, U. (1986). Sleepwalking: diagnosis and treatment through the life cycle. *Psychosomatics* 27:755–781.

Besana, R., Fiocchi, A., de Bartolomeis, L., et al. (1984). Comparison of niaprazine and placebo in pediatric behaviour and sleep disorders: double-blind clinical trial. *Current Therapeutic Research* 36:58–66.

Broughton, R. J. (1968). Sleep disorders: disorders of arousal? *Science* 159:1070–1078.

Brouillette, R. T., Fernback, S. K., and Hunt, C. E. (1982). Obstructive sleep apnea in infants and children. *Journal of Pediatrics* 100:31–40.

Burke, A. E., and Silverman, W. K. (1987). The prescriptive treatment of school refusal. *Clinical Psychology Review* 7:353–362.

Cameron, O. G., and Thyer, B. A. (1985). Treatment of pavor nocturnus with alprazolam. *Journal of Clinical Psychiatry* 46:504.

Carskadon, M. A., Anders, T. F., and Hole, W. (1988). Sleep disturbances in childhood and adolescence. In *Theory and Research in Behavioral Pediatrics*, vol. 4, ed. H. E. Fitzgerald, B. M. Lester, and M. W. Yogman. New York: Plenum.

Casas, J. M., Beemsterboer, P., and Clark, G. T. (1982). A comparison of stress-reduction, behavioral counseling and contingent EMG biofeedback with an arousal task. *Behaviour Research and Therapy* 20:9–15.

Cassisi, J. E., McGlynn, F. D., and Belles, D. R. (1987). EMG-activated feedback alarms for the treatment of nocturnal bruxism: current status and future directions. *Biofeedback and Self-Regulation* 12:13–30.

Cavior, N., and Deutsch, A. (1975). Systematic desensitization to reduce dream induced anxiety. *Journal of Nervous and Mental Disease* 161:433–435.

Czeisler, C. A., Richardson, G. S., Coleman, R. M., et al. (1981). Chronotherapy: resetting the circadian clocks of patients with the delayed sleep phase syndrome. *Sleep* 4:1–21.

Diagnostic and Statistical Manual of Mental Disorders (1994). 4th ed. Washington, DC: American Psychiatric Association.

Diagnostic Classification Steering Committee. (1990). *The International Classification of Sleep Disorders: Diagnostic and Coding Manual.* Rochester, MN: American Sleep Disorder Association.

DiMario, F. J., and Emery, E. S. (1987). The natural history of night terrors. *Clinical Pediatrics* 26:505–511.

Dinges, D. F., Shapiro, B. S., Reilly, L. B., et al. (1990). Sleep/wake dysfunction in children with sickle-cell crisis pain. *Sleep Research* 19:323.

Dollinger, S. J., Horn, J. L., and Boarini, D. (1988). Disturbed sleep and worries among learning disabled adolescents. *American Journal of Orthopsychiatry* 58:428–434.

Erman, M. K. (1987). Dream anxiety attacks (nightmares). *Psychiatric Clinics of North America* 10:667–674.

Ferber, R. (1985a). Sleep disorders in infants and children. In *Clinical Aspects of Sleep and Sleep Disturbance*, ed. T. L. Riley, pp. 113–157. Boston: Butterworth.

Ferber, R. (1985b). *Solve Your Child's Sleep Problems.* New York: Simon & Schuster.

Fisher, B., and McGuire, K. (1990). Do diagnostic patterns exist in the sleep behaviors of normal children? *Journal of Abnormal Child Psychology* 18:179–186.

Fisher, B., and Wilson, A. (1987). Selected sleep disturbances in school children reported by parents: prevalence, interrelationships, behavioral correlates, and parental attributions. *Perceptual and Motor Skills* 64:1147–1157.

Fisher, C., Kahn, E., Edwards, A., and Davis, D. M. (1973). A psychophysiological study of nightmares and night terrors: the suppression of stage 4 night terrors with diazepam. *Archives of General Psychiatry* 28:252–259.

Funch, D. P., and Gale, E. N. (1980). Factors associated with nocturnal bruxism and its treatment. *Journal of Behavioral Medicine* 3:385–397.

Glick, B. S., Schulman, D., and Turecki, S. (1971). Diazepam (Valium) treatment in childhood sleep disorders: a preliminary investigation. *Diseases of the Nervous System* 32:565–566.

Graziano, A. M., and Mooney, K. C. (1980). Family self-control instructions for children's nighttime fear reduction. *Journal of Consulting and Clinical Psychology* 48:206–213.

_____ (1982). Behavioral treatment of "night fears" in children: maintenance of improvement at 2 1/2- to 3 1/2-year follow-up. *Journal of Clinical and Child Psychology* 50:598–599.

Graziano, A. M., Mooney, D. C., Huber, C., and Ignaziak, D. (1979). Self-control instructions for children's fear reductions. *Journal of Behavior Therapy and Experimental Psychiatry* 10:221–227.

Guilleminault, C. (1986). Narcolepsy. *Sleep* 9:99–291.

Guilleminault, C., and Anders, T. F. (1976). Sleep disorders in children. *Advances in Pediatrics* 22:151–174.

Guilleminault, C., and Dement, W. C. (1988). Sleep apnea syndromes and related sleep disorders. In *Sleep Disorders: Diagnosis and Treatment*, ed. R. L. Williams, I. Karacan, and C. A. Moore, pp. 47–72. New York: Wiley.

Guilleminault, C., Korobkin, R., and Winkle, R. (1981). A review of 50 children with obstructive sleep apnea syndrome. *Lung* 159:275–287.

Guilleminault, C., Riley, R., Powell, N., et al. (1985). Obstructive sleep apnea syndrome in adolescents: diagnosis and treatment. *Sleep Research* 14:159.

Hagemann, V. (1981). Night sleep of children in a hospital: Part I. Sleep duration. *Maternal-Child Nursing Journal* 10:113.

Hartmann, E. (1989). Bruxism. In *Principles and Practice of Sleep Medicine*, ed. M. H. Kryger, T. Roth, and W. E. Dement. Philadelphia: Saunders.

Hewitt, K. E. (1981). Sleeping problems in pre-school children: what to ask and what to do. *Health Visitor* 54:100–101.

Horne, J. (1992). Annotation: sleep and its disorders in children. *Journal of Child Psychology and Psychiatry* 3:473–487.

Kales, J. D., Kales, A., Soldatos, C. R., et al. (1979). Sleepwalking and night terrors related to febrile illness. *American Journal of Psychiatry* 136:1214–1215.

Kales, J. D., Soldatos, C. R., and Caldwell, A. B. (1980). Nightmares: clinical characteristics and personality patterns. *American Journal of Psychiatry* 137:1197–2001.

Kales, J. D., Soldatos, C. R., and Kales, A. (1980). Childhood sleep disorders. *Current Pediatric Therapy* 9:28–30.

Kales, A., Weber, G., Charney, D. S., et al. (1977). Familial occurrence of sleepwalking and night terrors. *Sleep Research* 6:172.

Kardachi, B. J., Bailey, J. O., and Ash, M. M. (1978). A comparison of biofeedback and occlusal adjustment on bruxism. *Journal of Periodontology* 49:367–372.

Kardachi, B. J., and Clarke, N. G. (1977). The use of biofeedback to control bruxism. *Journal of Periodontology* 48:639–642.

Kellerman, J. (1979). Behavioral treatment of night terrors in a child with acute leukemia. *Journal of Nervous and Mental Disease* 167:182–185.

——— (1980). Rapid treatment of nocturnal anxiety in children. *Journal of Behavior Therapy and Experimental Psychiatry* 11:9–11.

Klackenberg, G. (1982). Somnambulism in childhood: prevalence, course and behavioral correlations. *Acta Paediatrica Scandinavia* 71:495–499.

Koe, G. G. (1989). Hypnotic treatment of sleep terror disorder: a case report. *American Journal of Clinical Hypnosis* 32:36–40.

Kramer, R. L. (1989). The treatment of childhood night terrors through the use of hypnosis – a case study: a brief communication. *International Journal of Clinical Hypnosis* 4:283–284.

Kravitz, H., and Boehm, J. J. (1971). Rhythmic habit patterns in infancy: their sequence, age of onset and frequency. *Child Development* 42:399–413.

Lask, B. (1988). Novel and non-toxic treatment for night terrors. *British Medical Journal* 297:592.

Mallory, G. B., Fiser, D. H., and Jackson, R. (1989). Sleep-associated breathing disorders in morbidly obese children and adolescents. *Journal of Pediatrics* 115:892–897.

Mauer, K. W., Staats, B. A., and Olson, K. D. (1983). Upper airway obstruction and disordered nocturnal breathing in children. *Mayo Clinic Proceedings* 58:349–353.

Mindell, J. A. (1993). Sleep disorders in children. *Health Psychology* 12:152–163.

Mindell, J. A., Spirito, A., and Carskadon, M. A. (1990). Prevalence of sleep problems in chronically ill children. *Sleep Research* 19:337.

Miser, A. W., McCalla, J., Dothage, J. A., et al. (1987). Pain as a presenting symptom in children and young adults with newly diagnosed malignancy. *Pain* 29:85–90.

Mitler, M. M., Nelson, S., and Hajdukovic, R. (1987). Narcolepsy: diagnosis, treatment, and management. *Psychiatric Clinics of North America* 10:593–606.

Noyes, R., Andreasen, N. O., and Hartford, C. (1971). The psychological reaction to severe burns. *Psychosomatics* 12:416–422.

Ollendick, T. H., Hagopian, L. P., and Huntzinger, R. M. (1991). Cognitive-behavior therapy with nighttime fearful children. *Journal of Behavior Therapy and Experimental Psychiatry* 22:113-121.

Palace, E. M., and Johnston, C. (1989). Treatment of recurrent nightmares by the dream reorganization approach. *Journal of Behavior Therapy and Experimental Psychiatry* 20:219-226.

Piccione, A., Coates, T. J., George, J. M., et al. (1982). Nocturnal biofeedback for nocturnal bruxism. *Biofeedback and Self-Regulation* 7:405-419.

Pietropinto, A. (1985). Children's reactions to illness and hospitalizations. *Medical Aspects of Human Sexuality* 19:129-136.

Popoviciu, L., and Corfariu, O. (1983). Efficacy and safety of midazolam in the treatment of night terrors in children. *British Journal of Clinical Pharmacology* 16:97-102.

Prugh, D., Staub, E., Sands, H., et al. (1953). A study of the emotional reactions of children and their families to hospitalization and illness. *American Journal of Orthopsychiatry* 23:70-106.

Reite, M. L., Nagel, K. E., and Ruddy, J. R. (1990). *Concise Guide to Evaluation and Management of Sleep Disorders.* Washington, DC: American Psychiatric Press.

Roberts, R. N., and Gordon, S. B. (1979). Reducing childhood nightmares subsequent to a burn trauma. *Child Behavior Therapy* 1:373-381.

Roth, T., Roehrs, T., and Zorick, F. (1988). Pharmacological treatment of sleep disorders. In *Sleep Disorders: Diagnosis and treatment,* ed. R. L. Williams, I. Karacan, and C. A. Moore, pp. 373-395. New York: Wiley.

Rugh, J. D., and Solberg, W. K. (1975). Electromyographic studies of bruxist behavior before and during treatment. *California Dental Association* 3:57.

Soldatos, C. R., and Lugaresi, E. (1987). Nosology and prevalence of sleep disorders. *Seminar in Neurology* 7:236-242.

Taboada, E. L. (1975). Night terrors in a child treated with hypnosis. *American Journal of Clinical Hypnosis* 17:270-271.

Tarnowski, K. J., Rasnake, L. K., and Drabman, R. S. (1987). Behavioral assessment and treatment of pediatric burn injuries: a review. *Behavior Therapy* 118:417-441.

Thorpy, M. M., Korman, E., Spielman, A. J., and Glovinsky, P. B. (1988). Delayed sleep phase syndrome in adolescents. *Journal of Adolescent Medicine* 9:22-27.

Wagner, M. T. (1981). Controlling nocturnal bruxism through the use of aversive conditioning during sleep. *American Journal of Clinical Biofeedback* 4:87-92.

Weissbluth, M. (1984). Is drug treatment of night terrors warranted? *American Journal of Diseases in Children* 138:1086.

White, M., Powell, G., Alexander, D., et al. (1988). Distress and self-soothing behaviors in hospitalized children at bedtime. *Maternal-Child Nursing Journal* 17:67-78.

White, M. A., Williams, P. D., Alexander, D. J. (1990). Sleep onset latency and distress in hospitalized children. *Nursing Research* 39:134-139.

Wittig, R., Zorick, F., Roehrs, T., et al. (1983). Narcolepsy in a 7-year-old child. *Journal of Pediatrics* 102:725-727.

13

PSYCHOPHYSIOLOGICAL DISORDERS

James W. Sturges
Ronald S. Drabman

INTRODUCTION

Although Axis III conditions are not necessarily associated with anxiety disorders of childhood, it is apparent that anxious children have a disproportionately high number of somatic complaints (Beidel et al. 1991). These complaints do not consist merely of problems commonly believed to be associated with anxiety, such as stomachaches and headaches (*Diagnostic and Statistical Manual of Mental Disorders* 1987, *DSM-III-R*), but include a variety of physical complaints such as heart palpitations, shakiness, flushes/chills, nausea, and dizziness (Beidel et al. 1991).

Strauss and colleagues (1988) studied the frequencies of symptoms in fifty-five children and adolescents diagnosed with overanxious disorder (OAD). They found that 73.9 percent of children under 12 and 77.4 percent of adolescents were rated by clinicians as having somatic complaints for which no physical basis could be established, one of the OAD criteria from the *Diagnostic and Statistical Manual of Mental Disorders*, third edition (*DSM-III*, 1980) and the revised third edition (1987).

In a sample of ninety-five children ages 6–12 with mixed diagnoses, on an inpatient psychiatric service for dangerous behavior or poor therapeutic progress, Livingston et al. (1988) found that the children reported an average of 4.7 somatic complaints. Separation anxiety and depression were associated with symptoms of gastrointestinal distress, common in the sample. A less common symptom was heart palpitations, which were also associated with separation anxiety. Somatic symptoms are so often identified with anxiety disorders that feeling very afraid and having four or more somatic symptoms that tend to occur unexpectedly is considered diagnostic of panic disorder

(*DSM-III-R* 1987). Similarly, responses to confrontations with feared objects in simple phobias are described as a feeling of panic along with somatic symptoms: tachycardia, perspiration, shortness of breath (*DSM-III-R* 1987).

Last (1991) used somatic subscales of the State-Trait Anxiety Inventory for Children (STAIC, Spielberger 1973, Fox and Houston 1983) and the Revised Child Manifest Anxiety Scale for Children (RCMAS, Reynolds and Richmond 1978) to determine if 158 inpatient children with anxiety disorders showed somatic symptomatology, finding that 60 percent of them did. For children under 13 years old, 50 percent reported somatic complaints; among adolescents, 69 percent did.

Prolonged physiological arousal in feared situations is common in children with anxiety problems (Beidel 1988, Beidel et al. 1985). Beidel (1988) studied fifty children 8–12 years old with high and low test anxiety (60 percent with diagnosed anxiety disorders). She measured their blood pressure and heart rate during a vocabulary test and oral reading test. Children with high test anxiety had larger heart rate increases than did children with low test anxiety, and their heart rates stayed high. (The low anxious children's heart rates rose initially but then declined, although this decline was not shown to be statistically significant.)

Sustained arousal may have debilitating effects on long-term health. Although controversial (cf. Angell 1985), especially with regard to linking particular psychological states with particular disease states, it is not going beyond the evidence to state that chronic psychological distress is associated with health problems (Friedman and Booth-Kewley 1987). Modulated by the neocortex, hypothalamus, and limbic system, the autonomic nervous system and the endocrine system influence stress-related responses of emotional distress, immune system function, and organ function such as heart rate and digestive processes.

Stress has been defined alternatively as a stimulus apart from the organism or as the combination of the stimulus and an individual's reaction to it. Although it is more straightforward and reliable to measure stress as a specific environmental event, we know that this has less impact on health than does the reaction to the stressor, such as whether it is perceived as controllable. There has also been controversy surrounding which events elicit undesirable reactions: Do major life changes affect health more than everyday stressors? This is difficult to measure because the two are often related to each other and to how well people take care of themselves, but daily events may be more directly linked to outcome (Rodin and Salovey 1989).

In addition to emotional distress, it appears that cognitive style is associated with health outcomes. In a thirty-five-year longitudinal study with ninety-nine men, stable and global perceptions of negative events were associated with future poor health (Peterson et al. 1988). That is, men who attributed negative events to stable and pervasive factors eventually had poorer health. Similarly, illness in reaction to environmental stressors has been attenuated when the environmental events were perceived to be positive (Cohen et al. 1982) or when the events were viewed as a challenge that could be coped with (Lazarus and Folkman 1984, Wilson et al. 1992). The cognitive interpretation of environmental events determines the effects of stressors, possibly by influencing the occurrences of the stressful events as well as such behaviors as personal health habits (Peterson et al. 1988). Regardless of the evidence for the impact of cognitive style on later health, therapeutic interventions that can reduce chronic psychological distress and increase perceived self-efficacy to cope with negative events can be argued to be beneficial purely for the desired outcome of alleviating psychological distress.

DIFFERENTIAL DIAGNOSIS

Psychological Factors Affecting Physical Condition

According to the revised third edition of the *Diagnostic and Statistical Manual of Mental Disorders* (*DSM-III-R* 1987), the diagnostic category "Psychological Factors Affecting Physical Condition" includes disorders that are referred to as both psychophysiological and psychosomatic. A number of examples of physical conditions are listed, many of which are likely to be stress related in some way (e.g., headache, asthma, gastric ulcer, duodenal ulcer).

The *DSM-III-R Case Book* (Spitzer et al. 1989) contains two cases with this diagnosis, both adults with duodenal ulcers apparently exacerbated by their interpretation of stressful environmental events. Ulcers can be affected by, but are generally not caused by, stress (Jackson and Grand 1991): "No data support a psychosomatic etiology in terms of stress, personality type, or psychiatric illness, although emotional or other psychosocial factors may affect the presentation and course of the disease" (p. 609).

Psychogenic factors were also once thought largely responsible for childhood asthma but are now viewed only as a trigger in children who already have the condition by changes in respiration (Sly 1987). The *DSM-IV* Criteria (1994) place psychological factors affecting physical condition in the category of "Other conditions that may be a focus of clinical attention," still to be coded on Axis I. The diagnosis was expanded to allow the differentiation of psychological and behavioral factors affecting physical condition. The types of contributory factors to be specified in a diagnosis are (a) disorders on Axis I or II, (b) psychological symptoms such as anxiety, (c) personality traits or coping style, (d) maladaptive health behaviors, (e) stress-related bodily responses or (f) unspecified psychological or behavioral factors. These factors are recognized to be important to health in terms of diet, exercise, disease prevention, adherence to medical regimens, coping, recovery from medical procedures, and so on. The breadth of this category is telling of the increasing importance of the role of behavioral medicine.

In order to receive one of these diagnoses, the following *DSM-IV* Criteria (1994) items would have to be met:

1. The presence of a general medical condition (coded on Axis III).
2. Psychological factors adversely affect the general medical condition in one of the following ways:
    (a) the factors have influenced the course of the general medical condition as shown by a close temporal association between the psychological factors and the development or exacerbation of, or delayed recovery from, the general medical condition,
    (b) the factors interfere with the treatment of the general medical condition,
    (c) the factors constitute additional health risks for the individual, or
    (d) the factors elicit stress-related physiologic responses that precipitate or exacerbate symptoms of a general medical condition (e.g., chest pain or arrhythmia in a patient with coronary artery disease). [p. 678]

Many referrals by pediatricians to mental health professionals will involve problems that fall into these categories. Adherence issues among chronically ill children, for example, are very likely to influence the course of the condition or at least interfere with treatment. When children must undergo painful medical procedures, their behavioral distress can make procedures difficult to manage. Taking a child's temperature, administering oral medication, venipuncture, bone marrow aspirations, and many other procedures can be associated with fear, anxiety, pain, and physical resistance. On an inpatient basis, we have seen many children whose behavior has at least temporarily precluded appropriate treatment.

Unfortunately, sometimes anxiety about a medical condition may itself precipitate a worsening of the condition, as when an asthmatic child who is worried about having an asthma attack increases the depth and rate of respirations, coughs excessively, or otherwise facilitates the onset of an episode (King et al. 1990). In the case of paniclike symptomatology, children's focus on bodily reactions to stressful events can induce or increase undesired physiological responses such as rapid heart rate (Hermecz and Melamed 1984).

Caution should be used in interpreting the directionality of the relation between disease or somatic symptoms and anxiety or depression. Because some ill children develop and need treatment for anxiety and depression, it may be erroneously concluded that the anxiety, depression, or certain personality characteristics were etiologic in the disease process. Furthermore, the current lack of complete understanding of the physiological events that comprise emotion and cognition, as well as the lack of complete understanding of the etiologic processes of disease, makes it extremely difficult to specify the relation between affective mood or psychological style and the origin and progression of disease, the functioning of the immune system, the experience of pain, and other somatic events. Meta-analytic findings suggest that the relation of anxiety, hostility, and especially depression with disease may range from a correlation of .10 to .25 or higher, indicating an important impact but one that is detectable only through large-scale epidemiological studies (Friedman and Booth-Kewley 1987).

There has been a general trend away from the simplistic tendency to try to categorize conditions as organic versus psychosomatic or psychophysiological, because the latter terms have been associated with unrealistic theories attributing specific physical disorders to specific psychological factors (Siegel 1990). There are still some intriguing possibilities of specific organ vulnerabilities to stress, however, such as in the case of recurrent abdominal pain (Gaffney and Gaffney 1987). It is now thought to be more useful to use the term *somatic disorders* regardless of etiology (Siegel and Richards 1978, Siegel 1990). Nonetheless, *DSM-IV* (1994) still discriminates between psychological factors affecting physical condition, which require the presence of a demonstrable medical condition believed to be exacerbated by psychological factors, and somatoform disorders "not fully explained by a general medical condition" (p. 445).

Somatoform Disorders

Somatoform disorders have symptoms that exceed what could be expected given the demonstrable pathology and are often associated with stress and anxiety (*DSM-III-R* 1987). In order to meet criteria for one of the somatoform disorders, the primary features are body-related[1] complaints that are not fully

---

[1]Gastric, pain, sexual, and pseudoneurologic in somatization disorder; motor/sensory in conversion disorder; illness-related in hypochondriasis; defects in appearance in body dysmorphic disorder; and pain-related in pain disorder.

explained by an existing medical condition or psychiatric diagnosis. For the diagnoses of pain disorder associated with psychological factors, pain disorder associated with both psychological factors and a general medical condition, and conversion disorder, a clinical judgment is also made that psychological factors are associated with the somatic symptoms (*DSM-IV* 1994).

In order to see whether or not the existing adult-oriented criteria for somatization disorder were appropriate, and to identify variables associated with somatization symptoms, Garber and colleagues (1991) developed the Children's Somatization Inventory (CSI). The CSI combined the Hopkins Symptom Checklist (Derogatis et al. 1974) and *DSM-III* criteria in a questionnaire for children to complete. Samples from grade school children indicated that although very few children had enough symptoms to likely receive a clinical diagnosis, roughly 15 percent had at least four somatic complaints. The complaints were greater among girls, especially for adolescents. They were positively related to anxiety and depression measures, and negatively related to self-esteem. Because (a) the adult criteria include items related to sexual activity and menstruation, (b) topology of somatization changes across development, and (c) frequent somatic complaints of children such as headaches are not included in the adult somatization criteria, gathering the information contained in the CSI may be more relevant to pediatric somatic problems than applying *DSM* criteria (Garber et al. 1991).

Researchers working with adults with somatic complaints have pointed to problems with the somatization label and concept, and have proposed redefining the problem in terms of the extent to which individuals tune into and amplify somatic experiences (Barsky and Klerman 1983). The somatic amplification construct has been explored with the chronic pain population, using a set of sensory, motor, and tenderness tests that should be negative even in chronic pain (Korbon et al. 1987). A conceptually similar measure has been to rate specific exaggerated pain behaviors occurring during physical examination (Keefe et al. 1984). These two measures were recently found to be correlated (Lofland 1994).

Other Diagnoses

The diagnosis of factitious disorder, the intentional production of physical symptoms in order to assume a sick role, is sometimes considered when inexplicable somatic complaints are reported. This includes factitious disorder by proxy, in which a child's caretaker is intentionally producing the symptoms in the child. In cases that involve apparent efforts to obtain benefits such as staying home from school (rather than an attempt to assume a sick role), malingering may be occurring, but that conceptualization may oversimplify the situation or be incorrect. Children with anxiety disorders such as social phobia and separation anxiety may experience somatic symptoms when faced with going to school (Beidel 1991), making the determination of malingering problematic.

ASSESSMENT PROCEDURES

Interviews

In order to obtain a valid assessment, the first consideration is establishing rapport with the child and the guardian(s) accompanying the child. In our experience, the ease with which this can be done varies depending on the way in which the referral process has occurred. If the therapist has been called in by a medical team as a last resort, the family may infer that their child's complaints have been labeled false and that the family is somehow being blamed for the condition. Neither of these perceptions is conducive to nondefensive information provision by the family or receptivity to interventions. If on the other hand the therapist is viewed as a part of the medical team from the initial arrival of the family at the facility, and if the psychosocial aspects of care are a routine concern of the team, then families feel less stigmatized by the involvement of the mental health professionals. The role of the clinician performing an assessment should be clarified at the onset of contact, and any concerns of the family should be addressed.

The goal of any assessment is to make decisions about treatment and recommendations. Therefore, the evaluation is not limited to an assessment of the particular problem and possible environmental contributions to the problem, but includes the potential for the success of the various possible treatment alternatives. Thus, a very useful source of information available from the family is what in the past has been successful at relieving distress or improving functioning. Building on the patient's and family's strengths and preferences allows a more viable treatment program to be developed.

Interviews or questionnaires can be used to determine the child's level of functioning in terms of daily living skills. This can be useful in determining needed areas of intervention as well as in monitoring practical indices of improvement. Structured interviews such as the Child Assessment Schedule (CAS, Hodges et al. 1982) can aid in diagnosis. Such structured interviews attempt to assess problems in social and family relations, anxiety and mood, and somatic problems, by asking parents specific questions to establish relative levels of problems in comparison to other children. Families can also be asked to collect data in diaries, observations can be conducted, assessment instruments can be administered, and physiological measures can be taken.

Self-Report and Parent-Report Measures

Somatic problems may be the presenting complaint or may turn up during diagnostic interviews with the child or parents. In addition to interviews related primarily to diagnostic criteria, several measures have been used to identify psychological factors that are likely mediators of the role of stress in illness and that may be responsive to intervention. For example, the evidence that daily stressors are associated with the health status of children with physiological disorders such as asthma, cardiovascular disease, diabetes, and sickle cell disease has provided the impetus for the development of scales such as the children's Daily Life Stressors Scale (DLSS, Kearney et al. 1993). The DLSS has thirty items tapping aversive events experienced by children, and has a correlation of .72 with the Children's Depression Inventory (CDI, Kovacs and Beck 1977), .67 with the Nowicki-Strickland Locus of Control Scale (Nowicki and Strickland 1973), .60 with the STAIC trait, .52 with the STAIC state (Spielberger 1973), and -.74 with the Piers-Harris Self-Concept Scale (Piers 1984). Among the findings in the initial sample were that male children reported greater daily stress than did female children, whereas among adolescents, females reported more stress than males. The authors hypothesized that although young males may experience gender role stress from a young age, they are socialized to deny this as they get older.

Rather than tap the aversiveness of negative events, the Child Anxiety Sensitivity Index (Silverman et al. 1991) asks children to rate how aversive they view anxiety symptoms. It was modeled after the anxiety sensitivity index for adults (Reiss and McNally 1985). The anxiety sensitivity construct makes sense given some clients' focus on bodily symptoms during anxiety, and the evidence that such a focus can be incorporated into exposure therapies (Rapee 1987).

Wisniewski, Naglieri, and Mulick (1988) have published a Children's Psychosomatic Symptom Checklist, which asks children how often they experienced headaches, backaches, stomach pain, trouble falling asleep, tiredness, sadness, nausea, stiffness, racing heart, eye pain, dizziness, and weakness, and how severe the problems are. Its authors found the items to be internally consistent and their scale showed the expected modest correlations with the CDI and the RCMAS.

Pain or symptom diaries kept by the child or family can be useful in determining the events that typically precipitate episodes, as well as the variables that appear to be associated with good levels of functioning. These, in combination with adaptive behavior scales, such as the revised Vineland Adaptive Behavior Scales (Sparrow et al. 1984) and the American Association on Mental Deficiency Adaptive Behavior Scales (Lambert and Windmiller 1981, Nihira et al. 1974), may allow an assessment of the severity of the problem in relation to same chronological or mental age peers (for a discussion of these measures, see Reschly 1990). In our clinic we make extensive use of the Child Behavior Checklist-Parent Report Form (CBCL), a well-known and reliable inventory that can be used to compare levels of behavior problems, and to some extent social competencies, to age-norms for children 4–18 (Achenbach 1991).

In a study of over- and underreporting of somatic symptomatology, Leikin and colleagues (1988) found that children who scored above the upper tertile of the Matthews Youth Test for Health (MYTH, Matthews and Angulo 1980), considered to have Type A personality characteristics such as hostility, competitiveness, and time-urgency (Matthews 1982), reported significantly fewer physical symptoms after surgery than did children who scored below the lower tertile on the MYTH, considered Type B. As in adults, the Type A children were more likely to continue their normal activities, ignore somatic sensations, and use medical services less than Type B children. Ironically, however, long-term avoidance of health issues by these children can lead to an increase in later problems (Leikin et al. 1988).

Measures of knowledge about the management of a disorder can tell the clinician whether specific information provision is needed. For example, in the area of asthma knowledge, several measures have been utilized including a seventy-seven-item checklist for parents by Spykerboer and colleagues (1986), a thirty-item questionnaire administered to children by Eiser, Town, and Tripp (1988), and a sixteen-item measure by Taggart et al. (1991). Taylor et al. (1991) developed videotaped scenarios involving diabetes management for families to view and discuss, in order to evaluate their responses. Parents' self-efficacy regarding management is associated with adherence to the recommended regimen (Radius et al. 1978).

Children's locus of control related to asthma can be assessed using the twenty-item Children's Health Locus of Control Scale (Parcel and Meyer 1978), and can help evaluate their initial and ongoing perceptions of their roles in management. Children's scores of state and trait anxiety according to the STAIC, and depression according to an instrument such as the CDI, are important aspects of self-report data in assessing somatic problems, as are reported fears, such as those measured by the Fear Survey Schedule for Children-Revised (Ollendick 1983).

Physiologic Measures

The measurement of physiologic symptomatology has been recognized as a useful component of the assessment of anxiety among children (King et al. 1990), such as in the evaluation of therapeutic progress during systematic desensitization, or in assessing distress responses during medical procedures. In reviewing findings of desynchrony even across only physiologic measures, King and colleagues (1990) point to the need for multiple data sources. In addition to heart rate and blood pressure, physiologic measures can include electrodermal activity and respiration. Electrodermal activity can be particularly sensitive to reactivity, and respiratory airflow can reflect therapeutic gains, as has been done with asthmatic children (King et al. 1990).

ESTABLISHING TREATMENT GOALS

Any reduction in somatic symptomatology or increase in functioning can be viewed as an improvement, and realistic expectations will explicitly acknowledge this. Goals that target small well-defined steps that may work toward these ends are helpful. These tasks include data collection by the parent or by the individual in the case of an older child or adolescent. One indication of rapport and motivation is whether an initial very simple monitoring assignment is completed between the first and second session. Such monitoring assignments include the number of headaches, stomachaches, or asthma episodes a child experiences. If the assignment is not completed, it may be necessary to re-address the rapport issue, to better explain what you are trying to accomplish, to find out more about what the parent views as a primary problem, and to design very simple strategies that are highly compatible with the normal routine. When the parents' goals are not congruent with the goals of the pediatric team, the therapist may be able to negotiate a better understanding between the parent and team. When a child's problems reflect a probable reaction to continuing inappropriate behavior by a parent, it may be necessary to refer the parent for treatment and sometimes involve the appropriate state agency concerned with neglect of children's care to ensure that the family will receive help.

Often, differential reinforcement of behavior that is incompatible with or at least an alternative to negative target behaviors is a useful strategy. The child may have learned to use somatic complaints as an attention-getting mechanism, and it may be undesirable to direct further attention to the complaints, even negative attention. The eventual goal is normal functioning. The steps toward that do not necessarily have to include a suppression of all somatic complaints, which, after all, can serve a purpose.

Of utmost importance is to keep a child in contact with the academic and social experiences in the school setting, which may be a focal point of difficulty for children with somatic problems. The explicit goal is usually the child's return to school, and it is sometimes suggested that behaviors such as crying and begging should be ignored (Hersen 1970). The steps toward accomplishing this vary from immediate return in acute situations to a more gradual approach with children who have more generalized anxieties (Stokes et al. 1989).

For children with chronic pain, goals may include reduction of medication use, with parent administration targeted to ensure gradual withdrawal and the use of time-contingent rather than pain-contingent administration. Individually tailored strategies of pain management, which depend on the therapist's resources and the inclinations and acceptance of the family, can be explored. These strategies may include relaxation, imagery, self-talk, thermal biofeedback, and specific well behaviors. A significant goal then becomes the performance of these strategies, and this is an important topic for discussion in therapy and phone contacts. Adjusting goals to accomplish as much as possible without surpassing the abilities or motivation of the family is a primary task of the therapist. The extent that suggestions are carried out is a function of the level of cognitive functioning of the family members, their perceptions of the therapist and the reason for referral, their belief in the need for and efficacy of the therapy, and extant concerns and problems in their daily life.

ROLE OF THE THERAPIST

Therapists often begin in the role of teacher, explaining biopsychosocial models of pain and illness in a developmentally appropriate fashion, setting appropriate behavioral goals and effective individualized strategies, and developing ways to promote adherence to the plans. Problem-solving and logistical planning sessions may be needed to maintain success. If obstacles are continuously placed in the path of success, extra issues may need to be addressed, such as poor relationships within the family or family members' reasons for resistance to change.

Many interventions, such as the ones that have been developed for pediatric headache, have usually been delivered directly by the therapist (Gagnon et al. 1992). Reducing the amount of direct patient contact via home-based and school-based treatment programs is a promising, more efficient alternative to this approach (Allen and McKeen 1991, Burke and Andrasik 1989, Larsson and Melin 1986). Utilizing parents in the amelioration of children's distress has been getting more attention in the literature (e.g., Blount et al. 1994). Parent training techniques, already used extensively for children with attention and conduct problems, can be effectively put to use for children with somatic complaints as well, especially when the home situation is judged to be integral to the problem.

Both a complicating factor and a benefit to therapists working with children who have somatic complaints is the relationship with the pediatrician. Some keys to success in working with pediatricians have been highlighted by Allen and colleagues (1993), summarized in Box 13-1.

TREATMENT STRATEGIES

Following a medical examination, the incorporation of behavioral interventions in the treatment of somatic problems can be highly effective (Siegel

Box 13-1. Working with Pediatricians

1. Learn about the training and the demand characteristics of pediatrics. Pediatricians take total responsibility for children for long periods of time. They are protective of the families with whom they work and find these relationships rewarding. By giving the pediatrician a source of effective short-term treatment packages without undermining the pediatrician-patient primary care relationship, therapists can become a valued ally of the pediatrician.

2. Learn about medical terminology and current research. Some time with a medical dictionary and some pediatric journals can go a long way toward making one more facile in communication with the pediatric team.

3. Be visible in the clinic regularly. Consultation requests increase when staff know you and see your involvement, and there will be less stigma attached to appointments with you if they are conducted in the pediatric clinic rather than a psychiatric facility. During discussions with staff, become familiar with their conceptualizations before making suggestions.

4. Make clear and simple presentations of behavioral techniques that can also be applied by the medical team, and develop protocols for them to follow.

5. Provide prompt written feedback that demonstrates competence, collaboration, and an understanding that the primary provider is the referring physician.

Source: adapted from Allen and colleagues. Copyright © 1993 by *Journal of Applied Behavior Analysis*, and used by permission of the authors.

1990). For example, in the case of asthma that appears to be exacerbated by emotional distress, treatments have included traditional psychotherapy, modification of behaviors that are related to asthma attacks, relaxation training, biofeedback, systematic desensitization, and practice of requisite skills. Electromyographic (EMG) biofeedback, airway resistance biofeedback, and hypnosis are some of the most promising interventions (Gagnon et al. 1992). No matter which strategies are taken, a step-by-step plan for asthma management should be established (Sheffer 1991).

In addition to training the family in these strategies, programs for families should involve daily data collection toward the goal of preventing asthma attacks. Mold and pollen, temperature changes, exercise, peak respiration flow values obtained with peak flow meters, and time of day can be predictive of asthma attacks (Creer and Bender 1993). A significant component of treatment is thus education of the family in the ways to define and measure antecedents to episodes. Knowledge of asthma, knowledge of skills, and performance of skills are all stressed.

Pediatric headache is another important problem. In one longitudinal study it was found that 53 percent of children with migraine headaches were still experiencing them thirty years later. Among the child and adolescent headache populations, consistent and positive effects of behavioral interventions have been found. Relaxation training has repeatedly been shown to be better than control conditions (Engel et al. 1992, Larsson et al. 1987a, Larsson and Melin 1986, Larsson et al. 1987b, Wisniewski, Genshaft, et al. 1988). However, comparisons of progressive relaxation with cognitive coping skills training and biofeedback have been equivocal (Fentress et al. 1986, Richter et al. 1986). Cognitive coping skills training has been shown to be more effective than control conditions when the coping skills were directed toward responding behaviorally to early signs of headache (Duckro and Cantwell-Simmons 1989). Children's headache improvement has been shown to be stable for three and four years after treatment with combinations of relaxation and biofeedback (Engel et al. 1992, Gagnon et al. 1992). The best documented improvements have been in headache frequency, with changes in headache intensity sometimes reported as well (Duckro and Cantwell-Simmons 1989, Engel et al. 1992). Skin temperature biofeedback may be appropriate for some patients, but not as a sole intervention (Duckro and Cantwell-Simmons 1989).

Concrete examples of ways that psychological factors are important can be very useful in helping people understand the reason for some of the types of issues that need to be addressed. In the context of introducing nonpharmacologic treatment to pediatric pain patients, McGrath (1990) suggested several good examples and analogies that can be used, such as how concentration on an interesting activity can make pain diminish or how some simple strategies such as rubbing a painful area sometimes block the pain signals to the brain. These examples are also accomplished via demonstrations. Biofeedback even as simple as hand warming to change a thermometer reading can break the ground for beginning treatment. It may also be helpful to remind families that the goal of treatment is not necessarily to accomplish a 100 percent resolution of the presenting problems, but to find ways that the extent of the problems may be reduced.

Evidence suggests that there are developmental differences in how children normally cope with stressors, and in how they interpret physiologic sensations. For example, they may not experience the cognitive component of panic disorder (Nelles and Barlow 1988). As children's level of cognitive development increases, so too does their focus on their emotional arousal and their ability to think through multiple-step plans of action. However, children at all ages seem to do little problem-focused coping, such as monitoring their behavior to control disease exacerbation (Compas et al. 1992). It is primarily this problem-focused coping that has been found to be beneficial (Peterson 1989). Thus interventions should involve building problem-focused coping skills. However, the way to teach the particular strategies must depend on the level of cognitive functioning of the child and involved family members. When it is found that procedures are too difficult, switch to simpler strategies.

Intervention complexity may vary across situations as well. For example, children are able to handle more complex coping strategies during periods of moderate physiological arousal than during periods of high levels of distress and pain, at which point they tend to rely on very simple strategies such as breathing exercises or calling out for a parent (Blount et al. 1989).

DEALING WITH COMMON OBSTACLES TO SUCCESSFUL TREATMENT

It is our philosophy that children should be treated in the most straightforward and least intrusive way first. The immediate environmental factors are addressed. Often this obviates the need for more complicated intervention, although it does not necessarily indicate that gains can be maintained if the situation is allowed to revert to the preintervention status. In cases where immediate environmental factors do not resolve presenting problems, family relationships, the child's early learning history, and the school situation are further assessed with an eye toward uncovering influential variables.

There is probably no more important time to carefully consider theoretical models than when dealing with somatic problems. There are many heuristics, but one of the most interesting involves an examination of attributions of responsibility for problems and their solutions, by Brickman and his colleagues (1982). We believe that one of the most valuable approaches to somatic problems is this compensatory model. In Brickman's model, individuals are not blamed for their illnesses, pain, or predicaments, as they implicitly are in a moral model. Also, unlike a medical model, which might cast them as passive recipients of treatment, they are considered to have the ability to improve their situations and to make positive changes. Believing one can make a change is not a sufficient condition for change (Folkman 1984), but self-efficacy can foster motivation to protect oneself from health dangers (Maddux and Rogers 1983). It should also be pointed out that measures of self-efficacy regarding disease management may be negatively correlated with depression (Creer and Bender 1993), and low levels of self-efficacy regarding disease management indicate the need for appropriate assessment for depression.

RELAPSE PREVENTION

Although behavior therapists have long searched for ways to enhance maintenance of change, it is not unreasonable to assume that continued change may take continued intervention, just as individuals who find relief with medical intervention may be required to continue to seek health care (Drabman et al. 1990). Certainly we should not expect maintenance to take care of itself, but instead take steps to increase the likelihood that behaviors will generalize over situations and time. The ways to do this have been outlined by Stokes and Osnes (1989) and in the now classic Stokes and Baer (1977) article. Either parents or preferably a professional should periodically assess a child who has experienced somatic problems related to psychological and behavioral factors. The return or increase in reports of somatic symptomatology will be an obvious indicator that the situation should be reevaluated. Monitoring also allows us to discover the problem when it is still small and therefore easier to treat.

Some physical problems are tied so closely to behavior that almost constant vigilance may be necessary to prevent relapse. In the case of obesity, for example, the return to prior eating and exercise habits can quickly and repeatedly reverse gains that have been accomplished during full or partial hospitalization or intensive outpatient treatment.

For cases in which difficult lifestyle change and adherence to medical regimen is required, therapy with older children and adolescents should address common difficulties that are likely to occur, such as negative affect, social pressure, and the abstinence violation effect (Marlatt 1985). Modeling, role-play, and rehearsal of appropriate behaviors in difficult situations is important for the behaviors to be sufficiently well learned to be likely to occur when needed. This should include self-statements rehearsed for particular high-probability scenarios.

Marlatt (1985) describes how infractions from recommendations may cause individuals to temporarily give up on adherence and to engage in further inappropriate behavior. This has also been described in the health promotion literature, in terms of lowered self-efficacy (Maddux and Rogers 1983). In the case of children with lifestyle-related problems such as obesity, or with difficult regimens such as those associated with diabetes management, there may be many situations in which a minor violation of regimen occurs. At that point it is important that the child or adolescent have a specific plan to get back on track without becoming discouraged. Parents can communicate their availability to help the child with these situations rather than demonstrate a punitive attitude, which could act to foster covert noncompliance.

TERMINATION

An important question at termination is whether coping skills have been mastered by the child and family. There is evidence, for example, that patients who continue to use relaxation-based coping strategies on a long-term basis report a greater reduction in chronic pain than patients who are less adherent. This could be due to differences in reporting styles or increased tendencies to use coping strategies when symptomatology is already lower, but appears to suggest the benefit of the continued use of cognitive-behavioral strategies (Young 1992).

If monitoring and contingency management has been utilized, it can be faded gradually and intermittently in order to help ensure that appropriate behaviors do not disappear. And although reinforcement should not cease, the child should be prepared for termination of therapy sessions. This may be especially important if the child and therapist have established a close relationship, such as during and after an inpatient hospitalization, or following many sessions at relatively short intervals. Casting termination in a positive light, as a graduation of sorts, may help make the experience more positive for the child. Spacing sessions out for longer intervals before terminating completely can also foster independence from the therapist and reduce the loss that might be experienced by the child with a sudden discontinuation of therapy sessions.

CASE ILLUSTRATION (TYPICAL TREATMENT)

Description and History

Delia was a 13-year-old white female with diabetes, kidney damage, and hypertension who lived with her parents in a rural part of the state. She had been diagnosed several years previously with diabetes, but her family had experienced difficulty in managing her disease. We were requested to help the diabetes nurse-educator develop a plan to deal with Delia's life-threatening problems with adherence to the medical regimen. When her family had attempted to help her make dietary and behavioral changes, they had met with resistance and become discouraged. Delia had two older brothers, who were concerned about her health but not happy about sharing in the responsibilities of diabetes management. Delia did not meet clinical criteria for depression but was unhappy about her situation. She had approximately low-average vocabulary according to the Peabody Picture Vocabulary Test-Revised (Dunn and Dunn 1981) but performed satisfactorily in school. She could administer her own insulin and check her blood sugar level with her glucometer.

At the same time that we were assessing Delia, other members of the team were developing meal plans and working with her school to ensure adherence in that setting as well. Administration of a diabetes knowledge test and observations of her attempts to monitor her blood sugar levels, administer her insulin, and identify appropriate ways to remain in metabolic control led to our conclusion that she had basic relevant knowledge. She correctly identified when she should check her blood sugar levels (four times each day) and that she should inject before her morning and evening meals. However, she had several skill deficits and needed better management goals. She was not able to readily categorize blood sugar readings as high, normal, or low without the glucometer, and she was unable to consistently state what she must

do following readings that were too high or too low in order to facilitate
return to appropriate levels.

Synopsis of Therapy Sessions

Delia's progress was monitored during an inpatient hospitalization
lasting two weeks. During the month following the inpatient stay,
Delia's mother was seen on three additional occasions. Delia was seen
during the second portion of these sessions. She explained that she
found it difficult to remember what she needed to do to manage her
diabetes, and she completed a Diabetes Assertiveness Test (Gross and
Johnson 1981). The assertiveness test identified some areas of strengths
in her willingness to try to stick to her program in the face of social
pressure, and she later enjoyed re-enacting these role-plays in the group
therapy sessions as a good example for the others. Delia also participated in a family session and participated for a year after discharge in
group sessions every other month. When the entire family was asked to
come in, they discussed their role in her day-to-day diabetes management and their willingness to join with her in a program of lifestyle
change. After Delia's first two group sessions, we met with her and her
mother again and helped them readjust their management program.

Between her first two group sessions she got into an argument
with her mother about whether or not she would be allowed to go on
a particular outing with friends. For two days she stopped recording her
adherence behaviors in her diary, ate some restricted foods, and did not
engage in exercise. In the following individual session, she was able to
realize that she was not hurting her mother through these actions so
much as herself, and identified some other ways she could communicate her anger to her mother and earn a greater degree of independence. We encouraged her mother to use noninflammatory statements
during disagreements and to allow Delia greater autonomy when she
demonstrated her ability to handle it responsibly.

With practice, Delia became able to readily categorize the blood
sugar readings and to take appropriate action when readings were
abnormal. At the same time, she became more aware of dietary and
exercise requirements and met other children who had diabetes with
whom she could join in a support group. The management program
that emerged from our sessions with Delia was one that combined
extensive self-monitoring and goal setting with an increased level of
change by other family members. Delia liked the idea of keeping a diary

and gained satisfaction in being able to record her efforts and successes along with other information about her thoughts and feelings.

To give a flavor of the support and information available from a group therapy approach with children who have chronic disease exacerbated by their behavior, the following excerpt was from her first group session.

Therapist: We've been practicing how to check blood sugars, and everybody seems to be good at that. What are some of the other things that you need to be doing to stay healthy?

John: Not eat much sugar and get enough exercise.

Delia: My mother wants me to get more exercise, but I don't like to do exercises.

Therapist: Has anyone else in the group had this problem?

John: Yeah, I used to watch a lot of TV instead of doing much else. When I stopped watching TV and got out on my bike more, I ended up getting a lot more exercise.

Leah: I still watch TV, but I am on a swim team, so I get a good workout from that.

Therapist: It sounds like you two get exercise in some fun ways.

Delia: I don't know.

Therapist: You're not sure you like that idea.

Delia: Yeah.

Therapist: What are some things that you enjoy doing?

Delia: I like to play with my dog.

John: That's exercise, isn't it?

Delia: I am going to start taking him for walks.

Therapist: When during your day do you think you could do that?

Delia: I can do that after school.

Therapist: What do you think will help you remember?

Delia: I can add that to the chart we made for my shots.

Therapist: That sounds good. Let's talk about when exercise can help and when it is important to stop and rest. . . .

As can be gathered from this small sample of the group discussion, the children tend to help each other find solutions to problems. At the same time, they voice some surprise that other children have the same concerns that they do. When they attend a summer camp specifically for other children with juvenile diabetes, they are often amazed at the number of other children who have the same medical problems and similar psychosocial sequelae. Parents remain very involved in the management strategies adopted by the younger children as well as in the more difficult cases.

Comments

In summary, the initial assessment, which included an evaluation of Delia's knowledge and skills, and an intervention that involved other family members, allowed changes in Delia's behaviors related to the management of her diabetes. Her self-monitoring indicated greater regularity of exercise, less consumption of restricted foods, more frequent glucometer readings, and more punctual insulin injections. Glycosolated hemoglobin readings at her clinic appointments reflected better metabolic control. We would recommend a group format for most children due to the social support available, especially for children who have difficulty with assertiveness and need practice in interacting with others regarding food refusal or explaining the need to stop an activity, use glucotabs, check blood sugar levels, and so forth. On the other hand, children with good social skills, such as Delia, may benefit from the teaching role that they can assume in the group setting.

CASE ILLUSTRATION (OVERCOMING OBSTACLES)

Description and History

Robbie, a 4-year, 10-month-old black male with sickle cell disease, had been admitted at least twenty-one times to our teaching hospital for pain crises or illnesses that involved pain crisis. He had also been admitted at least twice to a private hospital in the area. When he would begin to experience pain and refuse to bear weight on the affected joints, his mother would try to increase his fluid consumption at home for one to two days, without clinical benefit. Then she would take him to the pediatric emergency room, as she had on this admission (in February), where he would be admitted to the hospital for one to sixteen days with good response. Notes in the medical record reflected that he had a low tolerance to pain while awake but was able to sleep easily, and that he was usually slow to respond to intervention. Robbie was an only child, enrolled in a local grant-funded preschool program, and was happy and playful when not experiencing acute pain episodes.

Robbie's generally happy nature was apparent during our visits to his room, in which we were able to engage him in play and conversation. He indicated improvement in level of pain on a rating scale of facial expressions, choosing the smiling face rather than the sad face that he had chosen two days before. He demonstrated that he could count to seven and say the alphabet through the letter G, and stated that he was in the hospital when asked where he was. He could also state names of medications. When medicine was being administered by a nurse (orally with a needle-less syringe), he cheerfully complied.

The biggest obstacle in helping Robbie was that his mother appeared to be unable or unwilling to increase the amount of reinforcement available to Robbie for engaging in coping behaviors, and she was similarly unskilled or unmotivated in using distraction strategies with Robbie during his painful episodes. As a result, Robbie was not able to gain very much attention from his mother and was not generally encouraged to function at the highest level. Intervention thus was more difficult as it involved not only teaching the mother but repeated efforts to persuade her of the need for behavior change on her part.

Robbie's subjective level of experienced pain decreased in response to environmental stimulation, which served to functionally compete with the internal pain stimulus. A good example of this was that when we engaged him in a conversation about his favorite music, he stopped crying. Another indication was the repeated mention in the chart that he was consolable, or consolable by his mother. Although Robbie's level of coping could be increased by engaging him in activities such as singing, games, and conversation, it also appeared to be hindered by fear. He became very afraid of pain once the pain crises began. He was afraid to allow his mother to rub his legs gently when they hurt, and he was sometimes combative on examination by the physicians.

When he asked for pain medication and was told that he had recently received some and would not be able to have any more for some time, he began to cry very loudly for a long time. Unfortunately, as mentioned above, because of the chronic nature of Robbie's problems, the mother had apparently adopted the strategy of always ignoring Robbie rather than actively engaging him in distracting activities. When asked about how they cope with his pain, her responses (perhaps understandably) reflected more concern with her ability to tolerate his crying rather than attempts to relieve or distract him. Although knowledgeable in methods of distracting him, she had become frustrated with the frequency and duration of his complaints and crying. Regarding her own level of coping, she stated that she had substantially progressed in her ability to emotionally handle his condition. She indicated that she received social support from her family and friends, and assistance in child care from her sister and mother. A single parent, she remained employed at an office where she had worked since before Robbie's birth. Surprisingly to us, the mother mentioned the possibility of Robbie's premature death in his presence. However, Robbie and his mother appeared to have the ability to cope well with his disease and pain crises. He appeared to be a well-adjusted and happy child. His mother seemed to be resourceful and well intentioned.

Synopsis of Therapy Sessions

As is typical on our consultation service, we began with recommendations to the team and discussion of the recommendations. We recommended that he be administered medication regularly and prophylactically in a time-contingent fashion rather than on an as-needed basis. We stressed that early intervention during pain crises may also diminish his fear of pain over time. For future pain crises, we recommended that when Robbie was in the hospital we be contacted to teach him coping strategies that will increase in complexity as he gets older. For example, imagination-based distraction techniques and progressive muscle relaxation would be possible avenues, although the specific strategies would depend on what will be found to work best.

After being asked to follow through on our suggestion to involve the mother in parent training, we encouraged Robbie's mother to engage him in activities during pain crises. We demonstrated the benefit of varying her strategies and using repeated efforts, sometimes waiting for pain medication to reach therapeutic levels. The mother watched as we modeled these techniques, and rehearsed them while we observed, over the course of several sessions.

Age-appropriate patient and family education about sickle cell disease was already ongoing and we noted that it should be continued. Later we plan to use a videotape for families that demonstrates how to engage in progressive muscle relaxation and contains reminders about increased fluid intake and acetaminophen use in the home management of mild pain episodes.

Comments

This case illustrated a situation in which a child learned that he would be ignored if he engaged in normal activity when in pain but could obtain pain-relieving medication by increasing his overt distress. He had also become extremely fearful of pain crises, which tended to be severe. By intervening earlier in the process with noncontingent analgesics we found his distress could be reduced. By engaging him in distracting activities and encouraging a normal activity level to the extent possible, the focus on the pain was reduced as attention was diverted elsewhere. According to useful heuristics such as the gate control theory (Noordenbos 1959), this is not merely because children divert their attention, but potentially because of the limited receptive stimuli that can be processed simultaneously (i.e., there really is less experienced pain). Although parents are in the best position to provide therapeutic benefit for ill children, they may have found their previous attempts punishing and become discouraged in their efforts to help their children. Our greatest obstacle in this case was in helping Robbie's mother to rediscover the rewards of positive interactions with her child. By providing parent training and education, and by following through on developing some individual strategies with him on future visits, we hope to be able to continue to mitigate Robbie's pain crises.

SUMMARY

The area of somatic problems in children and adolescents has progressed from dualistic and unsupported hypotheses to a biopsychosocial model that recognizes physiologic reaction to perceived environmental stress as a response that can aggravate disease processes. Somatic problems are signficantly linked to stress and anxiety, and their management is a challenge. The area is difficult for clinicians because of the families' resistance to accepting the role that behavioral intervention can play. Thus, the way in which rapport is established and treatment is introduced can influence whether one has the opportunity to assist the child.

Similarities across differing topologies of somatic symptoms include the need to develop an understanding of the context and antecedents of the problems, an appreciation of the family's best potential methods of coping, and the development of a step-by-step plan that ensures the knowledge, skills, monitoring, and motivation necessary for effective management of the problem. Because of effective behavioral interventions that are available for stress management and relaxation in situations associated with physiological arousal, muscle tension, and breathing irregularities, mental health professionals have an opportunity to provide a valuable contribution to the pediatric arena.

REFERENCES

Achenbach, T. M. (1991). *Manual for the Child Behavior Checklist/4–18 and 1991 Profile*. Burlington: University of Vermont Department of Psychiatry.

Allen, K. D., Barone, V. J., and Kuhn, B. R. (1993). A behavioral prescription for promoting applied behavior analysis within pediatrics. *Journal of Applied Behavior Analysis* 26:493–502.

Allen, K. D., and McKeen, L. R. (1991). Home-based multicomponent treatment of pediatric migraine. *Headache* 31:467–472.

Angell, M. (1985). Letter to the editor: disease as a reflection of the psyche. *New England Journal of Medicine* 312:1570–1572.

Barsky, A. J., and Klerman, G. L. (1983). Overview: hypochondriasis, bodily complaints, and somatic styles. *American Journal of Psychiatry* 140:273–283.

Beidel, D. C. (1988). Psychophysiological assessment of anxious emotional states in children. *Journal of Abnormal Psychology* 97:80–82.

——— (1991). Social phobia and overanxious disorder in school-age children. *Journal of the American Academy of Child and Adolescent Psychiatry* 30:545–552.

Beidel, D. C., Christ, M. A. G., and Long, P. J. (1991). Somatic complaints in anxious children. *Journal of Abnormal Child Psychology* 19:659–670.

Beidel, D. C., Turner, S. M., and Dancu, C. V. (1985). Physiological, cognitive and behavioral aspects of social anxiety. *Behaviour Research and Therapy* 23:109–117.

Blount, R. L., Powers, S. W., Cotter, M. W., et al. (1994). Making the system work: training pediatric oncology patients to cope and their parents to coach them during BMA/LP procedures. *Behavior Modification* 18:6–31.

Blount, R. L., Corbin, S. M., Sturges, J. W., et al. (1989). The relationship between adults' behavior and child coping and distress during BMA/LP procedures: a sequential analysis. *Behavior Therapy* 20:585–601.

Brickman, P., Rabinowitz, V. C., Karuza, J., et al. (1982). Models of helping and coping. *American Psychologist* 37:368–384.

Burke, E. J., and Andrasik, F. (1989). Home- vs. clinic-based biofeedback treatment for pediatric migraine: results of treatment through one-year follow-up. *Headache* 29:434–440.

Cohen, F., Horowitz, M., Lazarus, R., et al. (1982). Panel report of psychosocial assets and modifiers of stress. In *Stress and Human Health: Analysis and Implications of Research*, ed. G. R. Elliot and C. Eisdorfer, pp. 147–188. New York: Springer-Verlag.

Compas, B. E., Worsham, N. L., and Ey, S. (1992). Conceptual and developmental issues in children's coping with distress. In *Stress and Coping in Child Health*, ed. A. M. La Greca, L. J. Siegel, J. L. Wallander, and C. E. Walker, pp. 303–326. New York: Guilford.

Creer, T. L., and Bender, B. G. (1993). Asthma. In *Psychophysiological Disorders*, ed. R. J. Gatchel and E. B. Blanchard, pp. 151–203. Washington, DC: American Psychological Association.

Derogatis, L. R., Lipman, R. S., Rickels, K., et al. (1974). The Hopkins Symptom Checklist. *Behavioral Science* 19:1–15.

Diagnostic and Statistical Manual of Mental Disorders (1980). 3rd ed. Washington, DC: American Psychiatric Association.

_____ (1987). 3rd ed., rev. Washington, DC: American Psychiatric Association.

_____ (1994). 4th ed. Washington, DC: American Psychiatric Association.

Drabman, R. S., Allen, J. S., Jr., Tarnowski, K. J., et al. (1990). Behavior modification with children: the generalisation trap. *Behaviour Change* 7:163–171.

Duckro, P. N., and Cantwell-Simmons, E. (1989). A review of studies evaluating biofeedback and relaxation training in the management of pediatric headache. *Headache* 29:428–433.

Dunn, L. M., and Dunn, L. M. (1981). *Peabody Picture Vocabulary Test-Revised*. Circle Pines, MN: American Guidance Service.

Eiser, C., Town, C., and Tripp, J. H. (1988). Illness experience and related knowledge amongst children with asthma. *Child Care Health Development* 14:11–24.

Engel, J. M., Rapoff, M. A., and Pressman, A. R. (1992). Long-term follow-up of relaxation training for pediatric headache disorders. *Headache* 32:152–156.

Fentress, D. W., Masek, B. J., Mehegan, J. E., and Benson, H. (1986). Biofeedback and relaxation response training in the treatment of pediatric migraine. *Developmental Medicine and Child Neurology* 28:139–146.

Folkman, S. (1984). Personal control and stress and coping processes: a theoretical analysis. *Journal of Personality and Social Psychology* 4:839–852.

Fox, J. E., and Houston, B. K. (1983). Distinguishing between cognitive and somatic trait and state anxiety in children. *Journal of Personality and Social Psychology* 45:862–870.

Friedman, H. S., and Booth-Kewley, S. (1987). The "disease-prone" personality: a meta-analytic view of the construct. *American Psychologist* 42:539–555.

Gaffney, A., and Gaffney, P. R. (1987). Clinical note: recurrent abdominal pain in children and the endogenous opiates: a brief hypothesis. *Pain* 30:217–219.

Gagnon, D. J., Hudnall, L., and Andrasik, F. (1992). Biofeedback and related procedures in coping with stress. In *Stress and Coping in Child Health*, ed. A. M. La Greca, L. J. Siegel, J. L. Wallander, and C. E. Walker, pp. 303–326. New York: Guilford.

Garber, J., Walker, L. S., and Zeman, J. L. (1991). Somatization symptoms in a community sample of children and adolescents: further validation of the Children's Somatization Inventory. *Psychological Assessment: A Journal of Consulting and Clinical Psychology* 3:580–595.

Gross, A. M., and Johnson, W. G. (1981). The diabetes assertiveness test: a measure of coping skills in preadolescent diabetics. *The Diabetes Educator* 7:26–27.

Hermecz, D. A., and Melamed, B. G. (1984). The assessment of emotional imagery training in fearful children. *Behavior Therapy* 15:156–172.

Hersen, M. (1970). Behavior modification approach to a school-phobia case. *Journal of Clinical Psychology* 26:128–132.

Hoch, T. A., Babbitt, R. L., Coe, D. A., et al. (1994). Contingency contacting:

combining positive reinforcement and escape extinction procedures to treat persistent food refusal. *Behavior Modification* 18:106–128.

Hodges, K., McKnew, D., Cytryn, L., et al. (1982). The Child Assessment Schedule (CAS) Diagnostic Interview: a report on reliability and validity. *Journal of the American Academy of Child and Adolescent Psychiatry* 21:468–473.

Jackson, W. D., and Grand, R. J. (1991). Ulcerative colitis. In *Pediatric Gastrointestinal Disease: Pathology, Diagnosis, Management*, vol. 1, ed. W. A. Walker, P. R. Durie, J. R. Hamilton, et al., pp. 608–618. Philadelphia: B. C. Decker.

Kearney, C. A., Drabman, R. S., and Beasley, J. F. (1993). The trials of childhood: the development, reliability and validity of the Daily Life Stressors Scale for children and adolescents. *Journal of Child and Family Studies* 2:371–388.

Keefe, F. J., Wilkins, R. H., and Cook, W. A. (1984). Direct observation of pain behavior in low back pain patients during physical examination. *Pain* 20:59–68.

King, N. J., Ollendick, T. H., and Gullone, E. (1990). Desensitisation of childhood fears and phobias: psychophysiological analyses. *Behaviour Change* 7:66–75.

Korbon, G. A., DeGood, D. E., Schroeder, M. E., et al. (1987). The development of a somatic amplification rating scale for low back pain. *Spine* 12:787–791.

Kovacs, M., and Beck, A. T. (1977). An empirical-clinical approach toward a definition of childhood depression. In *Depression in Childhood: Diagnosis, Treatment, and Conceptual Models*, ed. J. G. Schulterbrandt and A. E. Raskin, pp. 1–25. New York: Raven.

Lambert, N. M., and Windmiller, M. B. (1981). *AAMD Adaptive Behavior Scale-School edition*. Monterey, CA: Publishers Test Service.

Larsson, B., and Melin, L. (1986). Chronic headaches in adolescents: treatment in a school setting with relaxation training as compared with information-contact and self-registration. *Pain* 25:325–336.

Larsson, B., Daleflod, B., Hakansson, L., and Melin, L. (1987a). Chronic headaches in adolescents: therapist-assisted versus self-help relaxation treatment of chronic headaches in adolescents, a school-based intervention. *Journal of Child Psychology* 28:127–136.

Larsson, B., Melin, L., Lamminen, M., and Ullstedt, F. (1987b). School-based treatment of chronic headaches in adolescents. *Journal of Pediatric Psychology* 12:553–566.

Last, C. G. (1991). Somatic complaints in anxiety disordered children. *Journal of Anxiety Disorders* 5:125–138.

Lazarus, R. S., and Folkman, S. (1984). *Stress, Appraisal, and Coping*. New York: Springer-Verlag.

Leikin, L., Firestone, P., and McGrath, P. (1988). Physical symptom reporting in Type A and Type B children. *Journal of Consulting and Clinical Psychology* 56:721–726.

Livingston, R., Taylor, J. L., and Crawford, S. L. (1988). A study of somatic complaints and psychiatric diagnosis in children. *Journal of the American Academy of Child and Adolescent Psychiatry* 27:185–187.

Lofland, K. R. (1994). Somatic amplification in chronic low-back pain patients:

development of a multimodal assessment battery. *Dissertation Abstracts International* 55-02B:599.

Maddux, J. E., and Rogers, R. W. (1983). Protection motivation and self-efficacy: a revised theory of fear appeals and attitude change. *Journal of Experimental Social Psychology* 19:469–479.

Marlatt, G. A. (1985). Relapse prevention: theoretical rationale and overview of the model. In *Relapse Prevention: Maintenance Strategies in the Treatment of Addictive Behaviors*, ed. G. A. Marlatt and J. R. Gordon, pp. 3–70. New York: Guilford.

Matthews, K. (1982). Psychological perspectives on the Type A behavior pattern. *Psychological Bulletin* 91:293–323.

Matthews, K., and Angulo, J. (1980). Measurement of the Type A behavior pattern in children: assessment of children's competitiveness, impatience-anger, and aggression. *Child Development* 51:466–475.

McGrath, P. A. (1990). *Pain in Children: Nature, Assessment, and Treatment.* New York: Guilford.

Nelles, W. B., and Barlow, D. H. (1988). Do children panic? *Clinical Psychology Review* 8:359–372.

Nihira, K., Foster, R., Shellhaas, M., and Leland, H. (1974). *AAMD Adaptive Behavior Scale*, rev. ed. Washington, DC: American Association on Mental Deficiency.

Noordenbos, W. (1959). *Pain: Problems Pertaining to the Transmission of Nerve Impulses which Give Rise to Pain; Preliminary Statement.* Amsterdam: Elsevier.

Nowicki, S., and Strickland, B. R. (1973). A locus of control scale for children. *Journal of Consulting and Clinical Psychology* 40:148–154.

Ollendick, T. H. (1983). Reliability and validity of the revised Fear Survey Schedule for Children (FSSC-R). *Behaviour Research and Therapy* 21:685–692.

Parcel, G. S., and Meyer, M. P. (1978). Development of an instrument to measure children's health locus of control. *Health Education Monographs* 6:149–159.

Peterson, L. (1989). Coping by children undergoing stressful medical procedures: some conceptual, methodological, and therapeutic issues. *Journal of Consulting and Clinical Psychology* 57:380–387.

Peterson, C., Seligman, M. E. P., and Valliant, G. E. (1988). Pessimistic explanatory style is a risk factor for physical illness: a thirty-five-year longitudinal study. *Journal of Personality and Social Psychology* 55:23–27.

Piers, E. V. (1984). *Piers-Harris Children's Self-Concept Scale: Revised Manual 1984.* Los Angeles, CA: Western Psychological Services.

Radius, R. M., Becker, M. H., Rosenstock, I. M., et al. (1978). Factors influencing mothers' compliance with a medication regimen for asthmatic children. *Journal of Asthma Research* 15:133–149.

Rapee, R. (1987). The psychological treatment of panic attacks: theoretical conceptualization and review of evidence. *Clinical Psychology Review* 7:427–438.

Reschly, D. J. (1990). Adaptive behavior. In *Best Practices in School Psychology*, ed. A. Thomas and J. Grimes, 2nd ed., pp. 29–42. Washington, DC: National Association of School Psychologists.

Reiss, S., and McNally, R. J. (1985). Expectancy model of fear. In *Theoretical Issues in Behavior Therapy*, ed. S. Reiss and R. R. Bootzin, pp. 107–121. New York: Academic Press.

Reynolds, C. R., and Richman, B. O. (1978). What I think and feel?: a revised measure of children's manifest anxiety. *Journal of Abnormal Child Psychology* 6:271–280.

Richter, I., McGrath, P., Humphreys, P., et al. (1986). Cognitive and relaxation treatment of paediatric migraine. *Pain* 25:195–203.

Rodin, J., and Solovey, P. (1989). Health psychology. *Annual Reviews in Psychology* 40:533–579.

Sheffer, A. L. (1991). Guidelines for the diagnosis and management of asthma. *Pediatric Asthma, Allergy, and Immunology* 5:57–188.

Siegel, L. J. (1990). Somatic disorders of childhood and adolescence. *School Psychology Review* 19:174–185.

Siegel, L. J., and Richards, C. S. (1978). Behavioral interventions with somatic disorders in children. In *Child Behavior Therapy*, ed. D. Marholin, pp. 339–394. New York: Gardner.

Silverman, W. K., Fleisig, W., Rabian, B., and Peterson, R. A. (1991). Childhood Anxiety Sensitivity Index. *Journal of Clinical Child Psychology* 20:162–168.

Sly, R. M. (1987). Evolving views of asthma: past and present. In *Childhood Asthma: Pathophysiology and Treatment*, ed. D. G. Tinkelman, C. J. Falliers, and C. K. Naspitz, pp. 81–100. New York: Marcel Dekker.

Sparrow, S. S., Balla, D. A., and Cicchetti, D. V. (1984). *Vineland Adaptive Behavior Scales*. Circle Pines, MN: American Guidance Service.

Spielberger, C. D. (1973). *Manual for the State-Trait Anxiety Inventory for Children*. Palo Alto, CA: Consulting Psychologists Press.

Spitzer, R. L., Gibbon, M., Skodol, A. E., et al. (1989). *DSM-III-R Casebook: A Learning Companion to the Diagnostic and Statistical Manual of Mental Disorders*, rev. ed. Washington, DC: American Psychiatric Press.

Spykerboer, J. E., Donnelly, W. J., and Thong, Y. H. (1986). Parental knowledge and misconceptions about asthma: a controlled study. *Social Science and Medicine* 22:553–558.

Stokes, T. F., and Baer, D. M. (1977). An implicit technology of generalization. *Journal of Applied Behavior Analysis* 10:349–367.

Stokes, T. F., Boggs, S. R., and Osnes, P. G. (1989). Separation anxiety disorder and school phobia. In *Casebook of Child and Pediatric Psychology*, ed. M. C. Roberts and C. E. Walker, pp. 71–93. New York: Guilford.

Stokes, T. F., and Osnes, P. G. (1989). An operant pursuit of generalization. *Behavior Therapy* 20:337–355.

Strauss, C. C., Lease, C. A., Last, C. G., and Francis, G. (1988). Overanxious disorder: an examination of developmental differences. *Journal of Abnormal Child Psychology* 16:433–443.

Taggart, V. S., Zuckerman, A. E., Sly, R. M., et al. (1991). You can control asthma: evaluation of an asthma education program for hospitalized inner-city children. *Patient Education and Counseling* 17:35–43.

Taylor, G. H., Rea, H. H., McNaughton, S., et al. (1991). A tool for measuring the asthma self-management competency of families. *Journal of Psychosomatic Research* 35:483–491.

Wilson, G. T., O'Leary, K. D., and Nathan, P. (1992). *Abnormal Psychology.* Englewood Cliffs, NJ: Prentice-Hall.

Wisniewski, J. J., Genshaft, J., Mulick, J., et al. (1988). Relaxation therapy and compliance in the treatment of adolescent headache. *Headache* 28:612–617.

Wisniewski, J. J., Naglieri, J. A., and Mulick, J. A. (1988). Psychometric properties of a children's psychosomatic symptom checklist. *Journal of Behavioral Medicine* 11:497–507.

Young, L. D. (1992). Psychological factors in rheumatoid arthritis. *Journal of Consulting and Clinical Psychology* 60:619–627.

14

DEALING WITH COMORBIDITY

Sean Perrin
Cynthia G. Last

INTRODUCTION

The development of structured diagnostic interviews and improvements in
the *Diagnostic and Statistical Manual for Mental Disorders* (*DSM-III* and
DSM-III-R) (1980, 1987) over the last decade have led to increased interest in
psychiatric disorders (Maser and Cloninger 1990). As a result, efforts have
been made to establish the prevalence of psychiatric disorder in the community. Epidemiological studies now indicate that anxiety disorders are among
the most prevalent psychiatric disorders in children and adolescents in the
community (8.7–21 percent for any anxiety disorder) (Anderson et al. 1987,
Kashani and Orvaschel 1988). Moreover, between one-third and two-thirds
of the anxiety-disordered children suffer from comorbid behavior and depressive disorders (Anderson et al. 1987, Bird et al. 1993, Flament et al. 1988;
Kashani et al. 1987). Such findings are significant because children with
multiple disorders may be more disadvantaged in later life than children
without multiple disorders (Anderson et al. 1989).

Despite these findings and their implications for the treatment of
anxiety disorders, research on comorbidity is relatively new. The recency of
interest in comorbidity is due, in part, to hierarchical exclusionary rules,
present in *DSM-III*, that precluded the assignment of anxiety disorders in
combination with several other disorders (DiNardo and Barlow 1990). These
exclusionary rules received little empirical support and were largely removed
or modified in *DSM-III-R*, resulting in increased interest in comorbidity
(DiNardo and Barlow 1990). However, the extant research on this topic is
primarily of a descriptive nature (i.e., what disorders tend to co-occur).

Previous chapters in this book have discussed in detail issues related to
the treatment of the specific anxiety disorder subtypes. These chapters reflect

the considerable advancements made in the assessment and treatment of anxiety disorder over the last fifteen years. Yet, it is clear from the available research that anxious children rarely present for treatment with a single disorder. As there are few treatment-outcome studies of anxiety disordered children in general, our understanding of the impact of comorbidity on treatment is extremely limited. Still, comorbidity does have important implications for the treatment of anxious individuals (Brown and Barlow 1992). In this chapter, we briefly review some important conceptual issues in the study of comorbidity and provide some of the most recent findings on patterns of comorbidity among the anxiety disorder subtypes. We then offer some suggestions for modifying existing treatment approaches to anxiety disorders to account for comorbidity. As there have been no systematic studies of comorbidity with post-traumatic stress disorder (PTSD) in children, we do not discuss this disorder. Finally, the reader should note that while the majority of published studies have focused on the co-occurrence of anxiety, behavior, and depressive disorders, other Axis I and II disorders may be observed in anxious children.

DEFINING COMORBIDITY

Numerous definitions of comorbidity can be found in the psychiatric literature (see Brown and Barlow 1992 and Maser and Cloninger 1990 for a review). In its most general sense, psychiatric comorbidity refers to the co-occurrence of two or more distinct diagnostic entities at one point in time (i.e., cross-sectional comorbidity) (Brown and Barlow 1992). While most studies focus on cross-sectional comorbidity, comorbidity also can be examined from a longitudinal perspective (e.g., all disorders occurring over the lifetime) (Brown and Barlow 1992). Longitudinal or lifetime comorbidity rates are usually higher than comorbidity rates obtained from cross-sectional studies and provide a more complete picture of the relationships among disorders.

An additional distinction made among comorbid disorders is their primary or secondary status (Brown and Barlow 1992). The terms *primary* and *secondary* can refer to either the temporal or causal relationships among the disorders or their varying levels of symptomatology (Brown and Barlow 1992). Thus, in relationship to the secondary disorders, the primary disorder may be the one that came first, caused the others, or had the greatest level of severity and impairment.

Comorbidity as defined above should be distinguished from symptom comorbidity, or the co-occurrence of symptoms from distinct disorders. It has been suggested that emphasizing diagnostic comorbidity over symptom comorbidity results in a significant loss of information that may be useful to our understanding and treatment of anxious individuals (Brown and Barlow 1992). For example, a child with prominent symptoms of both separation anxiety disorder and major depression may be found to meet *DSM-III-R* criteria for the anxiety disorder only. Clearly, this categorical approach does not describe the full symptom profile of the child and therefore has limited utility in both a descriptive and prescriptive sense. A classification approach that accounted for several different dimensions of symptomatology simultaneously (see DiNardo and Barlow 1990) might be more useful to the clinician in the treatment process.

WHY DOES COMORBIDITY OCCUR?

Why comorbidity occurs has been the subject of much debate in the psychiatric literature recently. Briefly, this debate has focused on methodological and substantive interpretations of comorbidity (see Angold and Costello 1993 and Maser and Cloninger 1990). Methodological interpretations of comorbidity point to the considerable symptom overlap among different disorders, the varying methods of aggregating psychiatric data for assigning diagnoses, and the artificial nature of a categorical approach to classifying psychiatric disorders. In simpler terms, this approach suggests that comorbidity is simply an artifact of the way we define and assess the individual psychiatric disorders. Thus, the high rates of comorbidity found with anxiety disorders may not reflect any true relationship among co-occurring disorders, but their poor discriminant validity (Brown and Barlow 1992).

Alternative interpretations seek to explain comorbidity through an examination of the processes underlying the development of different psychiatric disorders (Angold and Costello 1993). From a substantive perspective, anxiety and depressive disorders may co-occur frequently because (a) they share similar risk factors (e.g., familial psychopathology), (b) they are alternative outcomes of one underlying disease process (e.g., emotional upset), (c) one disorder is actually part of the other, and/or (d) one disorder causes the other (Angold and Costello 1993).

Whether comorbidity is simply a methodological artifact of our current nosological system or is in fact an accurate reflection of the complex nature of psychiatric illness remains to be seen. Epidemiological, family-history, and prospective studies are needed to clarify this issue. While we await the outcome of additional research, a chapter on comorbidity is pertinent to clinicians working with anxiety-disordered children. Comorbidity can directly influence the selection of target behaviors for treatment, sequencing of interventions, the appropriateness of pharmacological interventions, and the need for placement in school-based programs for children with emotional and/or behavior disturbances. Unfortunately, the impact of comorbidity on the course and treatment of anxiety disorders has received scant attention.

EVIDENCE OF COMORBIDITY IN NONREFERRED CHILDREN WITH ANXIETY DISORDER

For the most part, epidemiological investigations have limited usefulness to researchers interested in comorbidity for the individual anxiety disorders. However, in nonreferred children with anxiety disorder, epidemiological studies indicate that between 15 and 38 percent meet criteria for at least one additional anxiety disorder (Kashani and Orvaschel 1988, McGee et al. 1990). In both studies, children with separation anxiety disorder and over-anxious disorder predominate, indicating considerable comorbidity among these disorders in the community. Flament and colleagues (1988) provide data on comorbidity for nonreferred children with obsessive-compulsive disorder. Half of the twenty subjects in their study were found to have a concurrent psychiatric disorder (75 percent lifetime). The most common additional disorders in this group of OCD children were major depression/dysthymia (30 percent), overanxious disorder (20 percent), and social and simple phobias (10 percent) (Flament et al. 1988).

In terms of comorbidity with other psychiatric disorders, estimates of the prevalence of depressive disorders in anxious children range considerably, from 7 to 17 percent (Anderson et al. 1987, Bird et al. 1993, McGee et al. 1990, Velez et al. 1989), to as high as 69 percent (Kashani et al. 1987). Consistently high rates of comorbid conduct and/or oppositional defiant disorders have also been reported in anxious children (i.e., 23–62 percent) (Anderson et al. 1987, Bird et al. 1993, Kashani et al. 1987). Finally, about one-quarter (22–24 percent) of anxiety-disordered children have been found to have a comorbid diagnosis of attention deficit hyperactivity disorder (ADHD) (Anderson et al. 1987, Bird et al. 1993). It should be noted that while rates of comorbidity vary considerably across epidemiological studies, they are often more than double that expected by chance, and are probably underestimates of the true rate of comorbidity in children (Caron and Rutter

1991). This has led some to conclude that comorbidity is the rule and not the exception in children with psychiatric disorders (Bird et al. 1993).

EVIDENCE OF COMORBIDITY IN CLINICALLY REFERRED CHILDREN WITH ANXIETY DISORDER

Very few studies have reported rates of comorbidity for children seeking treatment for anxiety disorder. Two of the most extensive investigations have been conducted by Last and colleagues (1987, 1992). In the first study, patterns of cross-sectional comorbidity were examined in fifty-seven children with separation anxiety disorder, overanxious disorder, social phobia of school, and major depression. More recently, longitudinal (i.e., lifetime) patterns of comorbidity among all the anxiety disorder subtypes were examined in 188 anxiety-disordered children. For the sake of clarity we present comorbidity data for the individual anxiety disorders from these two studies below. Additional studies of comorbidity with anxiety disorder are also presented where available.

Separation Anxiety Disorder (SAD)

Comorbidity with Other Anxiety Disorders

In a study of twenty-four clinically referred children with a primary diagnosis of SAD, Last et al. (1987) found 42 percent to meet criteria for a concurrent anxiety disorder. While this rate of additional anxiety disorders is high, it was lower than that found for children with a primary diagnosis of OAD (55 percent), social phobia (64 percent), or major depression (100 percent) (Last et al. 1987). The most common additional anxiety disorders in the SAD group were overanxious disorder (34 percent), simple phobia (13 percent), and avoidant disorder (13 percent). Panic and obsessive-compulsive disorders were infrequent (4–7 percent each) (Last et al. 1987, Last et al. 1992). The low frequency of panic disorder in SAD children cited above is consistent with previous studies that have failed to find support for the hypothesized relationship between the two disorders (see Thyer 1993 for a review).

Comorbidity with Depressive Disorders

Children with SAD often express symptoms of sadness, apathy, and difficulty concentrating during separation situations (Last 1992), and full-blown depressive disorders are not uncommon. Last and colleagues (1987) observed dysthymic disorder in 13 percent and major depression in 8 percent of twenty-four children with SAD. When considering a lifetime history of depression, the rate of depressive disorders among eighty-four children with SAD was 33 percent (Last et al. 1992). Children seeking treatment for school refusal and/or a primary mood disturbance have been found to have higher rates of concurrent SAD and depression (31-71 percent) (Ambrosini et al. 1989, Bernstein and Garfinkel 1986, Geller et al. 1985, Kovacs et al. 1989, Ryan et al. 1987). While this latter finding may reflect a referral bias, anxiety disorders, in general, are more common in nonreferred depressed children than the reverse (Angold and Costello 1993).

Comorbidity with Behavior Disorders

Approximately 17 percent of the children with SAD in the Last and colleagues' study (1987) met criteria for a concurrent diagnosis of oppositional defiant disorder or attention deficit hyperactivity disorder (ADHD). Again the lifetime rate of behavior disorders was slightly higher (23 percent) (Last et al. 1992). This latter finding is consistent with a recent study of 140 clinically referred children with ADHD, about 30 percent of whom were diagnosed with SAD (Biederman et al. 1993).

Overanxious Disorder (OAD)

Comorbidity with Other Anxiety Disorders

Of all the anxiety disorder subtypes, children with OAD have been found to have the highest rate of additional anxiety disorder (Last et al. 1987, Last et al. 1992). In a large sample of children with OAD (n = 51), Last et al. (1992) found that nearly all (96 percent) had an additional anxiety disorder at one time in their lives. The most frequent additional anxiety disorders in this group were social phobias (57 percent), simple phobias (43 percent), and SAD (37 percent) (Last et al. 1992). Rates of concurrent anxiety disorder were somewhat lower in a separate study: social phobia 36 percent, avoidant disorder 27 percent, and SAD 9 percent (Last et al. 1987).

Developmental differences in the expression of OAD were examined by Strauss and colleagues (1988b). In that study, SAD was found more frequently in younger children with OAD (70 percent) than those over the age of 12 (22 percent). By contrast, simple phobias were more common among older than younger children with OAD (41 percent vs. 9 percent, respectively) (Strauss et al. 1988b).

Comorbidity with Depressive Disorders

There appears to be a strong relationship between OAD and depression in children. In the Last and colleagues study (1992), a lifetime history of either major depression or dysthymia was found in nearly half (49 percent) of the fifty-one children with OAD. Only children with social phobias had a higher lifetime rate of depressive disorders (56 percent) (Last et al. 1992). Similar rates of comorbid OAD and depression (16–50 percent) have been found in children referred for a primary depressive disorder (Ambrosini et al. 1989, Kovacs et al. 1989, Ryan et al. 1987). Again, in terms of developmental differences in OAD, major depression was found more frequently among adolescents (47 percent) than younger children with this disorder (17 percent) (Strauss et al. 1988b).

Comorbidity with Behavior Disorders

A lifetime history of behavior disorder (i.e., oppositional defiant disorder, ADHD, and conduct disorder) was found in 20 percent of children with OAD by Last and colleagues (1992). Slightly higher rates of OAD (30 percent) have been found in children with ADHD (Biederman et al. 1993, McClellan et al. 1990). In terms of the specific behavior disorders, oppositional-defiant disorder appears more frequently than ADHD (36 vs. 18 percent, respectively) as a concurrent behavior disorder among children with OAD (Last et al. 1987). Not unexpectedly, ADHD is more common among younger children than adolescents with OAD (35 vs. 9 percent, respectively) (Strauss et al. 1988b).

Avoidant Disorder of Childhood and Adolescence (AD)

Comorbidity with Other Anxiety Disorders

The clinical features of AD overlap to some extent with generalized social phobic disorder, and there is some debate as to the distinctiveness of the two disorders (Francis et al. 1992). Almost two-thirds (65 percent) of the avoidant-disordered children in Last and colleagues' study (1992) were diagnosed with an additional social phobia (lifetime). Moreover, the onset of avoidant disorder either coincided or overlapped temporally with social phobia in all of the children with both disorders. After social phobias, OAD (60 percent) and SAD (35 percent) were the most frequent additional anxiety disorders (lifetime) in children with AD (Last et al. 1992).

Comorbidity with Depressive Disorders

Francis et al. (1992) observed concurrent depressive disorders in 27 percent of forty-one children with a current diagnosis of AD. A slightly higher rate of depression (35 percent) was found by Last et al. (1992) in a separate study of twenty children with a lifetime history of AD. By contrast, Ambrosini and colleagues (1989) observed AD, concurrently, in only 6 percent of sixteen children referred for an affective disorder.

Comorbidity with Behavior Disorders

There are few published reports that have examined patterns of comorbidity between AD and ADHD, oppositional defiant disorder, or conduct disorder. Last and colleagues (1992) found a lifetime history of these behavior disorders in 15 percent of twenty children with AD. Only children with social phobia had a lower lifetime rate of behavior disorders (i.e., 8 percent) (Last et al. 1992). While further studies are needed to determine if there is any relationship between AD and behavior disorders, this finding is consistent with the clinical presentation of AD children who are often shy and reserved in their behavior toward others (Last 1992).

Social and Simple Phobias

Comorbidity with Other Anxiety Disorders

Strauss and Last (1993) compared children with simple phobia (n = 38) and social phobia (n = 29) for rates of concurrent anxiety disorders. More than half the subjects in both groups met criteria for at least one additional anxiety disorder, mostly OAD and SAD. The two groups differed only in terms of the rate of concurrent OAD (social phobics 41 percent, simple phobics 16 percent), and avoidant disorder (social phobics 21 percent, simple phobics 3 percent).

Comorbidity with Depressive Disorders

In the Strauss and Last study (1993), concurrent depressive disorders were found more frequently among social phobic (17 percent) than simple phobic (5 percent) children (Strauss and Last 1993). In a separate study, a lifetime history of depressive disorders (any) was found in 56 percent of social phobics as compared to only 33 percent of the simple phobics (Last et al. 1992). Further examination of those children with a history of both major depression and social phobia found that in 74 percent of the cases, the social phobia preceded the onset of major depression. This finding suggests that social phobia may be a significant risk factor for the development of depressive disorders in children. Several studies of clinically referred children with a primary depressive disorder have found high rates (25–45 percent) of concurrent phobias (both simple and social) (Ambrosini et al. 1989, Ryan et al. 1987). However, the temporal relationships among these disorders were not specifically examined.

Comorbidity with Behavior Disorders

Behavior disorders were found more frequently among children with simple phobias than social phobias (15.4 percent vs. 6.8 percent, respectively) (Strauss and Last 1993). This pattern held true when examining the lifetime rates of behavior disorder in the two phobia groups (simple phobia 23 percent and social phobia 8 percent) (Last et al. 1992). Biederman and colleagues (1993) report similar findings for social phobia (13 percent) in clinically referred children with ADHD.

Panic Disorder (PD)

Comorbidity with Anxiety Disorders

The most frequent additional anxiety disorders (lifetime) in clinically referred children with PD were OAD (30 percent) and social phobias (26 percent) (Last et al. 1992). Of those children with a lifetime history of both OAD and PD, the OAD preceded the onset of PD in the majority of cases (90 percent) (Last et al. 1992). This temporal relationship between the two disorders is consistent with the hypothesis suggesting that generalized anxiety disorder (OAD in children) may increase the risk for panic disorder (Barlow et al. 1986, Lader and Matthews 1968). Interestingly, very few of the PD adolescents (13 percent) in the Last and colleagues study (1992) had a prior history of SAD, which does not support the previously hypothesized relationship between the two disorders (Last et al. 1992). While Alessi and Magen (1988) found SAD in five of seven children (86 percent) hospitalized with PD, this finding may be peculiar to this small sample of severely disordered children.

Comorbidity with Depressive Disorders

Few studies have examined patterns of comorbidity between depression and PD in adolescents. However, in the Alessi and Magen study (1988) of seven hospitalized children with PD, 57 percent were found to meet criteria for a concurrent depressive disorder. Last and Strauss (1989b) observed a much lower rate of concurrent depressive disorder (12 percent) in seventeen children and adolescents with PD referred to an outpatient clinic. This latter finding is consistent with the rate of concurrent depressive disorders found in panic disordered adults (see Brown and Barlow 1992). Similarly, Kovacs and colleagues (1989) observed very few cases (2 percent) of PD in children with a primary depressive disorder. However, there does appear to be a higher rate of comorbidity between the two disorders when viewed from a longitudinal perspective. Last and colleagues (1992) found a lifetime history of depressive disorders in 42 percent of PD children and adolescents, a finding consistent with a previous study examining the lifetime history of depression in adults with PD (Breir et al. 1984).

Comorbidity with Behavior Disorders

Last and Strauss (1989b) found concurrent behavior disorders in 12 percent of their sample of PD children and adolescents. Biederman and colleagues (1993) report a similar finding for the rate of concurrent PD in ADHD (i.e., 9 percent). When viewed from a lifetime perspective, the rate of additional behavior disorders in PD was somewhat higher (25 percent) (Last et al. 1992).

Obsessive-Compulsive Disorder (OCD)

Comorbidity with Other Anxiety Disorders

The most frequent additional anxiety disorders in children with OCD are OAD and simple phobias. In a study of clinically referred adolescents with OCD, Swedo and colleagues (1989) observed OAD in 16 percent and simple phobias in 17 percent. Last and Strauss (1989a) found slightly higher rates of concurrent simple phobias (35 percent), OAD (25 percent), SAD (20 percent), and social phobia (20 percent) in OCD children.

Comorbidity with Depressive Disorders

Last and Strauss (1989a) observed concurrent depressive disorders in only 10 percent of the children with OCD in their study. This relatively low rate of comorbidity between OCD and depression is consistent with that found in depressed children (2–13 percent) (Ambrosini et al. 1989, Kovacs et al. 1989). By contrast, Swedo and colleagues (1989) reported a much higher rate (i.e., 30 percent) of concurrent depressive disorders in seventy children who participated in a clomipramine treatment study at NIMH. This latter finding is consistent with lifetime rates of depressive disorder found in OCD (20–35 percent) by Last and colleagues (1987, 1992).

Comorbidity with Behavior Disorders

There are limited and conflicting findings for the rate of behavior disorders in OCD. Swedo and colleagues (1989) reported concurrent behavior and/or substance abuse disorders in one-third of their sample of severely impaired children with OCD. Moreover, in the majority of cases the behavior disorder preceded the onset of OCD. However, Last and colleagues (1992) reported a much lower lifetime rate of ADHD, oppositional defiant disorder, or conduct disorder (18 percent) in twenty-eight children with OCD. No cases of behavior disorder were found in children with ADHD by Biederman and colleagues (1993).

RISK FACTORS FOR COMORBIDITY

There are fairly consistent data across epidemiological studies suggesting a relationship between age, sex, and socioeconomic status, and the prevalence of certain psychiatric disorders (Costello 1989). In general, younger children and females show higher rates of anxiety and affective disorders than older children and males, while older children and males show higher rates of behavior disorder (Costello 1989). Children from low socioeconomic (SES) backgrounds show higher rates of all disorders compared to their higher SES counterparts (Costello 1989). There are, however, few and conflicting data regarding risk factors for the presence of multiple psychiatric disorders.

With regard to age, Anderson et al. (1987) observed that nonreferred children with multiple disorders tended to have an earlier age-at-onset of psychiatric disorder than children with a single disorder. Also, Kovacs and colleagues (1989) reported that clinically referred, depressed children with comorbid anxiety disorders tended to be younger than those with depression alone. However, Strauss and colleagues (1988a) observed the opposite finding in children referred for anxiety disorder (i.e., older children showed higher rates of comorbidity). The latter study also found no relationship between race and the rate of comorbid depression in anxiety. Finally, Bird and colleagues (1993) observed no relationship between sex and pubertal status and the rate of comorbid anxiety, affective, and behavior disorders in non-referred children.

Children with anxiety and affective disorders have been found to have higher rates of familial psychopathology in their relatives when compared to nondisordered children (Hammen et al. 1990, Kovacs et al. 1989, Last et al. 1991, Turner et al. 1987, Weissman et al. 1984). There is also evidence, albeit limited, that multiple anxiety disorders in the child may be associated with a history of multiple anxiety disorders in their first degree family members (Last et al. 1991). Also, Hammen and colleagues (1990) observed that children of mothers with unipolar depression were more likely to have multiple disorders than children of nondepressed mothers. While these findings suggest a link between familial psychopathology and multiple disorders in the offspring, direct comparisons between psychiatrically disordered children with and without multiple disorders are necessary to evaluate this relationship further.

COMMENT ON COMORBIDITY STUDIES

It is clear from the limited number of articles cited above that additional studies of comorbidity are needed. However, given the available data, a few preliminary conclusions can be drawn. First, among children clinically referred for anxiety disorder, approximately half will present with more than one anxiety disorder, and between one-fourth and one-third will present with a comorbid depressive disorder. Disruptive behavior disorders were found in roughly 25 percent. Phobias and OAD are the most common additional disorder among children with another anxiety disorder. These findings are consistent with comorbidity data for anxiety, depressive, and behavior disorders obtained from epidemiological studies. In terms of the specific anxiety disorder subtypes in clinically referred children, children with OAD and social phobias were most likely to present with an additional anxiety or depressive disorder. Children with SAD had the highest rates of concurrent behavior disorder and were least likely to present with an additional anxiety disorder. Significant rates of comorbidity were found between panic disorder and OAD, and avoidant disorder and social phobia. Children with simple phobias had high rates of SAD and social phobia. Finally, simple and social phobias and OAD were common among children with OCD, but findings for depressive and behavior disorders in this group were mixed. Additional epidemiological investigations of the prevalence and risk factors associated with comorbidity for the specific anxiety disorder subtypes are needed.

DIFFERENTIAL DIAGNOSIS

Previous chapters have discussed differential diagnoses with the specific anxiety disorder subtypes; however, a few comments are warranted based on the above review of comorbidity and several changes in *DSM-IV*. The considerable symptom and syndrome overlap between avoidant disorder and social phobia have made differential diagnosis between these two disorders difficult at best. This problem should be alleviated in the fourth edition of the *DSM* (*DSM-IV*). Changes for avoidant disorder in *DSM-IV* (1994) include its removal from the child section of the manual and its incorporation with the criteria for social phobia (social anxiety disorder) in the main anxiety disorders section.

OAD was one of the most frequently assigned comorbid anxiety disorders in clinically referred children with SAD, avoidant disorder, social and simple phobias, panic disorder, and OCD. This finding is not unusual given that the somatic complaints and frequent worrying seen in OAD are not entirely unique to this anxiety disorder and are not uncommon in nonreferred children (Bell-Dolan et al. 1990). Some have even suggested that the symptoms of OAD may serve as a prodromal phase for the development of other anxiety disorders (i.e., social phobia) (Beidel 1991). In our study of clinically referred children with OAD, almost all (96 percent) had a lifetime history of at least one additional anxiety disorder (mostly social phobias) (Last et al. 1992). However, while OAD preceded the onset of social phobia in 59 percent of the children with both disorders in this study, this prodromal hypothesis was not supported for the anxiety disorders overall (i.e., OAD preceded the onset of all other anxiety disorders only 49 percent of the time). While symptoms of OAD may be seen in the other anxiety disorders and depression, OAD can be distinguished from these disorders by its hallmark symptom, worries about future events.

Still, there is considerable debate over the validity of OAD as a distinct diagnostic entity. In DSM-IV (1994), OAD is incorporated under generalized anxiety disorder (GAD) in the adult section of the manual. In contrast to DSM-III-R, where a child could meet criteria for OAD without evidencing somatic complaints or a marked inability to relax, DSM-IV requires the presence of at least three symptoms indicative of persistent autonomic arousal (e.g., restlessness, difficulty concentrating, muscle tension, fatigability, irritability, and sleep disturbance). Whether these more stringent criteria for OAD will lead to a reduction in the rates of comorbidity with OAD awaits further investigation.

Like OAD, simple and social phobias also were frequently diagnosed in children with another anxiety disorder. Again, this finding is not surprising given that circumscribed fears are common in nondisordered individuals as well (Bell-Dolan et al. 1990). Thus, the clinician must ascertain whether these symptoms are of sufficient severity and distinctiveness from other anxiety disorders to warrant diagnosis of simple or social phobia. DSM-III-R (1987) specifies several criteria for evaluating the clinical significance of fears that can help in this distinction: (a) the fear must be persistent, (b) the phobic stimulus almost invariably elicits an immediate anxiety response, (c) the phobic situation is avoided or the person has a compelling desire to avoid due to intense anxiety, (d) the individual recognizes that the fear is excessive or unreasonable (may be absent in children), and (e) there is significant impairment and/or marked distress about having the fear. For example, a child with SAD who refuses to sleep alone may additionally report a fear of the dark that appears to be related to separation anxiety. In such cases, if fear of the dark results in significant distress and avoidance, even in the presence of an attachment figure, an additional diagnosis of simple phobia may be warranted.

The developmental appropriateness of fears and other anxiety symptoms also should be considered in distinguishing between normal or subclinical anxiety and clinically significant anxiety disorders (Last 1992). Morris and Kratochwill (1983) have provided normative data on fears in children from birth to age 12 that may be useful in distinguishing fears from phobic disorders. In general, fears of loud noises, strangers, separation, and animals are common in children under 9 years of age, while social-evaluative fears are found more frequently in children 9 years and up (Morris and Kratochwill 1983). The prevalence, gender distribution, and developmental expression of symptoms of SAD, avoidant disorder, OAD, and phobias in nonreferred children also have been examined (see Bell-Dolan et al. 1990). Subclinical symptoms of OAD were equally prevalent (10–30 percent) among children of all ages, while symptoms of SAD and avoidant disorder are more common (roughly 20 percent) in younger children (i.e., less than 13 years of age) (Bell-Dolan et al. 1990).

Finally, a frequent presenting complaint of children and parents seen at our anxiety clinic is school refusal. School refusal is especially common among children with SAD, but children with other disorders (e.g., OAD, phobias, oppositional defiant disorder, and major depression) may also exhibit this problem (Last and Strauss 1990). In distinguishing school refusal resulting from SAD versus a circumscribed fear of some aspect of the school environment (e.g., being called on in class), it is often helpful to inquire where the child is when not in school (Last 1992). Children with SAD will want to remain at home or with an attachment figure, while the phobic child will be comfortable in any environment other than school. Also, children with an oppositional defiant disorder may also report a fear of school; however, further assessment usually finds that school refusal is part of a much larger pattern of noncompliant behavior. Depressed children who exhibit school refusal often show a general lack of interest in all activities.

ASSESSMENT

The assessment of multiple psychiatric disorder requires a comprehensive psychiatric interview and referral to the *specific inclusion and exclusion criteria* for psychiatric disorders outlined in the *DSM* (Last 1992). A comprehensive psychiatric assessment should include (a) interviews with both the child and parents, (b) all relevant *DSM-IV* criteria for the major Axis I categories, and

(c) some method for assessing the severity and impairment associated with symptoms and/or disorders. Interviews with both the parent and child are essential because their reports are often discrepant. Parents often emphasize the external aspects of their child's symptoms and may be unaware of particular fears or negative emotions. Children often minimize the extent and severity of their own disruptive behaviors. Rating the severity and impairment of individual symptoms and/or disorders is particularly important in assessing comorbidity. The decision to assign more than one diagnosis often depends upon the clinical significance of secondary or additional diagnoses.

In addition to semi-structured interviews, self-report questionnaires that address a wide array of symptomatology and adaptive functioning also are useful in diagnostic decision making. When completed prior to the psychiatric interview, these questionnaires can serve as helpful prompts to both parent and child to clarify vague, negative, and discrepant responses during the interview. This is especially true of children and adolescents who are often shy and/or reluctant to voice certain complaints to a stranger (e.g., "I think about killing myself"). Finally, as discussed in previous chapters in this book, direct behavioral observation of the anxious child by the therapist (where possible) also is invaluable in the assessment process. Direct observation of avoidant or disruptive behaviors, and the appearance of the child (e.g., happy or sad), may supplement both interview and questionnaire data. Teachers, while not unbiased in their reports, are also important sources of behavioral data.

ESTABLISHING TREATMENT GOALS

Comorbidity bears directly on the establishment of treatment goals and the focus of treatment. However, it is usually the case that individual symptoms and not disorders are incorporated directly into treatment goals. In the case of a child with multiple disorders, there are likely to be several prominent symptoms. Thus, an important first step in establishing treatment goals is to have the patient (and parent) rate which symptoms are most distressing and/or impairing. Active client involvement in the establishment of treatment goals is an important prerequisite to treatment compliance and successful outcome.

The decision as to which of the client-rated symptoms should be the focus of treatment bears on the issue of treatment modality and timing of interventions. Pharmacological interventions often produce a diminution in a wide variety of emotional and behavioral disturbances simultaneously. However, the long-term side effects of psychotropic drugs may outweigh their usefulness in therapy. Kendall and colleagues (1992) have suggested that a cognitive-behavioral approach provides a useful framework for integrating treatments developed separately for anxiety and depression. The same is true for certain symptoms of behavior disorder. However, at the present time, there are no empirical studies to guide treatment planning issues in children with comorbid disorders, and the clinician must rely on the available literature for the treatment of individual disorders.

ROLE OF THE THERAPIST

The role of the therapist in the treatment of anxious children with comorbid disorders is similar to that of the therapist dealing with a single disorder. These issues have been discussed in detail in previous chapters in this book. However, Kendall and colleagues (1992) have pointed out that therapists working with comorbid disorders must be aware of the potentially incompatible or synergistic effects of various treatments. For example, while relaxation training has been shown to be effective in reducing symptoms of both anxiety and depression, it may not be useful in reducing disruptive behaviors. A second consideration is the particular symptom profile of the child (Kendall et al. 1992). Two children with major depression and SAD may have vastly different symptom profiles and require different treatment approaches. Finally, the therapist should consider the developmental level of the child in treatment planning (Kendall et al. 1992). Very young children with anxiety and depression may not have the cognitive ability to engage in problem-solving and cognitive-restructuring treatments, and may not be appropriate for pharmacological interventions. Thus, the therapist working with comorbid disorders must be flexible in the use of standardized treatment packages (Kendall et al. 1992). Moreover, he or she should discuss the limitations of treatment designed for specific disorders so that the parent and the child understand that all symptoms may not remit simultaneously.

TREATMENT STRATEGIES FOR COMORBID DISORDERS

In treating anxious children with multiple disorders, we have found that it is helpful to first establish which disorder is primary and which are secondary. In a clinical sense, the term *primary* refers to the disorder with the greatest level of severity and/or impairment. The remaining disorders are designated as secondary based on their lower levels of severity and/or impairment. Targeting the most severe disorder is often necessary because of the disruption to school and family activities associated with the primary disorder. Following successful treatment of the primary disorder, secondary disorders may be treated sequentially, again depending on their associated level of severity and impairment.

As stated above, it is often useful to consider the temporal and/or causative relationships among comorbid disorders in treatment planning. Comorbid disorders may have different ages-at-onset that suggest that the earlier disorder is causing or maintaining the second. Take, for example, the case of an adolescent with a long-standing history of social phobia who develops a major depressive episode. An analysis of the relationship between the two disorders might suggest that social-evaluative anxiety has led to withdrawal from a large number of reinforcing activities, resulting in the present depressive episode. In such a case, reducing social anxiety may produce a corresponding reduction in depressed mood. Alternatively, if the disorder with the earliest age-at-onset is stable in its symptom presentation, the more recently developed disorder may be the focus of treatment. Such might be the case in a child with ADHD who is being effectively treated with stimulants but who has recently developed SAD.

Once issues of severity and temporality have been addressed, the therapist must choose the appropriate treatment(s) for the existing disorders. Unfortunately, there are no studies that have directly evaluated the simultaneous or sequential treatment of multiple disorders in anxious children. Thus, the clinician must rely on the available treatment-outcome literature on specific disorders in treatment planning. Previous chapters have discussed treatment approaches to the individual anxiety disorder subtypes. In terms of depressive disorders, treatment-outcome studies have focused primarily on the effectiveness of such pharmacological agents as tricyclic antidepressants, monoamine oxidase inhibitors, and lithium (Reynolds 1992). Findings for all three drugs are mixed, and additional clinical trials are needed (Reynolds 1992). As with the anxiety disorders, cognitive-behavioral treatment (CBT) packages developed for depressed adults have been modified for use with children with some success (see Reynolds and Coats 1986, Stark et al. 1987). Such packages typically include coping and social skills training, awareness of the relationship between mood-states and activities, and self-reinforcement. Often, the primary goal of CBT for depression is increasing the frequency of positively reinforcing experiences and the use of coping skills for reducing stress.

In terms of the disruptive behavior disorders, several studies (Dulcan 1986, Tannock et al. 1989) have demonstrated the effectiveness of stimulant medications in the treatment of ADHD. Behavior modification and CBT have yielded more mixed results (Abikoff and Klein 1992). However, behavior modification packages for ADHD typically include parent-training and classroom management procedures designed to increase on-task and prosocial behaviors, and to improve academic performance. Alternatively, CBT approaches to ADHD focus on the development of self-control strategies. Parent-training procedures that focus on reinforcement of positive and/or compliant behaviors, and CBT packages focusing on problem-solving and social skills training have received limited support for the treatment of both conduct disorder and oppositional defiant disorder (see Abikoff and Klein 1992, Wicks-Nelson and Israel 1991).

DEALING WITH COMMON OBSTACLES TO SUCCESSFUL TREATMENT

Many obstacles involved in the treatment of anxious children have been described in detail in previous chapters. Also, treatment obstacles linked with comorbid anxiety and depression have been mentioned above and described elsewhere (see Kendall et al. 1992). Briefly, the presence of comorbid disorders implies a variety of symptoms, all of which may or may not be the focus of treatment at any one point in time. When the clinician decides to target one disorder or cluster of symptoms, it is possible that the symptoms of the other comorbid disorders remain the same or get worse during treatment.

In children with both an anxiety disorder and major depression, it is often necessary to stabilize the depression before addressing the anxiety, especially if suicidal ideation is present. Severe depression can reduce the child's energy level and motivation to comply with treatment interventions. Also, children with severe depression may focus too much on the negative aspects of their own behavior and minimize the positive effects of treatment. Referral for a medication evaluation may be necessary. While there is some evidence that tricyclic antidepressants reduce symptoms of anxiety, there is only limited evidence to suggest that cognitive-behavioral treatment of an anxiety disorder may lead to a corresponding decrease in comorbid symptoms of depression.

In children with both behavior and anxiety disorders, parents are often more interested in reducing the frequency of disruptive behaviors, even when anxiety is the most severe feature of the child's symptom profile. Such a situation is not uncommon in children with anxiety-based school refusal and oppositional defiant disorder. While the primary focus of treatment may be graduated exposure to the school environment, the parents are concerned with noncompliant behaviors across a wider variety of settings. Moreover, they often assume that if the child can get back into school, he or she should automatically behave at home. Thus, they may begin to question the effectiveness of treatment and drop out. However, noncompliant behaviors and hyperactivity can interfere with standardized treatments for anxiety disorder. Thus, ensuring treatment compliance may require that disruptive behaviors be targeted first. As stated above, parent training and CBT may be used in the treatment of oppositional defiant disorder.

Another obstacle to successful treatment of anxiety arises when an untreated comorbid disorder leads to the re-emergence of previously mastered fears and anxiety. This is not an unusual occurrence in a child with a primary anxiety disorder who develops a full-blown depressive episode during treatment. The parent and the client may interpret the depression and the re-emergence of anxiety as evidence of the ineffectiveness or iatrogenic effects of therapy. In such cases, the therapist must make immediate efforts to stabilize the depression and keep the client in treatment. Often a medication evaluation is required and treatment goals should be modified to address current symptomatology.

Finally, as discussed above in the section on risk factors for comorbidity, there is evidence of an increased risk of psychopathology in the first-degree family members of children with anxiety and depressive disorders. Thus, it is not uncommon for a clinician to encounter psychopathology in the parents and siblings of children with an anxiety disorder. While no studies have directly examined this issue, anxiety and/or major depression in the parent(s) can represent a significant obstacle to the successful treatment of the anxious child.

More specifically, parental involvement is a major component of many treatment approaches for childhood anxiety disorders. An anxious parent who has similar fears and avoidant behaviors as the child may be unable or unwilling to assist in treatment. Alternatively, the parent may recall his or her own distressing experiences with the same fears and reinforce the child's avoidant behaviors. In such cases, the therapist must help the parent recognize his or her contribution to the child's anxiety. Also, it is useful to have the parent weigh the temporary nature of the child's discomfort during treatment against the long-term consequences of anxiety.

RELAPSE PREVENTION AND TERMINATION

Relapse prevention is an important issue in the treatment of children with comorbid disorders. As stated above, untreated disorders can result in the loss of previous treatment gains. Additionally, there is no empirical evidence that untreated disorders will remit during treatment. Thus, the child may be at risk for relapse or continued psychiatric disturbance following treatment of the primary disorder. In order to reduce the risk of relapse, the therapist must first consider the status of all psychiatric disorders prior to the termination of treatment. Readministration of a semistructured interview can assist in determining the status of untreated disorders. When possible, treatment should continue until all comorbid disorders have been successfully treated. In the event that the parent or child chooses not to continue in treatment, the therapist may recommend booster sessions. Booster sessions typically involve a brief review of gains and losses since termination and problem solving around continued areas of difficulty. Portions of the treatment package may also be re-administered. Making efforts to ensure that gains made in treatment have generalized to the real world setting may also reduce the risk of relapse.

SUMMARY

In this chapter, we have reviewed findings from several studies that indicate that anxiety-disordered children frequently present with multiple anxiety disorders and with comorbid depressive and behavior disorders. However, research on comorbidity is relatively new and there have been no studies examining the efficacy of treatments for multiple disorders. Thus, there are few empirical data to guide treatment planning decisions for anxiety-disordered children with comorbid disorders. For the present, cognitive-behavioral approaches to treatment may offer the best framework for dealing with comorbid disorders. Future studies will need to address this issue, as well as the impact of comorbidity on the selection and timing of disorder-specific interventions and the effectiveness of existing treatments for multiple disorders.

Finally, it has been suggested that the prevalence of comorbidity in children and adults calls into question the validity of our current diagnostic nomenclature. At present, there is an underlying assumption in the *DSM* that individual psychiatric disorders reflect distinct disease processes. However, this assumption is undermined by the considerable symptom overlap among the different psychiatric disorders and our limited understanding of their etiology. The current categorical approach to diagnostic classification is, at best, artificial and only loosely based on empirical research. While symptom or dimensional approaches to psychopathology may be more useful to therapists and researchers, it is unlikely that they will be adopted in the near future. Still, it is inevitable that the *DSM* will be modified in accordance with future studies of comorbidity.

REFERENCES

Abikoff, H., and Klein, R. G. (1992). Attention-deficit hyperactivity and conduct disorder: comorbidity and implications for treatment. *Journal of Consulting and Clinical Psychology* 60:881–892.

Alessi, N. E., and Magen, J. (1988). Panic disorder in psychiatrically hospitalized children. *American Journal of Psychiatry* 145:1450–1452.

Ambrosini, P. J., Metz, C., Prabruki, K., and Lee, J. C. (1989). Videotape reliability of the Third Revised Edition of the K-SADS. *Journal of the American Academy of Child and Adolescent Psychiatry* 28:723–728.

Anderson, J. C., Williams, S., McGee, R., and Silva, P. A. (1987). *DSM-III* disorders in preadolescent children. *Archives of General Psychiatry* 44:69–76.

_____ (1989). Cognitive and social correlates of *DSM-III* disorders in preadolescent children. *Journal of the American Academy of Child and Adolescent Psychiatry* 28:842–846.

Angold, A., and Costello, E. J. (1993). Depressive comorbidity in children and adolescents: empirical, theoretical, and methodological issues. *American Journal of Psychiatry* 150:1779–1791.

Barlow, D. H., DiNardo, P. A., Vermilyea, B. B. et al. (1986). Comorbidity and depression among the anxiety disorders: issues in diagnosis and classification. *Journal of Nervous and Mental Disease* 174:63–72.

Beidel, D. C. (1991). Social phobia and overanxious disorder in school-age children. *Journal of the American Academy of Child and Adolescent Psychiatry* 30:545–552.

Bell-Dolan, D. J., Last, C. G., and Strauss, C. C. (1990). Symptoms of anxiety disorders in normal children. *Journal of the American Academy of Child and Adolescent Psychiatry* 29:759–765.

Bernstein, G. A., and Garfinkel, B. D. (1986). School phobia: the overlap of anxiety and affective disorders. *Journal of the American Academy of Child and Adolescent Psychiatry* 25:235–241.

Biederman, J., Faraone, S., Spencer, T., et al. (1993). Patterns of psychiatric comorbidity, cognition, and psychosocial functioning in adults with attention deficit hyperactivity disorder. *American Journal of Psychiatry* 150:1792–1798.

Bird, H. R., Gould, M. S., and Staghezza, B. M. (1993). Patterns of diagnostic comorbidity in a community sample of children aged 9 through 16 years. *Journal of the American Academy of Child and Adolescent Psychiatry* 32:361–368.

Breir, A., Charney, D. S., and Heninger, G. R. (1984). Major depression in patients with agoraphobia and panic disorder. *Archives of General Psychiatry* 41:1129–1135.

Brown, T. A., and Barlow, D. H. (1992). Comorbidity among anxiety disorders:

implications for treatment and *DSM-IV*. *Journal of Consulting and Clinical Psychology* 60:835–844.

Caron, C., and Rutter, M. (1991). Comorbidity in child psychopathology: concepts, issues and research strategies. *Journal of Child Psychology and Psychiatry* 32:1063–1080.

Costello, E. J. (1989). Developments in child psychiatric epidemiology. *Journal of the American Academy of Child and Adolescent Psychiatry* 28:836–841.

Diagnostic and Statistical Manual of Mental Disorders (1980). 3rd ed. Washington, DC: American Psychiatric Association.

Diagnostic and Statistical Manual of Mental Disorders (1987). 3rd ed. revised. Washington, DC: American Psychiatric Association.

Diagnostic and Statistical Manual of Mental Disorders. (1994). 4th ed. Washington, DC: American Psychiatric Association.

DiNardo, P. A., and Barlow, D. H. (1990). Syndrome and symptom co-morbidity in the anxiety disorders. In *Comorbidity of Mood and Anxiety Disorders*, eds. J. D. Maser and C. R. Cloninger, 1st ed., pp. 205–230. Washington DC: American Psychiatric Press.

Dulcan, M. K. (1986). Comprehensive treatment of children and adolescents with attention deficit disorders: the state of the art. *Clinical Psychology Review* 6:539–569.

Flament, M., Whitaker, A., Rapoport, J., et al. (1988). Obsessive compulsive disorder in adolescence: an epidemiological study. *Journal of the American Academy of Child and Adolescent Psychiatry* 27:764–771.

Francis, G., Last, C. G., and Strauss, C. C. (1992). Avoidant disorder and social phobia in children. *Journal of the American Academy of Child and Adolescent Psychiatry* 31:1086–1089.

Geller, B., Chestnut, E., Miller, D., et al. (1985). Preliminary data on *DSM-III* associated features of major depressive disorder in children and adolescents. *American Journal of Psychiatry* 142:643–644.

Hammen, C., Burge, D., Burney, E., and Adrian, C. (1990). Longitudinal study of diagnoses in children of women with unipolar and bipolar affective disorder. *Archives of General Psychiatry* 47:1112–1117.

Kashani, J. H., Beck, N., Hoeper, E., et al. (1987). Psychiatric disorders in a community sample of adolescents. *American Journal of Psychiatry* 144:584–589.

Kashani, J. H., and Orvaschel, H. (1988). Anxiety disorders in mid-adolescence: a community sample. *American Journal of Psychiatry* 145:960–964.

—— (1990). A community study of anxiety in children and adolescents. *American Journal of Psychiatry* 147:313–318.

Kendall, P., Kortlander, E., Chansky, T., and Brady, E. U. (1992). Comorbidity of anxiety and depression in youth: treatment implications. *Journal of Consulting and Clinical Psychology* 60:869–880.

Kovacs, M., Gatsonis, C., Paulauskas, S. L., and Richards, C. (1989). Depressive disorders in childhood. IV: A longitudinal study with and risk for anxiety disorders. *Archives of General Psychiatry* 46:776–782.

Lader, M. H., and Matthews, A. M. (1968). A physiological model of phobic anxiety and desensitization. *Behaviour Research and Therapy* 6:411–421.

Last, C. G. (1992). Anxiety disorders in childhood and adolescence. In *Internalizing Disorders in Children and Adolescents*, ed. W. M. Reynolds, 1st ed., pp. 61–106. New York: Wiley.

Last, C. G., Hersen, M., Kazdin, A. E., et al. (1991). Anxiety disorders in children and their families. *Archives of General Psyhiatry* 48:928–934.

Last, C. G., Perrin, S., Hersen, M., and Kazdin, A. E. (1992). *DSM-III-R* anxiety disorders in children: sociodemographics and clinical characteristics. *Journal of the American Academy of Child and Adolescent Psychiatry* 31:1070–1076.

Last, C. G., and Strauss, C. C. (1989a). Obsessive-compulsive disorder in childhood. *Journal of Anxiety Disorders* 3:295–302.

———— (1989b). Panic disorder in children and adolescents. *Journal of Anxiety Disorders* 3:87–95.

———— (1990). School refusal in anxiety disordered children and adolescents. *Journal of the American Academy of Child and Adolescent Psychiatry* 29:31–35.

Last, C. G., Strauss, C. C., and Francis, G. (1987). Comorbidity among childhood anxiety disorders. *Journal of Nervous and Mental Diseases* 175:726–730.

Maser, J. D., and Cloninger, C. R. (1990). Comorbidity of anxiety and mood disorders: introduction and overview. In *Comorbidity of Mood and Anxiety Disorders*, eds. J. D. Maser and C. R. Cloninger, 1st ed., pp. 3–12. Washington, DC: American Psychiatric Press.

McClellan, J., Rubert, M. P., Reichler, R. J., and Sylvester, C. E. (1990). Attention deficit disorder in children at risk for anxiety and depression. *Journal of the American Academy of Child and Adolescent Psychiatry* 29:534–539.

McGee, R., Feehan, M., Williams, S., et al. (1990). *DSM-III* disorders in a large sample of adolescents. *Journal of the American Academy of Child and Adolescent Psychiatry* 29:611–619.

Morris, R. J., and Kratochwill, T. R. (1983). *Treating Children's Fears and Phobias*. New York: Pergamon.

Reynolds, W. M. (1992). Depression in children and adolescents. In *Internalizing Disorders in Children and Adolescents*, ed. W. M. Reynolds, 1st ed., pp. 149–254. New York: Wiley.

Reynolds, W. M., and Coats, K. I. (1986). A comparison of cognitive-behavioral therapy and relaxation for the treatment of depression in adolescents. *Journal of Consulting and Clinical Psychology* 54:653–660.

Ryan, N., Puig-Antich, J., Ambrosini, P., et al. (1987). The clinical picture of major depression in children and adolescents. *Archives of General Psychiatry* 44:854–861.

Stark, K. D., Reynolds, W. M., and Kaslow, N. J. (1987). A comparison of the relative efficacy of self-control therapy and behavioral problem-solving therapy for depression in children. *Journal of Abnormal Child Psychology* 15:91–113.

Strauss, C. C., and Last, C. G. (1993). Social and simple phobias in children. *Journal of Anxiety Disorders* 7:141–152.

Strauss, C. C., Last, C. G., Hersen, M., and Kazdin, A. E. (1988a). Association between anxiety and depression in children and adolescents with anxiety disorders. *Journal of Abnormal Child Psychology* 16:57–68.

Strauss, C. C., Lease, C. A., Last, C. G., and Francis, G. (1988b). Overanxious disorder: an examination of developmental differences. *Journal of Abnormal Child Psychology* 16:433–443.

Swedo, S. E., Rapoport, J. L., Leonard, H., et al. (1989). Obsessive compulsive disorder in children and adolescents: clinical phenomenology of 70 consecutive cases. *Archives of General Psychiatry* 46:335–341.

Tannock, R., Schachar, R. J., Carr, R. P., et al. (1989). Effects of methylphenidate on inhibitory control in hyperactive children. *Journal of Abnormal Child Psychology* 17:473–491.

Thyer, B. A. (1993). Childhood onset separation anxiety disorder and adult onset agoraphobia: review of evidence. In *Anxiety across the Lifespan: A Developmental Perspective*, ed. C. G. Last, pp. 128–147. New York: Springer.

Turner, S. M., Beidel, D. C., and Costello, A. (1987). Psychopathology in the offspring of anxiety disorder patients. *Journal of Consulting and Clinical Psychology* 55:229–235.

Velez, C. N., Johnson, J., and Cohen, P. (1989). A longitudinal analysis of selected risk factors for childhood psychopathology. *Journal of the American Academy of Child and Adolescent Psychiatry* 28:861–864.

Weissman, M. A., Leckman, J. F., Merikangas, K. R., et al. (1984). Depression and anxiety disorder in parents and children. *Archives of General Psychiatry* 41:845–852.

Wicks-Nelson, R., and Israel, A. C. (1991). *Behavior Disorders of Childhood*. Englewood Cliffs, NJ: Simon & Schuster.

Part III

RELATED
INTERVENTION
STRATEGIES

15

PSYCHODYNAMIC PLAY THERAPY

Donna M. Cangelosi

REVIEW OF THE LITERATURE

The use of psychoanalytic treatment for children presenting with anxiety disorders began as early as 1909 when Sigmund Freud described the case of "Little Hans," a 5-year-old boy with a horse phobia. While Freud did not maintain a direct ongoing therapeutic relationship with the child (because he believed that only the child's father could elicit the authority required for a positive transference), he conducted psychoanalysis vis-à-vis the parents. Freud's description of this analysis demonstrated that the boy's phobia was a symptom of unconscious conflict.

Historically, the case of Little Hans was very significant because it portrayed an in vivo example of the Oedipus complex and castration anxiety. It also highlighted the importance of the instinctual life, psychic conflicts, and resulting neurotic symptoms that operate in young children. In describing this case, Freud attempted to educate adults regarding the needs of children when he wrote: "It seems to me that we concentrate too much upon symptoms and concern ourselves too little with their causes" (p. 143).

Sigmund Freud was also the first psychoanalyst to observe the therapeutic functions of play. Freud (1920) noted the repetitive quality of play in young children. He proposed that play allows children to transpose events that happen to them into experiences in which they are in charge. Play, therefore, enables children to assimilate distressing experiences and gain mastery over anxiety and other affective states. This premise set the stage for psychoanalytically informed play therapy, which has been used in the treatment of anxiety since the early 1920s.

Herta von Hug-Hellmuth (1921) employed play as a therapeutic technique to uncover the anxieties and thoughts of children. The psychoanalytic play technique was expanded by Melanie Klein (1932) who, like Sigmund Freud, distinguished between objective anxiety and neurotic anxiety. Objective anxiety arises from the child's complete dependence on the mother for need gratification and the relief of tension. Neurotic anxiety, on the other hand, is a result of instincts and distressing unknown emotions being projected onto external objects or experiences. In describing neurotic forms of separation anxiety, Klein concluded that children fear they will never see their parent again due to their fantasy that they have destroyed the parent through intense emotions such as anger and rage.

Klein used play as the equivalent of free association. In working with anxious and other symptomatic children, she strictly interpreted not only play behavior but also interruptions and inhibitions that were noted during play. Klein interpreted play as having symbolic meaning and used it to uncover underlying instincts, oedipal issues, oral themes, and resistance.

Anna Freud also applied psychoanalytic principles to play therapy. However, she did not interpret play in a strict symbolic sense nor did she see it as the equivalent of free association. Anna Freud focused on the ego rather than unconscious id impulses (A. Freud 1936). She used play to elicit dreams, daydreams, and discussions of difficulties in order to understand how the ego deals with conflicts stemming from id impulses and superego demands. She attempted to identify and understand which defense mechanisms were being used by symptomatic children. This information was used, together with a strong therapeutic alliance, to direct anxious children toward healthier coping mechanisms. Anna Freud worked collaboratively with parents in treating children.

Within the field of psychodynamic play therapy, Anna Freud and Melanie Klein continue to have a tremendous influence. Their early work has provided the foundation for all subsequent developments in the psychoanalytic treatment of children. Since the early 1920s, countless case studies have demonstrated the value of psychodynamic therapy in the treatment of a wide variety of anxiety disorders in children. These include separation anxiety (Boersma et al. 1991, Erikson 1976, Glenn 1978, Thompson 1991); school phobia (Bornstein 1949, Dellisch 1991, Klein 1923); psychophysiological disorders (Ablon 1988, DeFolch 1988, Gavshon 1987); elective mutism (Chethik 1977); obsessive disorders (Klein 1932, Kulish 1988); post-traumatic stress disorder (Brandell 1992, Furman 1986); overanxious disorder (Lush et al. 1991); and anxiety-induced thought and behavior problems (Barros 1992, Miller 1992, Watson 1990). This list of case studies primarily includes recent publications and is not exhaustive of work that has been done in the field. However, a general theme is highlighted throughout the literature; namely, that the goal of psychodynamic play therapy is to understand *both* the internal and the external factors that contribute to the symptom and to address these in the context of a therapeutic alliance with the child as well as the parents.

EGO PSYCHOLOGY TECHNIQUES FOR TREATING CHILDHOOD ANXIETY

The remainder of this chapter will focus primarily on the tenets of ego psychology that were outlined and applied to the treatment of children by Anna Freud (1936, 1965). Within this paradigm, anxiety is seen as an expression of delayed or incomplete development of ego control. The symptom may result not only from psychopathology but also from the child's inability to cope with stressors that are inherent in normal development. For this reason, a thorough developmental assessment of the child is conducted early on. Focus is on understanding the psychodynamic makeup of the child, the interaction of environmental forces, and the underlying causes of the child's difficulties.

Following the assessment phase, psychodynamic treatment with children requires a period of preparation. The initial focus is on establishing a therapeutic alliance and imparting to the child insight and motivation for change. The therapist uses play to engage the child and to enhance the child's wish to come to sessions. In some cases, the therapist needs to resist rushing in with feedback that may frighten the child. In other cases, quick interpretations may be necessary to make the child feel understood and engaged. Parental support may be needed during this preliminary stage of treatment to facilitate the child's wish to return (Kennedy and Moran 1991, p. 196).

In psychodynamic play therapy, the therapist allows the child to play spontaneously without interruption, encourages elaboration of play themes, and joins the child's play fantasies. The therapist verbalizes and clarifies observable themes or behaviors to increase the child's awareness of preconscious material. An example is provided by Solnit (1987) in his work with a 5-year-old child who cuddles a teddy bear and offers it to him. The therapist cuddles the teddy bear and says, "Oh, the teddy bear wants to be cuddled because it feels left out of what mama and daddy bear are doing" (p. 210). Interpretation is later used to "widen the child's consciousness." The therapist helps the child to understand the source, history, and meaning of defenses and behaviors so as to counteract unconscious activity. This process of putting unconscious thoughts into words transfers them from primary process to secondary process, thus placing them in the hands of the conscious ego. A stage of working through follows and results in increased maleability in the defensive structure. This, in turn, opens up the opportunity for the child to adapt more useful ways of coping.

As noted by A. Freud (1965), in treating children the therapist is called upon to verbalize much more than with adults, due to the cognitive and verbal limitations of children. Other aspects of the therapeutic relationship include making direct educational suggestions to the child, providing a corrective emotional experience by way of becoming a "new object," providing reassurance to the child when necessary, and working with parents. With regard to the latter, focus is on educating and supporting parents to help the child develop ego resources and to make any necessary environmental changes that will further this process (A. Freud 1965).

ASSESSMENT PROCEDURES

Anna Freud (1965) proposed that various types of anxiety disorders in children are invariably related to four consecutive stages of development: biological union with mother (e.g., separation anxiety), object relatedness (e.g., fear of loss of love), the Oedipus complex (e.g., castration anxiety), and superego formation (e.g., guilt). According to her, mental health throughout the lifespan is best predicted by the ego's ability to deal with anxiety. As such, the psychodynamic assessment addresses the child's reactions to developmental challenges and his/her ego development.

It entails gathering information from the child's parents before beginning treatment. Gaining an understanding of the child's overall developmental history, his/her way of coping with external and internal stressors, and how parents and other environmental factors influence this process is crucial. This assessment must include information about the various areas and layers of the child's personality including organic, psychic, environmental, innate, and historical aspects. Environmental factors such as traumatic and growth-enhancing events, past and present development, and behavior and symptoms are addressed. The psychic makeup of the child is assessed by analyzing clinical information. The therapist looks at drive activity; ego resources; id, ego, and superego forces and conflicts; and defense mechanisms. It is very important that the therapist be mindful of the interaction between these factors so as to avoid analyzing single influences in isolation from the total picture.

In assessing anxiety disorders, particular focus is placed on the child's frustration tolerance, sublimation potential, overall attitude to anxiety, and progressive developmental forces versus regressive tendencies. Level of frustration tolerance maintains psychic equilibrium. Accordingly, when it is low the child is faced with excessive anxiety. This often results in regression, defense activity, and symptoms. Likewise, the child who is unable to tolerate anxiety has to deny and repress external and internal triggers or project internal states onto the environment, making the world a frightening place. Understanding how these processes contribute to the child's symptomatology is done through the assessment process.

In addition to assessing the child's development, it is helpful for the psychodynamic play therapist to obtain background regarding the parents. Relevant information includes their experience of being parents, parenting styles, co-parenting issues, their own family backgrounds, information regarding how they were parented, their individual relationships with the child (and the child's siblings), and information regarding their marital relationship (or issues that led to divorce).

During this part of the assessment process, clinical information is gathered regarding the parents' personalities, as well as their motivational level, expectations, and resistances regarding treatment. It is helpful to meet with the child after this information is gathered to conduct a play assessment. During the latter, focus remains on assessing the child's personality vis-à-vis his/her mode of interacting with the therapist, play themes, affective states, and overall reaction to the therapeutic situation. Following one or two sessions with the child, information gathered throughout the assessment process is integrated and analyzed prior to a feedback session with the parents. At this time, specific recommendations for treatment are discussed.

ESTABLISHING TREATMENT GOALS

Within the psychodynamic framework, it is useful for the therapist to divide treatment goals into two broad categories: process goals and outcome goals. Outcome goals are static in nature and are developed directly from information gathered during the assessment process. Process goals, on the other hand, are fluid and change as the treatment progresses. The latter have a direct impact on choice and implementation of therapeutic techniques (Kennedy and Moran 1991).

In the treatment of anxiety, process goals might include establishing and maintaining a therapeutic alliance with the child as well as the parents; addressing the child's phase-specific developmental needs (e.g., respecting the latency-age child's need to distance from internal conflicts); and adapting techniques that are attuned to developmental delays or deficits (e.g., setting external limits to instill a sense of internal safety in extremely fearful or anxious children) (Kennedy and Moran 1991). In addition, the therapist must be prepared to address environmental changes or stressors in the child's life.

The outcome goals of psychodynamic play therapy involve relieving internal conflicts by bringing them into consciousness and helping the child to achieve better ego resources such as intellectual understanding, logical reasoning, changing of external circumstances, and mastery instead of retreat (A. Freud 1965). These approaches are aimed at enhancing the child's ability to cope with anxiety, which will simultaneously have the effect of decreasing excessive defense activity and symptomatology. This process paves the way toward a normal developmental pathway (A. Freud 1965).

ROLE OF THE THERAPIST

Conducting psychodynamic play therapy requires that the therapist be flexible enough to fulfill two distinct roles for the child. On the one hand, the therapist must serve as a "new object" to satisfy the child's need for a healthy, new experience. Equally important, the therapist must serve as a transference object to fulfill the child's urge to repeat and work through internal conflicts. The therapist is called upon to move carefully between these two roles, which can run contrary to one another and effect the therapeutic alliance. S/he must simultaneously be "an active participant, an astute observer, and an objective interpreter" (Despert 1976, p. 465).

With children, transference material can take a number of different forms and it is necessary for the therapist to understand and interpret it accordingly. Children's transference may reflect emotions and defenses experienced toward parents not only in earlier periods of development but also in the present. With regard to the latter, the therapist must always keep in mind the ongoing influence of parents in the child's everyday life.

Transference material may also reflect externalization wherein the child puts onto the therapist that which is inside of him/her. Externalization allows the therapist an understanding of the child's inner world and is treated differently than transference proper (Furman 1980). Here, the role of the therapist is to verbalize and neutralize anxiety. The therapist becomes an auxiliary (external) ego to help the child deal with overwhelming and frightening internal states and the resulting feelings that the world is a dangerous place. Through identification and internalization of the therapist's soothing functions, the child gradually takes on these ego functions.

PLAY THERAPY STRATEGIES

Erik Erikson (1976) wrote, "To play it out is the most natural self-healing measure childhood affords" (p. 475). Based on this premise, the psychodynamic play therapist attempts to foster play that will provide an understanding of the child's difficulties and coping mechanisms. The therapist is called upon to develop a play language with which to communicate with the child. The most useful toys for engaging the child in this process are those that are inherently interesting or "fun," stimulate fantasy play, have communication value for the child, and elicit a wide range of information that can be interpreted by the therapist (Beiser 1976).

Lebo (1976) offered a list of twenty-eight toys that were empirically found to have expressive value for children involved in nondirective play therapy. Hierarchically, from most expressive to least expressive, these include: doll house, family and furniture; poster paints, brushes, paper, easel, and jars; sandbox; blackboard and colored chalk; cap guns and caps; coloring books; hand puppets; balloons; nursing bottles; films and viewer; water in basin; pop guns; bubble gum; coffee pot; rope; animals; wood; balls; crayons; baby dolls; bow and arrows; clay; cars; checkers; shovel; masks; toy soldiers; and water colors. In addition to this list, building materials have been found to have significant value in psychodynamic play therapy.

The play therapist follows the child's lead and focuses on material that is most accessible to elaboration and interpretation at the moment. Sometimes this requires having to hold off on making an interpretation that the child is not ready for, even though it might bring out a conflict and relieve anxiety. In other words, it is inadvisable for the therapist to devise and stick to a static treatment plan. Instead, the therapist must be attuned to changes in the child's communications, behavior, and affect (Despert 1976).

Emotional responses that do not fit with circumstances are used both diagnostically and therapeutically. For example, if a child reacts with anxiety where anger or sadness would be expected, it is important to address this issue. The child's ego may be defending against emotions that are perceived as unsafe. This strategy of defense analysis was demonstrated in a classic case described by Berta Bornstein (1949), which involved Frankie, a 5 1/2-year-old school-phobic boy.

Bornstein noted that Frankie's aggression and anxiety were ego defenses against intense sadness about his mother's absence during the birth of his sister two years earlier. By sympathizing with the sadness of a play character who was also left alone, the analyst helped Frankie to confront his own feelings of sadness, which eventually led to an awareness of feelings of abandonment. Bornstein observed that Frankie experienced being sent to school as a repetition of the traumatic abandonment that he had experienced passively earlier in life. Through play therapy and the analyst's efforts at connecting Frankie's recent experience to the past, both the hostility he had demonstrated toward his mother and the school phobia subsided.

Successful treatment of anxiety disorders requires that the therapist incorporate ego supportive strategies and carefully timed interpretations. Both are offered in a manner that is attuned with the child's needs and level of readiness. These strategies are effective only inasmuch as they are provided within the context of a strong treatment alliance.

DEALING WITH COMMON OBSTACLES TO SUCCESSFUL TREATMENT

Anna Freud (1965) noted that children tend to externalize inner conflicts so as to shift their focus from internal processes to external battles. Thus, children tend to seek environmental solutions rather than internal change. They commonly look to the therapist to fix environmental problems. When the therapist does not meet this need or demand, as the case may be, it is not uncommon for the child to lose motivation for continuing treatment and to view it as unhelpful. In some cases, the child may come to see the therapist as someone who is not on his/her side because the therapist did not help. While this is undoubtedly a very difficult issue to address, it is possible to engage most children in treatment provided that parents do not join or collude with the child by focusing on quick environmental fixes. However, when this obstacle does present itself it can be addressed in several ways.

An assessment of the parents' motivational level and hopes for treatment is always recommended before treatment actually begins. When parents lack insight regarding the child or therapy, the therapist may need to provide ongoing education and/or parent counseling. The parents' understanding and ongoing involvement in the therapeutic process is essential for treatment to be successful. Anna Freud (1965) wrote: "It is not the patient's ego but the parents' reason and insight on which beginning, continuance, and completion of treatment must rely. It is the task of the parents to help the child's ego to overcome resistances and periods of negative transference without truanting from analysis. The analyst is helpless if they fall down on this task and side with the child's resistances instead" (p. 48).

Another approach for addressing the child's focus on environmental solutions is to prepare the child for treatment and take the time to develop a therapeutic alliance. It is only in a trusting relationship that children (and most adults) feel safe enough to look at their inner world. In many cases, the therapist must serve as an ancilliary ego until the child's own ego is safe and strong enough for this process to unfold.

Sometimes as treatment progresses the child becomes attached to the therapist and experiences loyalty conflicts between the therapist and his/her parents. This can result in increased anxiety or resistance. A working alliance between the therapist and parents is needed to assist the parents in helping the child deal with conflictual feelings and to prevent parents from feeling alienated from the therapeutic process. With regard to the latter, the therapist may need to help parents to address their own feelings about the child's attachment to the therapist. Through this process the therapist helps parents channel their feelings so that they are not unconsciously acted out with the child.

Another, more extreme, obstacle to successful treatment occurs when a parent behaves in ways that serve to maintain the child's symptom so as to fulfill their own pathological needs. While it is hoped that this will be picked up during the assessment, it is not uncommon for the therapist to be fooled initially by passive compliance. However, when a pattern of resistance and/or sabotage is detected, the therapist may have to recommend separate treatment for the parent. In this situation it is best for the child and parent to be treated simultaneously by different therapists who can consult together. When this is not possible, some of the more extreme situations may require that the parents be treated alone for the child's disturbance (A. Freud 1965).

RELAPSE PREVENTION

Perhaps the biggest frustration experienced by psychodynamic therapists is that parents very commonly discontinue treatment when the child's symptoms are relieved. This is sometimes unavoidable. However, relapse prevention requires that the child's internal conflicts be adequately addressed and worked through and his/her ego adequately developed to cope with normal developmental challenges and everyday stressors. To simply reduce the child's anxiety would only result in symptom substitution, premature termination, and ongoing developmental delays.

Even when treatment seems to be successful, the issue of relapse prevention is very difficult when it comes to treating children. Their internal and external worlds are not firmly delineated, their intrapsychic world is very much affected by new objects, and hence they are vulnerable to pathological input (Kennedy and Moran 1991). For these reasons, relapse prevention is ensured not only when the child demonstrates internal changes and improved coping skills but also when external supports are in place. This, once again, points to the important role that parents play in the therapeutic process.

TERMINATION

The termination process is a very important part of psychodynamic play therapy and proceeds based on the child's individual needs. In general, working through feelings of loss, abandonment, and/or separation as well as related defenses against these feelings serves to consolidate the therapy. During this process the therapist must be sensitive not only to the child's transferential issues of loss but also the child's reaction to separating from and losing the "real object" (i.e., the therapist) (Ablon 1988). In general, children tend to feel abandoned even when they are actively involved in the decision to leave. The therapist needs to keep this in mind regardless of the child's conscious actions and verbalizations.

The therapist also needs to be aware of his/her own feelings regarding separating from the child so that these feelings do not impact the termination process. McCarthy (1989) highlighted the important role that countertransference plays in psychodynamic therapy with children. The therapist must be careful not to overestimate the child's progress and terminate too quickly or underestimate the child's process and contribute to the treatment becoming interminable. Termination, like psychodynamic play therapy in general, requires the therapist to be attuned to the child's needs. The therapist follows the child's lead and provides a safe arena for the child to work through and master separation issues that perhaps were not worked through in earlier stages of development. This is particularly true of separation anxious children. Through psychodynamic play therapy they are provided an opportunity to rework separation issues vis-à-vis the therapeutic alliance and termination process.

CASE ILLUSTRATION (TYPICAL TREATMENT)

Description and History

Terri was 9 years old when she was brought for treatment by her mother and stepfather. One month prior to the initial parent consultation, Terri had become very anxious about separating from her mother, began to have nightmares and difficulties falling asleep, and subsequently developed a pattern of becoming tearful and agitated to the point of having tantrums each night before bedtime. The symptoms were first noted while Terri was visiting her natural father during a weekend. This was the first time that Terri was spending the night at his house since his girlfriend Kathy had moved in with him (two weeks earlier). Terri was so upset at that time that Kathy decided to sleep with her to comfort her. When Terri returned home after the weekend her symptoms continued and began to generalize to the point that she sometimes followed her mother around the house. Mrs. G. was so upset by Terri's panic and fear that she set up a cot in her bedroom. At the time of the initial consultation, Mrs. G. had not slept in her own bedroom for over three weeks.

Several weeks before Terri became symptomatic, Terri's mother and stepfather told her that they were going to have a baby. She reportedly took the news very well and verbally welcomed the idea of being a big sister. Nonetheless, Mrs. G. noted that Terri had become increasingly withdrawn since she was told about the baby.

Terri was an only child who was described as an early bloomer in terms of achieving developmental milestones. Her mother noted that Terri had never demonstrated any difficulties with separations earlier in her life. Her parents divorced when she was 3 years old and she had lived alone with her mother for over five years. Mrs. G. dated Mr. G. for over four of those five years and he developed a very close relationship with Terri during that time. Nonetheless, when they married (eight months before treatment began) Terri became somewhat withdrawn and complained of not liking it when her stepfather told her what to do. At the same time she was described as being very affectionate toward him. Terri's relationship with her natural father was described as "consistently inconsistent." There was no set visitation pattern and he frequently did not call Terri for weeks at a time. In spite of this, Mrs. G. noted that she made sure to maintain a relationship with her ex-husband so that she would always be able to talk with him about Terri.

Throughout the parent consultations Terri's mother presented with a tremendous amount of anxiety and guilt. She stated that she felt terrible for "putting Terri through so much change." Mr. G. was also sympathetic in this regard, but he disagreed with his wife's tendency to try to make up for Terri's difficulties by buying her everything she wanted. He argued that Terri had entirely too much control over her mother and in the household in general. Terri frequently heard her mother and stepfather disagree about this issue.

Synopsis of Therapy Sessions

Terri arrived for her first session accompanied by her mother. When I greeted them in the waiting room, Mrs. G. was extremely anxious and confided that Terri did not want to come to the session but that they had worked out "a deal." Terri then came into the therapy room without hesitation. She seemed very tense and uncomfortable and informed me that she had nothing to talk about and only came because she wanted to go to the mall afterward. I commented that it must be hard when parents make so many decisions. Terri nodded and looked down. I sensed that she had made her mind up not to talk about this matter further and proceeded to show Terri the cabinet of toys and art supplies. I told her that even though she didn't choose to come to see me, she could choose what to do. Terri sheepishly took out paper and a pencil and began to draw a house.

Terri became absorbed with the drawing and embellished it with meticulous detail. She added fancy doorknobs, curtains, windowpanes, a cobblestone walkway, and then a flower-trimmed garage and mailbox. A smiling girl, with the same degree of detail, was drawn with a letter in her hand ready to mail. The girl was trimmed with lace and topped off with a flowered hat. Even her shoes and the letter had bows on them. Scenery was added behind the house. Snowcapped mountains, trees, birds, and sun filled the sky. A raccoon with disproportionately large eyes (and eyelashes) was drawn peeking out of one of the trees. Throughout the time that Terri drew this picture I periodically commented and/or asked questions. For instance, when the raccoon was drawn I noted that raccoons stay up at night. No interpretation was made.

Terri became increasingly relaxed and animated as the session and the drawing progressed. The session closed on a much more positive note than it had begun. Afterward, I noted to myself that Terri was dressed in much the same way as the girl in her picture, that is, with meticulous detail. This was, in fact, noted as a pattern in the weeks that followed. Terri arrived each week with a different outfit with matching socks, shoes, purses, belts, and hair pieces. While some of this concern with appearance was seen as age appropriate, it was Terri's obsessive defense and extremely high standards that stood out as ongoing themes throughout her treatment. The latter reflected superego demands that are inherent in the latency period. Based on Terri's developmental history and overall presentation it was suspected that Terri's fears and anxieties were at least in part a result of harsh, externalized superego demands.

Terri used many sessions to draw or make craft projects. She consistently demonstrated a need to include obsessive detail to her projects and frequently concealed them from me to make sure that they turned out the way she wanted. When they did not, Terri became frustrated and complained vehemently that it was "stupid coming to therapy." These instances were used to address Terri's use of externalization. I frequently remarked that Terri thought that everyone expected as much from her as she did. Throughout the first few months, the focus was on helping Terri to discriminate between what she expected of herself and what others expected of her.

By the second month of treatment Terri demonstrated more and more anger toward me. She routinely started each session by complaining about having to come to therapy and then proceeded to discuss concerns while becoming involved in art projects. Therapy provided a safe arena for her to express anger. During one session she used rubber stamps to make a picture of a family walking together. A baby was in the picture, separated from the rest of the family and suspended in the air. Terri then added an airplane and directed it toward the baby. She spontaneously said, "It looks like it's gonna hit it!" No interpretation was made, but this session marked a turning point in the treatment. Terri's anger and resentment toward "a baby" surfaced for the first time, indicating a shift in her defensive structure.

Terri's parents noted a decrease in Terri's clinginess and an increase in her anger during this period. They responded very intuitively to these behaviors and understood them as Terri's first open admission that she had some feelings about the baby. Mr. and Mrs. G. used their bimonthly sessions with me very productively to discuss helpful ways of addressing Terri's needs. Terri's natural father and his fiancé were also seen for periodic consultations for the same purpose. Simultaneously, the focus of Terri's sessions shifted to helping her discriminate between feelings and actions. As it became clearer that her thoughts and wishes could not hurt others, she was freer to express her feelings of fear about being displaced by the baby. Connections were made between being left alone at night and being left alone in general. By this time, Terri's anxiety symptoms had subsided.

Terri was sleeping alone at night for several months by the time her brother was born (seven months into the treatment). She adjusted very well to his birth and was able to express both positive and negative emotions about him (i.e., being "a pain" but at the same time "so cute"). With her parents' help Terri became involved in helping with the baby, yet both her mother and stepfather made sure to spend time alone with her. One month after the birth of her brother, Terri requested family sessions to help her talk to her parents. Her parents welcomed this request and used their bimonthly sessions for this purpose. Weekly sessions of individual therapy with Terri continued for three more months. During this time she addressed changes in her household, peer relationships, and her frustration about never having time with her father. Terri used one of her last sessions to write her father a letter in which she discussed her feelings and needs. While she decided not to mail the letter, it somehow helped her to make sense of her inner experience. I was struck at the time by the strides Terri had made. She progressed from the position of being an anxious, withdrawn child who drew smiling "perfect" girls to becoming a child who was free and capable of acknowledging and expressing frustration, anger, and needs.

Comments

At the close of Terri's treatment she was in the midst of dealing with several environmental stressors including adjusting to sharing her custodial parents with the new baby, preparing for the transition to middle school, preparing for her father's wedding, and addressing issues about her relationship with her father. While these issues were certainly not resolved, Terri was better equipped to deal with them. Internally, Terri's ego was freed up to confront problems instead of defending against them. She had a better understanding of her needs, greater tolerance of her internal states, and increased ability to cope with environmental stressors as well as the high standards of her superego. In addition to these changes, Terri's ego was supported by her parents, who had also made great strides during the treatment. Mrs. G. worked through much of her own guilt and anxiety during the initial phase of treatment, which helped her to stop acting in ways that gratified Terri's id impulses (i.e., endless shopping and sleeping in her room). Instead, she and Mr. G. had taken on the role of helping Terri in ways that supported ego mastery and fostered healthy development.

CASE ILLUSTRATION (OVERCOMING OBSTACLES)

Description and History

Carol's treatment began shortly after her fourth birthday. Her parents were separated seven months earlier and Carol had become increasingly clingy since that time. Her mother (Mrs. R.) reported that Carol "would not let her out of her sight" and that Carol cried hysterically at bedtime and calmed down only when her mother joined her. This resulted in a pattern of Mrs. R. staying in Carol's room every night until she feel asleep. More recently, Carol cried each day before her mother left for work and "begged" her not to leave. This symptom caused Mrs. R. a tremendous amount of guilt and discomfort and prompted her initial consultation with me.

Carol was born in Florida and resided there with her mother and father until she was 3 1/2 years old. At that time, Mrs. R. separated from her husband and relocated to New Jersey to move home with her parents. She felt that the marriage was at a dead end and found herself depressed and using drugs to "escape." Mrs. R. was in counseling with a certified drug counselor to address these issues. She reportedly had not used any drugs in over six months. Throughout the treatment Carol resided with her mother and both maternal grandparents. Mrs. R. was unhappy with this arrangement because her parents reportedly "told her what to do" and undermined her in front of Carol. Mrs. R. also felt that they spoiled Carol and neglected to set appropriate limits with her because she was their only grandchild.

Carol's developmental milestones were within the norm but Carol was described as "very attached" to her mom "from day one." Mrs. R. noted that Carol was "precocious" and attempted to be like her mom. She imitated her voice, wanted to dress like her, and so on.

Carol's parents' separation had been a bitter one. Mr. R. accused his wife of taking Carol away from him. She, in turn, was angry at him for not calling on a consistent basis and for not visiting Carol since they had left Florida seven months earlier. Despite her apparent anger, Mrs. R. noted that she was still entertaining the possibility of returning to the marriage. She struggled with not letting Carol know how angry she was because she wanted her to have a positive relationship with her father. While Mrs. R. had some discomfort about taking Carol from Florida, she thought it was best for Carol to be "near family" during the separation. Her insight regarding Carol's attachment to her father

seemed limited and she felt strongly that it was her husband's responsibility to maintain a relationship with Carol "no matter where she
lived." Mrs. R. did not see herself as having any role or responsibility
regarding this process. She expressed concern that Carol was feeling
rejected by her father as he had not phoned in several weeks. Nonetheless, Mrs. R. had not taken any action to serve as a liaison for Carol.
Mrs. R. noted that Carol often asked questions regarding her father,
presented with a lot of anger toward him, and often spoke of "hating
him." Mrs. R. suspected that this was her daughter's way of "acting
tough" when in fact she was very hurt. Mrs. R. believed that Carol "got
this brave soldier routine" from her, as this had been her way of coping
with stress and pain throughout her life.

Synopsis of Therapy Sessions

During the initial phase of treatment, Carol was seen once a week for
play therapy and her mother was seen once a week for supplemental
parent counseling. Carol was dressed very stylishly, albeit in a somewhat precocious manner, during the first session and consistently
demonstrated a stolid expression and very serious demeanor. She had
arranged with her mother that she would come to the session only if her
mother accompanied her. This was permitted and Carol spent the
entire first session exploring toys and showing them to her mother.
Periodically she looked up at me but she communicated verbally only
to her mother. Upon leaving the session she seemed significantly less
tense and looked back at me before exiting.

During the second play therapy session Carol was able to communicate directly to me. She asked me for assistance while building an
airplane out of fiddle sticks. Upon completing the structure, she
commented to her mother that she wished the plane could bring daddy
to New Jersey. She then became agitated, took the plane apart, and
said, "That's a make believe plane not a real one." I did not make any
interpretation, as the primary goal during this phase of treatment was
to establish an alliance and help Carol see that expressing her wishes,
fantasies, thoughts, and feelings could be safe in the playroom. Mrs. R.
became very anxious after this session and called to say that she was
going to discontinue treatment because it was "making Carol too
upset." She was asked to come in for a session to discuss her concerns.
Support and education was provided; however, it was only after she
spoke with her own counselor that she was able to feel comfortable
enough to commit to further treatment.

By the third session Carol was able to come into the playroom without her mother, provided that the door remained open so that she could not only see her mother from the distance but move freely between me and her mother. She lined up two rows of dinosaurs and explained that one row was following the daddy and the other was following the mommy. I commented that it must be hard for them to choose which one to follow. Carol then decided that the baby would have to ride on the mommy's back and attempted to place it in a sturdy position. After several unsuccessful attempts at doing so, Carol placed clay on the mother dinosaur's back and stuck the baby on top. Carol repeated this play theme several times in the weeks that followed. I highlighted the baby dinosaur's wish to ride on the mommy's back to address its fear, anxiety, and anger about being separate and alone. Throughout this initial phase of treatment Carol was able to play for short periods of time but became panicky when she realized she was alone (i.e., without her mom). She had to check in with her mother in the waiting room every few minutes. However, by the sixth session she showed increased ability to become involved in imaginary play and checked in with her mother only twice. At about this time Mrs. R. informed me that she had to cut back on parent counseling sessions due to financial difficulties. Although a fee adjustment was offered, she asked to come for parent counseling on an as-needed basis. With some encouragement she agreed to come a minimum of once every three weeks. Carol would continue her weekly sessions.

Major shifts took place in terms of Carol's separation anxiety during this initial phase of treatment. While she became increasingly tolerant of being away from mom for longer periods of time, she became increasingly anxious and at times intolerant of separating from me. Initially, Carol became very angry at me at the end of sessions for "making her go." In the weeks that followed she developed a pattern of asking me, "Is it time to go?" from five minutes into the session until it was in fact time to leave.

By the third month of treatment Carol was able to stay in the therapy room without her mother and with the door closed. While she periodically expressed a need to show her mother what she had made or to simply check in with her, there was a sense that Carol was significantly more comfortable with being separate. This, in turn, allowed her the freedom of becoming absorbed in imaginary play. Carol became very interested in playing with a family of figures that she had made out of clay (which were put aside in a special place for her each week). The family included a mother, father, brother, and baby. During a session nearly four months into the treatment, the mother was "too tired to hold the baby" but the baby was able to seek comfort from the father. Interestingly, it was during this time that Carol's mother was planning a trip to Florida to bring her to see her dad and to see if there was any possibility for a reconciliation. It was clear by this point in the treatment that Carol's defensive structure was beginning to change. She was safe enough to wish for a comforting father and had the freedom to play without having to remind herself that it was "only make believe" (i.e., as she had done with the airplane during the first session). This session seemed to be her way of preparing for her visit with dad. There also seemed to be transferential meaning to Carol's play because it paralleled the increased comfort she was experiencing with me. There was evidence that she was beginning to internalize the idea of being able to attain comfort from other sources when mother was not available.

Carol returned from Florida with a smile! It was the first smile that I had seen on her face in the four months that we had been working together. Upon entering the playroom she went directly to the toy closet and proceeded to play peek-a-boo with me. She then attempted to scare me by repeatedly hiding and jumping out. I played with Carol and made statements reflecting the theme of disappearance and reappearance (e.g., "just when I think I'm alone I realize you're still there" and vice versa). After several repetitions of this, Carol asked if I still had the family figures that she had made. I reminded her that her basket of toys was still in her special place even though we were separated for a few weeks. Interestingly, Carol did not play with the figures after finding them. She clearly was happy to be reunited with me and relieved to see that she had not been forgotten.

In the sessions that followed, Carol became very interested in playing house. She repeatedly took on the role of a very busy mother who ironed clothes, talked on the phone, and made coffee while feeding the baby. She was frequently impatient with the baby, saying things like, "Can't you see I'm busy?" Likewise, Carol repeatedly staged a nighttime routine—feeding, changing, and then laying the baby down to sleep, telling it to go to sleep while shutting the lights off, lying down herself, and instructing me to go to sleep. She then would sigh in a relieved manner that it was "lights out" and proceed with her role of the busy mother. I used these sessions to address how the baby was feeling alone, with the lights out, and so on. It is noteworthy that during this time Carol continued to demonstrate a great deal of anxiety about leaving. During sessions she continually asked, "Is it time to go yet?" However, her mother noted that while bedtime was still a difficult time, Carol was significantly more comfortable with separating from her during the day.

Two weeks after returning from Florida (four and a half months into the treatment), Mrs. R. called and left a message on my answering machine informing me that she had decided to pursue a divorce from Carol's father. She also informed me that she had decided to terminate treatment so that she could save money for an apartment. She thanked me for my help and noted that Carol was doing much better. When I called Mrs. R. back she was not open to discussing the possibility of a fee adjustment and was set on terminating the treatment. When I alerted her that terminating so abruptly might be upsetting to Carol in light of her history and difficulties with separation and attachment to me, she agreed to come in for one last session so that Carol could have the opportunity to say good-bye.

During the last session Carol became closed and angry when I attempted to talk about it being our last session (i.e., saying good-bye). She played with the baby doll and repeatedly told it not to cry while she (the mother) got ready to go to work. Throughout this session Carol seemed extremely anxious. She walked in and out of the room and in and out of the toy closet and repeatedly started sentences and "forgot" what she was going to say. In an attempt to make the therapy real (and not something that disappears), I gave Carol the clay figures that she had made. Mrs. R. was asked to join us during the last few minutes of the session so that we could all say good-bye.

Comments

Throughout this treatment, attempts were made to educate and involve Carol's parents in the therapeutic process. While Mr. R. approved of his daughter's treatment, he was not involved in therapy because of his physical distance and his related sense of being an outsider and helpless regarding Carol's fate. Although Mrs. R. sought treatment, she was very anxious that therapy would add to Carol's problems and mark her as "problemed." Furthermore, Mrs. R. was continually attempting to ward off guilt about being responsible for her daughter's difficulties. To come to treatment was to her admitting that something was wrong and that she was the cause. She struggled with her anger toward Carol's father and her concern that it might not be in Carol's best interest to be so far away from him. The more I attempted to address these issues during parent counseling sessions the more she withdrew from treatment and the more fearful she became that Carol's treatment would somehow hurt her. I attempted to address these fears throughout the four-and-a-half-month treatment. However, Mrs. R. was clearly too frightened to address her own internal conflicts and resorted to her "soldier routine" when she terminated treatment so abruptly. Her visit to Carol's father and the emotions it provoked gave her the impetus to push forward in a manner that allowed her to push aside any related thoughts or feelings (i.e., about a separation). Unfortunately, Carol's repeated message to the doll during her last session ("Don't cry") reveals that she was in fact attempting to be a brave soldier as well.

SUMMARY

The two cases described in this chapter illustrate how similar symptoms can stem from very different dynamics and conflicts. While both children manifested symptoms associated with separation anxiety, their causes were very different, as was the focus of their treatment. Terri's anxiety stemmed from rigid superego demands that made it impossible for her to express and work through anger related to her mother's pregnancy and her father's lack of availability. Terri's ego was not capable of negotiating id impulses, superego demands, and the realities of her environment that resulted in these defenses. Carol's anxiety, on the other hand, was caused by panic about actually losing her mother (as she had her father) and unneutralized internal fear that her angry impulses could actually destroy her mother.

In addition to addressing internal dynamics, careful consideration must be given to developmental issues when treating children with anxiety disorders. Based on Terri's history it seemed that she was working hard to defend against sexual fantasies and impulses. These were not addressed due to her age-appropriate developmental need to, in fact, repress sexual impulses. Likewise, Carol's need to repeatedly check with her mother was seen as a developmental issue related to the rapproachment crisis.

Another aspect that has been repeatedly highlighted as a cornerstone for successful treatment involves work with parents. Anna Freud (1965) proposed that unlike adult treatments, psychotherapy with children requires a period of preparation to increase the child's insight and motivation, impart confidence in the therapist, and foster the child's sense of the therapist as someone who can be helpful. I would go as far as to say that in treating children with anxiety disorders it might be equally important to involve parents in this same process. A period of preparation may be helpful for all parents, but more specifically those who enter treatment with hesitations or conflicts that can interfere with the therapeutic process. Terri's parents were able to address their own anxieties and her therapeutic gains were supported and enhanced by them. Carol's treatment, on the other hand, was hindered by her mother's anxiety and related conflict. These cases demonstrate the tremendous difference that parent involvement can have in the therapeutic process and how very important it is for the therapist to be attuned not only to the child's internal world but to the dynamic interplay between the child and the environment.

REFERENCES

Ablon, S. L. (1988). Developmental forces and termination in child analysis. *International Journal of Psychoanalysis* 69:97–104.

Barros, E. L. (1992). Psychic change in child analysis. *International Journal of Psycho-Analysis* 73:303–311.

Beiser, H. (1976). Play equipment. In *Therapeutic Use of Child's Play*, C. E. Schaefer, ed., pp. 423–447. Northvale, NJ: Jason Aronson.

Boersma, F. J., Moskal, R., and Massey, D. (1991). Acknowledging the wind and a child's unconscious. *Arts in Psychotherapy* 18:157–165.

Bornstein, B. (1949). Analyses of a phobic child. *Psychoanalytic Study of the Child* 3–4:181–226.

Brandell, J. R. (1992). Psychotherapy of a traumatized 10-year-old boy: theoretical issues and clinical considerations. *Smith College Studies in Social Work* 62:123–138.

Chethik, M. (1977). Amy: the intensive treatment of an elective mute. In *Psychiatric Treatment of the Child*, eds. J. F. McDermott and S. I. Harrison, pp. 117–135. New York: Jason Aronson.

DeFolch, T. E. (1988). Communication and containing in child analysis: towards terminability. *International Journal of Psycho-Analysis* 69:105–112.

Dellisch, H. (1991). Illness causing anxiety within the family. *Praxis der Kinderpsychologie und Kinderpsychiatrie* 40:126–133.

Despert, J. L. (1976). Play therapy. In *Therapeutic Use of Child's Play*, ed. C. E. Schaefer, pp. 463–474. New York: Jason Aronson.

Erikson, E. (1976). Play and Cure. In *Therapeutic Use of Child's Play*, ed. C. E. Schaefer, pp. 475–485. New York: Jason Aronson.

Freud, A. (1936). *The Ego and the Mechanisms of Defense. The Writings of Anna Freud, Volume II.* New York: International Universities Press, 1966.

———— (1965). *Normality and Pathology in Childhood: Assessments of Development. The Writings of Anna Freud, Volume VI.* New York: International Universities Press, 1970.

Freud, S. (1909). Analysis of a phobia in a five-year-old boy. *Standard Edition* 10:5–149.

———— (1920). Beyond the pleasure principle. *Standard Edition* 18:3–64.

Furman, E. (1980). Transference and externalization in latency. *Psychoanalytic Study of the Child* 35:267–284. New Haven, CT: Yale University Press.

———— (1986). Aggressively abused children. *Journal of Child Psychotherapy* 12:47–59.

Gavshon, A. (1987). Treatment of an atypical boy. *Psychoanalytic Study of the Child* 42:145–171. New Haven, CT: Yale University Press.

Glenn, L. (1978). *Child Analysis and Therapy.* New York: Jason Aronson.

Hug-Hellmuth, H. von (1921). On the technique of child analysis. *International Journal of Psycho-Analysis* 2:286–305.

Kennedy, H., and Moran, G. (1991). Reflections on the aim of child analysis. *Psychoanalytic Study of the Child* 46:181–198. New Haven, CT: Yale University Press.

Klein, M. (1923). The development of a child. In *Contributions to Psycho-Analysis 1921–1945.* London: Hogarth Press, 1948.

———— (1932). *The Psychoanalysis of Children.* London: Hogarth Press.

Kulish, N. (1988). Precocious ego development and obsessive compulsive neurosis. *Journal of the American Academy of Psychoanalysis* 16:167–187.

Lebo, D. (1976). Toys for nondirective play therapy. In *Therapeutic Use of Child's Play,* ed. C. E. Schaefer, pp. 435–447. New York: Jason Aronson.

Lush, D., Boston, M., and Grainger, E. (1991). Evaluation of psychoanalytic psychotherapy with children: therapists' assessments and predictions. *Psychoanalytic Psychotherapy* 5:191–234.

McCarthy, J. B. (1989). Resistance and countertransference in child and adolescent psychotherapy. *American Journal of Psychoanalysis* 49:67–76.

Miller, L. (1992). The difficulty of establishing a space for thinking in the therapy of a 7-year-old girl. *Psychoanalytic Psychotherapy* 6:121–135.

Solnit, A. J. (1987). A psychoanalytic view of play. *Psychoanalytic Study of the Child* 42:205–219. New Haven, CT: Yale University Press.

Thompson, T. C. (1991). The place of ego building work in psychotherapy with children. *Child and Adolescent Social Work Journal* 8:351–367.

Watson, A. (1990). On his brother's blindness. *Journal of Child Psychotherapy* 16:127–134.

16

FAMILY THERAPY

Richelle N. Moen

FAMILY THERAPY IS AN effective approach to intervening with anxiety-disordered children. Information about family structure is used to conceptualize the etiology of a problem, and the family is the focus for direct intervention and an ally of the therapist in maintaining individual changes (Kendall 1985). Within this shift toward family in therapy in the past four decades, the systems models of family therapy have enjoyed extraordinary growth and increasing popularity. Systems models refer broadly to those models of family therapy that have been influenced by, or based in part on, the concepts of the general systems theories of von Bertalanffy (e.g., 1950, 1968). These theories introduced a shift from the linear thinking of individual therapy to the circular thinking of family therapy, which considers the whole to be greater than the sum of its parts.

It is the belief of family therapists that the behavior of an individual will change if there is change in the system of interpersonal relationships of which they are a part. Unlike the traditional individual psychotherapist, the family therapist views a child's problems within the context of the family. The family therapist begins the exploration of the child's difficulties by examining the nuclear family (i.e., everyone living in the household). The family becomes the patient.

This chapter will focus on the integration of the structural and strategic models of family therapy as approaches to working with anxiety-disordered children and their families. Relevant components of each family therapy model will be presented, including generation of hypotheses and intervention strategies that give direction to family treatment. Family therapy is a valuable adjunct to the individual therapies such as cognitive-behavioral therapy that have been found to be effective in working with persons with anxiety disorders.

Special thanks to Jody Regan, M.A., C.M.F.T., for all of her wisdom and support in preparing this manuscript.

LITERATURE REVIEW

Etiology of Anxiety Disorders in Children

The long-standing nature versus nurture controversy among mental health professionals regarding the etiology of psychological diagnoses is especially relevant in family therapy. Research can be found to support both sides of the argument. Evidence of familial patterns of anxiety disorders is shown in a number of reports (Beardslee et al. 1983, Bernstein and Garfinkel 1988, Crowe 1983, Last et al. 1987b). Torgerson (1983) in particular suggests that genetic factors appear to influence the development of certain anxiety disorders, namely panic disorder and agoraphobia with panic attacks.

Other researchers examining biological vulnerability to anxiety disorders, however, have highlighted the likely contribution of environmental forces as well (Last et al. 1987a, Oppenheimer and Frey 1993, Roth 1959, Raskin et al. 1982). Some researchers, for example, have found that exposure to an agoraphobic parent who models caution and fearfulness is a possible factor in predisposing a child toward developing anxiety. Some reports indicate that agoraphobic patients were often reared in overprotective families (Raskin et al. 1982, Roth 1959, Solyom et al. 1974). Solyom and colleagues (1973, 1974) noted that mothers of agoraphobic patients scored significantly higher on measures of maternal control and concern than overprotective mothers on whom the scale norms were based. Thus, parents of agoraphobic children may foster an anxious attachment in the child.

Other studies focusing on families with a child exhibiting school phobia with symptoms of anxiety have emphasized various disturbances in family interactions, including poorly resolved dependency needs between mother and child, difficulty of the child separating from the mother, family conflict due to the lack of clarity regarding parent–child roles, ambiguous messages due to poor communication skills among family members, and inhibited expression of painful feelings (Bernstein and Garfinkel 1988, Waldfogel et al. 1959). Mothers of children with school phobia have been described as overprotective, controlling, ambivalent, and providing their children with contradictory messages regarding independence (Eisenberg 1958, Waldron et al. 1975).

The family therapist must consider individual traits, family history, family dynamics, and the social context in which the family lives, among other things. The intent is not to lay blame anywhere for the child's problem, but to expand the vision of the problem in order to expand the avenues for intervention. So while the family therapist may choose to work with parents to improve their parenting skills, this is done to empower the parents rather than blame them for the child's problem.

Systems Models of Family Therapy

Family therapy in general suggests that the most effective method for alleviating anxiety in the child is by working within the family system (McDermott et al. 1989). The child's symptom is conceptualized by the family as an individual problem and then reformulated by the therapist in terms of how the child's disorder is consistent with family dynamics. After the therapist observes the child within the context of family, the relationships among individuals are examined for dysfunctional patterns. The primary goal of family intervention is to replace dysfunctional, anxiety-producing patterns with new, more functional patterns.

Recent decades have witnessed the development of numerous models of family therapy that utilize general systems theory to explain family functioning. Differences among approaches are based less on varying interpretations of family functioning from a systemic perspective and more on the characteristics of families, which each model emphasizes in its conceptualizations of the problem and interventions. In addition, some family therapy models borrow techniques from other theories such as cognitive restructuring and behavioral modification interventions. The interventions, however, are implemented within the context of the family.

Because a comprehensive review of all systemic approaches to family therapy is not possible here, two well-known models have been selected because of their effectiveness in helping families with anxiety disorders. The two models that will be outlined in this chapter are (1) structural family therapy, most closely identified with Salvador Minuchin, Braulio Montalvo, and associates, and (2) the problem-solving, strategic family therapy approach of Jay Haley.

Structural Family Therapy

The structural family therapy model was developed by Salvador Minuchin and his associates, first at the Wiltwyck School for Boys and later at the Philadelphia Child Guidance Center. The principles and techniques of structural family therapy appear in three books (Minuchin 1974, Minuchin et al. 1978, Minuchin and Fishman 1981). Minuchin's theory is based on a normative model of family functioning that is used as a basis of comparison for how well families delegate responsibilities and roles to the marital, parental, and sibling subsystems. According to the structural family therapy model, an appropriately organized family will have clearly delineated boundaries and a hierarchy with rules that prescribe who should be in contact with whom about what (Minuchin 1974). Thus, the goal of structural family therapy is to change the underlying family structure so that problematic patterns of interaction (transactions) can be exchanged for more functional patterns of interaction.

The structural family therapy model suggests that for optimal functioning the marital subsystem will have closed boundaries that protect the privacy of the spouses while the parental subsystem will have clear boundaries between it and the children, but not be so impenetrable as to limit the access necessary for good parenting. The sibling subsystem will have its own boundaries and will be organized hierarchically so that children are given tasks and privileges consonant with sex and age as determined by the family's culture. Finally, the boundary around the nuclear family will also be respected, although its permeability will depend on cultural, social, and economic factors that the therapist must take into consideration (McGoldrick et al. 1982).

The hierarchical arrangement of a family is expressed by rules that prescribe different degrees of decision-making power for various individuals and subsystems. While some form of hierarchical arrangement is a condition of healthy family functioning, different families function with different kinds of hierarchies. Generally, in a well-functioning family, the parents are hierarchically positioned above the children, that is, they are in charge (not in the sense of arbitrary authoritarianism, but in the sense of leadership and protection).

Triangulation is a hierarchy problem in which generational boundaries are breached. There are two kinds of triangulation: (1) cross-generational coalitions in which a child is aligned with one parent against the other parent (weak generational hierarchy), or (2) the detouring of conflict through joint parental focus on the child (strong generational hierarchy). A factor such as chronic illness may provide a catalyst for such family patterns. For example, in weak hierarchy triangulation, overprotection of a child by one parent may activate the other parent to be firmer in expecting the ill child to assume responsibility for his/her physical and psychosocial well-being. This triangulation provides multiple stressors for the child, who becomes unable to please both parents.

Alternatively, the child may enter a coalition with one parent against the other parent. Or the child may shift back and forth in coalition, first with one parent and then with the other. In strong hierarchy triangulation, family members avoid conflict by concentrating on, worrying about, or caring for the ill child. Excessive family worry of this sort, with the primary focus of the family on the child, increases the child's stress level.

From a structural perspective, the problems that are faced by families with children who develop anxiety disorders are a result, in part, of boundaries that are excessively blurred (enmeshment) or excessively rigid (disengagement). Enmeshment is characterized either by subsystem boundaries that can easily be intruded upon by other family members or by a heightened emphasis on clannishness that promotes the sacrifice of autonomy and suggests a "we are all one" mentality. An example of the former is the school-age child who consistently becomes involved in his/her parents' marital disagreements. The child either overtly or covertly makes attempts to distract or interrupt the parents by diverting attention onto him/herself. Another example is the single parent who, under the stresses of daily life, becomes overcontrolling due to a sense of helplessness. In this type of enmeshed family, any evidence of loss of control over her children makes the mother anxious and she develops an overwhelming need to overprotect and control her children.

Disengagement, on the other hand, is characterized by a family's inability to alter or cross subsystem boundaries when necessary or by a lack of involvement among family members; that is, the emphasis is on autonomy to the exclusion of support and intimacy.

Enmeshment and disengagement represent different strategies for avoiding conflict—in the one case by curtailing contact and in the other by denying differences and disagreement. Even the constant bickering in which some couples engage serves the purpose of avoiding conflict, inasmuch as it allows for the chronic expression of each party's hostility without pressing for either to change. When a third party, such as a child, is present, cross-generational coalitions result. The child is put in the middle of the couple and has to take sides, which can create internal turmoil and anxiety. Witnessing domestic violence can have a similar effect on a child.

Structural family therapy is sensitive to the role external stressors play in creating family dysfunction. Unlike the strategic family therapist who sees the symptom as an adaptive solution (i.e., the symptom-bearer sacrifices himself to maintain family homeostasis), the structural therapist regards the family as an organism in which this adaptation is not a helpful response, but a reaction to stress. All family members are viewed as equally symptomatic. Dysfunctional family structures result from a combination of stressors impinging on the family and the inability of the family to cope with them. Stressors may be external (the family faces financial hardship or lives in a violent neighborhood) or internal (children reach adolescence, a parent or grandparent dies). They may be universal, such as the developmental transitions of the family life cycle (Carter and McGoldrick 1988), or idiosyncratic, such as an accident, chronic or catastrophic illness, or loss of a job.

Within the structural family therapy model, the first task of the therapist is to observe interactional patterns and boundaries as they are revealed in the therapy session. This includes spatial relationships within the therapy room (e.g., where family members sit in relation to one another), which are considered a valuable index of structural relationships. Various techniques are used to enable the therapist to see family members' typical patterns of relating to one another. One of these techniques is the assignment of in-session tasks (enactment) that reveal organizational features of the system and established patterns of functioning. A typical task assignment might be to have one parent deal with the behavior of a fidgety 7-year-old. As the parent and child begin to interact, the family will play out their typical patterns and the therapist will gain insight into parameters such as hierarchies, power, and support in the family.

The second task of the therapist is to generate hypotheses and define goals for therapy while "joining with the family" (Aponte and Van Deusen 1981, Minuchin 1974). When the therapist joins with the family, he/she becomes a participant in the system that he/she is attempting to transform by adopting the family's style of communication and interactions and then observing what happens as he/she begins to vary the pattern. The emphasis on joining and becoming involved in the family's interactions is to test for areas of flexibility in the system. As the therapist experiences the family transactions, he/she begins to form an experiential diagnosis of family functioning, noting coalitions, affiliations, explicit and implicit conflicts, and the role various family members play (i.e., some family members may operate as detourers of conflict and others operate as "switchboards" with most of the family's communication coming through them) (Minuchin and Fishman 1981). The experiential diagnosis leads to the generation of working hypotheses on which the therapist bases interventions. It should be noted that the therapist identifies areas of strength as well as dysfunction.

As the therapist gathers data on the symptoms and examines the ways the family system participates in producing and maintaining the symptoms, he/she looks for methods to reframe the anxiety disorder into interactional terms to alter family dynamics. The therapist operates on the assumption that the planned restructuring will free the family from the pattern of interactions that has been dysfunctional. The structural therapist does not necessarily discuss these structural goals with the family, but assigns tasks and offers reframes that allow the family to experience a change in structure.

Finally, the restructuring phase of therapy consists of the therapist's attempts to dismantle, reinforce, or reorganize the old hierarchical structures and build new structures as needed. The techniques employed are grouped into three categories: (1) systems recomposition, (2) symptom focusing, and (3) structural modification (Aponte and Van Deusen 1981). An example of system recomposition would be inclusion of the youngest daughter in an established, close female sibling subsystem so that she can benefit from her older sisters' knowledge about how to negotiate with the parents, her siblings, and the outside world. An example of symptom focusing would be the relabeling of a symptom in such a way that it has new meaning for the family and allows them to see problems in a new light. Another technique in this category is symptom exaggeration in which the symptom is repeated to such an extent that the function it had in the family is diminished (i.e., a son is asked to complain louder regarding his anxiety so that his father can hear him). The structural modification techniques, on the other hand, emphasize differences among family members to dispel the need for detouring coalitions (i.e., if individual differences are viewed as natural, no one has to be blamed for being different) and blocking established interactional patterns to guide family members toward finding new ways of interacting with one another. An example of this would be for the therapist to intervene with the family to prevent a 7-year-old from interrupting the parents when they are discussing a problem either in session or at home.

In summary, the structural model of family therapy assumes that a symptom (i.e., anxiety) is the product of a dysfunctional family system, and that if the family organization becomes more functional, the symptom will disappear. The therapist's task is to respectfully challenge the family's definition of the problem and reframe the symptoms in transactional terms to facilitate the restructuring of the family system.

Strategic Family Therapy

Strategic family therapy is defined by Jay Haley (1973) as a problem-solving approach in which the therapist focuses on the process of change rather than a normative model of families such as that presented by Minuchin. Several books and articles by Haley (1973), Madanes and Haley (1977), and Stanton (1981a, 1981b) provide a theoretical overview of the strategic approach.

A basic tenet of strategic therapy is that therapeutic change comes about through the "interactional processes set off when a therapist intervenes actively and directly in particular ways" in a family system (Haley 1971, p. 7). The therapist works to substitute new behavior patterns or sequences for unhealthy sequences that exist in the family (Weakland et al. 1974). The goal of the strategic therapist is to change dysfunctional sequences of behavior presented by the family appearing for treatment.

The strategic approach emphasizes a distinction between creating a problem by applying a diagnosis or characterizing an individual or family in a certain way and identifying a problem as it is presented by the family in therapy. As with most family therapy models, psychiatric and psychological diagnostic criteria are seldom used as the focus of therapy. The first task of the strategic therapist is to define a presenting problem in such a way that it can be solved. The approach is sensitive to the wider social network of the family, including other professionals who have involvement with the person with the presenting problem (Laing 1967, 1969).

Strategic therapy focuses on resolution of the presenting problem. A problem is defined as "a type of behavior that is part of a sequence of acts between several people" (Haley 1976). The symptom or symptomatic situation is closely investigated. The family's previous methods of failing to solve the problem are briefly discussed. These previous methods have all failed because they were first-order solutions that did not promote a healthy rebalancing of family homeostasis but simply rearranged the existing dysfunctional behavior patterns.

Another goal of strategic family therapy is to help people past a crisis to the next developmental stage of family life. The stages of the family life cycle have been described by Haley (1973) and Carter and McGoldrick (1988). Strategic family therapy emphasizes the importance of the stages of the family life cycle and the presence or absence of age-appropriate behavior in families (Haley 1976, 1980).

The therapist's choice of a particular intervention strategy is based on how he/she conceptualizes the problem brought into therapy. That conceptualization is based on the specific characteristics of the problem and the people who present it. Furthermore, the way the therapist thinks about the problem—the way that problem resonates with him or her—determines which strategy will be used to solve it. For example, an adolescent son who refuses to go to school may be thought of as being either disobedient and out of control or as misunderstood and mistreated. He may be thought of as a pawn in a struggle between the parents or as overly concerned about and protective of the parents, resulting in the sacrificing of himself to keep mother company while father is preoccupied with other endeavors. He might also be thought of as the victim of an oppressive school system that does not recognize his sensitivity and talents. All of these hypotheses may fit the situation equally well. The hypothesis that is chosen from among the many different ways to view a problem is the one that makes the most sense to the therapist at a particular time; it is the one that elicits his/her sympathy and interest in the family.

Madanes (1991) suggests that the many different ways of thinking about a problem cluster around a set of six concepts used in strategic therapy. Each of these concepts encompasses a range or continuum that goes from one extreme to another. For example, a therapist might think about relationships in a family in terms of hostility and love, with a range of emotions falling between the two extremes. The strategy for therapy will be chosen based on the therapist's conceptualization of the problem, whether that be in terms of love and hostility, or in terms of another continuum such as equality and hierarchy.

The six dimensions for conceptualizing a problem in strategic family therapy outlined by Madanes (1991) include:

1. *Involuntary versus voluntary.* "Sometimes the first step in resolving the presenting problem is to redefine it as voluntary rather than involuntary behavior" (Madanes 1991).

2. *Helplessness versus power.* A symptomatic person appears helpless in that he/she presents unfortunate or involuntary behavior that is out of his/her control; the person cannot change even though he/she wants to. This very helplessness, however, is a source of power in relation to the family members whose lives are limited and dominated by the unreasonable demands, fears, and needs of the symptomatic person. The therapist may choose to view the helpless, symptomatic child as either powerful or victimized, and the parents may be seen as either exploited or tyrannical.

3. *Metaphorical versus literal sequences.* A child who refuses to go to school may be thought of as being a disobedient child, and the problem may be understood in terms of getting the child back in school. In contrast, the refusal to go to school may be viewed as an allusion to another problem in the family; the therapist may connect it, for example, to mother's depression and difficulty in finding a job. The child's behavior in relation to the parents may be considered similar to the mother's behavior in relation to the father, that is, the symptom of the child's school refusal may be a metaphor for the struggle between the mother and father regarding mother's refusal to go to work in spite of the father's efforts to convince her she should.

4. *Hierarchy versus equality.* When the child acts to help the parents in indirect ways with adult issues, the child takes a position of leadership in the family that is incongruous with the notion that the parents are to be in a superior position and help and support the child. The therapist's task is to correct this hierarchy and reorganize the family.

5. *Hostility versus love.* A person's action can be seen as being motivated by either emotion. The strategic therapist tends to think of and redefine people as being benevolently motivated. It is the therapist's task to both provide the attribution of meaning and reframe the problem, for example, "Yelling is father's way of showing that he cares and is very concerned about your future."

6. *Personal gain versus altruism.* A symptomatic person may be motivated by personal gain or altruism. If the symptomatic person is hostile, his/her motivation is most likely viewed by the family as being for personal gain. With the help of the therapist's redefinition of the problem, the symptomatic child may be seen as being concerned about helping others or as needing more affection.

Strategic therapy incorporates paradoxical techniques to facilitate the solving of problems. For example, a therapeutic double bind is set up when the therapist instructs the family not to change, thereby turning family resistance to advances. If the family does change, the therapeutic goal has been reached, but if the family does not change, its members are cooperating with the therapist's instruction, a sign of engagement with the treatment. Strategic prescriptions might be quite ordinary, for example, telling a child to be anxious for a few hours each day to keep his/her parents busy so they are unable to focus on their own issues (Fisch et al. 1982), or quite outlandish, for example, directing the child to spill milk on dad and then apologize for it. The therapist's goal is to figure out how the symptom works in the system and then determine the particular strategy, tactic, or countermove that might undo the symptom.

In summary, strategic family therapy is symptom focused and goal oriented with less emphasis on boundaries and subsystems. The goal of therapy is to create change as expeditiously as possible by reframing a problem in a solvable way and introducing new behavioral patterns. Paradoxical techniques are used to shift the responsibility for change from the therapist back to the individual and family. Stanton (1981c) identified numerous similarities between the structural and strategic approaches to family therapy, which aids in their integration. As with structural family therapy, strategic therapy emphasizes the present rather than the past; highlights the repetitive behavioral sequences that need to change; emphasizes the use of directives, which requires the therapist to be extremely active in the therapy sessions; and promotes the use of interpretation to relabel or reframe the problem rather than produce insight. The assignment of behavioral tasks and the use of techniques that unbalance the family system and move the family from a dysfunctional to a functional stage are also components of both the structural and strategic approaches. Last, both models of family therapy utilize the practice of brief rather than long-term therapy, and there is an emphasis on the importance of joining with the family to reduce defensiveness. The technical aspects of integrating the structural and strategic models will be highlighted later in this chapter under Focus of Treatment.

DESCRIPTION OF TECHNIQUES

Primary Techniques of Structural Family Therapy

Structural family therapy techniques are used to assess the structure of the family, probe for areas of flexibility, examine coalitions and dysfunctional transactions among family members, and facilitate the reorganization of family structure around healthier ways of communicating. These structural techniques include joining, completing a family-of-origin genogram, developing working hypotheses, implementing enactments, reframing, stating the problem in a solvable form, giving homework assignments, and developing rules/chores in families.

Joining

Joining a family is as much attitude as it is technique, and is the umbrella under which all therapeutic transactions occur. Joining conveys to the family that the therapist wants to understand them and is working with and for them. Only under this protection can the family have the security to explore alternatives, try the unusual, and change. Joining is a part of each family session and calls for the therapist to connect with family members on an ongoing basis by emphasizing "the aspects of his personality and experience that are syntonic with the family's" (Minuchin 1974).

There are several ways to join a system. These include exploring areas of interest of the various members and spending time identifying with some of the family values. A parent might refer nostalgically to the good old days when parents knew how to teach their kids respect and how things were better then. Appropriate reinforcement of such recollections might be part of the joining process. Just how one joins is less important than the fact that the therapist finds a way to connect with the family. The goal of joining is to help the family to feel comfortable, less threatened, and confident that the therapist understands and, therefore, can help. Joining is a necessary condition of trust, and without trust significant change in the family system cannot occur.

Genogram

The genogram is a format for drawing a family tree that records information about family members and their relationships over at least three generations (see McGoldrick and Gerson 1985). Although neither structural nor strategic family theorists have included this family-of-origin map in their models, the genogram is generally viewed in practice as an essential tool for assessment and treatment planning. The genogram is extremely useful for organizing information and tracking shifts that occur around births, deaths, and other transitional life events. This information aids in the development of hypotheses regarding coalitions, roles, grief and loss, and the family's adaptive style (McGoldrick and Gerson 1985). The genogram illustrates current and historical family patterns and dysfunctional family structures. In addition, the genogram, which maps relationships and patterns of functioning, helps the therapist to think systematically about how events and relationships in the family's life are related to patterns of mental and physical illness.

Through the construction of a genogram, the clinician and family members can visualize the overall family system—including past marriages, unwed pregnancies, births, deaths, and tragic accidents in the parents' families of origins—and the positions of various members and subsystems in relation to others. The genogram allows the children and family an opportunity to "see" how they are all connected. It can assist the therapist in sorting out a complicated network of relationships, noting conflictual relationships and cross-generational replication of dysfunctional patterns, identifying potential resources, and determining who should be involved in intervention plans.

Working Hypotheses

This is the therapist's conceptualization of a problem based on information from the family and revised as treatment progresses. For example, the structural family therapist might hypothesize that a son's disrespect toward his father is a reaction to the father's anger toward mother and to the license mother has given the son to fight her battles for her. The therapist works with this hypothesis as he/she begins to probe the system. Each hypothesis is revised or discarded based on its viability as a tool for producing effective interventions. The therapist may use several working hypotheses simultaneously.

Enactment

This is a technique designed to bring conflict and the presenting problem into the family session, so the therapist's office becomes a laboratory in which to examine dysfunctions within the system. The therapist constructs an inter-actional scenario in the session in which dysfunctional transactions among family members are played out. While facilitating this transaction, the therapist observes family members' verbal and nonverbal ways of interacting. The therapist intervenes in the process by increasing the intensity, pro-longing the time of the transaction, involving other family members, sug-gesting alternative transactions, and introducing experimental probes that give both the therapist and the family information about the nature of the problem, the flexibility of the family's boundaries, and possible alternative ways of coping with the problem.

Minuchin and Fishman (1981) describe an enactment as a "dance in three movements." In the first step, the therapist observes the spontaneous transactions of the family and decides which dysfunctional areas to highlight. In the second step, the therapist organizes the scenario in which the family members dance their dysfunctional dance in his/her presence. In the third step, the therapist suggests alternative ways of interacting.

A common enactment is one in which a parent states that a child is unmanageable. Simply talking about the child's problem is not always helpful, since the child may be quiet during the discussion or begin com-plaining about being in the therapy room and request to leave the room as a way of distracting the parent from discussing the behavior. Hearing a verbal account of behavior that occurs at home leaves it up to the therapist to imagine what the dynamics may be. The best approach is to have the child enact the behavior in the session so it can be observed by the therapist and so structural interventions can be made. The goal of a successful enactment is to exacerbate conflict within the therapy session so that behaviors and family structures can be studied and modified in a way that reduces the potency of the presenting problem.

Stating the Problem in a Solvable Form

The definition of the problem should be agreed upon by the therapist and the family. It should focus on behaviors that can be observed, counted, or measured, so that one can assess whether change has occurred. This is a concept borrowed from behavioral therapy. The statement, "Jim is an anxious child," with the goal of decreasing his anxiety is not solvable. If the problem is reframed as, "Jim needs to learn to speak up for himself and make requests so that other children won't tease him for being quiet," the problem would be solvable. The goal then can be to increase his assertiveness, which can be broken down into concrete tasks and homework assignments.

Reframing

Reframing is the art of attributing new meaning to a behavior so the behavior will be seen differently by the family (Haley 1976, Minuchin and Fishman 1981). Reframing is a method of cognitive restructuring in which the therapist provides a new perspective to the family, rather than soliciting it from the identified patient. By redefining, or reframing, the therapist challenges the meaning attributed to the symptomatic behavior. This usually has a powerful effect on family attitudes, responses, and relationships. It is not the goal of reframing to impart insight.

One type of reframing is the "positive connotation" of the paradoxical schools of family therapy. It is employed as a precursor to assigning the family the paradoxical task of maintaining the symptomatic behavior (Selvini Palazzoli et al. 1978). An overprotective mother may be redefined by the therapist as a "concerned mother," or the symptomatic child with incapacitating anxiety as "the holder of all the feelings in this family." Such positive connotations, or noble ascriptions, are intended to convey to the family that there is good intention underlying the problem behavior.

Reframing is also an effective form of joining (Minuchin 1974) that (1) reduces resistance, (2) revises the family's present view of the problem behavior, (3) allows the therapist entrance into the family, and (4) strengthens the potential influence of the therapist. As the therapist helps the family see alternate ways of perceiving the problem and conveys the hope that solutions can be found, his/her power and influence will be enhanced.

Homework Assignments

These are tasks the therapist assigns to family members to be carried out at home between sessions to facilitate the achievement of the therapy goals. Homework assignments of various kinds allow therapists the efficient use of time and promote positive change in real-life family situations outside the treatment room. The tasks are designed to restructure the family and reinforce changes discussed in the sessions or create a situation that causes spontaneous change to occur within the family. Homework assignments or tasks can be specific, such as, "Jim will take out the trash every other day and Father will be in charge of making sure he does it," or as vague as, "Mother will help Dad deal with Jonathan," depending on what the therapist wishes to achieve. The therapist may also ask the family to keep track of how often certain behaviors occur—that is, how many arguments family members have each week—to gather baseline data and elevate the family's level of awareness.

Tasks are a useful measure of the level of motivation and cooperation in therapy. The therapist may need to reassign a task or assign an easier or more specific task to noncompliant family members. A paradoxical message (such as labeling change as "too dangerous" or the family as "moving too fast") may be included with the reassigned task.

Rules and Chores

Families need rules and chores to guide and organize them. A particular family's rules are based on the beliefs of the individuals within the family. Families under stress may either become chaotic and abandon all sense of order or become extremely rigid. The family therapist strives to make the rules overt and helps the family to reestablish a functional sense of order.

Primary Techniques of Strategic Family Therapy

The strategic techniques were developed from treating rigidly homeostatic families and are effective for dealing with resistance. These techniques emphasize the use of directives, taking the path of least resistance, paradoxical interventions, strategic disengagement, unbalancing, and positive connotation (the latter as described under the structural techniques). The focus is on symptom management, not contextual changes in family relationships.

Directives

These directives may be straightforward behavioral instructions or requests for the family to change. It is important to suggest rather than order tasks. If the patient or family appears reluctant, the therapist backpedals and takes the path of least resistance. For example, the therapist may tell the family, "It is too early to do that," or, "Think about it, but don't take any action yet."

Taking the Path of Least Resistance

The therapist uses implicit or indirect ways of turning the family's investment in the problem to positive use (as in reframing). The therapist strives to avoid power struggles with the family members (Weakland et al. 1974).

Paradoxical Interventions

Paradoxical interventions are used with the expectation that the patient or family will rebel or react against the prescription (Jessee and L'Abate 1980). Paradoxical interventions include paradoxical instruction and restraining methods. Paradoxical instruction involves "prescribing the symptom," or prescribing behavior that appears to be in opposition to the goals of treatment to generate movement toward change. Compliance-based paradoxical interventions are based on the premise that by complying with the paradoxical prescription of continuing the symptom in an altered form, the patient will change and the symptom will cease. For example, the therapist may direct a child to have a stomachache and feel anxious for one hour each day, at the same time. Complying with the task implies the child has control of his/her symptom (Jessee and L'Abate 1980).

Restraining is a method used to deal with resistance, to solidify behavioral change, and to keep the therapist from working harder than the family to achieve the goals of treatment. There are various ways of restraining. Many therapists use a restraining strategy early in the therapeutic process to avert the problem of family resistance and unbalance their established homeostasis. Three major restraining strategies include (1) exploration of the negative consequences of change, that is, giving up the anxiety; (2) predicting a relapse; and (3) prescribing a relapse.

The exploration of the negative consequences of change can be used after the initial session and goal setting. The family is told that change can have both good and bad effects. Before the therapist can agree to help the family make their stated desired behavioral changes, the therapist makes sure they understand the cost or negative consequences of change. For example, the therapist cautions the family to think carefully about giving up the anxiety symptoms because the child may become more independent and the parents may feel less needed.

Predicting a relapse is essential to most paradoxical work. In general, this intervention is used after a paradoxical prescription has been given and resulted in the cessation of symptoms. The next step is to predict a relapse. The family is told that the symptom will suddenly reappear. By predicting a relapse the therapist is placing the client in a double bind (Weeks and L'Abate 1982). If the symptom does occur again, the therapist has predicted it, so it is under his control. If it does not occur again, it is under the client's control. The symptom has been defined in such a way that it can no longer be perceived as uncontrollable or spontaneous. A therapist, thus, prescribes a relapse on the rationale that it further increases control over the symptom. "Now that you have managed to turn the symptom off, if you can manage to turn it back on during the next week, you will have achieved even more control over it."

Prescribing a relapse is used to help families see how easily they can fall back into the old dysfunctional patterns and to discover ways to prevent this from happening. To facilitate a relapse prescription, the therapist may ask the child to pretend to have a symptom (Haley 1976). For example, a child could be instructed to have the symptom of stomachaches and panic attacks whenever the parents look angry at each other but aren't talking. If the child begins to relapse in the future, the parents are forced to consider their part in the problem. The use of restraining techniques requires careful timing and delivery. The general rule is that as soon as change begins, a restraining statement should be given to the client.

Strategic Disengagement

This is a technique the therapist uses to distance him/herself from the family when it is clear that a family is resisting change or trying to place the responsibility for change on the therapist. The therapist might respond with a calm, withdrawing statement such as, "I can see you've got a problem." When the family agrees and asks what to do about it, the therapist might say, "It's a tough one." If they pursue further, asking for instruction, the therapist might respond with, "I don't know what you should do." This technique can have at least two effects: (1) it shifts the responsibility for change back onto the family; and (2) it may unite the family against the therapist, placing them in a position where they are no longer diverting their energies toward triangulating the outsider but must turn to each other for cooperation, problem solving, and change.

Unbalancing

Unbalancing is a technique the therapist uses to help challenge the homeostatic status quo within the family. The therapist may choose to side with one parent against the other to force members to assert themselves and practice a more direct form of communication. Unbalancing facilitates the dissolution of dysfunctional behaviors. This is followed by a period of reorganization within the family involving healthier ways of communicating. The intervention focuses on the family structure (content) and the manner in which people respond to one another (process), not on the issues discussed.

ASSESSMENT PROCEDURES

Assessment procedures within the structural and strategic models of family therapy are part of the therapy itself. By closely observing the family's interactions and focusing on process rather than content, the therapist gains valuable diagnostic information. It is this information that allows the therapist to assess the structure of the family and begin to plan strategies for the constructive reorganization of this structure. The development of working hypotheses begins with the first phone call from the family. Continued adding and modification of hypotheses is done throughout the duration of therapy.

At least three family members are required for the therapist to be able to observe coalitions, detours and protection, or invasion of subsystem boundaries. The ideal assessment unit is everyone who is relevant in the case; all members residing in the home plus extended or estranged family members. It is important to have the involvement of all persons who play an important part in opening or obstructing avenues for change—without them, the therapist cannot access potentially valuable resources and critical roadblocks. Data from school personnel and other professionals involved with the family should be accessed either by phone consultation or from written summaries.

The genogram is constructed in one of the first two sessions and revised as new information becomes available. As mentioned previously, the genogram is viewed as an essential tool for assessment and treatment planning. It is used to organize data on family history—including physical health, mental health, chemical dependency, loss issues, and transitional life events in the family. The genogram is also used to diagram current, historical, and cross-generational patterns of family interactions, and to identify dysfunctional family structures.

Beginning with a more structural approach, the therapist's assessment is based on the direct observation of a family's behaviors during spontaneous transactions that occur while gathering the genogram data or getting a definition of the problem. The therapist evaluates the observable transactions (process) more than the verbal accounts (content) of the family's stories. When one family member is talking, the therapist notices who supplies information, who interrupts or completes the information, and who gives help (Minuchin and Fishman 1981). This process data gives the therapist a tentative picture of who is close to whom, and what the affiliations, coalitions, and overinvolved dyads or triads are in the family. It reveals patterns that express and support the structure. In addition to tracking and observing spontaneous transactions among family members, the structural family therapy assessment includes the creation of enactments to help the therapist identify the strengths and weaknesses of the family.

Another part of the assessment process is the incorporation of the collected data into the treatment process. The therapist selectively chooses to highlight certain transactions and content while ignoring or downplaying others. This technique of punctuation is used by the therapist to feed back to the family members a transactional version of their conversations and behaviors in the session: "You are a close family"; "This family is grieving the loss of their protector, Grandpa"; "It's easier for your son to talk to Mother than to you." Because these statements are comments on transactions, they challenge the family's notion that individual behaviors are a straightforward expression of the desire for personal gain. They help each family member see his/her own behavior as affecting the whole, and lay the groundwork for a change in the perceptions of the problem from an individual to a family problem.

FOCUS OF TREATMENT

An integrated model of structural-strategic therapy in working with anxiety disorder families specifies a three-stage focus of treatment. Following Stanton's (1981c) general rules for the integrated model of family therapy, the therapist starts by using a structural approach—joining, testing boundaries, and restructuring hierarchy and patterns (General Rule Number 1). The therapist assumes a directive role vis à vis the family. The initial goal of family therapy is to change the underlying family structure so problematic interactional patterns can be exchanged for more functional ways of relating to one another (Minuchin 1974).

If the therapist finds that structural techniques are not succeeding or are unlikely to succeed, the next strategy of the integrated model is to switch to a predominantly strategic approach with the goal of changing the dysfunctional sequence of behaviors in the family (General Rule Number 2). This "switching to a more strategic focus" is done when the somewhat confrontational structural approach leads to the escalation of defensiveness in family members.

The third phase of therapy in this integrated model suggests that "following success with strategic methods, and given that a family continues in therapy, it may be advisable to revert once again to a structural approach" (General Rule Number 3). This is the "restructuring phase" (Andolfi et al. 1980). In this phase of family therapy the identified patient becomes less central and all family members start to behave more as individuals with separate boundaries rather than as a group. At this point structural techniques such as creating boundaries and use of enactment are appropriate.

Within the structural-strategic model, treatment goals exist on two levels. On one level goals are negotiated between the therapist and the family. Usually these goals focus on a specific complaint with an identified patient. The agreed-upon goal for the family would be to eliminate the source of the complaint, such as (1) Mary should quit turning off all the lights and locking all the doors in the house, or (2) Jim should control his temper and make some friends. Concern about the complaint may or may not be shared by all family members. Mary may view her behaviors as normal safety precautions, and Jim might not see anything wrong with his temper and may feel he has enough friends. It may also be that Jim's father doesn't see anything wrong with his son's anger outbursts and tendencies to be a loner, but mother is concerned. So the therapist listens, encourages discussion among family members, explores what each person wants, and identifies congruencies and incongruencies among the respective goals, helps the family formulate common goals when possible, and points out areas of dispute when it is not.

On another level the therapist may have an additional set of goals based on the family assessment process, which may not coincide with the way in which the family views themselves. Parents may, for example, want a closer relationship with their son when, developmentally, the adolescent should begin the process of individuating from his parents and family. To help the family, the therapist will challenge them on the locus of the problem and how it should be solved. The difference between the family and family therapist in terms of structural goals is inherent in the process of structural family therapy. The therapist does not necessarily share his/her goals with the family.

ROLE OF THE THERAPIST

Although some theoretical approaches encourage the therapist to be reflective, passive, and generally nondirective, the structural-strategic approach to family therapy necessitates that the therapist be directive, assertive, and at times use his/her role as the expert to facilitate systemic changes. The therapist interrupts conversations, pushes for conflict through enactment, and may support one family member over another to unbalance the system. The therapist controls the rhythm of the session and sometimes may act in an inconsistent manner. For example, he/she may initially support an obnoxious 16-year-old to join with the youngster to gain some leverage, but support the parents in setting limits and encouraging them to be firm with their son later in the session.

The therapeutic alliance between the therapist and parents as well as that between the therapist and children must be respectful and affirmative for the therapist to join with the family and develop the trust needed for therapeutic change. As Bergin and Lambert (1978) and others have suggested, the therapeutic alliance is a necessary but not sufficient condition for change.

The therapist must operate flexibly. He/she has to join the system but also must retreat quickly when necessary, lest he/she be inducted by the power of the system. The therapist must have a game plan prior to the start of each session. This plan is based on knowledge of the family structure as well as hypotheses concerning the family and the relationship between the presenting problem and the dynamics of the system.

TREATMENT STRATEGIES

The integrated model of structural-strategic therapy incorporates ongoing modification of the treatment strategy. This approach maintains, as outlined under the focus of treatment, that the therapist must continually assess and reassess hypotheses and techniques to ascertain their effectiveness and determine whether a change of focus is necessary.

Within the overall framework of the structural-strategic model, there is flexibility regarding who attends the treatment sessions. While most sessions may be attended by the whole family (including parents and children, and sometimes grandparents or others who live in the same household), others may be reserved for selected members, depending on the need to concentrate on the development of specific subsystems. The children, or the parents, may be excused from a session in order to work on subsystem issues, create boundaries, realign the hierarchy, or work toward conflict resolution within a dyad.

Although the current state of the economic pressures and managed mental health care may influence the duration of therapy, the structural-strategic model does not prescribe a standard regarding the length of treatment, number of sessions, or duration of the session. The length of treatment is negotiated between therapist and client. The structural and strategic family therapy sessions, however, tend to be fewer than those of other models of psychotherapy. The strategic therapist in particular prefers to keep therapy brief and terminate as soon as possible following positive change in the presenting problem (Stanton 1981c). The structural viewpoint would suggest that although a symptom drops off after a few sessions, structural change must occur to prevent a recurrence. The structural therapist works toward symptom reduction as quickly as possible, while at the same time looking to restructure the family system so changes will endure over time.

DEALING WITH COMMON OBSTACLES TO
SUCCESSFUL TREATMENT

The Absent-Parent Family

The term *absent parent* is used here to describe a family in which one parent must carry out all parental obligations and ongoing involvement when the other parent is precluded from doing so, as in unwed pregnancies, death of a parent, abandonment, or cases of serious abuse. Current estimates suggest that nearly 50 percent of all new marriages will end in divorce (U.S. Bureau of the Census 1989), and that divorce will affect nearly one-third of the minor children in this country (Bane 1979). Other data indicate that over 80 percent of these postdivorce single-parent families are headed by women (U.S. Bureau of the Census 1989).

Following divorce, a large number of children grow up without the continuing involvement of their biological father. Many fathers are left in conflictual or cutoff positions and do not provide ongoing financial or emotional support to their children and the custodial mothers. Weitzman's (1985) investigation of divorce in California revealed that despite changes in the divorce laws to promote no-fault divorce and joint custody, 23 percent of fathers did not see their children at all after divorce. In a national study, 50 percent of the children had not seen their nonresidential father in the past 5 years. Of the 50 percent who had contact, 20 percent had not seen their fathers within the past year and only 16 percent saw their fathers weekly (Furstenburg et al. 1983).

For the therapist working with anxiety disorders in children, it is important to be cautious regarding the use of the term *single parent* so as not to reinforce a dysfunctional cutoff by the absent parent. Secondhand reports of father's unwillingness or inability to be involved should not be relied on without exploration of his past, current, and potential contributions to the family. Imber-Black (1991) suggests that presumptions that an absent parent is uncaring, destructive, crazy, or hopeless should be examined along with the potential benefits of a reunion with the estranged parent. She suggests that attempts should be made to change the situation and incorporate estranged parents into the family structure if appropriate and possible. These steps may help to ameliorate a mother's burden and to improve the well-being of the children.

Other issues involved in absent-parent and divorced families include the overload of parental duties on the custodial parent. When overload occurs, a distressed parent may be unable to provide emotional support and set appropriate limits for a confused, anxious, or demanding child. The child's upset exacerbates parental distress. As pressures mount, the custodial parent may become punitive, less affectionate, and more erratic in discipline (Weiss 1979). Children often develop myths and fantasies regarding the absent parent that can elevate the absent parent to the role of hero. Children may also develop a fear that the custodial parent will quit loving them and abandon the family.

It is important for clinicians to be aware of nontraditional family structures within many single-parent or absent-parent families. Many single parents, especially poor, minority women, live with their own mothers. The executive or parental subsystem that requires validation consists of these two women who are raising the children. The clinician must assess the role of other significant members of the household, especially grandparents, other extended family members, or the new partner of the custodial parent.

Economic Barriers

Families that are poor generally lack access to adequate health care and competent educational systems and are required to interact with the welfare system. Interaction with the system is often intimidating. Stresses of poverty are compounded by stresses in dealing with numerous agencies and professionals. Welfare system requirements may fragment families through practices and policies that ignore diverse family organizations—such as households headed by two women—or may require fathers to leave for the family to receive aid.

As the financial problems play out, children may become overly knowledgeable and involved in adult issues. Developmentally, the children would ideally be free of these worries to focus on school and the development of peer relationships. In reality, children living in poverty tend to internalize their parents' worries and resentments regarding the struggles of meeting basic needs for food, clothing, and shelter.

It is important for the family therapist to be aware of the impact of poverty on families and know how to facilitate the development of boundaries and hierarchies when children may be participating in the economics of the family. Some modification in interventions will be necessary to accommodate the family's economic reality.

Economic limitations also interfere with a family's participation in therapy due to the lack of money or insurance to assist in the cost. Another barrier may arise in terms of scheduling family therapy appointments. Many low-income parents work two or three low-paying part-time jobs. Parents may work opposite shifts to avoid the expense of child care. Finding time for therapy sessions will call for flexibility on the part of both therapist and family.

The Coordination of Services with Multiple Providers

A family with multiple problems may be involved with a variety of professionals (Coppersmith 1985, Selig 1976). The family therapist must be informed about the involvement of doctors, school counselors, the welfare system, and so on. Consultation among collateral professionals can help avoid further chaos for the family and assist all involved in moving the family toward autonomy.

One barrier to treatment can be mixed messages given to individuals and families when various therapists and agencies are involved. There can be loyalty issues, duplication of services, and the external mirroring of patients' internal confusions and anxieties. Imber-Black (1991) suggests that within some multiproblem families resistances may arise that need to be examined in terms of the wider social context of relationships. She refers to this as the "family-larger-system." She describes how the family therapist may serve as negotiator between the family and the larger systems to reduce anger and misunderstanding. The therapist may mediate, translate obscure policies, and facilitate conflict resolutions through coordination of services.

The family's involvement with social services or child protection provides a unique form of family-larger-system relationship that has an intense impact on family therapy. When a larger system, such as child protection, cannot get information from a family, it may use a family therapy referral in an attempt to gain greater access. The referring agency may expect the therapist to furnish reports on the family and provide crucial information for its decision-making process. It is important for the therapist to be vigilant regarding his/her part in the macrosystem. Boundaries need to be defined and the family therapist's role clearly addressed to prevent inadvertent alliances with child protection that might sabotage family therapy.

Families often do not tell the therapist they are involved or have been involved with other systems or professionals. Some families, however, may prefer multiple helpers due to their belief that their problems are too big for one professional to handle. The danger is the lack of coordination of services.

Upon discovering that a family is involved with larger systems, the therapist may establish phone contact with the other professionals to discern their roles in the case. A release of information must be signed by the family. Freeman (1992) suggests that care should be taken regarding the sharing of information that emphasizes the negative, dysfunctional aspects of the family in order to respect the family's confidentiality, to promote positive change, and to allow the other professionals to create their own opinions regarding the family. Subjective impressions about family members should not be provided. Only the sharing of goals and treatment plan is recommended. A case conference or staffing with the family and other helpers present may be helpful to clarify roles and expectations.

If reports or memos are requested by other professionals, it is recommended that the family participate in providing the data, and the parents are also given the opportunity to read the written reports before they are sent. This will allow the therapist to reduce the ominous nature of the family being talked about by others and continue to cultivate trust, which is part of the on-going joining process.

Open communication and respect among professionals is the key to the coordination of services. Differences among helpers, and the effects of these differences on the family and individual, need to be discussed. One area of concern for some family therapists is the use of medications for anxiety disorders. It is important that the family therapist understand and support the prescribing physician's work and recommendations with the family. A sharing of goals and treatment plan will help the child stabilize.

Family Secrets

Secret keeping is probably one of the most negative processes that occurs in a family system. Secret keeping involves collusion and exclusion. Although excluded family members are often, in fact, aware of the secret, they feel unable to address the issues of the secret directly (Freeman 1992). Family secrets can become a major obstacle to the family therapy process. Anderson and Stewart (1983) outline four categories of secrets that create obstacles to therapy. These include (1) family members have secrets from each other that interfere with the free and open use of the family therapy sessions; (2) family members have secrets from each other that they attempt to share with the therapist; (3) family members have secrets that they share with each other but not with the therapist; and (4) family members are afraid that the therapist will share their secrets with the world.

Secrets may involve facts about the family's history such as depression, mental illness, or suicide attempts. Secrets may also involve more current events such as one family member having an extramarital affair, a young person taking drugs, alcoholism in a parent, or physical or sexual abuse. Sometimes the withholding of information involves a collusion between family members. For example, the mother may not tell the father or the therapist about a child's misbehavior because she feels the response will be negative. By withholding this information from the other adults, the mother and child keep the father at a distance and, at times, the therapist as well.

Family members who keep secrets will usually attempt to involve the therapist in the secret-keeping process. It is critical that the therapist avoid becoming a party to secrets. At times, it is necessary for the therapist to state clearly to the family in the beginning phase of therapy that he/she will not be a party to information that is kept from other family members. The family needs to understand that the therapist who participates in secret keeping restricts his/her freedom to ask those questions that help family members to understand their problems clearly. Occasionally a family member will telephone a therapist and proceed to tell him/her something in confidence. Before this process can be halted the therapist may find him/herself in the middle of a secret. When this happens, it is best handled by the therapist telling the family member that the secret cannot be kept. For parents to discuss with the therapist parental or marital issues without the children present is not considered secret keeping, in fact, the structural-strategic model encourages such subsystem boundaries. The children may be asked to leave the therapy room while the adult issues are discussed.

RELAPSE PREVENTION

Symptom improvement may not be accompanied by long-term changes in family functioning. In a study examining family therapy with adolescent school refusers with obsessional symptoms and depression, Bryce and Baird (1986) suggested therapeutic contact with the families well beyond the child's initial return to school to prevent a relapse. Others (Berg et al. 1976, Berg 1982) have also identified a high incidence of persistent emotional and social difficulties in their longitudinal studies of school refusing adolescents. These problems occurred in one-third of the teenagers three years after treatment. They suggest that the best predictor of outcome is the actual clinical state at termination. Valles and Oddy (1984) reported that the resolution of family conflicts played a crucial role in the outcome of school refusal in children. This supports the three-phase structural-strategic integrated family therapy model, outlined earlier in this chapter, which suggests that the therapist shifts back from strategic to structural interventions following symptom reduction to assure that hierarchical and subsystem boundaries are in place prior to termination. This may be done in less frequent follow-up sessions.

It is recommended that the family be involved in at least two monthly follow-up sessions prior to termination to allow for the solidification of contextual and symptomatic changes. During these follow-up sessions the therapist focuses on the gains the family has made and encourages continued flexibility around problem solving. The therapist supports each family member's functioning within his/her subsystem. As outlined under paradoxical techniques, either prescribing a relapse or predicting a relapse will help in relapse prevention. It is also suggested that when a problem child begins to obey parents and the parents are sufficiently united to take charge, there may be a reaction from other people involved in the family. A common reaction is that of other siblings. A sibling may begin to act out when the hierarchy begins to stabilize with the parents in charge; this is one of the reasons for having all children in the family present for the first few sessions (at minimum) to observe which child is at risk to develop difficulties. The correction of the hierarchy with the parents in charge is a change, one that the siblings do not necessarily welcome. The goal is to persuade the siblings to stay out of the problem and shift the responsibility back to the parents prior to termination (Haley 1976).

TERMINATION

There are various signs that it is time to terminate family therapy. A major indicator of the readiness of a family to stop formal therapy sessions is the ability of the family members to deal with anxiety and tension without developing coalitions or scapegoating a family member, and the ability to communicate more directly with one another. As mentioned earlier, the structural-strategic model of family therapy suggests that structural changes are needed in addition to the cessation of symptoms in the identified patient to maintain long-term changes.

When the therapist senses the family therapy is coming to a close, it is important to schedule a session to evaluate the treatment process and goals. This final evaluation session is an important part of the overall process for both the therapist and family (Freeman 1992). It provides family members with an opportunity to evaluate what they have learned about themselves and the family. The family members are the experts on what has worked for them. During this termination session the therapist reviews the course of treatment, has the family identify their gains, and gives the family and individuals credit for their achievements. The therapist also notes any unresolved issues and remarks on the probable future beyond termination.

A helpful exercise in the termination session is for the therapist to raise possible future scenarios and ask how the family members would use their new learning to deal with these scenarios differently. The scenarios will involve issues with which family members have traditionally had difficulty. It is helpful to remind families that treatment is not intended to solve all of their problems and that they will not be problem-free. They will need to continue working on finding creative ways to respond to ongoing problems using their new problem-solving and communication skills.

In some cases, families who make progress seem unsure of themselves and are concerned about termination. One way of dealing with this problem is by terminating without terminating. That is, let the family know that they seem ready to go on their way and that change can only be really judged by how the family deals with life experiences outside of therapy. The family is then told that the plan is to take a break from treatment and if they should encounter some difficulty later they may return for a follow-up session. Usually, the family departs more at ease and does not call upon the therapist further.

As mentioned in the section of treatment strategies, the therapist works toward symptom removal quickly while at the same time looking to restructure the family so that changes endure. Rosenberg (1983) suggests that this should occur within three to six months. In this time frame, family structures can be successfully modified. Rosenberg (1983) suggests that changes that do not occur within this amount of time are not likely to occur. Rather than continue indefinitely with therapy, it is suggested that the therapist terminate at the point where the presenting problem has been alleviated and the family structure has been altered sufficiently to allow for more effective problem solving. At termination, families are encouraged to be self-reliant and to depend on their own resources, which have been identified during the course of treatment. The door is left open for them to resume therapy in the future if necessary. When families return after an absence from therapy, they most often require only a few sessions to regain their confidence and ability to function satisfactorily.

CASE ILLUSTRATION (TYPICAL TREATMENT)

Description and History

The identified patient is a 10-year-old boy named Mark who was referred to therapy due to a history of panic attacks and refusing to go to school. He was given a full psychiatric evaluation and diagnosed with separation anxiety and overanxious disorders. He was initially referred for individual therapy, although the system-oriented therapist requested that the entire family come for at least two intake sessions. The family consisted of Mark (10), Julie (8), Mother (41), and Father (45). The psychiatric report indicated that the son had a two-year history of school refusal and that he had been described as a "clingy" child since approximately age 4. There was a positive history of mental illness in the family, including a maternal grandmother diagnosed with a delusional disorder and the mother who had dealt with bouts of depression for the past twenty years. "Excessive drinking" and chemical dependency treatment of two paternal uncles were identified. Other medical conditions included Mother's treatment for breast cancer three years prior, which included a bilateral mastectomy. She also had a history of asthma and numerous allergies. Father had not participated in any of the identified patient's treatment or evaluation.

It was Mother who made the initial phone call to the therapist. When the requirement for the entire family to attend the first two sessions was indicated, she replied, "I don't think that his father can take off of work." The therapist provided several therapy time options and outlined the importance of the involvement of the entire family. She offered to speak to the father directly to answer any questions he might have. Mother sighed and in a reluctant tone of voice offered to try to get Dad to come and scheduled an evening appointment. The therapist's initial working hypotheses: Mother either feels hopeless in the pursuit of getting her husband involved in their son's treatment or she prefers not to be bothered by having him involved.

Synopsis of Therapy Sessions

Sessions 1–3

The initial goal was to join with the family while getting a clear definition of the problem from each family member. The family's agenda was to cure their "sick" member, Mark. The therapist's task was to explore the function and reactions of each family member to his problem. In other words, in viewing the system, the therapist must find out how each one responds to Mark and his anxiety and what impact this anxiety has on the entire family. A behavioral sequence of the problem (i.e., episodes of anxiety or panic attacks) and a family-of-origin genogram were completed to develop an interactional context for the anxiety.

Mother was unsuccessful in getting Father to attend Session 1 but with coaching from the therapist was able to find ways to persuade her husband to attend subsequent sessions. The therapist began Session 1 by asking the children their ages, grade in school, and how they felt about being at the therapy session. Once the therapist engaged with everyone, got a history of previous therapy, and asked for any initial questions, she moved on to get a clear definition of the problem by asking, "What brings the family here for therapy?" This was repeated in

Session 2 when Father was present. The working hypotheses were: Both children were enmeshed with Mother; Julie appeared to also be overly close to Father, which indicated a father–daughter coalition that left Mother out. Therapist wondered about marital conflict. Father was ambivalent regarding his involvement in therapy.

Homework assignments included: The children were to allow Mother to have privacy when she goes into the bathroom, and to follow her around the house less. So the children knew that they would get Mother's undivided attention each day without following her to the bathroom, a daily time was set for the children to talk to Mom about school and homework. Dad could be involved in this, too, if he wasn't busy.

As the family came in and sat down at the beginning of Session 2, the therapist observed the family's structural configuration in the seating arrangement. Mother was sitting closest to Mark, then Father, and then Julie. The therapist explained the importance of having the entire family involved, since Mark's anxiety was affecting the entire family and the family was the primary support system for Mark. She highlighted the need to investigate how each person in the family participated in the anxiety. She described that, "Often the entire family can have anxiety or anger or disappointment that they have problems." She then made an attempt to solicit Dad's help in decreasing the symptoms in both of the children. The therapist explained:

> Therapist: After the last session, it became clear that both Mark and Julie have separation anxiety. Mother also appears to have a great amount of fear that Mark won't get better and may possibly get worse.
> Therapist: [Turning to Dad] Do you have the same fears that Mom does regarding your son? Have you noticed how both children refuse to let Mom out of their sight even to the extent that Mom can't use the bathroom by herself?
> Father: No, I don't worry about my son as much as my wife does. In fact, he seems to be handling it better when the children tease him at school now. My son simply refuses to go to school or if he goes he sometimes just lets the kids get to him. It does bother me that he falls behind in his schoolwork. . . . And yes, both kids follow Mom around the house.

The parents disagreed on their son's condition. The therapist made a mental note that Father may indeed see the son as healthier than Mother does, but he appears to be angry at the son for being defiant and refusing to go to school.

Later in the interview, Mother and the children reported that when Dad gets upset he leaves to go to his brother's house. Using a piece of paper and drawing arrows between each transaction in the sequence, the therapist diagrammed the events before, during, and after Dad leaving the house. By diagramming these transactions in a circular way, the therapist was reframing the problem from being an individual problem to being a family problem—no event happens independently and is in fact a reaction to an event that precipitates it. While gathering this transactional data regarding typical interactions among family members, the therapist noted how they communicated with one another and with her while telling their story. The therapist asked for the family to describe the events that lead up to Dad leaving. They told the therapist that Dad had come home from work at 4:00 P.M. and Mom at 5:30 P.M.

Julie: My mom has a picture of me on her steering wheel so she can see it every day when she drives to work and home [changing the subject but providing information about her closeness to Mom].

Mother: Both Mark and Julie ran out to the car when I drove up. They gave me a big hug and helped me carry groceries. Then they followed me around the kitchen as I made dinner. [With a sigh] I wish their Dad would cook but he never does!

Therapist: After the children came and helped you carry things inside and then followed you around the house, what happened next to lead toward Dad getting upset and going to his brother's house?

Mother: I went to the bathroom. As usual both children sat outside the bathroom door and continued to talk to me. I got so upset that I told their Dad about this after dinner. Then Dad threatened to kill the dog!

Therapist: What does the dog have to do with this?

Mother: I don't think he would really do it.

Julie: [Tearful] It's my favorite dog.

Mark: All summer Dad said that he'd put the dog to sleep and threatened to take him to the vet "for shots."

Mother: In May the family put our eighteen-year-old cat to sleep. [Defending Dad] Dad doesn't communicate well sometimes.

Therapist: [Turning to Dad, who has been distant and quiet throughout this dialogue] So when your wife complained to you regarding the children sitting outside of the bathroom again you got upset and said that perhaps you would put the dog to sleep?

Father: Well, our dog is getting old. The kids don't seem to play with it much and no one wants to feed it.

Therapist: When did you leave and what triggered you to leave to go to your brother's house?

Father: I just get tired of all the fighting and noise. The children whine and complain all the time. It gets too crazy so I leave.

Therapist: [Turning to Dad] Is this your release—take a break and leave so that you don't get too angry or continue to yell?

Father: Sorta. My brother and I get along well and he lives down the road.

The therapist was careful not to get sidetracked or introduce a new focus, but took note of additional data regarding the way this family communicated. Since Father was tentative at best regarding his involvement in therapy, it was important not to challenge him or suggest that he make changes until the joining process was more complete.

As the therapist gathered genogram data during Session 3, she looked for reframes and an interactional definition of Mark's anxiety problem. The therapist requested information regarding any history of worrying or events that would trigger family members to worry. Using a blank piece of paper, the therapist drew symbols for each person and asked for dates, ages, and so on. The therapist observed who provided information, what information was unknown, and looked for communication and transactional patterns while collecting the data. Content and process were both important here. Hypothesis: Mark's anxiety was the family's anxiety and a reflection of the fears of Mother's mortality due to her history of cancer. The family was not ready to talk about Mother's health problem yet. At the beginning of the session the therapist reviewed the homework assignment from the previous session. An example of the dialogue: "To let Mom go to the bathroom without either child bugging her, which would provide increased privacy." Improvements were praised. The separation anxiety symptoms were reframed in terms of a "bad habit" rather than defiance, uncontrollable fears, or anxiety. The therapist asked them to continue to work on this for the following week.

Genogram Information

Father's Family: Dad is the second youngest of seven children. His diabetic father died when he was 12 years old. According to Mother, his father was alcoholic, but Dad denied this. Mother also reported that his next older brother went through chemical dependency treatment and, "All of his brothers and sister drink a lot." "His oldest sister is also an alcoholic but doesn't admit it," Mother said. Dad eventually described his family. "They all have tough attitudes, are kinda like fighters and know what to do to survive." He reported that all six of his siblings and his mother live within a five-mile radius of each other in their small town.

Hypothesis: Father could be uncertain about his role as a father due to losing his father at such a young age. He seems to be the protector of his family-of-origin and it's not acceptable to talk about problems such as alcoholism. He also has allowed his wife to be his translator and communicator.

Mother's Family: Mother is the second youngest of four, with one brother and two sisters. Her mother has a delusional disorder and, "Had a breakdown when I was 11." Her mother also was and is addicted to prescription drugs. "Both of my parents are alive, my Dad takes care of my mother twenty-four hours a day and is an alcoholic due to the stress." "My older sister had emotional problems and I was officially diagnosed with major depression five years ago although I've coped with it since I was about twenty years old. I also had a bilateral mastectomy two years ago and then had replacement nonsilicone implants put in one year ago." Her family all live out of state, but within a twelve-mile radius of one another. She is the only one who left the area, so she has only her husband's family around her.

Hypothesis: Mother's history of cancer, double mastectomy, and replacement surgery affects the anxiety level in this family in some ways.

After completing the genogram in Session 3:

Therapist: Both Mother and Father come from very large families and each of them I imagine had to function as very responsible children when they were young due to only having one parent

each of them could count on. In Dad's family his father was
very sick for many years and then died when Dad was 12; about
your age [looking at Mark and then at Dad]. I don't know if
Dad has ever talked about how difficult it was for him not
having a dad [planting a seed regarding the importance of
fathers in families].

Father: It was so long ago.

Therapist: [Turning to Mother, and then to the children] Then for
your Mom; your Mother's mom has been very sick since your
Mother was 11 years old. It must have been very scary for her
and her brothers and sisters having a mother who had to leave
to go to the state hospital for two years at a time and never
knowing what to expect from her.

Mother: Yes it was. She really didn't function like a mother. My
older sister and I ran the family and took care of everything
while my dad and brothers worked.

Sessions 4-5

Goals: To examine the cross-generational coalitions, especially that
between Mother and son. A mother's excessive closeness to a child may
indicate lack of closeness in the marriage. The treatment strategy was to
increase the closeness between Father and son, allowing Mother and
son to separate. The goal was to eventually move the parents back to
the marital subsystem, and to strengthen the marital and parental
subsystems. The therapist began to push gently for structural change to
allow Mark to communicate his concerns to Dad and re-establish the
father–son relationship. The therapist focused on the concept of family
time and each child needing special time with each parent.

Homework assignments included one-to-one time between father–son and mother–daughter subsystems (i.e., playing games, going
on outings). Father was asked to teach his son to be less sensitive. Mom
was asked to take deep breaths and count to ten whenever she felt the
need to step in and protect her son from becoming frustrated or angry.
Mark was to be in charge of his own homework. Julie was asked to stay
out of conflicts and bake cookies with Mom once a week.

At the beginning of Session 4 the parents initiated the agenda.
Mother stated, "Mark had another anxiety attack at school." A description of the sequence was taken around the events leading up to the
onset of the anxiety. Mother started:

Mother: Mark told me it started before gym when he realized he didn't have his gym clothes and had had a schedule change which upset him.

Therapist: Okay, let's back up a bit . . . what happened the night before and in the morning before school?

Mother: When I got home from work Mark was upset. Dad and Mark got into some disagreement about something like Mark not listening to Dad well enough—Mark refused to eat the food that was on the table.

Mark: Dad pushed the table!

Mother: Oh, yes, Dad did hit the table with his hand. Mark had an anxiety attack shortly after this and then Dad left to go to his brother's. The only time that my husband is in a good mood is when he goes to Uncle Gary's cabin in Wisconsin!

Mark: Dad is in a good mood when the other kids are over for Boy Scouts [changing the focus but commenting on his relationship with Dad indirectly].

Mother: Mark and his Dad really don't talk in Boy Scouts but all the other kids get along with his Dad great.

Therapist: The anxiety or Mark's moodiness, or "anxiety attack" if you will, appears to have started the night before with unre-solved conflicts between him and Dad. Each of you including Mark and Dad, plus Mother and sister, all seem to be walking on eggshells and uncertain how to get over conflicts. The children seem uncertain how to get along with Dad and not clear what his standards are. Mom seems to function as the "switchboard" and "fixer" in this family. She comes home from work and tries to smooth everything over when, really, the conflict was between Mark and his dad.

Mother: Right.

Father: [Nodded affirmatively]

Later in Session 4:

Therapist: [Turning to Dad] As long as we have you here today, Dad, I would really like to get an idea how your son and daughter get along with you. [Then turning to Mark] How would you describe your relationship with Dad?

Mark: I don't know.

Father: [Interrupting] We really aren't as close as I'd like to be [glancing toward his son], we don't seem to get along very well.

We always seem to be on a different plane, whenever I want to go someplace Mark doesn't want to go with me.

Therapist: At what age did you last get along well together?

Father: I don't really know, maybe age 6 or 7, Mark used to really enjoy being with me and would go anywhere and everywhere with me.

Julie: [Interrupting therapist] Mark really likes to play Nintendo but this is something that Dad doesn't do as well.

Mother: [Interrupting daughter] I don't think Mark understands Dad, and he doesn't know when Dad is yelling or not and takes it very personal because he is so sensitive.

Therapist: [Turning to Mark] Would you like to go more places or do more things with your Dad?

Mark: [Tearfully] I don't know.

Therapist: [Addressing his affect change] You seem to be upset about this, your eyes are watering.

Mark: I'm just sensitive, I cry at school a lot also. I'm emotionally developing faster than the other kids my age.

(The therapist made a mental note of this 10 year old's adultlike language.)

Dad: It's okay for Mark to cry but maybe he doesn't understand my sarcasm. Julie knows when I am joking and when I am just being sarcastic, but Mark often thinks I am yelling or in a grouchy mood.

Halfway through this session the therapist had Julie and Mark switch places so that Mark and Dad were next to each other (structural rearrangement of seating to set up an enactment).

Therapist: Dad, could you tell your son how you would like your relationship to be with him?

Father: It's hard to describe . . . [glancing at therapist]. I miss how he used to want to be with me.

Therapist: Tell your son.

Father: [Turning to his son] I miss how you used to want to drive around with me in the truck and follow me to the garage when I would work on the car. I realize that you are older now, and this is probably boring to you, but we used to have some good talks and laughs.

Therapist: Do you remember those times, Mark?

Mark: Yeah, a little.

Therapist: [Turning toward Dad] Could you describe for your son what your relationship was with your dad?

Father: [Looking toward Mark] When I was real little we used to be close, but from when I was 7 up until he died when I was 12, he was so sickly all he'd do was yell if we were loud, made messes, or didn't help our mother enough. He was bedridden in the living room for the last one or two years.

Therapist: So you may be uncertain how to have a close relationship with a son who is 10 years old with different interests, yet you would like to be closer.

Father: Yes.

Therapist: And you're a yeller just like your dad.

Father: I guess so.

Therapist: [Toward Mark] Would you like to be closer to Dad?

Mark: Yeah.

As the discussion continued, the sarcasm was reframed as Dad's way of getting close to people.

Therapist: [Turning to Dad] Do you think you could teach Mark to be less sensitive and to understand when you are joking and being sarcastic versus yelling and moody?

Father: I don't know. How?

After discussing possible ways, the therapist presented the homework assignment and a closing comment.

Therapist: At his point I won't ask Mom to stay completely out of father–son and father–daughter arguments, that's too big, but I'd like for the family to just notice how often this happens. So another part of the homework assignment is for each of you to keep track of how often Mom tries to step in and solve your conflicts.

Session 5 was the first session in which there was an alignment switch with Mark letting Mother know that it was not okay for her to call his friends without his permission. This appeared to be threatening to Mother, who put so much energy into protecting her son from any upset. The system was being unbalanced so it could realign in a healthier way. The therapist continued to challenge the family and positively reframe Mother's behaviors. The role of anxiety of other family members was revealed. An example of the dialogue:

> Therapist: Dad on one hand is able to see Mark as much healthier and able to handle the stress of schoolwork and coping with friends but Mom does not trust this and isn't able to kind of let go of Mark and let him be a 10 year old. It is very important to Mom to be a good parent and see that her son gets absolutely all the help that he needs so he doesn't get any sicker.
>
> Mother: I do get afraid. When he panics, I panic. In fact, sometimes I get on edge and get butterflies before he gets upset because I anticipate his tantrums or frustration.
>
> Therapist: So you become anxious even before your son becomes frustrated.
>
> Mother: Yes.

The therapist discussed with the family the need for both individual and subsystem boundaries with the need for children to stay out of adult issues including mother–father disagreements. The therapist reframed the family's behaviors as Mark needing to learn that it's okay to make mistakes without Mother interfering; Mother does too much; and Mother learned to become a worrier from her family-of-origin.

Session 6

Goal: To move the parents closer together in order to continue to dismantle the cross-generational coalitions and to encourage the parents to begin to function as a parental subsystem "united front." The therapist began the session with the entire family but then later met with the parents only. The therapist reinforced a subsystem boundary by asking for the children to leave the room for part of the session so she could talk about "adult issues." She then directed the parents to talk directly to each other (enactment).

The therapist reviewed the homework from the previous session. The family received an "A-plus," with everyone completing their parts. Dad initiated the agenda by stating, "Mark had another hissy fit."

> Therapist: What does this mean?
>
> Father: He has a tantrum and runs around calling me names!
>
> Mark: You yell and yell—it's not me. I got mad, yeah. You chased me to my bedroom again and I wouldn't go this time!
>
> Therapist: [To the parents] Before we go any further I need to meet

with you two alone to find out how you would like your family to operate. Would you mind if the children go to the waiting room while we discuss "adult issues"?

Parents: Sure, that's okay.

The children were asked to leave the office while the therapist talked to the parents.

Therapist: There appears to be a great deal of yelling and name-calling that is different from the sarcasm and joking you are helping to teach your son [looking toward Father]. This may be a bad habit or it may be the way the two of you want your family to function. As you have mentioned earlier, Chuck's father was a yeller [Looking toward both parents]. I will follow your lead. How do the two of you want the communication to be like between you and your children? Between the two of you? Would the two of you talk to each other now and let me know?

Mother: [Looking at therapist] There's too much yelling in our family. No one listens to each other.

Therapist: Talk to your husband. Does he agree?

Mother: [Looking at her husband] Chuck, don't you think you yell too much and the kids yell back too much also?

Father: [Looking at therapist—then looking at wife] I guess.

Mother: Don't you?

Father: Maybe, yes—but how else can we get the children to listen?

Therapist: Those are other issues for us to talk about: How else to reinforce children for positive behavior and how family members can learn to communicate with each other.

Mother: [Turning to husband] No one ever yelled in my family, they weren't sarcastic and they didn't yell.

Father: I'd like it more quiet too. I work in a machine shop all day, I'd like it more peaceful.

Therapist: So both of you are in agreement about wanting the family to decrease yelling and increase positive communication?

Mother: Yes.

Father: Yes.

The children were asked back into the session. The parents together explained the plan for everyone to decrease yelling. This maneuver was done not only to set boundaries around the parental subsystem but also to give the parents the opportunity to present a united front and to show the children that their parents were in agreement and neither child needed to step in to take sides.

Sessions 7–9

Goal: Continue strengthening subsystems through the exploration of Mother's history of cancer. After Mother reported that she has been sickly due to allergies and a cold, the therapist chose to punctuate this and push the family to address the unspoken issue of Mother's cancer. An example of the dialogue:

> Therapist: It seems like both children and Dad along with Mom have fears and anxieties about Mom getting sick. I wonder how each of you handled Mom's cancer operation three years ago and then another operation this past year. When Mom gets sick or upset no one seems to know what to do or say so each of you have a lot of built-up feelings inside. Other than during the intake session I have never heard anyone even mention Mom's history of cancer.
>
> Mother: The children are more attached to me than to their dad. I'm also very close to them, I pace back and forth if either of my children stay overnight somewhere.
>
> Therapist: Are you wondering if your husband can take care of the children if you get sick again?
>
> Mother: Oh, I know he can't. When I was sick with the cancer, I had to have my girlfriend come and take care of the kids.
>
> Therapist: Why? [looking toward Dad]
>
> Father: I'm just not very good at those household things.

As the discussion continued, Father's peripheral role was a focus as well as his lack of understanding of his parenting role. He talked about his desire to get closer to his children and learn to help out more, but was uncertain whether his wife wanted this. All family members became tearful while talking about Mother's cancer and the five years of fears they will hold until she gets a clean bill of health. This was a very moving session with all family members showing a great deal of love, kindness, and sensitivity to one another.

Sessions 8 and 9 were held with the whole family to encourage the continued sharing of feelings and talking about unspoken concerns. During session 9 the family discussed how Mark had been in school for five weeks without any absences and three weeks without panic attacks.

Both Mark and Julie had made several friends at school in the past month, which made both parents very happy. Mark had even joined the wrestling team at school. The therapist then requested to meet with the parents to focus on parenting issues and helping parents act as a united front. The plan was set up to have a one-month follow-up session with the whole family after two sessions with the parents.

Sessions 10–11

The parents were seen alone. The parenting sessions initially addressed specific ways of setting limits with the children and how to continue to keep the children out of adult issues. Eventually they both spoke more openly regarding their marital problems, including lack of intimacy, poor communication, and fears of growing apart. Homework assignments were given for the parents to begin to go out on dates without the children and to have private conversations each day.

Sessions 12–13

One follow-up and then the termination session. The therapist reviewed the progress with the family, including increased boundaries with the children staying out of adult issues and a decrease of each child's attempt to fight their parents' battles; an increase of direct communication; and increased parent–children interactions and quality time together. The therapist also discussed the role anxiety has played in the family, with each family member's earlier responses and the walking on eggshells. The possibility of tension and anxiety returning to this family was discussed along with potential red flags that would indicate a relapse. Preventive strategies were outlined including calling a family meeting in the home when conflict arises or if family members find that they have fallen back into old patterns of yelling or indirect communication, or the children try to function like adults again. The family was somewhat reluctant to terminate, so the therapist left the option of returning for a follow-up session in three months.

Comments

The family was involved in thirteen sessions over a six-month period. Phone contact was made after the three-month period; continued progress was noted with no need for additional therapy sessions. This case illustrates the use of several of the structural-strategic model assessment and intervention tools described earlier in this chapter. This case also illustrates the importance of addressing individual and family fears regarding health problems (e.g., cancer). Parents are often uncertain how to or whether they should discuss these issues openly with their children. It is the therapist's task to facilitate open communication regarding fears and concerns of each family member while helping parents to set boundaries, based on the age and developmental level of their children, to avoid transferring their own fears onto their children.

CASE ILLUSTRATION (OVERCOMING OBSTACLES)

Description and History

A male/female co-therapist team was requested to work with this family due to the absence of any male role models and the reported chaotic nature of the family. This information came from the initial phone contact with the mother and from the consultation with the referring child psychiatrist. Although co-therapist teams are often a luxury in mental health settings, in this teaching hospital a male resident was available to join the therapy team.

This was a single-parent family consisting of Andy (12), diagnosed with separation anxiety and overanxious disorder, Mary (11), diagnosed with separation anxiety with symptoms of panic disorder, and mother, Martha (45). The family was referred because the children were acting out and being overtly defiant with their mother. Child protection had been involved with the family intermittently over the past ten years. There had been a brief foster placement of both children when they were 2 and 3 years old, according to Mother due to "my ex-husband's abusive behavior to me, not the children." There had also been one reported incident of the children being left unattended while Mother went to work. Mother had been divorced for eight years and the children had no contact with their biological father. The mother had recently threatened to place the children in voluntary foster care due to her own frustration and feelings of inadequacy in parenting, and there was a continued increase of violence by the children and toward her.

Synopsis of Therapy Sessions

Sessions 1–3

The typical course of treatment was begun using the structural approach of joining, gathering data regarding transactions, and collecting family-of-origin data using the genogram. As family resistances created roadblocks to treatment, the therapists switched to a more strategic approach with the plan of returning to hierarchical and boundary issues in the later stages of therapy. The initial working hypotheses were: This family might lack trust in professionals due to previous involvement with child protection services. The separation anxiety symptoms of both children might be a function of Mother's ongoing threats of foster care placement, which triggered abandonment issues in them. Hypotheses (formulated during the first two initial assessment sessions): The children might be playing out Mother's ambivalence toward therapy and discomfort with men. The task of the male therapist was to join with Mother, which would ultimately result in the joining with the children because of their overprotection and enmeshment with Mother. The children's distractions in session served some function in the family.

Genogram Information

Mother's Family: Mother was the oldest of five siblings. Her parents divorced when she was 16 years old, which left her to care for her siblings. She described her father as extremely authoritarian and controlling and her mother as "an emotionally abusive woman who didn't like children." Mother also described her parents as "perfectionists—I never could do things good enough for them." Mother briefly described herself as being "physically, sexually, and emotionally abused all my life by my parents and my ex-husband." She was diagnosed with major depression and was seeing an individual psychotherapist on a biweekly basis. Mother left home when she was 22 and never returned. She moved to the Midwest "to get away from my family and ex-husband." Both parents were dead and she had not seen any of her siblings for over two years. She had one female friend whom she trusted but who "doesn't like to be around my children because they fight too much."

Although the biological father was not present and had been absent from the family for several years, data was still gathered using the genogram to determine (1) whether he was accessible, (2) the impact his absence had on the family, and (3) whether there was any contact with the parental side of the family.

Father's Family: He also was the oldest of five siblings. All of his siblings were divorced or remarried. He was a lawyer by profession but the family heard four years ago that he was working as a mail clerk at a post office. There was a question raised as to whether he was an alcoholic. His father and two brothers were all "heavy drinkers." Mother reported that he had been extremely violent with her to the point she had suffered broken bones. There was an active restraining order in place although Mother believed that he had no knowledge of which state the family lived in. There had been no contact with the paternal side of the family for six years.

The goal of Session 3 was to look for ways to reframe and redirect the children's chaotic behaviors. Throughout the session the children threatened to leave, called each other names, rocked their chairs over, and made animal noises. The family had not completed the homework assignment for the second consecutive week. They were to keep track of the number of fights between family members in one week. The family did, however, go for one week without threatening each other with knives or other objects.

Halfway through Session 3, the female therapist (F-therapist) inquired about the way in which the children communicated with Mother and how Mother responded to their whining, begging, and sarcasm. The therapists viewed this behavior as disrespectful and wondered if Mother did, too.

> Mother: I listen to my children and ask their opinion. My parents, as I told you before, were authoritarian and believed that "children are to be seen and not heard." I think it's important to run the family in a more democratic way.
>
> Andy: Yeah. My mom shouldn't be told what to do. I don't want to be here, this is stupid! [He continued to rock his chair and make noises.]
>
> Mary: Yeah, this is stupid! Mom, why do we have to come here? [She then fell over in her chair.]
>
> Mother: Be quiet, you two! [Turning to Mary] Are you okay?
>
> M-Therapist: That's a good question, Mary. Why do we need family therapy? [Glancing at all three family members.] What needs to change? We're not here to change your mother or either of you for that matter, we are here to help with problems. Often families aren't certain how they want help.
>
> Mother: That's true, sometimes it's confusing to me also. It's so hard to get the kids to come here, I have to beg them and then promise to buy them candy or a snack. I get so frustrated, hopeless, and depressed.

F-Therapist: Does it sometimes seem like family therapy and coming here makes things worse? This is common, things often get worse before they get better . . . and sometimes therapy doesn't help, especially if we aren't sure what you want help with.

The children started laughing at each other, pushing each others' chairs, and telling their mother over and over they wanted to leave. Mother continued to ignore this behavior and talked as if it weren't happening. She again made reference to her authoritarian parents, who had extremely strict rules for behavior that interfered with her having an emotionally close relationship with them.

M-Therapist: It seems like you are wanting to do things very differently in your family with your children. You have done a very good job of instilling the values of open communication with your children and giving your children permission to come to you and talk about anything. It has been important for you not to overpower your children, and to teach them the importance of cooperation in a family.

Mother: Yes, yes I have. My children can come to me and tell me everything and anything. And I am very open with them also. They know who I'm dating when I am dating someone, when I work, who my friends are, and most everything. When a mom is all alone like I am, it's important that we get emotional support from our children. It's a two-way street!

M-Therapist: That is true, when there isn't another adult around, often a single parent will turn to their children until they get a chance to get in contact with another adult.

The therapists, while continuing the joining process, begin to shift to a more strategic approach, abandoning the attention to hierarchy. Reframes were provided regarding Mother's permissive behaviors. The therapist praised her encouragement of open communication and the way in which she was being different from her emotionally distant and abusive parents. It was important to meet the parent at her belief system, mirror her language, and agree with her on several different levels while keeping the option for change open. To make attempts to change Mother's view on "democratic" parenting would be futile.

Session 3 ended with the therapists requesting to have an individual session with Mother regarding how she would like her family to operate and to assure the children that they listen to Mother. A paradoxical prescription was provided, restraining them from changing. The family was asked "not to change anything." They were also told, "This is a very close family who care about each other very much. Even the hitting and teasing between the children and of Mother appears to be a way to stay close and perhaps avoid anxiety. We as therapists do not want to interfere with this or increase the anxieties in this family by asking you to make any changes this week until Mother provides us with more information. The only changes we are looking for initially are safety and to stop violence with dangerous weapons such as the knives and this has already been accomplished."

Session 4

Meeting with Mother alone. Goal: Join with Mother, take a "one-down position" and apologize for not listening to her well enough. Elicit from her an option to work as a team with us to help her children and stress the importance of her being the head of the team. Hypothesis: If Mother joins with the male therapist, the children will become less suspicious and more cooperative with therapy. Strategic plan: The male therapist's task during this and subsequent sessions was to align with Mother and look for opportunities to provide encouragement. The female therapist was to do any challenging on issues that were necessary until the joining process was more complete. An example of the dialogue:

> M-Therapist: I really appreciate your willingness to come in for a session without the children. I also like your assertiveness with me. I can see how you might have gotten the message that I was trying to change your style of parenting. I admit that the way I have helped families in the past is with more of a "parents are in charge" model, but that doesn't always have to be. There are different arrangements families make, and yes, in single-parent families like the one you grew up in, the oldest children are often put in charge and look after their younger siblings and provide emotional support. Are there any left-over issues from last session from you?
>
> Mother: No, not really except to say that I am glad that you realize this . . . and that I don't have to put down the law like my parents did. It's too hard for me, I need to treat my children more like friends. My depression does get in the way.

M-Therapist: I'm glad you brought that up. Your depression is something we wanted to get a clearer idea about—how it is for you, how your children react to your depression. What symptoms do they know about? I realize that you are in individual therapy to cope with the specifics and other nonchildren issues, but just generally speaking.

Mother: As I mentioned, my children know a lot. They know a lot about my health, my depression, the pills for my depression, the pills for my diabetes, and my irregular heartbeat I dealt with a couple of years ago.

F-Therapist: How do your children handle this information and your health conditions?

Mother: Andy will sometimes tell me, "Go take your happy pills!"

F-Therapist: Is that okay?

Mother: I think it gives my kids a sense of security when they know I am taking my pills. One thing that's helpful as a single parent, if something should happen, I get run over by a car or something, my children will know what to do. They know what pills I need to take, at what time, and what my diagnoses are. I don't threaten and don't try to instill fear in my children like my mother did . . . she would tell me to change my underwear daily in case we were in a car accident. It's nice to know my kids care and they are concerned. I don't want Andy or Mary to be overly worried.

F-Therapist: Do you ever use this as ammunition for the children, your health conditions to keep them in line with their behaviors?

Mother: [Abruptly] No! [Then a deep breath] Well, I have caught myself at times, like when I totally freaked out when I was screened for the heart murmur. I have also been concerned about reducing stress because of my diabetes and also when they thought I had that heart murmur. I have probably said things that could have been called "scary."

M-Therapist: Could you give us an example of what you have said?

Mother: Oh, that I may have a shorter life because of them and their acting out . . . but generally I keep this to myself. Stress does increase diabetic symptoms, you know.

M-Therapist: I see that you have been keeping the boundaries with your children yet sharing some important information with them on your safety. When you're angry or very frustrated you

may have slipped a few times, telling the children you may die
or blame them for causing or increasing your diabetic symptoms—but generally you are clear that your health conditions
are separate from them.

Mother: Yes, because I know it is very frightening. My parents did
that and I don't want to. They were emotionally abusive.

M-Therapist: You're right, it is very frightening for children, especially in a single-parent family when you are the only person
they can rely on. It sounds like you're real clear on this. Great.

Mother: In desperation, when I'm feeling at a loss for what to do and
trying to keep them from hurting me or hurting each other, I
have said, "What if you two cause me to have a heart attack
right now? Um . . . I did something this past week that worked.
Andy started acting out and I feigned that I was fearful of him
and he stopped. I cringed and told him I was afraid of him.

F-Therapist: Did this work?

Mother: Yes, he stopped. He never apologized, but he stopped.

Later in Session 4:

M-Therapist: It will be helpful for us to have a clearer idea of what
your tolerance level is. We've been impressed by how you can
pay attention to us, provide us with information during the
session, and ignore or rather be so patient with your children
who either are teasing each other or bantering back and forth.
At some point you do tell them to stop and then even after
telling them five to ten times to stop you maintain your
composure for a very lengthy period of time. It's confusing to us
how it gets to a level when you become emotional, tearful, and
then they stop without you asking them.

Mother: I never could cry when the children were growing up. Now
I can cry, which is healthy. I have come a long way.

F-Therapist: You have come a long way. You have your individual
therapist who you seem to work well with and you seem to get
support and guidance with your depression and emotions.
We're wondering about your role as the parent—in our sessions, how many times or how many minutes can you tolerate
their interruptions? That would be helpful. We are not, as we
said earlier, going to enforce our guidelines of perhaps three
warnings and then take a break from the therapy room for five
minutes. You are the parent and have your own tolerance level.

Mother: I do follow the adage that if you ignore behavior it will go away. I know my children are looking for attention — it's never enough, they always need more than I can give.

M-Therapist: That fits with their separation anxiety symptoms.

Mother: I have something to bring up. Mary doesn't like men and has a problem with [M-Therapist]. She's kind of afraid of him, Andy is uncertain of him also. They're never around adult males.

M-Therapist: So this is an added variable. Thank you for bringing this up. I will try not to be threatening and also be clear with both of them that I am in no way here to take the power away from their mother. I like your notion of egalitarian relationships. I see the three of us, in working with your children who struggle with anxiety, are all working together at the same level although you're the expert on your children. You know them better than anyone. About the interruptions — how should we handle them? I have a harder time listening to more than one person at a time.

Mother: Maybe five warnings. This may seem like a lot, but they get so wrapped up in it they forget that I've told them to stop.

M-Therapist: Okay, that's fine. Who gives the warnings?

Mother: All three of us.

M-Therapist: We will take your lead though, okay?

Mother: Okay.

The session ended with the plan for Mother to present this five-warning plan to the children at the beginning of the following family session. Mother also agreed to monitor her anger and blaming of the children regarding her health problems.

Sessions 5–6

The whole family. Goal: To focus on symptoms of anxiety and find out how each child responds to Mother being absent from the home while running errands or working. To work directly with symptom management and set up paradoxical double binds that will encourage flexibility within the family and free the family from the need for the symptom. The therapist attempted to get detailed information on the problem of somatic complaints and map a sequence of how each person responds to sickness in the family. Hypotheses included: Stomachaches and staying home sick may serve a function in the family of keeping Mother busy or of protecting Mother in some way. A tentative plan to incorporate a strategic intervention was agreed upon by the therapists prior to Session 5. The paradoxical technique of prescribing the symptom was used.

Mother began Session 5 by explaining the five-warning rule as planned. Andy took out a paper and pencil and became the monitor of the interruptions. Mother approved his role as the recorder, so the therapist pointed out that he was the "big brother."

M-Therapist: When we first met, Andy and Mary both described nightmares and fears. Each of you [looking at the children] get stomachaches and headaches a lot. Could you tell us how this past week has been with these problems?

Andy: Mother's never home!

Mary: I got a stomachache in school before I came home and went to see the nurse.

M-Therapist: [Turning to Andy] When Mother's not home you feel sick inside?

Andy: Not really, but she's never home.

Mother: I have to work! As a nurse I have long hours—even though I work part-time they are weird shifts. The children have to be left alone. They are old enough.

Andy: But then you sometimes go to your friend's and don't tell us!

F-Therapist: So you have some concerns about your mother. Do you worry about her?

Andy: Yes—she's not a good driver.

Mother: I am too!

Andy: How come our car has so many dents?

Mother: [Turning to the therapists] The kids don't understand fender benders or dents from the parking ramps.

The children have openly provided some new information that appeared to have startled Mother. Hypothesis: Mother appeared defensive around the amount of time she spent away from the children. The therapists chose to wait until a more solid foundation of trust was built before addressing the issue. The therapists changed the topic. [Taking the path of least resistance] The therapists continued to join with the parent and make sure she got the message that she was not viewed as pathogenic but as doing the best she could. The session continued:

F-Therapist: Has anyone missed school this week?

Mother: No, surprisingly enough. Usually when I have a day off I'm taking care of a sick kid. I'm always playing nurse at home.

M-Therapist: Is your mother a good nurse?

Mary: Yes, she knows everything about medicine . . . old remedies from her grandma so we don't have to take drugs that cost a lot.

F-Therapist: Not this week, but in past weeks each of you had missed school. The plan was not to change anything. How does your mother usually know that you are sick?

Mary: I tell her I have a stomachache.

F-Therapist: When does it usually happen?

Mary: When I wake up in the morning.

Mother: I can't get her to get out of bed.

M-Therapist: What triggers this?

Mary: I don't know.

M-Therapist: Andy, how about you? Do you get sick on the same or different days?

Andy: Usually different.

M-Therapist: Do you ever stay home together?

Mother: [Speaking for Andy] No, not usually.

M-Therapist: This is going to sound strange but—we've found through research on anxiety that quite often children can have anticipatory anxiety or stomachaches just thinking about going to school or just thinking about a mom being home alone and thinking she's lonely.

Andy: What?

M-Therapist: Stomachaches can be related to anxiety and your thoughts about Mother or thoughts about school.

Andy: [Pushing at his sister after she stuck out her tongue] Stop it, Mary!

Mother: Quit it, you kids. Listen to the doctors.

Andy: Can we leave?

The therapists seemed to have gotten too close to the issue so they retreated in an effort to detour the resistances and defensiveness and to keep the session safe for the family.

M-Therapist: Just a second. I'm not saying anyone's faking it. The stomachaches are real—ask your mother, the nurse.

F-Therapist: We'll need to find ways to stop the stomachaches before

they happen—or stop the anxiety or thoughts before they
happen.

Mother: How?

M-Therapist: We don't know for sure. We'll need your help [looking
at Mother and then the children].

F-Therapist: Do you want them to stop?

Mary: Yes.

Andy: Of course! Can we go now?

M-Therapist: [Turning to Mother] Several approaches can be taken.
It's like trying new medications, some work better for certain
people. What we've found, for example, is that getting up thirty
minutes before the stomachache usually starts and having
breakfast and playing a game can be helpful. This allows the
focus to be on fun instead of school or Mom being alone.
[Looking at the children] This will confuse your stomach, calm
you down, and bring you joy.

A plan was outlined for Mother to get the children up thirty
minutes earlier on days she had off from work to play board games or
cards with the children. The other part of the plan was also described:

M-Therapist: The other part is that on the days Mother does work—
sometime after she gets home, we want the two of you to let
Mom pretend to nurse you. Mom will go through her "nurse
duties" for thirty minutes.

Mary: What if I really have a stomachache?

M-Therapist: Either way Mom is to nurse you the same. We would
like for you not to tell Mom if it is a real or pretend stomachache. Remember—we're not saying you don't have real stomachaches!

The family persisted to be a bit bewildered regarding the assignment. Mother wondered how this could possibly work, since the
stomachaches and panic attacks in the children became so overwhelming that she felt that they "couldn't possibly not let me know real
versus pretend." The therapists focused on the high level of intelligence
in the children and their ability to act out plays since they were very
little. The therapists also assured the family that, although this task
might be too difficult, at least if they tried it for a week, all would gain
more understanding regarding their anticipatory anxiety. Each per-

son's role and tasks in the assignment were clearly written out on paper and sent home with the family.

A paradoxical prescription always includes a rationale, such as, "for us to gain more information regarding the anticipatory anxiety," and specifies each person's part very clearly. Bewilderment and confusion unbalance the system that is part of the paradoxical intervention. An added note: Session 5 was the first session in which neither child left the room or became so disruptive that a time-out was needed. There was no hitting, yelling, or sarcasm toward the therapists or Mother. Mother also voluntarily sat next to the male therapist for the first time. Hypothesis: A transition has occurred in the trust level in Mother, which has had a calming effect on the children. The children are taking Mother's lead in therapy — Mother is more committed to therapy.

Session 6 began with Andy coming in the room stating that he had fooled his mother so well that, "She never knew when I was faking it!"

M-Therapist: What did you say, Andy?
Mother: I did, too!
Andy: No you didn't, Mom. You never knew when I was faking it!
M-Therapist: [Turning to Andy] How many times did you have a real stomachache, panic attack, or feel anxiety this past week?
Andy: Not at all.
M-Therapist: [Looking puzzled] What?
Andy: I faked it every time! This was a week that I felt okay.

Mother didn't agree with this and went into a long description of three incidents when she "knew for a fact" that Andy had a stomachache related to his anxiety. When the therapists explored the issue further, Mother did agree that Andy hadn't missed school and had a friend over to the house over the weekend, which "probably distracted him." One episode of physical complaints reportedly occurred shortly before the friend came over — Mother was adamant that this was "real anxiety." Andy maintained that it was "pretend." As for Mary, she made the same case for herself and reported that this was a good week for her also. She reported no real stomachaches but that she had two times complained of stomach pains to Mother. Mother agreed and stated, "It was easy to tell Mary was faking, she kept cracking a smile!"

The therapists appeared to remain puzzled and perplexed throughout the entire session. They suggested that this must be a fluke and to expect the real stomachaches to return but possibly be shorter and not so painful as before. The session ended with the therapists asking the family to repeat the assignment with one small change; each morning the children were to give Mom a hug and tell her that they loved her. If, by chance, either child had been in an argument with Mom for some reason or Mom was in a bad mood, he/she was to simply draw a heart on a piece of paper and put it by the front door before he/she left for school.

Session 7

Goal: If symptoms were absent again, begin to gently introduce structural concepts such as rules and boundaries. The family reported that the decrease in anxiety had continued and all family members were in agreement that neither child had stomachaches or panic attacks. Mother suggested that the change in symptoms was due to her decrease in stress at work and having a couple of days off from work so she was home when the children came home from school. Mother then complained about receiving numerous phone calls at work from the children and about some fighting between the children, which seemed to have become violent again. A sample of the dialogue:

F-Therapist: [Looking toward Mother] Is there a rule around phone calls to your work?

Mother: Yes, sorta. I tell them not to call me, but they do.

M-Therapist: How often do they call?

Mother: Oh, Andy calls sometimes as many as five times a night.

Andy: Some of those are Mary telling me to call!

M-Therapist: [Looking toward the children] Are there certain questions or reasons you call your mom about?

Andy: When we can't find anything to eat, when there's no money to go to the store. Things like that.

Mother: Oh, yeah, each of them will call me regarding what to eat. Then they'll call me back to tattle about the other one hitting or name-calling. It's terrible!

M-Therapist: [Looking toward Mother] Do you think it would be helpful to outline what specific reasons to call you at work are okay, and perhaps make a list of other things to do instead of calling you. For example, deciding what's around for snacks or dinner the night before or in the morning when you're home.

Mother: Sure, that would be great!

Mother appeared to be more trusting and able to talk about rules at this session. During this session, the issue of the children sleeping in Mother's bed (a family secret until Session 6) was addressed and the issue of boundaries was introduced. Mother's lack of privacy and personal space was emphasized. Mother also raised the issue of the children not liking anyone she dated but this could not be addressed directly due to Mother's current lack of involvement with a male.

The family cancelled the next three sessions for various reasons including illness and the children not wanting to miss school. The therapists were in contact with Mother throughout a two-month period. Eventually Mother reported by phone that the children were doing so well that she wanted to reward them by honoring their request of not returning to therapy. There had been no violence for two months, both children had not missed school, and in fact, Andy made the A honor roll and Mary received all Vs (Very good) and Os (Outstanding) on her report card.

The therapist complimented Mother on her children's progress and the caring in the family and outlined briefly all the progress they had made. Mother declined the therapist's suggestion for a termination session for closure. The therapists sent a letter to the family outlining the strengths of each child, congratulating them on their excellent school performance and on the completion of all the family therapy goals.

Comments

Three months later the therapists received a handwritten note with school pictures of each child. The note stated that they were all doing well and were planning a summer vacation together. There had been periodic stomach-aches and some clinging behaviors off and on, but Mother was proud of their age-appropriate behaviors and how the children were making friends. Mother closed with a brief statement regarding herself and her new romantic relationship with a man whom the children really liked.

This family was involved in seven sessions over a three-month period. This case illustrates the need for therapists to remain flexible and to have the ability to detour resistances and deal with obstacles that may interfere with therapy. The therapists began with the structural family therapy approach and quickly shifted to a more strategic focus. It was important to acknowledge the impact and role of the absent father, previous involvement with child protection and foster care, as well as Mother's beliefs in a nontraditional family structure. It is the therapist's responsibility to find ways to join and engage with families who have had life experiences that have resulted in a lack of trust and suspiciousness of professionals.

SUMMARY

Family therapy is an essential primary or adjunct therapy for the treatment of any child diagnosed with a mental illness. An integrated structural-strategic family therapy approach has been presented as a straightforward and effective method of treatment for children with anxiety disorders. Grounded in the principles of systems theory, the structural-strategic family therapy approach focuses primarily on the relationship between the symptom (anxiety) in the individual and the function it serves in the family. The exploration of the impact the anxiety has on the entire family and how the family operates to maintain the symptomatic behavior are essential features of this approach. As presented in this chapter, it is important to examine the context in which the child lives. Using the structural family therapy approach as a first step, the therapist examines the family in terms of roles, subsystems, boundaries, and hierarchical structure to determine rigidity, enmeshment, or disengagement among family members. Directives and enactments are used in assessment and intervention. The goal of the structural component of this model is to establish a functional hierarchy so as to permit the family to deal in a competent and cooperative manner with the tasks of the family life cycle stage that are most salient at the particular time.

In order to avoid conflict with the family and cope with resistance to therapy and change, the structural-strategic model requires that the therapist remain flexible and be able to switch from a structural approach to a more strategic approach when needed. The strategic focus is on the resolution of the presenting problem—the anxiety disorder—and the examination of the presence or absence of age-appropriate behaviors. This phase of treatment incorporates paradoxical techniques, such as therapeutic double binds, in order to use family resistance to aid in problem resolution.

The last phase of treatment as suggested by Stanton (1981c) is the return to the structural tasks of establishing appropriate subsystem boundaries and the delineation of a more functional family hierarchy in order to facilitate permanent change and prevent relapse. Treatment is brief (eight to ten sessions) and the coordination of services among multiple professionals is essential.

The family therapist has an important role to play in the treatment of children with anxiety disorders. The inclusion of the family in treatment provides valuable information that is needed to design effective interventions. In addition, the family is empowered to assist the identified patient, who is in turn relieved of the entire burden of the diagnosis. The usual course of family treatment has the advantage of being brief. This is less time consuming for busy families, allows the therapist to treat more clients in need, and is cost effective for today's managed mental health care insurance companies.

REFERENCES

Anderson, C. M., and Stewart, S. (1983). *Mastering Resistance: A Practical Guide to Family Therapy*. New York: Guilford.

Andolfi, M., Menghi, P., Nicoló, A. M., and Saccu, C. (1980). Interaction in rigid systems: a model of intervention in families with a schizophrenic member. In *Dimensions of Family Therapy*, eds. M. Andolfi and I. Zwerling. New York: Guilford.

Aponte, H. J., and Van Deusen, J. M. (1981). Structural family therapy. In *Handbook of Family Therapy*, ed. A. L. Gurman and D. P. Kniskern, pp. 310–368. New York: Brunner/Mazel.

Bane, M. J. (1979). Marital disruption in the lives of children. In *Divorce and Separation: Context, Causes, and Consequences*, ed. G. Loevinger and O. C. Moles. New York: Basic Books.

Beardslee, W. R., Bemporad, J., and Keller, M. B. (1983). Children of parents with major affective disorder: a review. *American Journal of Psychiatry* 140:825–832.

Berg, I. (1982). When truants and school refusers grow up. *British Journal of Psychiatry* 141:208–210.

Berg, I., Butler, A., and Hall, G. (1976). The outcome of adolescent school phobia. *British Journal of Psychiatry* 128:80–85.

Bergin, A. E., and Lambert, M. J. (1978). The evaluation of therapeutic outcomes. In *Handbook of Psychotherapy and Behavior Change: An Empirical Analysis*, 2nd ed., ed. S. L. Garfield and A. E. Bergin. New York: Wiley.

Bernstein, G. A., and Garfinkel, B. D. (1988). Pedigrees, functioning and psychopathology in families of school phobic children. *American Journal of Psychiatry* 145:70–74.

Bertalanffy, L. von (1950). An outline of general systems theory. *British Journal of the Philosophy of Science* 1:134–165.

———— (1968). *General Systems Theory*. New York: Braziller.

Bryce, G., and Baird, D. (1986). Precipitating a crisis in family therapy and adolescent school refusers. *Journal of Adolescence* 9:199–213.

Carter, B., and McGoldrick, M. (1988). *The Changing Family Life-Cycle: A Framework for Family Therapy*, 2nd ed. New York: Gardner.

Coppersmith, E. I. (1985). Families and multiple helpers: a systemic perspective. In *Applications of Systemic Family Therapy*, ed. D. Campbell and R. Draper. New York: Grune & Stratton.

Crowe, R. R. (1983). A family study of panic disorder. *Archives of General Psychiatry* 40:1965–1969.

Eisenberg, L. (1958). School phobia: a study of the communication of anxiety. *American Journal of Psychiatry* 114:712–718.

Fisch, R., Weakland, J. H., and Segal, L. (1982). *The Tactics of Change: Doing Therapy Briefly*. San Francisco: Jossey-Bass.

Freeman, D. S. (1992). *Multigenerational Family Therapy*. New York: Haworth.

Furstenberg, F., Nord, C. W., Peterson, J. L., and Zill, N. (1983). The life course of children of divorce: marital disruptions and parental contact. *American Sociological Review* 48:656–668.

Haley, J. (1971). *Changing Families*. New York: Grune & Stratton.

—— (1973). *Uncommon Therapy: The Psychiatric Techniques of Milton H. Erickson*. New York: Ballantine.

—— (1976). *Problem-solving Therapy*. San Francisco: Jossey-Bass.

—— (1980). *Leaving Home*. New York: McGraw-Hill.

Imber-Black, E. (1991). A family-larger-system perspective. In *Handbook of Family Therapy*, vol. 2, ed. A. S. Gurman and D. P. Kniskern. New York: Brunner/Mazel.

Jessee, E., and L'Abate, L. (1980). The use of paradox with children in an inpatient setting. *Family Process* 19:59–64.

Kendall, P. C. (1985). *Cognitive-behavioral Therapy for Impulsive Children*. New York: Guilford.

Laing, R. (1967). *The Politics of Experience*. New York: Pantheon Books.

—— (1969). *The Politics of the Family*. New York: Random House.

Last, C. G., Hersen, M., Francis, G., and Grubb, H. J. (1987a). Psychiatric illness in the mothers of anxious children. *American Journal of Psychiatry* 144:1580–1583.

Last, C. G., Phillips, J. E., and Statfeld, A. (1987b). Childhood anxiety disorders in mothers and their children. *Child Psychiatry and Human Development* 18:103–112.

Madanes, C. (1991). Strategic family therapy. In *Handbook of Family Therapy*, vol. 2., eds. A. S. Gurman and D. P. Kniskern, pp. 396–443. New York: Brunner/Mazel.

Madanes, C., and Haley, J. (1977). Dimensions of family therapy. *Journal of Nervous and Mental Disease* 165:88–98.

McDermott, J. F., Werry, J., and Petti, T. (1989). Anxiety disorders in childhood or adolescence. In *Treatments of Psychiatric Disorders*, vol. I, pp. 401–446. Washington, DC: American Psychiatric Association.

McGoldrick, M., and Gerson, R. (1985). *Genograms in Family Assessment*. New York: W. W. Norton.

McGoldrick, M., Pearce, J., and Giordano, J. (1982). *Ethnicity and Family Therapy.* New York: Guilford.

Minuchin, S. (1974). *Families and Family Therapy.* Cambridge, MA: Harvard University Press.

Minuchin, S., and Fishman, H. C. (1981). *Family Therapy Techniques.* Cambridge, MA: Harvard University Press.

Minuchin, S., Rosman, B., and Baker, L. (1978). *Psychosomatic Families: Anorexia Nervosa in Context.* Cambridge, MA: Harvard University Press.

Oppenheimer, K., and Frey, J., III (1993). Family transitions and developmental processes in panic-disordered patients. *Family Process* 32:341–352.

Raskin, M., Peeke, H. V. S., Dickman, W., and Pinsker, H. (1982). Panic and generalized anxiety disorders: developmental antecedents and precipitants. *Archives of General Psychiatry* 38:687–689.

Rosenberg, J. B. (1983). Structural family therapy. In *Handbook of Family and Marital Therapy,* eds. B. Wolman and G. Stricker, pp. 159–185. New York: Plenum.

Roth, M. (1959). The phobic anxiety-depersonalization syndrome. *Proceedings of the Royal Society of Medicine: Section of Psychiatry* 52:587–595.

Selig, A. (1976). The myth of the multi-problem family. *American Journal of Orthopsychiatry* 46:526–531.

Selvini Palazzoli, M., Prata, G., Cecchin, G., and Boscolo, L. (1978). Hypothesizing — circularity — neutrality: three guidelines for the conductor of the session. *Family Process* 19:3–10.

Solyom, L., Beck, P., Solyom, C., and Hugel, R. (1974). Some etiological factors in phobic neurosis. *Canadian Psychiatric Association Journal* 19:69–78.

Solyom, L., Heseltine, C. F. O., McClure, D. V., et al. (1973). Behavior therapy versus drug therapy in the treatment of phobic neurosis. *Canadian Psychiatric Association Journal* 18:25–31.

Stanton, M. (1981a). Marital therapy from a structural/strategic viewpoint. In *The Handbook of Marriage and Marital Therapy,* ed. G. Sholevar. New York: S.P. Medical and Scientific Books.

——— (1981b). Strategic approaches to family therapy. In *Handbook of Family Therapy,* ed. A. L. Gurman and D. P. Kniskern. New York: Brunner/Mazel.

——— (1981c). An integrated structural/strategic approach to family therapy. *Journal of Marital and Family Therapy* 7:427–438.

Torgersen, S. (1983). Genetic factors in anxiety disorders. *Archives of General Psychiatry* 40:1085–1089.

U.S. Bureau of the Census. (1989). *Statistical Abstracts of the United States,* 109th ed. Washington, DC: Government Printing Office.

Valles, E., and Oddy, M. (1984). The influence of a return to school on the long term adjustment of school refusers. *Journal of Adolescence* 9:199–213.

Waldfogel, S., Tessman, E., and Hahn, P. (1959). A program for earlier intervention in school phobia. *American Journal of Orthopsychiatry* 29:324–332.

Waldron, S., Shrier, D. K., and Stone, B. (1975). School phobia and other childhood neuroses: a systematic study of the children and other families. *American Journal of Psychiatry* 132:802–808.

Weakland, J., Fisch, R., Watzalawick, P., and Bodin, A. M. (1974). Brief therapy: focused problem resolution. *Family Process* 13:141–168.

Weeks, G. R., and L'Abate, L. (1982). *Paradoxical Psychotherapy.* New York: Brunner/Mazel.

Weiss, R. S. (1979). *Going It Alone.* New York: Basic Books.

Weitzman, L. (1985). *The Divorce Revolution: The Unexpected Social and Economic Consequences for Women and Children in America.* New York: Free Press.

17

COGNITIVE-BEHAVIORAL GROUP THERAPY

Golda S. Ginsburg
Wendy K. Silverman
William S. Kurtines

INTRODUCTION

This chapter describes group cognitive-behavioral treatment (GCBT) for children with anxiety and phobic disorders. GCBT is currently being evaluated with the support of the National Institute of Mental Health at the Child Anxiety and Phobia Program (CAPP) at Florida International University. Overall, the activities at CAPP aim to develop and test approaches to assessment and intervention that integrate and combine the most efficacious features of the cognitive-behavioral approach. These assessments and interventions are targeted for problems and populations that have historically been neglected in the empirical literature, children and adolescents with phobic and anxiety disorders and their families.

The chapter begins with a brief review of the literature on group treatment for children with anxiety and phobic problems, followed by a description of GCBT – its conceptual rationale, assessment procedures, and treatment techniques. The methods for establishing treatment goals, the role of the therapist, specific treatment strategies, obstacles to treatment success, relapse prevention, and termination issues are also discussed. The chapter closes with case vignettes of GCBT that illustrate various aspects of implementation.

Completion of this chapter was supported by NIMH grant #49680 awarded to Dr. Silverman and Dr. Kurtines.

LITERATURE REVIEW

Research literature on the effectiveness of group treatment for children with anxiety and phobic disorders is limited. Moreover, the literature that does exist is fraught with methodological problems that thereby render it difficult to draw conclusions regarding treatment efficacy. Many of the methodological problems are similar to those found in the individual childhood anxiety/phobia treatment literature and have been discussed in detail elsewhere (e.g., Silverman and Kearney 1991, Silverman and Rabian 1993). A brief mention of these methodological issues is worth noting here. Treatment outcome studies for childhood anxiety and phobic disorders are characterized by a failure to employ controlled experimental procedures, clinical samples, formal diagnostic approaches, multimethod-multisource assessment procedures, and systematic follow-ups (Silverman and Rabian 1993). In addition, research in this area has inadequately addressed the issue of the relative efficacy of one treatment technique (e.g., modeling vs. systematic desensitization) or format (individual vs. group) over another.

Another important limitation, specific to the group treatment literature, is that the majority of the studies conducted were not designed specifically to evaluate a group approach per se. Rather, in most of the studies, it appears that children with excessive fears or anxieties just happen to receive a particular procedure (e.g., systematic desensitization) in a group format. The reasons for the group-administered procedure appear to be guided more by practical than by conceptual considerations. It should also be noted that the early group treatment literature is vague, and it is not always clear precisely how the treatment procedures were implemented. With the above limitations noted, a brief review of the studies that have used a group format for treating childhood anxiety and phobias now follows.

One of the earliest studies to employ a group approach for the treatment of childhood anxiety was conducted by Kondas (1966). In this study, the effectiveness of three different group-administered treatments was compared to a no-treatment control in reducing test anxiety and stage fright in twenty-three 11- to 15-year-old children. The three specific treatments, which varied in duration, were (1) relaxation training only (ten sessions, three of which included practice of relaxation in the classroom), (2) systematic desensitization (seven sessions of relaxation training plus five sessions of group-administered systematic desensitization), and (3) imaginal exposure (four sessions, which included imagining items on a fear hierarchy with no relaxation training). The children, obtained from a large school, were selected for treatment based on their scores on self-report measures (e.g., an adapted version of the Fear Survey Schedule, Wolpe and Lang 1964), an interview, and teacher descriptions of symptoms and degree of stage fright. The identified children were randomly assigned to the four groups (five to six children per group). Pre- and posttreatment assessments and a five-month follow-up assessment included the adapted version of the Fear Survey Schedule and the clinical interview, as well as a measure of palm perspiration during a staged examination. On each of the post- and follow-up assessment measures, improvement was greatest for the children in the systematic desensitization group (Group 2). Children in the relaxation and hierarchy groups (Groups 1 and 3) also showed some improvement, but these gains were not maintained at follow-up. The children in the control group did not evidence any improvement on any of the assessment measures.

Another study, targeting test anxiety in 12- to 14-year-old children, compared the effectiveness of individual versus group-administered vicarious and direct counterconditioning treatments relative to a no-treatment control group (Mann and Rosenthal 1969). Fifty children served as experimental subjects and twenty-one children served as control subjects. All children were referred to the study by school counselors after being counseled for reported test anxiety on at least one occasion. The experimental subjects were ranked according to their initial scores on a scale designed to assess test anxiety (Emery and Krumboltz 1967) and were then assigned by stratified random sampling to one of the following groups: (1) individual direct desensitization—child constructed fear hierarchy and practiced desensitization; (2) individual vicarious desensitization—child observed another child being desensitized; (3) group direct desensitization—group constructed a fear hierarchy and practiced desensitization; (4) vicarious group desensitization—group observed another group undergoing desensitization; (5) vicarious group desensitization, observing direct desensitization of a peer model—group observed an individual peer undergoing desensitization. Pre- and post-assessments were based on the test anxiety scale and a reading test.

Relevant to the present discussion are the results indicating that children in the treatment conditions all evidenced greater reductions in test anxiety and significant improvements in reading relative to the children in the no-treatment control group. With respect to the efficacy of one treatment condition over another, the authors concluded that "the major treatment variations (individual vs. group X direct vs. vicarious) had accomplished roughly equivalent outcomes" (Mann and Rosenthal 1969, p. 363). In summary, then, individual and group formats using either vicarious or direct counterconditioning were equally effective in reducing test anxiety.

Additional studies using a group format to target children's fears or anxieties have since been conducted. The fears or anxieties targeted across these studies have varied and include snakes (Ritter 1968), fires (Jones et al. 1989), reading (Muller and Madson 1970), tests (Barabasz 1973, Deffenbacher and Kemper 1974a, 1974b), public speaking (Johnson et al. 1971), and hospital procedures (Cofer and Nir 1975, Peterson and Shigetomi 1981); the treatment techniques have also varied and include systematic desensitization (e.g., Barabasz 1973, Deffenbacher and Kemper 1974a, 1974b), behavioral rehearsal (Jones et al. 1989), direct exposure (Johnson et al. 1971), relaxation training only (Laxer et al. 1969), and modeling (Ritter 1968). Although these studies have also varied widely in terms of their rigor and control, taken all together, the results have generally supported the efficacy of using these techniques in a group format.

As noted earlier, however, none of these studies provide any conceptual basis with respect to the role that group processes may play in facilitating the reduction of fears and anxiety in children. Below we address this issue with respect to GCBT for children with anxiety and phobic disorders.

CONCEPTUAL RATIONALE FOR GCBT

GCBT builds on the growing consensus that an exposure-based treatment that incorporates cognitive-behavioral components is most efficacious for anxiety and phobic disorders (Morris and Kratochwill 1983, Silverman and Eisen 1993). However, GCBT extends this approach in several important ways: first, in the conceptualization of the key content of the treatment; second, in the conceptualization of the sequence in which the contents of the treatment are administered; third, in the conceptualization in which the treatment is administered (i.e., group). Each of these points is briefly elaborated below.

As currently being tested, GCBT targets 8- to 12-year-old children who meet *DSM-III-R* criteria for overanxious disorder (OAD), social phobia (SOP), and avoidant disorder (AVD). The reason for targeting these disorders is that children who present with OAD, SOP, and AVD share common clinical features (e.g., social evaluation/performance concerns). In terms of the content of the treatment then, exposure—primarily to social evaluation/performance stimuli—is key. Such exposure is based on two key premises: (1) that OAD, SOP, and AVD share common symptomatology (i.e., excessive concern about social evaluation/performance) and (2) that due to this common symptomatology, treatment for these disorders involves a common therapeutic ingredient (i.e., exposure to social evaluation/performance stimuli).

It should be noted that these two key premises are equally applicable to the revisions in *DSM-IV* (1994). Moreover, the revisions provide further support for the recognition that these disorders share common symptomatology. For example, because AVD shares features with social phobia, AVD was eliminated in *DSM-IV*. Because the symptoms of OAD are viewed as being nonspecific across all the anxiety disorders, in *DSM-IV*, OAD is subsumed under the previous adult category of generalized anxiety disorder.

In terms of the sequence in which the contents of the treatment are administered, this reflects our conceptualization of the process of effective, long-term behavioral change in children. This process, based on the notion of transfer of control, is that effective child behavior change efforts, in general, and childhood anxiety/phobic problems, in particular, involve a gradual transfer of control where the sequence is from the therapist to the parent to the child. According to this conceptualization, exposure results in immediate, short-term clinical change, but effective long-term change requires a transfer of control to the child. This proposition provides the rationale for the sequence of the administration of the behavioral and cognitive components of GCBT. Briefly (see Treatment Strategies section for more detail), this sequence involves first training parents in child management skills and then teaching them to use these skills to encourage their child's exposure to anxious/phobic situations (parent control). This is followed by a gradual fading of parental control while the child is taught to use cognitive self-control strategies as a way to help manage his or her own exposures (child control). Thus, the transfer of control shifts from external agents (i.e., therapist to parent) to an internal agent (i.e., child).

To facilitate transfer of control, the children and parents are seen in separate, concurrent sessions led by two different therapists. In the parent sessions the focus is on instilling in parents the notion and the skills necessary for them to control or manage their child's fearful or anxious behaviors, and to train them in how to gradually transfer this control to their child. In the child sessions the focus is on teaching the children how to gradually make the transition from parental control to self-control of their fearful or anxious behaviors.

The third extension of GCBT involves the use of cognitive-behavioral procedures in a group format. The group format appears to be a valuable means for facilitating child behavior change for several reasons. First, the group approach is beneficial with respect to our conceptualization of transfer of control. For example, the group approach provides peer reinforcement to the child for successful change efforts, thereby assuming some of the functions provided by the parents and thus facilitating the fading of parental control. Second, the group format provides the therapist with access to natural group processes that are not available in the individual approach. These processes include peer modeling, peer reinforcement, feedback, support, and social comparison. For example, when the child in the group observes a group peer perform a successful in vivo exercise, it provides the opportunity for positive modeling to occur. The successful completion of the exposure task, in turn, results in peer reinforcement for the child who completed the exercise. The group also provides a context for corrective or instructive peer feedback (e.g., as when a child shares with the other youngsters his/her method for approaching an anxiety-provoking situation). Moreover, when one child discusses his or her success between session experiences, the sharing of these experiences provides positive support because all of the children observe that progress is being made. The group format also facilitates social comparison processes, in that hearing about how other children handle situations involving various fearful or anxious events contributes to the child's adjustment of how he or she handles particular events. Finally, the group process itself provides support for the members. The continuing and ongoing interactions among the group members contribute to the experience of group cohesion, rendering the therapy experience less isolating (e.g., children and parents feel they are not alone with this problem) and more enjoyable.

DESCRIPTION OF TECHNIQUES

The techniques used in GCBT include gradual exposure (imaginal and in vivo), peer modeling, contingency management and contracting, relaxation training, cognitive self-control strategies, and social skills training. Each of these techniques and their rationale are discussed respectively below.

As noted, exposure is currently viewed as an essential component of any successful fear and anxiety reduction program (Marks 1969). Gradual exposure involves having the children approach or confront fearful or anxious stimuli in a gradual fashion, thereby providing the child with step-by-step success experiences with the anxious or phobic event or object. Gradual exposure is introduced in treatment through a fear hierarchy. Each child in the group develops a hierarchy specific to his or her fear/anxiety problem. Each hierarchy consists of specific situations that elicit only very slight fear/anxiety in the child to situations that elicit extreme or excessive fear/anxiety. During the course of GCBT, each child moves up the hierarchy as he or she engages in gradual exposure tasks (i.e., each step on the hierarchy). As discussed later, contingency contracting and management as well as cognitive self-control strategies serve to facilitate the child's movement or progress up the hierarchy.

Modeling techniques involve the child learning to be less fearful by observing how others handle the feared object or situation. The modeling technique used in GCBT is the "tag along" procedure (Ollendick and Cerny 1981). In this procedure, the therapist first models the appropriate fearless or coping behavior when in the presence of the feared object or event. The child then "tags along" or follows the behaviors of the therapist, with the therapist providing feedback and encouragement. As noted, GCBT also utilizes natural group processes that provide the opportunity for peer modeling.

The third technique, contingency management and contracting, is based on the principles of operant conditioning and stress the importance of the causal relationship between stimuli and behavior (Morris and Kratochwill 1983). These procedures involve rearranging the environment to ensure that positive consequences follow exposure to the fearful or anxious stimuli, and to ensure that positive consequences do not follow avoidant behavior (i.e., extinction).

In GCBT, parents and children are taught these concepts and a list of rewards is generated. To ensure that approach behavior is followed by a positive consequence, written contracts are devised each week between each child–parent dyad in the group. Each contract details the specific behavior (i.e., step on the hierarchy) to be performed by the child that week (between sessions) and the specific reward to be provided by the parent, contingent on successful completion of the exposure task. It is critical that the contract devised between the parent and child be written with explicit and specific terms. For example, it is not enough to indicate that a child's reward for successful confrontation with a feared object is "to go to the park." Such nonspecificity opens the door to later conflict and disagreement. Rather, the reward on the contract should indicate the child will "go to the park on Saturday for two hours with parent." An example of a written contract appears in Table 17–1. As noted, contingency contracting procedures are faded out during the course of treatment and are replaced by cognitive self-control procedures, described next.

Cognitive self-control techniques stress the important contribution of cognitive processes to behavior change with each child directly involved in regulating his or her own behavior. In GCBT, the children are taught specific thinking styles that they are to apply when confronted with the fearful/

Table 17-1.

Parent–Child Contract

Let it be known that on this Thursday day, the 9th of December
                        (day of week)   (date)   (month)
in the year 1993, a contract between Anthony and mother/father
                                   (child's name)
   Mom   concerning the child's fear of sleeping alone was signed,
(parent's name)   (phobic object)
witnessed by Dr. Silverman .
          (therapist's name)
The above parent and child hereby agree that if Anthony successfully
                              (child's name)
stays in his room 20 minutes, without T.V., and only the closet and hall
                         (approach task)
light on, without calling to his mother,

then he will be taken to the amusement park for 30 minutes. This task is to
             (reinforcement child will receive)
be done by the child on Saturday, and the parent is to give child the
               (when)
above mentioned reward on Saturday.
            (when)

anxious stimulus. In addition, each child is taught to examine the specific cognitions that play a role in maintaining his or her fear. Using the STOP acronym (S stands for scared?; T stands for thoughts; O stands for other thoughts or things I can do; and P stands for praise), the child learns to recognize feelings of fear or anxiety, to identify maladaptive or negative anxious/fearful thoughts and behaviors, to generate and use adaptive or positive nonanxious/nonfearful coping thoughts and behaviors, and to praise him- or herself for doing so.

The fifth technique, relaxation training, is included in GCBT in order to teach the children how to decrease the aversive physiological arousal frequently associated with excessive fear or anxiety. Each child is taught how to relax his or her body when fearful or anxious through a progressive muscle relaxation and a deep breathing exercise (cf. King 1980). The progressive muscle relaxation exercise that we use in GCBT involves teaching the child that "just as he/she can make his/her body tense, he/she can make his/her body relax," thus emphasizing the notion that one can learn to control bodily or physiological feelings of fear or anxiety. A deep breathing exercise is also included in relaxation training. Using a balloon as a metaphor, the child pretends that his or her body is like a balloon that expands when it fills with air and deflates when the air is let out. The child is instructed to place one hand on the stomach and the other on the chest and to inhale through the nose (blowing up like a balloon), and to exhale through the mouth.

The final technique used in GCBT is social skills training. Because the participants in GCBT share common clinical features (i.e., concerns about social evaluation/performance), specific social skills (e.g., smiling/laughing, greeting others, joining activities, extending invitations, conversational skills, verbal complimenting, and physical appearance/grooming) are taught as a way to help them handle their fear and anxiety in social evaluation/performance situations. The main procedures used in teaching social skills are modeling, coaching, and behavioral rehearsal.

ASSESSMENT PROCEDURES

The assessment procedures for GCBT are based on a tripartite or multi-channel conceptualization of anxiety (Lang 1977, Rachman 1977) and involve the measurement of three domains: (1) cognitive/subjective, (2) behavioral/motoric, and (3) physiological. Before proceeding with a description of the various measures to assess each domain, it should be noted that the utility of these measures for diagnostic purposes has not been clearly demonstrated. For example, it has not been found to be the case that a particular questionnaire (for the cognitive/subjective domain), behavioral task, or physiological measure can differentiate a child with simple phobia versus SOP versus OAD (Silverman and Rabian 1993). In addition to lacking discriminant validity, there is also the issue of construct validity (i.e., whether these instruments are indeed measuring the constructs they were designed to measure, such as anxiety and fear). With respect to the questionnaires, for example, recent reviews of the literature suggest that these measures may be assessing a diffuse global state of "negative affectivity" (Finch et al. 1989, King et al. 1991). Despite the above limitations, the assessment procedures used in GCBT are designed to provide a comprehensive picture of how anxiety and phobias manifest themselves in each child and thereby serve as useful indices of treatment outcome.

With respect to the cognitive/subjective domain, clinical interviews, self- and parent-report questionnaires, and self-monitoring procedures are typically employed. Specifically, in terms of the clinical interview, respective versions of the Anxiety Disorders Interview Schedule for Children (ADIS-C/P, Silverman and Nelles 1988, Silverman and Eisen 1992) are administered to child and parent. The ADIS-C/P is a structrured interview that parallels the DSM criteria for childhood and adult anxiety disorders.

The interview uses a Fear Thermometer to obtain severity ratings of fear experienced by the child on a five-point scale (0–4). In addition, the child and parent are asked to rate the degree to which the child's fear interferes with or "messes up" the child's daily functioning (in terms of friends, school, and family). Based on the endorsement of symptoms and the ratings of interference, separate child, parent, and composite diagnoses are assigned. (See Silverman 1991 for further details in how composite diagnoses are derived using the ADIS-C/P.)

The assessment of the cognitive/subjective domain also includes child self-report questionnaires of anxiety symptoms. These questionnaires include the Fear Survey Schedule-Revised (Ollendick 1983), the Children's Manifest Anxiety Scale-Revised (Reynolds and Richmond 1978), and the State-Trait Anxiety Inventory for Children (STAIC, Spielberger 1973). (For a review of the psychometrics of these measures, see Silverman and Rabian in press.) Because the children in GCBT share social evaluation concerns, specific measures assessing children's friendships (Bierman and McCauley 1987), social skills (Gresham and Elliot 1990), and social anxiety (La Greca and Stone 1993) are also administered.

A final procedure used to assess the cognitive/subjective domain is self-monitoring. Children in the group are asked to keep a "Daily Diary" of their encounters with the fearful or anxious object or situation. For each entry on the Daily Diary the child is asked to describe the situation in which fear/anxiety has been experienced, whether the child confronted or avoided the feared object/situation, accompanying cognitions, and degree of fear (using the fear thermometer rating scale of 0 to 4). Self-monitoring begins two weeks prior to the initiation of treatment and continues throughout the treatment, thereby providing some indication of the child's progress from pre- to posttreatment. Based on our clinical experiences there is much variability in the quality of the children's self-monitoring. Our general impressions are that older children seem to be better (i.e., more accurate and thorough) self-monitors than younger (for the younger children parents often assist in the completion of self-monitoring); verbal children seem to be better than less verbal; and highly motivated children seem better than poorly motivated children (Silverman and Rabian 1993).

To assess the behavioral domain, an in vivo behavioral task is used. For the children in GCBT, the task involves having each child talk about him- or herself for five minutes in front of a group of strangers. From a clinical perspective it is informative to observe what a child actually does in this situation (rather than just hear about it through self- or parent-report). Typical responses observed include crying, silence, refusal, hesitant speech, and so on.

Our assessment of the physiological domain is conducted simultaneously with the assessment of the behavioral domain, that is, during the in vivo behavioral task. The physiological measure we assess is the child's heart rate via a Computer Instruments Heart Watch (a watch that is placed on the child's wrist to record heart rate). Recent data from our research clinic indicate that this procedure yields reliable test-retest heart rate scores in phobic children (Chapinoff 1992). Moreover, preliminary results from our ongoing treatment study indicate positive changes in heart rate from pre- to posttreatment (Silverman 1993).

In summary, a multichannel assessment is conducted with all participants and provides a comprehensive picture of each child's pretreatment strengths and weaknesses. Information from this assessment is used to assign diagnoses, assure appropriateness for GCBT, set treatment goals, and compare with the information obtained at the posttreatment and follow-up assessment sessions.

ESTABLISHING TREATMENT GOALS

The primary goals of GCBT include (1) increasing child approach behavior toward social evaluation/performance situations or events, (2) improving parental management of their child's approach/avoidance behaviors via contingency contracting, (3) improving child social skills, (4) developing child cognitive self-control skills, and (5) decreasing aversive states of bodily arousal (e.g., jumpiness, tenseness) when faced with phobic/anxious situations or events. These goals are addressed directly in GCBT via the specific strategies described below.

With respect to increasing approach behavior, as noted earlier, a fear hierarchy is constructed for each child. The specific approach behavior to be targeted in the hierarchy varies for each child (although there is often overlap across children) and is determined from information obtained during the assessment phase. Specifically, children and their parents identify fearful objects or situations that the child avoids and that interfere most with the child's daily functioning. Each child (with parent and therapist assistance) constructs a list of these situations ranging from mildly fearful to extremely fearful. The child is expected to gradually expose him- or herself to each of these situations.

With respect to improving parental management of their child's approach/avoidance behaviors, this is accomplished via contingency management and contingency contracting procedures. As noted earlier, in the beginning of GCBT, the parent sessions primarily focus on teaching the parents basic principles of effective child management, including principles of positive reinforcement, extinction, the importance of consistency, and so on. In addition, the parents obtain experience in practicing these principles through the contingency contracts that they devise each week with their child. (As indicated earlier, these contracts are gradually faded out as the child learns to use self-control strategies during the exposure exercises.)

With respect to establishing specific goals for social skills, the children (with parental, therapist, and group input) decide on two skills to be targeted. These skills are then modeled and rehearsed in session. Based on the in-session rehearsal and role-plays, individual skills are further targeted for each child to practice (e.g., eye contact, voice tone, etc.). Additional practice outside of the treatment sessions is also expected. These out-of-session tasks may involve having the children apply their newly acquired social skills in real situations such as initiating a conversation with a peer or asking a peer for his or her phone number.

With respect to developing cognitive self-control skills, all children are instructed in how to recognize their negative or scary/anxious thoughts and in how to generate positive, coping thoughts and/or actions that will help them handle their fear/anxiety. The specific goals for each child are established based on the particular maladaptive thinking patterns indicated on the Daily Diaries as well as those that are brought out during the group discussions in session. Each child generates his or her own list of coping thoughts and action plans and then practices the plans—both during the sessions with the other group members and as out-of-session activities.

Finally, with respect to decreasing aversive states of bodily arousal (e.g., jumpiness, tenseness), the children are taught two types of relaxation exercises, progressive muscle relaxation and deep breathing exercises (see Description of Techniques for details on these procedures). Once the therapist has modeled the exercises, the group practices weekly in session as well as out of session.

In summary, GCBT has several major treatment goals that include increasing child approach behavior, improving parental management of their child's approach/avoidance behaviors, improving child social skills, developing child cognitive self-control skills, and decreasing child tenseness or negative bodily arousal. The specific behaviors to be targeted are established based on the particular needs of each child, thereby rendering GCBT a flexible, individually tailored treatment modality.

ROLE OF THE THERAPIST

The therapist in GCBT fulfills several roles and must attend to both individual and group processes. In the beginning of treatment, the role of the therapist is analogous to that of a teacher and consultant. For instance, during the first several sessions the therapist "teaches" (i.e., introduces and explains) the cognitive-behavioral concepts and treatment techniques. The children's role is analogous to that of "student"—listening and learning. Because GCBT is based on the notion of "transfer of control," the role of the therapist as teacher gradually shifts to a more consulting and supportive role. Specifically, once the children have learned the skills (e.g., relaxation, self-control), the therapist "consults" in how to improve these skills and provides guidance, feedback, and encouragement.

Another primary role of the therapist is to establish group cohesion and facilitate group processes such as peer modeling, reinforcement, feedback, support, and social comparison. This is accomplished through highlighting similarities and differences among group members, encouraging interactions and structuring exercises (e.g., working in dyads), fostering trust among group members, and establishing a sense of working together for a common goal.

TREATMENT STRATEGIES

As noted, the treatment strategies used in GCBT are based on our conceptualization that effective behavior change efforts in childhood involve a gradual transfer of control where the sequence is from the therapist to the parent to the child. The sequence of the treatment techniques is designed to promote this transfer of control with group processes being used to further facilitate this transfer. Children and parents are seen weekly in separate groups for forty-five minutes, followed by a conjoint meeting for fifteen minutes with the therapists, for a total of twelve weeks. Below is a brief session-by-session description of the specific treatment strategies.

The first session of GCBT in both child and parent groups is devoted to establishing group cohesion, discussing the benefits of group treatment, and explaining group rules (e.g., confidentiality, respect, sharing, etc.). The group format lends itself to a discussion of how helpful it is to know that "one is not alone," that other children/parents share similar problems, and that each group member can learn from one another in overcoming their problems. The notion that the program is a joint effort between the therapist, the parents, and the children is also emphasized.

Three other key concepts are also explained during the initial session. These include the cognitive-behavioral conceptualization of anxiety/fear, the fear hierarchy, and the out-of-session activity. With respect to the conceptualization of anxiety, it is explained that fear or anxiety usually shows itself in three ways: (1) bodily reactions, such as heart beating faster than usual, stomachaches, sweating, and so forth, (2) talking to oneself ("I might get hurt"), and (3) actions or behaviors, that is, avoiding the feared object or event. GCBT addresses each of the above, as all three components interact and affect one another.

With respect to the fear hierarchy, children and parents are informed that learning how to handle their fears or anxiety involves exposure – "facing your fear/anxiety." It is made clear that the program uses a gradual approach to "facing one's fear"; taking just the "right size steps" up a fear hierarchy. An example of a hierarchy for a social phobic child might include first saying hello to a peer at school, then starting a conversation with a peer at school, asking a peer for his or her phone number, inviting a peer to play, going to a party, going to a sleep over party at a friend's house, and so on.

To introduce out-of-session activities, Show-That-I-Can (STIC, Kendall, Kane, Howard, and Siqueland 1989) jobs are introduced as assignments given each meeting. It is explained to both children and parents that just as the teacher at school gives homework, there is homework in GCBT. However, it is not exactly the same as school homework because there are no right or wrong answers with STICs. The emphasis is on trying and doing one's best. The weekly STIC task is generally an exposure task that the children should attempt, that is, it is a step on the hierarchy. Another STIC task that the children are expected to perform each week is self-monitoring via the Daily Diaries.

Sessions 2, 3, and 4 begin the relaxation and behavioral components of GCBT. In terms of relaxation training, both progressive muscle relaxation and deep breathing exercises are modeled for the children and practiced weekly (see Description of Techniques for details on these procedures). The behavioral component of GCBT emphasizes exposure exercises and the use of contingency contracting, which begin in Session 3. The importance of exposure or approach behavior is explained to both children and parents in the following way: When individuals engage in avoidance of the phobic/ anxious objects or events, their phobia/anxiety is maintained because the individuals never learn that "there is really nothing to be afraid or anxious of." The best way to learn that "there is really nothing to be afraid or anxious of" is to gradually expose oneself, that is, to approach the fearful object/event or to perform the anxious behavior. (The analogy of "getting back on a bicycle after falling off" is made.)

Basic learning principles (e.g., reinforcement, punishment, and extinction) and their role in the development and maintenance of fearful and avoidant behavior are discussed with both children and parents. In GCBT, reinforcement and extinction are used to reduce fearful/avoidant behavior and increase approach behavior. Toward this end, approach behavior is followed by a positive reinforcer, the children (with parental and therapist assistance) devise a list of rewards (social, tangible, activity) that will be used in the subsequent weeks, following completion of the STIC tasks. The reinforcer is provided contingent upon completion of the desired behavior. That is, if the child performs X (the desired behavior), then Y (the reinforcer) is given; if the child does not perform X, then Y is not given.

The behavioral component demarcates the initial transfer of control from therapist to parent. As indicated earlier, in the parent groups, an emphasis is placed on teaching parents specific child behavior management strategies and learning principles that will enable them to modify their role in maintaining their child's fearful and anxious behaviors. For example, parents are instructed in how to assist in decreasing these behaviors via the use of rewards, placing fearful/avoidant behavior on extinction, and eventually encouraging child self-control.

In addition, two common traps that parents often fall into that influence the maintenance of their children's fearful/anxious behaviors are discussed with the parents. The first is referred to as the criticism trap and occurs when parents reinforce their children's fearful or avoidant behavior by providing negative attention (e.g., yelling, criticizing). This type of reinforcement may be rewarding for the parent in the short run because the child complies. However, in the long run the child's fearful or avoidant behavior is being reinforced (as parental negative attention is "better" than no attention at all). Thus, parents become trapped into providing negative attention.

The second trap is referred to as the protection trap and occurs when the parents reinforce their children's fearful or anxious behavior by providing positive attention, such as comfort or reassurance. This type of reinforcement may also be rewarding for the parent in that feeling that one is nurturing and protecting one's offspring is positive in nature. It is also most certainly rewarding for the child, as parental nurturance and protection is craved by most. Unfortunately, however, it also serves to escalate children's fearful or avoidant behavior patterns. Strategies for avoiding the criticism and protection traps include placing fearful/avoidant behavior on extinction and following approach or brave behavior with positive rewards.

In Sessions 5, 6, and 7 the group-based social skills training is implemented. Because the children in GCBT tend to have concerns about social evaluation/performance, specific skills that will help them handle social evaluative/performance situations are taught. The therapist describes each social skill (e.g., conversation skills), gives examples of appropriate and inappropriate behavior in each area, and then models the skills. The children practice the skills with one another in session, role-play situations based on their reported anxiety-provoking social interactions indicated on their Daily Diaries, and receive coaching and feedback from the therapist and other group members. Children are also encouraged to critique or self-evaluate and modify their own performance. Parents assist children with social skills by role-playing at home and monitoring social exposure exercises.

The cognitive self-control component of GCBT treatment is presented in Sessions 8, 9, and 10. To facilitate the children's and parents' understanding of cognitions, an approach recommended by Kendall et al. (1989) is used in which stick figures with "thought bubbles," similar to those seen in comic strips, are drawn on a blackboard to illustrate different types of self-talk. During the cognitive self-control training, the children are taught how to recognize and change their thoughts by filling in thought bubbles from fearful/anxious thoughts to nonfearful/nonanxious thoughts. The therapist models several coping thoughts by questioning out loud whether or not these thoughts are realistic, by asking "Is that really likely to happen?" "Has it actually happened before?" "Do I really need to worry about it?" and so on. Each child practices this with one of the anxious situations from his or her hierarchy, receiving feedback and support from the group and therapist. The therapist also encourages the group to think about what might happen if each child's worst anxiety or fear actually came true. The aim of this procedure is to help the children realize that constructive alternatives are available even in the worst of situations.

Another key element of self-control training is the idea of self-evaluation and self-reward, referred to as praise within the STOP acronym. It is the final step in the plan for coping with anxiety and phobias. Self-evaluation is based on deciding whether or not you are pleased or satisfied with your own work. This is followed by self-reward for those positive aspects of your work. A list of possible self-rewards that each child might do or give to him- or herself (with an emphasis on verbal praise) is then generated within the group. Examples might include: "Great job!" "I really handled that well," "I can handle it if I try," "Good going," "I'm really proud of myself," "I am a brave boy/girl," and so forth. The importance of using self-reward or praise even for partial successes, not just for reaching the final goal (i.e., the highest step on the hierarchy), is emphasized. Each member of the group takes turns practicing self-evaluation and praise, while the other group members provide feedback and suggestions.

The cognitive self-control component demarcates the final phase in the transfer of control, i.e., from therapist to parent to child. Parental rewards, used previously, are faded out as the child is expected to reward him- or herself using praise. In addition, during this period in which the child is mastering self-control skills, it is being emphasized to the parents, in their meetings, that they encourage their children's use of self-control. Difficulties that parents face in doing this are discussed (e.g., the protection trap). It is stressed to the parents that they need to convey to their child that they have confidence in the child's ability to handle his or her anxiety/phobia by him- or herself, without parental involvement.

A summary of the concepts taught to the child to help him or her handle fear/anxiety is presented to both the children and the parents as a four-step plan that, as noted, follows the acronym STOP (Scared? Thoughts? Other thoughts or actions that will help? Praise). The objective of using the STOP acronym is to help make recall of the four-step plan easier and to facilitate successful self-control. Each child makes a small wallet-size card of STOP to take home.

The final sessions of GCBT (11 and 12) are used to review the children's progress, practice their skills, present the concepts of relapse prevention, and address termination issues. Each of these areas is described in separate sections below.

OVERCOMING OBSTACLES TO SUCCESSFUL TREATMENT

The interventions described above may not always be implemented as smoothly as one might like. Obstacles that interfere with successfully carrying out a group treatment can be placed into two general categories—those applicable to most clinical treatment cases and those specific to GCBT and its implementation (Silverman and Eisen 1993). Both sets of obstacles will be discussed respectively below.

As Silverman and Eisen (1993) delineated, obstacles applicable to most clinical treatment cases include poor child and/or parent motivation, competing demands on the child and/or family, and concomitant emotional problems. The most problematic obstacle of these is a lack of motivation. Without adequate motivation on the child's and/or parents' part, it is unlikely that any treatment program will be successful. In GCBT, lack of motivation typically manifests itself in noncompliance with STIC tasks (i.e., exposures and failure to complete the Daily Diaries) and repeated canceled appointments. In group treatment, such noncompliance is particularly problematic, as it interferes with the development and maintenance of group cohesion.

In GCBT, the importance of motivation is emphasized prior to treatment. Specifically, following the initial assessment, it is explained to the child and parent that successful treatment depends on adherence to the prescribed steps of GCBT. Moreover, it is made clear that there is no "magic wand" that will make the child's phobia go away and that for treatment to work, it is important for the children to practice the various things that they learn in the sessions, just as they would practice any other skill that they are learning, such as tennis or piano. If the child and/or parent appear hesitant about participating in GCBT (i.e., motivation appears lacking), postponing treatment may be suggested. Fortunately, this has rarely occurred in our experience because the majority of our clients are highly motivated. This is primarily because the child's anxiety or phobia significantly interferes with the child and/or family's daily functioning.

In addition to assessing motivation levels, it is important to assess and ensure that the child's anxiety or phobia is the primary problem. In those cases where other comorbid conditions (e.g., depression, conduct disorder, attention deficit/hyperactivity) are more severe than the child's anxiety or phobia, referrals to appropriate service providers are made so that these other problems may be addressed prior to the child's participation in GCBT. If these competing problems are not first addressed they will likely interfere with treatment success.

Similarly, evidence for severe parental pathology must also be assessed. Parents with severe symptomatology may be limited in their ability to participate in the parent group and/or to assist in their child's change efforts. Moreover, if the parent has several other competing demands such as extensive child care responsibilities, occupational, economic, or marital difficulties, and so forth, commitment to treatment may also be compromised.

The second set of obstacles to treatment success, those attributed to the treatment techniques and/or their implementation, usually occur when constructing the fear hierarchy and performing the STIC tasks. In terms of constructing a fear hierarchy, it is important that the steps on the hierarchy reflect fearful/anxious situations that the therapist and parent have some control over. For example, it is not uncommon for many children with OAD to report worries that do not lend themselves to exposure (e.g., getting kidnapped). Thus, to address worries such as these, the child is instructed to think of where they are and what they are doing when they worry about each particular situation or event. A step on the hierarchy is then constructed for that situation.

In terms of actually performing the exposure tasks, children may find it difficult to carry out (either in session or between sessions) a specific task prescribed in the hierarchy. There are several reasons why this might occur. The most common reason is that the step in the fear hierarchy is "too big." In other words, the exposure task evokes too much fear or anxiety in the child, suggesting that the steps composing the hierarchy are not gradual enough. Another reason children have difficulty carrying out the exposure tasks is that the parent(s) may not be supporting (and may be discouraging) the child's efforts to do so. As noted earlier, in our work we call this the protection trap. That is, some parents find it difficult to watch their child confront the feared stimulus during in vivo exercises. Such parents are concerned that their child will become too uncomfortable or distressed. Thus, the parents' instincts are to protect their child from these uncomfortable feelings either by not encouraging or by actually discouraging the child's exposure efforts. We handle the protection trap by dealing with it directly with all parents as soon as the exposure phase of treatment begins. We explain to parents that although it is not unusual for some parents to behave in ways indicated above, we also remind them how countertherapeutic such behavior is, as it contradicts the entire premise of our program. That is, rather than supporting and reinforcing the child's approach/exposure, the parents' protective behaviors are actually supporting and reinforcing the children's avoidance. With many parents, our explanation and discussion of the protection trap appear to be sufficient. Unfortunately, however, there are always a few parents who, no matter how much we emphasize the dangers of engaging in the protection trap, disregard our warnings. In such cases, progress in GCBT is unlikely to occur.

RELAPSE PREVENTION

Relapse prevention is an important aspect of treatment and it is stressed throughout the group via the concept of practice. Because one cannot assume that the progress observed during treatment will automatically be maintained, strategies to prevent relapse are explicitly programmed and structured into the final phase of GCBT. Specifically, an entire session is devoted to relapse prevention and the major ideas behind it are reviewed in part of another with both the children and parents. The approach that we use to explain relapse prevention in GCBT is described briefly below.

When addressing relapse prevention we begin with a review of the children's progress made thus far in the GCBT. We reinforce this progress and provide the expectation that progress will continue; there is no reason why it should not, especially if the children continue to practice the skills they learned during treatment. We also indicate, however, that sometimes slips (i.e., feeling excessively anxious or fearful again) are not uncommon. However, a slip does not mean that the children are back where they started prior to treatment. An analogy of changing one's eating patterns correctly and losing weight on a diet, but then going off the diet on one occasion, such as a party, and gaining some weight back, is used as an illustration. That is, it is illustrated that going off the diet one time does not mean that the whole diet was a waste and that the whole weight loss effort is now "blown." Most children readily grasp the parallel between the diet analogy and their own experience in overcoming their own fears/anxieties.

A discussion of strategies that help to prevent slips (i.e., continued exposure and practice using STOP) then ensues. The children are reminded that they were taught a skill—how not to be afraid or anxious. Like any other skill, such as playing the piano, if one practices regularly one will get better and better, the skill will get easier, and one will not get rusty and forget the things learned. In other words, practice will make it less likely that a slip will occur. If a problem or slip does occur, the group discusses ways of handling it. For example, if the children find that they slip, they should not despair and they should "pick themselves up" again and continue making progress (just as one can go back on a diet). The children are instructed to try the same step on the hierarchy again, and if necessary, to try something a little lower on the hierarchy and work their way back up.

The importance of not despairing if slips occur is critical to emphasize to the parents as well. Parents need to be made aware that to the extent that they feel that their child has failed because of the slip, so too will the child. Conversely, to the extent that they feel confident that the child's slip is merely that—a slip that can be readily overcome—so too will the child. Taken all together, relapse prevention is an important component of GCBT that can serve to improve the maintenance of treatment effects.

TERMINATION

Two primary objectives are involved in the termination phase of treatment. The first is to review and summarize GCBT, focusing on the children's progress. The second is to bring closure to the group and the therapeutic relationship. With respect to the first objective, each child's progress is reviewed and strengths and weaknesses are assessed by all group members. The children's increased ability to handle fears and anxiety is emphasized. Group members are given a handout that reviews the key concepts of GCBT—the importance of exposure, nonavoidance, and STOP. The process of transfer of control is also reviewed in order to emphasize that the children now can handle their phobia/anxiety themselves by using STOP. The therapist conveys confidence that they will be able to succeed at managing their phobia/ anxiety and stresses that the progress that has been made has been primarily due to their own efforts. Now that they have all of the tools to handle their phobia/anxiety, the children (and parents) are ready to go out on their own.

With respect to the second objective, bringing closure to the group, children are encouraged to express their feelings about ending the group. Each child discusses his or her experience in the treatment program, commenting on which aspects of treatment were found to be most (and least) helpful and in what ways. The therapist shares with the group that it can be sad to end. Children often report they will miss the shared support and assistance of other group members. A discussion is focused on how each member of the group was helped by other members of the group and how the group as a whole helped each child achieve his or her individual goals. During the final moment of treatment, therapist and group members share highlights of the group experience. In our experience with GCBT, both the children and parents have formed close relationships with their fellow group members, which have occasionally continued posttreatment.

CASE ILLUSTRATION

Description and History

Jane, an 8-year-old Caucasian female, was referred to CAPP because of her excessive worrying, pervasive fearful behavior, and extreme need for reassurance. During the assessment session, Jane reported on the ADIS-C that she worried a great deal about "not being good enough" in her school performance and in making friends. She also indicated that she worried about "making mistakes," "being teased by others," and "being in accidents" in which she or her parents would be hurt. In addition, Jane reported several specific fears including sleeping alone in the dark, injections, and blood. Concurrent with these fears and worries, Jane reported various somatic complaints such as headaches, stomachaches, and increased heart rate. Both Jane and her parents indicated that her anxieties and fears were adversely affecting her ability to develop and maintain friendships, disrupting the family life, and interfering with her daily functioning. Jane was assigned a primary diagnosis of overanxious disorder.

Juan, a 9-year-old Hispanic male, was brought to CAPP by his mother, who felt her son was "overly sensitive." On the ADIS-P, the mother reported that her son gets "anxious easily" (e.g., if parent is late picking him up) and needs a great deal of reassurance. In addition, the mother indicated that Juan often had trouble being alone and usually resisted sleeping alone at night. Juan described himself on the ADIS-C as not having friends and feeling as though other children did not like him. He was extremely preoccupied with what others thought of him and felt very nervous in social situations. Due to his anxiety in social situations, he avoided going to parties or social events. He also often complained of stomachaches or headaches before going to school in the mornings. Juan and his mother both felt his symptoms were significantly interfering with his academic and social life. Juan was assigned a primary diagnosis of social phobia.

Sally, a 9-year-old Caucasian female, was referred for treatment due to her excessive worrying and concurrent physiological symptoms including stomachaches, increased heart rate, and muscle tension. Although Sally reported on the ADIS-C having many friends, she felt very nervous meeting new people and was extremely concerned about the evaluation of others. She reported numerous worries about natural disasters, personal safety, and "making God angry." Sally was assigned a primary diagnosis of overanxious disorder.

John, a 10-year-old Caucasian male, was referred for treatment by his school counselor because of his school refusal behavior. John's parents reported on the ADIS-P that John had few friends, avoided going to parties or other social activities with peers his own age, refused to eat in public, and clung to his parents when out in the community.

On the ADIS-C, John concurred with his parents that he had few friends, avoided social situations, and described fears of being humiliated in front of others. John was assigned a primary diagnosis of social phobia.

Synopsis of Therapy Sessions

The initial sessions of GCBT introduced the cognitive behavioral concepts (i.e., the nature of fears and their concomitant reactions) and provided an overview of the program. The children readily disclosed their fears and worries with one another and began constructing their individual fear hierarchies. The items composing each of the children's fear hierarchies reflected fears and anxieties that they shared, as well as those unique to each. Below is a portion of the dialogue occurring during the initial session in which the therapist encouraged the children to share with the group their fears and worries.

Therapist: What are some of the things that make you feel scared or worried?

Jane: I worry about being left alone. It scares me when no one is with me because anything can happen. I'm also afraid of the dark. I saw on the news these big holes underneath the ground that fill up with water and the ground crumbles in little by little. It scares me that we might be living on ground that might cave in and our house will sink into the ground. It scares me whenever I'm lying in bed.

Juan: We have an alarm system at my house and we lock all the doors and windows. I worry whether other kids will insult me or not like me. I don't have any friends.

Sally: Yeah, being left out. I'm scared of getting teased and not having any friends to play with and not being invited to other peoples' parties. I'm also afraid of cats.

John: Going to school and being with the kids at school. I hate it if I have to eat in the cafeteria.

Juan: Being up high, in high places.

Jane: I'm afraid of being teased by my brother or friends too. I'm also worried that something will happen to my parents because they're going skiing and I've never seen snow before.

The children were instructed to rank order their fears and worries from the least scary or anxious to the most, like a "ladder," in order to construct the fear hierarchy. It was suggested that the children begin by first placing the two extremes, that is, the most and then the least scary, on the ladder. Once each child's fear hierarchy was completed, the use of contingency contracts was initiated. The concepts of positive reinforcement and extinction were explained to the children (and the parents during the concurrent parent group session) and a list of rewards (social, tangible, and activities) was devised. It was explained to the parents and children how contingency contracts were to be generated, that is, how very specific rewards were to be given by the parent to the child contingent on the child's successful completion of each exposure task (i.e., one step on the hierarchy). Contingency contracts were also used to target specific social situations that the children were anxious or worried about. As illustrated below, the children shared their successes and/or failures and received support, encouragement, and corrective feedback from the other members of the group.

> Therapist: Let's remind each other what our STIC job was this past week and talk about how it went.
>
> Juan: I had to ask another kid at school for their phone number. I asked five kids for their phone numbers but they all said no, but I still received my reward because at least I tried. My mother took me to the Discovery Zone.
>
> Group: Awesome!! [all applaud].
>
> Sally: Um, I had to go up to a house by myself and ask if they wanted to buy Girl Scout cookies. I did that while my mom stayed in the car. My reward was that I was able to have a friend sleep over that night and we watched a video.
>
> Group: Yeah!! [all applaud].
>
> John: I had to go to a party and start a conversation, without wiggling, and I had to keep the conversation going by asking questions. I did it but my mother didn't get me the reward . . . I get it tonight. Some baseball cards.
>
> Group: Great job! [all applaud].
>
> Jane: I was supposed to ask someone at school to play with me but I didn't do it.
>
> Therapist: Can you tell us what happened and why you couldn't do the STIC?
>
> Jane: I don't know, because people might not like me.
>
> Sally: If there are kids you don't know and you want to play with them you could walk up to them and show them a game.

Juan: Yeah, you can go up to them and start talking about a subject until it leads to another subject and it will keep going on and on.

John: You can talk to them just like you talk to us. I'll practice with you what to say.

The succeeding sessions introduced the cognitive component. The children were taught to examine their cognitions when faced with situations or objects that they fear or worry about. Using the STOP acronym described earlier, the children were helped to recognize when they were anxious or scared and to modify their anxious thoughts with more adaptive coping thoughts and behaviors. They were also taught to evaluate their ability to control their anxiety and fear and to praise themselves for doing so. Next are excerpts from these sessions.

Therapist: Let's practice O–changing our scary thoughts to *other* coping thoughts and actions that will help you handle the situation.

Jane: First when I think I might not see a car coming at me and it might run over me or I might get robbed and that there are crazy people out there I change my thoughts so "if a car comes I'll be able to see it and what's the chance that a robber would break into my house tonight; it's never happened before and I know the doors and windows are locked."

Sally: My scary thought is I'll fall in the pool and die but my O is "it's a million to one that I'll fall in the pool and even if I do my mom is right there to help me."

John: I think the jellyfish are going to sting me and the crabs are going to bite me so I don't like to go to the beach but my O is, "I've never been bitten by a jellyfish before and even if I do I won't die and the beach is fun too."

Jane: But I don't like it when people laugh at me, then everyone will laugh at me and I want to leave school.

Sally [to Jane]: So what if they tease you, they aren't going to kill you!

Juan [to Jane]: If they tease, you can ignore it.

John [to Jane]: You have to say "I'm going to face it. I'll just try as hard as I can. I'm brave."

Jane: I'll try it. I can tell myself I have to roll with the punches, tell myself I can handle it and they may not be laughing at me.

Juan: Yeah, and if one kid doesn't want to play with me I can make other friends. Another O is no one has everyone liking them.

Comments

During the twelve weeks of GCBT, each of the children in the group progressed up their fear hierarchies and demonstrated an increased ability to handle fearful/anxious situations. Improvement on several of the assessment measures was apparent as well. Most notable was that at posttreatment none of the children met criteria for their primary diagnosis (OAD and SOP) on the ADIS-C and ADIS-P, and scores of social anxiety, particularly on the fear of negative evaluation subscale of the Social Anxiety Scale for Children-Revised, decreased. In addition, both the children and parents reported that the previous symptoms no longer interfered with the child or family's daily functioning and improvements in peer relations were also reported.

SUMMARY

A group cognitive-behavioral treatment program (GCBT) was described in this chapter. GCBT contributes to the treatment research literature in three important ways. First is the conceptualization of the content of treatment, that is, the premise that children with OAD, SOP, and AVD share the common symptomatology of excessive concern about social evaluation/performance. Thus, the key content of treatment involves exposure to primarily social evaluation/performance stimuli. Second is the conceptualization of the sequence of treatment, that is, that long-term behavior change results from a gradual transfer of control from external agents (therapist to parent) to an internal agent (the child). Third is the format in which the treatment is administered, that is, the group.

All children who participate in GCBT are assessed in each of three domains: cognitive/subjective (e.g., structured interviews), behavioral/motoric (i.e., an in vivo behavioral approach task), and physiological (i.e., heart rate monitoring). The specific treatment techniques used in GCBT include gradual exposure (imaginal and in vivo), modeling, contingency management and contracting, relaxation training, cognitive self-control strategies, and social skills training.

Treatment goals for GCBT include increasing child approach behavior toward social evaluation/performance situations, improving parental management of their child's approach/avoidance behaviors (via contingency contracting, improving child social skills, developing child cognitive self-control skills, and decreasing aversive states of bodily arousal (e.g., jumpiness, tenseness) when faced with phobic/anxious situations or events. The therapist in GCBT performs several roles including teacher, consultant, and facilitator. Several critical treatment issues, such as obstacles to successful treatment, relapse prevention, and termination issues were discussed. The chapter concluded with several case vignettes that illustrate some of the treatment techniques.

REFERENCES

Barabasz, A. (1973). Group desensitization of test anxiety in elementary schools. *Journal of Psychology* 83:295–301.

Bierman, K., and McCauley, E. (1987). Children's descriptions of their peer interactions: useful information for clinical child assessment. *Journal of Clinical Child Psychology* 18:9–18.

Chapinoff, A. (1992). *Test-Retest Reliability of Heart Response in Children with Phobic Disorder.* Unpublished master's thesis.

Cofer, D. H., and Nir, Y. (1975). Theme-focused group therapy on a pediatric ward. *International Journal of Psychiatry in Medicine* 6:541–550.

Deffenbacher, J. L., and Kemper, C. C. (1974a). Counseling test-anxious sixth graders. *Elementary School Guidance and Counseling* 7:22–29.

_____ (1974b). Systematic desensitization of test anxiety in junior high students. *The School Counselor* 21:216–222.

Diagnostic and Statistical Manual of Mental Disorders (1987). 3rd ed. revised. Washington, DC: American Psychiatric Association.

_____ (1994). 4th ed. Washington, DC: American Psychiatric Association.

Emery, J. R., and Krumboltz, J. D. (1967). Standard versus individualized hierarchies in desensitization to reduce test anxiety. *Journal of Counseling Psychology* 14:204–209.

Finch, A. J., Jr., Lipovsky, J. A., and Casat, C. D. (1989). Anxiety and depression in children and adolescents: negative affectivity or separate constructs? In *Anxiety and Depression: Distinctive and Overlapping Features,* eds. P. C. Kendall and D. Watson, 2nd ed., pp. 171–196. San Diego: Academic Press.

Gresham, F. M., and Elliot, S. N. (1990). *Social Skills Rating System.* Circle Pines, MN: American Guidance Service.

Johnson, T., Tyler, V., Jr., Thompson, R., and Jones, E. (1971). Systematic desensitization and assertive training in the treatment of speech anxiety in middle school students. *Psychology in the Schools* 8:263–267.

Jones, R. T., Ollendick, T. H., McLaughlin, K. J., and Williams, C. E. (1989). Elaborative and behavioral rehearsal in the acquisition of fire emergency skills and the reduction of fear of fire. *Behavior Therapy* 20:93–101.

Kendall, P. C., Kane, M. T., Howard, B. L., and Siqueland, L. (1989). *Cognitive-Behavioral Therapy for Anxious Children: Treatment Manual*. Philadelphia: Temple University.

King, N. J. (1980). The therapeutic utility of abbreviated progressive relaxation: a critical review with implications for clinical practice. In *Progress in Behavior Modification*, vol. 10, eds. M. Hersen, R. E. Eisler, and P. M. Miller. New York: Academic Press.

King, N. J., Ollendick, T. H., and Gullone, E. (1991). Negative affectivity in children and adolescents: relations between anxiety and depression. *Clinical Psychology Review* 11:441–459.

Kondas, O. (1966). Reduction of examination anxiety and 'stage-fright' by group desensitization and relaxation. *Behaviour Research and Therapy* 5:275–281.

La Greca, A. M., and Stone, W. L. (1993). The Social Anxiety Scale for Children-Revised: factor structure and concurrent validity. *Journal of Clinical Child Psychology* 22:17–27.

Lang, P. J. (1977). Imagery in therapy: an information processing analysis of fear. *Behavior Therapy* 8:862–886.

Laxer, R. M., Quarter, J., Kooman, A., and Walker, K. (1969). Systematic desensitization and relaxation of high test-anxious secondary school students. *Journal of Counseling Psychology* 16:446–451.

Mann, J., and Rosenthal, T. L. (1969). Vicarious and direct counterconditioning of test anxiety through individual and group desensitization. *Behaviour Research and Therapy* 7:359–367.

Marks, I. M. (1969). *Fears and Phobias*. New York: Academic Press.

Morris, R. J., and Kratochwill, T. R. (1983). *Treating Children's Fears and Phobias: A Behavioral Approach*. New York: Pergamon.

Muller, S. D., and Madson, C. H. (1970). Group desensitization for anxious children with reading problems. *Psychology in the Schools* 7:184–189.

Ollendick, T. H. (1983). Reliability and validity of the revised fear survey schedule for children (FSSC-R). *Behaviour Research and Therapy* 21:395–399.

Ollendick, T. H., and Cerny, J. A. (1981). *Clinical Behavior Therapy with Children*. New York: Plenum.

Peterson, L., and Shigetomi, C. (1981). The use of coping techniques to minimize anxiety in hospitalized children. *Behavior Therapy* 12:1–14.

Rachman, S. (1977). The conditioning theory of fear acquisition: a critical examination. *Behaviour Research and Therapy* 15:375–387.

Reynolds, C. R., and Richmond, B. O. (1978). What I think and feel: a revised measure of children's manifest anxiety. *Journal of Abnormal Child Psychology* 6:271–280.

Ritter, B. (1968). The group desensitization of children's snake phobias using vicarious and contact desensitization procedures. *Behaviour Research and Therapy* 6:1–6.

Silverman, W. K. (1991). Diagnostic reliability of anxiety disorders in children using structured interviews. *Journal of Anxiety Disorders* 5:105–124.

_____ (1993). Behavioral treatment of childhood phobias: an update and preliminary research findings. In *Psychosocial and Combined Treatment for Childhood Disorders: Development and Issues*. Symposium conducted at the meeting of the new clinical drug evaluation unit program, ed. E. Hibbs, Boca Raton, FL, June.

Silverman, W. K., and Eisen, A. R. (1992). Age differences in the reliability of parent and child reports of child anxious symptomatology using a structured interview. *Journal of the American Academy of Child and Adolescent Psychiatry* 32:117–124.

_____ (1993). Overanxious disorder in children. In *Handbook of Behavior Therapy with Children and Adults: A Developmental and Longitudinal Perspective*, eds. R. T. Ammerman and M. Hersen. Needham, MA: Allyn & Bacon.

Silverman, W. K., and Kearney, C. A. (1991). The nature and treatment of anxiety in school-aged children. *Educational Psychology Review* 3:335–361.

Silverman, W. K., and Nelles, W. B. (1988). The Anxiety Disorders Interview Schedule for Children. *Journal of the American Academy of Child and Adolescent Psychiatry* 27:772–778.

Silverman, W. K., and Rabian, B. (1993). Simple phobias. In *Handbook of Phobic and Anxiety Disorders of Children*, eds. T. H. Ollendick, N. J. King, and W. Yule. New York: Plenum.

_____ (in press). Rating scales for anxiety and mood disorders. In *Assessment in Child Psychopathology*, eds. D. Schaffer and J. Richters. New York: Guilford.

Spielberger, C. (1973). *Manual for the State-Trait Anxiety Inventory for Children*. Palo Alto, CA: Consulting Psychologists Press.

Wolpe, J., and Lang, P. J. (1964). A Fear Survey Schedule for use in behaviour therapy. *Behaviour Research and Therapy* 2:27–30.

18

PHARMACOTHERAPY

Jovan G. Simeon
Doreen M. Wiggins

INTRODUCTION

In dealing with anxiety disorders of children and adolescents, nonpharmacological interventions should always be used initially. Even chronic and severe degrees of anxiety can respond markedly and rapidly to psychotherapy. Pharmacotherapy should be considered when anxiety symptoms are either severe, chronic, or persistent, and do not respond to psychosocial interventions. The possibility that childhood or adolescent anxiety may be associated with other disorders such as depression, attention deficit hyperactivity, or conduct disorders is important when making diagnostic assessments and treatment plans. When anxiety is symptomatic of another psychiatric disorder, the primary disorder should be treated first (Simeon 1990). However, the presence of severe anxiety may interfere with the overall case management, and anxiolytics may facilitate the treatment of the primary disorder. Comorbidity raises additional questions for the clinician: Does the primary drug for one disorder have an effect on the symptoms of the other, and does the presence of another disorder alter drug response? (Gadow 1992). Care should be taken that combined drug treatment does not lead to polypharmacy. For example, drug-induced adverse effects may be mistaken for worsening of anxiety or of agitation. Adverse effects to tricyclics are occasionally exhibited as irritability or aggression. Such symptoms can be difficult to distinguish from anxiety, panic, or depressive dysphoria and may be incorrectly treated with an increase in dosage (Kutcher et al. 1992). Behavioral disturbances may be caused by benzodiazepines in a minority of patients representing exacerbation of disinhibition in an underlying ADHD (Biederman 1990).

There are no established indications for the use of anxiolytic medications in children and adolescents, and no established pharmacologic treatments for childhood anxiety disorders apart from those for obsessive-compulsive disorder (Popper 1993). Nearly all research in this area has focused on the treatment of adults, with few controlled drug studies in children and adolescents with anxiety disorders. The psychopharmacology of childhood anxiety has also been hindered by the lack of reliable quantitative evaluations and by fluctuations in the manifestations of the type and degree of anxiety in many of the patients, making the assessment of drug effect difficult (Simeon and Ferguson 1985). Measurements of anxiety in children have been largely limited to checklists of symptom observations and clinical global impressions. Although self-ratings have been used to assess levels of anxiety, their clinical value remains uncertain. It has been found that the symptoms have been checked contradictorily on the same sheet, and that the symptoms checked were inconsistent with the clinical global impression (Hoehn-Saric et al. 1987). Children may underrate or overrate their anxiety for secondary gain or manipulation, or out of fear or embarrassment. Children not only lack self-awareness, they also tend to externalize their feelings, denying the symptoms they perceive as signs of weakness in order to present a "brave face." However, a skillful semistructured clinical interview usually allows the child to disclose symptoms more readily, and the use of clinical ratings and checklists improves reliability. Situational factors also require a comprehensive evaluation for social behavior, family dynamics, and school environment. Manipulation of these environmental and psychological variables is a necessary first step before initiating pharmacotherapy. The evaluation of these variables, which in adults may be considered nonspecific, can have a more pronounced influence on outcome in childhood.

Anxiety disorders are as much a public health problem in children as they are in adults (Popper 1993). The aggregate burden of suffering for a disorder is defined as the burden placed on individuals and communities from the incidence, duration, and severity of the disorder, its impact on the community, and the pain and suffering experienced by the individual with the disorder (Beitchman et al. 1992a). When the aggregate burden of suffering is known, then the cost to the community of the disorder can be estimated. Although anxiety disorders are common in childhood, and individuals may suffer a great deal, most indicators suggest that the aggregate burden is small when compared to other major childhood psychiatric disorders (Beitchman et al. 1992b). However, there is greater concern when anxiety disorders are associated with other disorders, as this increases the demand on the allocation of community resources. It is essential to keep a longitudinal view of the child's development and future liabilities when making decisions about treatment plans and goals. Many children with long-term impairment in functioning and persistent underachievement may have extra medical and dependency costs, possibly due to an overly targeted approach to the treatment of the complex problems associated with anxiety (Popper 1993).

REVIEW OF SPECIFIC PHARMACOLOGICAL AGENTS

Benzodiazepines

Of all psychotropic drugs, benzodiazepines are the most widely prescribed and extensively researched in adults. They are also frequently used in children, but conclusive data on efficacy in child psychiatry are limited. Early studies using low-potency chlordiazepoxide indicated some treatment effect for school refusal (D'Amato 1962, Kraft 1965). However, these studies did not use diagnostic ratings, and other methodological shortcomings make interpretation difficult. A number of single cases and of preliminary studies of the high-potency benzodiazepines have been reported in various anxiety disorders in children and adolescents. Biederman (1987) described three cases of paniclike symptoms in children successfully treated with clonazepam. An open clinical trial of clonazepam in adolescents with panic disorder indicated successful short-term treatment outcome (Kutcher and Mackenzie 1988). The average rate of panic attacks dropped from three to one per week. Preliminary results from a double-blind study also suggested a significant improvement in the frequency of panic attacks and overall anxiety (Kutcher 1990).

Alprazolam has been used in the treatment of anticipatory and acute situational anxiety in children (Pfefferbaum et al. 1987). The brief intervention in this open trial demonstrated a positive treatment effect. A preliminary open study of alprazolam effects in overanxious and avoidant disorders also indicated a favorable outcome (Simeon and Ferguson 1987). However, in a double-blind, placebo controlled study on the efficacy and safety of alprazolam in adolescents and children with anxiety disorders, thirty outpatients (twenty-three boys and seven girls) aged 8.4 to 16.9 years (mean, 12.6 years) diagnosed with overanxious (n = 21) or avoidant (n = 9) disorders, the difference between alprazolam and placebo treatment outcome did not reach statistical significance (Simeon et al. 1992). Initial daily dose was either 0.25 mg for patients under 40 kg body weight, or 0.50 mg for those over 40 kg body weight. The average maximum daily dose was 1.57 mg (range, 0.5 mg to 3.5 mg) by the end of the fourth week. Alprazolam was well tolerated, and adverse effects were mild and transient. Clinical findings indicated a treatment effect for both alprazolam and for placebo. While the data indicated that alprazolam was safe to use in children, this lack of statistically superior efficacy of alprazolam relative to placebo is in contrast to the clinical effects of alprazolam reported in adult studies. The general significance of the clinical data obtained was limited by the small number of patients, the short duration of drug administration, and the relatively low drug dosages. In addition to clinical evaluations, quantitative EEGs were undertaken to determine if clinical effects were related to the pharmacological effects and dosage of alprazolam, or to nonspecific placebo effects. Relative to baseline, the effects of acute alprazolam administration on brain functions measured by quantitative EEG showed a significant increase in beta power in the right occipital lobe; chronic alprazolam administration increased beta EEG power in both lobes.

The available information on the benzodiazepines in the treatment of childhood anxiety disorders is still quite limited, and therefore it is difficult to give specific prescribing guidelines. Pharmacokinetic and pharmacocynamic differences of various benzodiazepines between children, adolescents, and adults may be very relevant to their clinical effects. Children absorb and metabolize benzodiazepines faster than adults and therefore the medications are nontoxic in therapeutic doses. In addition to their anxiolytic effect, benzodiazepines also have hypnotic, anticonvulsive, disinhibitive, sedative, and muscle relaxant properties. While children and adolescents may have a greater tolerance for the sedative and motor discoordinating effects of benzodiazepines, they may be more susceptible to the disinhibiting effects (Reiter et al. 1992).

In children the probable indications for the use of benzodiazepines are insomnia, night awakening, night terrors, and somnambulism. Possible indications are separation anxiety, overanxious disorder, and panic attacks (Coffey 1990). Benzodiazepines should be used with caution in children and adolescents with impulsivity and aggressivity, as disinhibitory effects may aggravate these behaviors (Simeon 1993). In treating anxiety disorders with benzodiazepines, initial doses should be subtherapeutic and increased gradually. Maximum dosage should be determined by monitoring the clinical response and any emergent side effects. Common side effects include drowsiness and ataxic and behavioral disturbance. These tend to occur early in treatment and may be dose related. Side effects tend to subside with chronic administration or dose adjustment. Treatment periods should be short term, usually not to exceed about three to four months. For a number of adolescents, however, optimal academic and psychosocial functioning appears possible only if benzodiazepine therapy is maintained on a long-term basis. Withdrawal symptoms or rebound anxiety are a potential hazard, and it is important to taper dosages very gradually at the end of the treatment period. While there is a potential risk for abuse and dependence in adults, there are no published data on the frequency of any physical or psychological dependence in children or adolescents.

The clinical use of benzodiazepines is made simpler by their relative safety and low side effect profile. Thus, they frequently appear the drug of choice in the treatment of uncomplicated juvenile anxiety disorders, or in combination with other appropriate pharmacotherapy when anxiety accompanies other psychiatric disorders.

Antidepressants

The therapeutic effects of antidepressant drugs have been evaluated in a broad range of child and adolescent psychiatric disorders, including behavioral disorders, depression, separation anxiety, panic attacks, obsessive-compulsive disorder, eating disorders, enuresis, and sleep disorders. The usefulness of antidepressants in the management of childhood anxiety disorders has been established for obsessive-compulsive disorder. Data for overanxious disorder, separation anxiety, and school avoidance are inconclusive or conflicting, while there are no controlled studies as yet for panic disorder.

An early imipramine treatment study of elementary school children with school phobia indicated that drug therapy was superior to placebo (Gittelman-Klein and Klein 1971); a later study with clomipramine did not replicate these results (Berney et al. 1981). A more recent, double-blind study of imipramine in separation anxiety in children aged 6 to 15 years also failed to obtain significant drug treatment effects (Klein et al. 1992). A comparative study of imipramine, alprazolam, and placebo in school refusal indicated a trend for clinical improvement with medication over placebo, but these differences were not statistically significant (Bernstein et al. 1990).

In controlled studies clomipramine has been shown to be effective in the treatment of childhood and adolescent obsessive-compulsive disorder (Flament et al. 1985, Leonard et al. 1989). A recent multicenter trial indicated treatment effect with significant improvement in 37 percent of the clomipramine group compared to 8 percent in the placebo group (DeVeaugh-Geiss et al. 1992). Studies with fluoxetine, a nontricyclic, have also suggested its usefulness in the treatment of children and adolescents with obsessive-compulsive disorder, either alone (Jenike et al. 1989, Liebowitz et al. 1990, Riddle et al. 1992) or in combination with clomipramine (Simeon et al. 1990) or buspirone (Alessi and Bos 1991).

Widely ranging concentrations of antidepressants are found in patients receiving the same dose, potentially leading to markedly different outcomes. Adverse effects such as dry mouth, blurred vision, and constipation are not generally related to drug serum levels. However, serum drug concentrations have been associated with adverse cardiovascular effects. When a clinician decides to prescribe tricyclic antidepressants to children or adolescents, serum drug levels and ECG monitoring should be used to guide dosage adjustments. Such monitoring is recommended not only to assess clinical response but also to determine the limits of serum concentration and the associated cardiovascular effects. Sinus tachycardia is one of the most frequently reported side effects of tricyclic antidepressant treatment. A report in the early 1970s described the unexplained death of a 6-year-old following an increase in the dosage of imipramine higher than what is now the recommended maximum daily dose (Saraf et al. 1974). Two other reports of death in prepubertal children were due to a multidrug ingestion that included imipramine, and a combination of imipramine and physical trauma (Popper and Elliott 1990). Recent reports of sudden deaths in children treated with desipramine have caused concern (Popper and Elliott 1990, Riddle et al. 1991); a direct causal relationship, however, between tricyclic treatment and sudden death has yet to be established (Reiter et al. 1992).

The suggested daily dose of tricyclic antidepressants ranges from 3 mg/kg to 5 mg/kg in divided doses. Treatment should be initiated at a low dose of 10 mg to 25 mg/day, and titrated gradually. Daily doses of fluoxetine are not clearly established for children and adolescents. Clinical experience suggests a dose range of 0.5 mg to 1 mg/kg in the morning. If patients improve significantly while receiving antidepressant treatment, it is advisable to continue drug treatment for up to six months before gradually reducing the dosage to determine whether further treatment is needed (Reiter et al. 1992). If there is no therapeutic response, antidepressants should be tapered gradually. Flu-like symptoms with gastrointestinal upset and vomiting may occur if the drug is discontinued abruptly.

Of the available tricyclic antidepressants, only clomipramine, in controlled clinical trials, has been shown to be significantly effective in the treatment of obsessive-compulsive disorder. Other selective serotonin reuptake inhibitors (SSRIs) such as fluoxetine and fluvoxamine also appear effective. Indications for tricyclic antidepressants together with the newer, reversible monoamine oxidase inhibitors (MAOIs) and SSRIs in the treatment of panic disorder, separation anxiety, or school avoidance have not been clearly established as yet. While preliminary findings are encouraging, specific recommendations on treatment with antidepressants for these disorders cannot be made. The variable response of children and adolescents with anxiety disorders to antidepressant treatment may reflect the fact that the frequent comorbid states represent distinct pathological disorders with unique pharmacological profiles (Ambrosini et al. 1993). This area of pediatric psychopharmacology research is quite promising, both in its potential for more effective therapy and in the elucidation of the biological substrates of these disorders.

Buspirone

Basic requirements in the pharmacotherapy of young patients are that the drug should be effective, safe, cause no phsysiological dependence, and should not interfere with vigilance or cognitive functioning. Despite a lack of conclusive findings related to clinical efficacy in children and adolescents, buspirone, a new anxiolytic, appears to meet these requirements. Buspirone appears to be as effective as the benzodiazepines in treating adult anxiety disorders, but with no significant clinical withdrawal problems (Coffey 1990, Rickels et al. 1988). Current data also suggest that buspirone does not result in abuse or dependence (Lader 1987) or adversely affect psychomotor functioning (Mattila et al. 1982). In a comparative study of buspirone and diazepam in adults (Bond et al. 1983), subjects reported feeling calmer with both drugs, while cognitive performance was not impaired by buspirone, a favorable indication for its use in children and adolescents who attend school.

There have been no controlled studies on the efficacy of buspirone in children and adolescents with anxiety disorders. An open study comparing buspirone with fenfluramine and methylphenidate in hyperactive autistic children showed that buspirone was more effective in controlling the hyperactivity and aggression (Realmuto et al. 1989). A single-case study of a 13-year-old boy with overanxious disorder, school refusal, and physiological symptoms showed response to desipramine treatment, but side effects were intolerable. Treatment with buspirone provided significant symptomatic relief (Kranzler 1988). There is also a single report on the use of buspirone to augment fluoxetine in the treatment of a child with obsessive-compulsive disorder (Alessi and Bos 1991). A series of single-case trials in adolescents diagnosed with generalized anxiety or overanxious disorder indicated a treatment effect for buspirone over a period of six weeks (Kutcher et al. 1992).

In single-case trials, thirteen adolescents 12 to 20 years old (mean, 16 years) with diagnoses of attention deficit and/or conduct disorder (n = 4), anxiety and/or depressive disorders (n = 5), obsessive-compulsive disorder (n = 2), and psychosis (n = 2) received buspirone alone or in combination with other drugs (Simeon 1991). These adolescents had shown poor or no clinical response to prior drug therapy. The daily dosage of buspirone ranged from 10 mg to 40 mg (mean, 25 mg) from 1 to 4 months (mean, 2.5 months). With the addition of buspirone to the prior medication, clinical global improvement became marked in seven cases, moderate in three, mild in two, and none in one. Regardless of diagnosis, the greatest improvement was in mood (n = 9), anxiety (n = 6), social interaction (n = 6), sleep (n = 4), aggression (n = 3), concentration (n = 3), and irritability (n = 1). These preliminary data suggested the usefulness of buspirone in the treatment of a variety of adolescent psychiatric disorders characterized by significant degrees of affective and anxiety symptoms. In an open clinical trial of childhood and adolescent anxiety disorders, fifteen patients (ten male, five female) 6 to 14 years old were treated with buspirone (Simeon et al. in press). All had DSM-III-R (1987) diagnoses of one or more anxiety disorders. Two also had a comorbid attention deficit hyperactivity disorder, and one had a comorbid obsessive-compulsive disorder. The study consisted of a two-week single-blind placebo phase, followed by a four-week buspirone administration. At admission clinical global severity was rated as severe in seven patients, marked in five, and moderate in three. At the conclusion of the trial, clinical global improvement was marked in three patients, moderate in ten, and minimal in two. Connor's (1993) rating scales for parents and teachers showed a statistically significant improvement on anxiety and behavioral factors. There was also significant improvement in the anxiety and worry factors of the self-report scales. Side effects were mild and transient, and tended to occur after the weekly increase in dosage. These consisted of sleep difficulties or tiredness reported by seven patients, nausea or stomach pains by four, and headaches by three. To prevent possible clinical relapse at the conclusion of the trial, thirteen patients continued to receive buspirone (10 mg twice daily) while two patients received no further medication. The two patients with comorbid attention deficit hyperactivity were prescribed concomitant d-amphetamine. One patient, who had initially presented with severe and persistent overanxious symptoms, was becoming withdrawn and was prescribed concomitant fluvoxamine 50 mg twice daily. Buspirone administration, either alone or in combination with other psychotropic drugs, was well tolerated and associated with significant clinical improvements. These overall preliminary results suggest that buspirone is a safe and effective treatment. Further clinical trials are needed to determine the clinical usefulness of buspirone in the treatment of childhood anxiety disorders.

A secondary objective of this study was to investigate the use of quantitative EEG to determine buspirone's effect on brain function as an index of brain bioavailability. Analyses of the quantitative EEG data failed to show a statistically significant drug effect on background electrocortical activity. While there were no significant correlates between the quantitative EEG and clinical outcome criteria, this may have been due to the relatively low dosages used and the wide variability in the patients' clinical response to buspirone.

Due to lack of controlled studies and conclusive data, there are no established indications and dosage regimen for buspirone in children and adolescents. However, published findings suggest that buspirone may be beneficial for various anxiety disorders. For adolescents, recommended dosage guidelines are 5 mg to 10 mg twice daily. Increments can consist of 5 mg or 10 mg every four to five days, and should not exceed the maximum adult daily dose of 60 mg. For prepubertal children it is more prudent to initiate buspirone therapy at 2.5 mg to 5 mg twice daily, or at bedtime, with dosage increase of 2.5 mg after five to seven days. This dosage level should be maintained for approximately two weeks; any additional increases should be gradual and based on therapeutic response. The most common side effects of buspirone are gastric upset, dizziness, headache, and insomnia. These tend to be dose related and can be alleviated by an adjustment in dosage or by taking the medication with food. At therapeutic levels buspirone generally has a low rate of sedation. It has been reported that buspirone may increase the blood level of haloperidol, and may result in increased blood pressure when combined with monoamine oxidase inhibitors (Kutcher et al. 1992, Sussman 1987). Therefore, the effect of such drug combinations should be carefully monitored.

Due to its slow onset of action, buspirone is not indicated for emergency use or for the relief of situational anxiety. Its primary role appears to be in the treatment of persistent and chronic forms of anxiety (Popper 1993). As long-term efficacy has not been established, periodic reassessments are recommended.

Other Anxiolytics

Barbiturates and propanediols are now infrequently used. Their efficacy as anxiolytics in children is unproved, and they are unsafe and lethal in high doses, as they depress a wide range of central nervous system and motor functions. Barbiturates are addictive and withdrawal may result in distressing symptoms. Antipsychotics have various autonomic, extrapyramidal, endocrine, cognitive, and other adverse effects. Prolonged use in children has frequently resulted in severe and chronic tardive dyskinesia.

Despite the widespread use of antihistamines in childhood and adolescence there are no clear indications for their use in the treatment of anxiety disorders. They are generally used for the control of sleep problems in children, as their sedative effect is similar to that of the antipsychotics. The sedating side effects of antihistamines can be used to decrease sleep latency and midsleep awakenings without prolonging total sleep time (Russo et al. 1976). Dosage should be titrated slowly to minimize the potential for excessive sedation. The use of antihistamines is also indicated in the emergency treatment of agitation and preoperative sedation.

The anxiolytic properties of beta blockers in children and adolescents have not been established. The most frequent use of such blocking agents in children has been for the treatment of migraines (Coffey 1990). While beta blockers have been used successfully to treat aggression in adults, there have been no controlled studies in a young population. Though conclusions cannot be made at present, case studies suggest that aggressive children and adolescents may also respond to beta blockers (Connor 1993). In an open study of children with post-traumatic stress disorder, it was demonstrated that propranolol had a significant effect (Famularo et al. 1988). Propranolol also had a positive effect on adolescents suffering from hyperventilation attacks possibly associated with panic disorder (Joorabchi 1977). Although these studies suggest the usefulness of beta blockers, their well-described side effects in adults such as sedation, bradychardia, faintness, dizziness, and bronchoconstrictor qualities do not support their routine use in childhood anxiety disorders.

CASE ILLUSTRATION (TYPICAL TREATMENT)

Description and History

Eileen, a 9½-year-old girl, was referred to the clinic by a school social worker for very severe fear of separation from her parents, in particular her mother. The situation had been developing gradually over the previous three to four months. The patient was also becoming unhappy when away from her house and became withdrawn from her friends and any social activities. Eileen could attend school only when one of her parents took her there and stayed in school all day. Eileen's mother gave up a university course and took a part-time evening job to be with Eileen in school. This was causing considerable concerns for both school personnel and Eileen's parents.

Eileen's birth and milestones were normal. Her health was generally good, though she had experienced chronic sleep difficulties with initial insomnia. At the age of 6 years she hurt her head falling off her bike, resulting in a hospital emergency visit. Eileen's parents described her as a nervous child who always clutched a security blanket. They also reported that she was particularly nervous in elevators. Eileen was easily intimidated, though this had not been a problem at school until the previous year when Eileen was the victim of some bullying. This problem seemed corrected by school staff. Eileen was good at sports, particularly gymnastics, and liked to ride her bike with her friends.

Both parents were in good physical health. There was a history of alcoholism on both sides of the family, anxiety and panic disorder on the father's side, and depression in the mother's family. Throughout the initial diagnostic interview Eileen clung to her mother and had to sit on her lap. The preliminary diagnosis was separation anxiety with school refusal, and a possible comorbid overanxious disorder.

Treatment Course and Outcome

The treatment plan included pharmacotherapy, combined with behavior modification and family therapy. Buspirone was initiated at 5 mg twice daily and increased weekly by 2.5 mg to 10 mg twice daily. After two weeks of medication Eileen's mood had improved and her parents reported that she appeared more relaxed. She was sleeping better with less initial insomnia. Reported side effects to buspirone were headaches and nausea. These appeared to be related to each dose increase and generally lasted only for a day or two. A behavior modification program was established with the cooperation of school personnel. A parent would take Eileen to school, leave her with a teacher, and return home. They would come back to be with Eileen at recess, take her home at lunch time, return again at recess, and collect her at the end of the afternoon session. A reward system was set up for the days Eileen was able to stay in school alone. One specific goal established was for Eileen to take the bus to school. While Eileen was aware of her problem, and stated she wished to overcome it, she showed little motivation and tended to manipulate her parents. Progress in implementing this program was slow at first, and the parents needed a great deal of encouragement to be firm and consistent. After two weeks of buspirone maintained at 10 mg twice daily, Eileen was able to let her mother stay away from school for much longer periods of time, although she still worried that her mother might not return at the end of the morning or afternoon session.

Following six weeks of combined pharmacotherapy and behavior modification there was a marked clinical improvement. Eileen was more spontaneous during clinical sessions. Mother reported that she only needed to take Eileen to school in the morning and meet her again at the end of the day. Eileen had also started to play with her friends after school. Plans were then implemented for Eileen to take the bus to and from school, and if this was achieved successfully to discontinue the medication.

Eileen received buspirone therapy for a total of twelve weeks, with an optimal daily dose of 10 mg twice daily. There were no withdrawal symptoms following the discontinuation, and Eileen continued to attend school. Although her mood remained cheerful she still tended to worry, and she still had some insomnia. Her parents, however, were satisfied with the outcome. At a follow-up appointment set three months later, Eileen appeared happy and functioning well. Her school report card was good and she was playing with friends after school. Physically she appeared healthy and her sleep and appetite were good. Although she still would not go far from home or her parents, overall she was much improved. Eileen was aware of her fears and was making a conscious effort to control them. No prescription and no further appointment were given.

Comments

This case illustrates many of the typical management issues of children with separation anxiety and school refusal. The diagnostic evaluation should include a clear understanding of the development of the disorder in relation to any medical, psychological, family, school, and social problems. It is important to determine how the child views these problems in contrast to the parents, how each member of the family responds, the relative severity of the child's anxiety, parental concerns, interference with psychosocial functioning, and factors associated with improvement or worsening. Bedtime events and their management also often represent special difficulties and should be differentiated from sleep problems. As in all such cases, treatment should be comprehensive with specific goals and strategies. The treatment plan and its implementation must be reviewed with the parents, the child, and teachers. Early during the course of therapy the child should understand that secondary gains from illness and symptoms may normally occur, but that such behaviors are maladaptive; the child's motivation and determination to overcome the handicaps caused by the symptoms are essential. Pharmacotherapy should be viewed by the parents and the patient as facilitating this goal by reducing the fear that the child cannot help.

The progress and any strengths the child shows during the course of therapy should be credited to the child and parents for their efforts; further strategies are offered as challenges, not as demands, and any necessary firmness by the parents or therapist should be presented as an optimal therapeutic tool, not as a power struggle. Expectations should be realistic and clear, and when these are achieved, therapy should be terminated. The therapist's message should be that he or she is unlikely to be needed, but will be available if problems recur.

CASE ILLUSTRATION (DIFFICULT TREATMENT)

Description and History

Michael, a 13-year-old boy, was referred by his family doctor for assessment and treatment of possible panic attacks. Michael had suffered three attacks in the previous two months with weakness, dizziness, and palpitations, and his parents were very apprehensive that these attacks would occur again. Similar, though less severe, attacks had occurred sporadically during the previous two years. The family doctor had examined Michael and ruled out possible physical causes. Due to his anxiety Michael was beginning to avoid public places such as shopping malls, restaurants, and church. Michael reported getting depressed, as he did not understand what was causing his attacks. In addition he was developing severe anticipatory anxiety due to a planned trip for a family wedding that involved flying from Ottawa, Ontario, to and from Saskatchewan, a flight of about four hours' duration. His parents expected some rapid management to deal with the problem of Michael's fear before and during the flights. As the family was due to leave two weeks following the initial interview, Michael was prescribed alprazolam 0.25 mg/day, gradually increasing to 0.25 mg four times a day. An appointment was made following the family's return for a full diagnostic assessment and comprehensive management. On their return the mother reported that even with alprazolam, Michael was extremely tense and nervous and had to leave part way through the wedding reception. His mother did admit that she was expecting worse. Michael took alprazolam 0.25 mg four times daily for one week, with no apparent drug withdrawal. Following his return Michael suffered two panic attacks at school, felt overwhelmed by school work, and felt that his classmates picked on him; thus he became very tense on Sunday evenings.

Michael's birth and milestones were uneventful, though he had some coordination difficulties. Hyperextension of the joints seemed to affect both fine and gross motor skills. At the age of 6 years he received occupational therapy for about one year with no obvious improvement. Michael was always an overcautious child who was reluctant to play with other children. He dropped out of Cub Scouts and avoided all group sports activities. Michael admitted he still disliked athletics and other sports, but he did enjoy riding his bike. Physically he was in good health. Michael was very concerned about his symptoms of shaking, sweating, and palpitations. He said he felt "out of control" and desperately needed to remove himself from the situation related to these attacks.

Initially Michael had no difficulty in school, and his marks were average to above average. By grade six he was the target of some teasing by peers. Currently in grade eight, teachers were aware of his problems and he had permission to leave the classroom when he felt the need. Generally his peers ignored or avoided him. Family history revealed both nervousness and tenseness in the father's family, but no reported emotional problems. Michael's mother suffered from a high level of anxiety but had never been treated. There were also traits of agoraphobia in her family and high levels of anxiety but no one had received therapy.

Treatment Course and Outcome

Preliminary diagnoses for Michael were panic disorder with agoraphobia and overanxious disorder. The treatment plan was for pharmacotherapy with buspirone together with individual and family therapy, and referral to a social skills group. Buspirone was initiated at 5 mg twice daily. During the next few days Michael suffered a severe panic attack and was unable to return to school for four days. His anticipatory anxiety was also increasing. Over the next two weeks buspirone was gradually increased to 10 mg twice daily. While both Michael and his parents reported less severe panic attacks, he still remained extremely anxious and tense. Michael also felt tired and sleepy. He was going to bed early, falling asleep almost immediately, and his mother said it was difficult to wake him in the morning. After four weeks of buspirone therapy (10 mg twice daily), Michael felt his mood had improved somewhat. Dosage was adjusted to 5 mg in the morning, 5 mg at noon, and 10 mg at bedtime. Michael still worried about school, particularly end-of-term exams, but in the evenings and on weekends his parents stated that he seemed more relaxed and happier. Michael reported he felt more "in control." His sleep patterns became more normal. It was then planned to gradually involve Michael in trips to the mall, museums, restaurants, and other public places. Unfortunately there had been no openings for Michael in the current social skills group.

During the Christmas holidays and six weeks into the new term, Michael's improvement remained relatively stable. Then the school guidance counselor informed us that Michael's teachers were becoming increasingly concerned, as he was becoming more withdrawn and his academic work was deteriorating. They were recommending placement in a day treatment program in high school for the following academic year. At home Michael appeared to be coping, although he still had anxieties and fears. Fluvoxamine 50 mg at bedtime, increasing to 50 mg twice daily, was added to the buspirone 10 mg twice daily. Michael was also referred for relaxation therapy. After an initial improvement Michael again relapsed; panic attacks returned, his anxiety level increased, and he was failing his school grade. Fluvoxamine was reduced to 25 mg twice daily, while buspirone therapy was maintained. Michael remained relatively unstable until the end of the school year, with occasional panic attacks, although relaxation therapy seemed to help.

During the summer vacation Michael again improved: he accompanied the family on a trip and visited with friends. It was decided not to follow the recommendation for special placement when Michael started at high school in the fall. He appeared more relaxed and better able to cope. Although still very anxious, he had no panic attacks. Pharmacotherapy (buspirone 10 mg + 5 mg, and fluvoxamine 25 mg twice daily) was maintained until after the winter exams. As the anxiety of Michael's mother was having a negative effect on Michael's progress, it was discussed in family session how best to handle this problem. Michael was encouraged to continue with his relaxation techniques. At the start of Michael's second semester in high school he seemed more stable overall. He appeared, however, to be developing a social phobia related to eating; whether at home or in a restaurant Michael would feel his anxiety level rising and his breathing getting out of control.

Fluvoxamine was increased to 25 mg three times daily. Michael again improved; he was able to go to public places, though he remained oversensitive. His school work became satisfactory, but he asked to be excused from compulsory gym classes. He was very conscious of his apparent clumsiness and complained that his peers picked on him, particularly during team activities. By early summer Michael continued doing well in school. Panic attacks were mild, and he did not seem to suffer from side effects. Mild mood swings and variability in sleep patterns persisted. Further maintenance therapy with buspirone and fluvoxamine was recommended, but Michael's mother discontinued fluvoxamine at the end of the school year. Michael had some withdrawal symptoms and reported that he felt weak, tired, and rather bizarre. Buspirone (10 mg twice daily) treatment was maintained. Michael remained in control of his anxiety during the summer and was able to take a four-week trip with his family. He reported periods of tenseness but no major anxiety. He was confident about returning to school.

When last seen, Michael was in good physical health. He reported several bouts of anxiety that were generally related to school stress. His appetite was good, but he still had a mild initial insomnia. To maintain this level of functioning buspirone was adjusted to 10 mg in the morning, 5 mg at noon, and 10 mg at bedtime. To date, Michael has been receiving buspirone for a total of twenty-four months.

Comments

Many of the comments about the previous case are also applicable in this one. The challenge to the therapist in such cases is to develop an integrated and flexible case management approach to manage comorbidity and pathological changes over the course of the illness. Family pathology and dynamics must also be addressed. Parents may require referral to therapy for their own anxiety and/or depression. It is essential to obtain parents' cooperation when their pathology interferes with the child's therapy. Teachers should also be involved actively in dealing with the problems, as academic and social functioning is usually significantly affected.

Pharmacotherapy should be symptomatic and flexible. Medications, in addition to any direct effect on symptom alleviation, should also be used as tools to facilitate other types of therapy and develop a positive rapport with the child and the parents. Multiple symptoms and comorbid conditions may require combined pharmacotherapy. Care must be exercised to change only one drug or dosage at a time; parents often will exert pressure on the therapist for more rapid changes of medications, and this must be resisted.

Parents may also be overly anxious about the drugs' risks or side effects, and the therapist must be frank about the present-day knowledge and limitations of drug effects. A balanced approach is needed between the therapist's optimism and encouragement on one hand, and giving false expectations on the other; this is especially relevant to pharmacotherapy. Even when significant improvements are obtained, it is not certain that ongoing drug therapy is needed; this can be determined only if a drug is gradually decreased. If improvement persists, pharmacotherapy could be discontinued. The therapist, however, should be alert to early signs of relapse, as a significant relapse can reverse months of therapeutic efforts. Complicated cases such as the one illustrated may require long-term management. The child and family should learn to deal with the patient's symptoms as handicaps to be compensated, and to focus on optimal psychosocial functioning and quality of life rather than get preoccupied with the complete elimination of symptoms. In chronic cases it is important that pharmacotherapy and psychosocial interventions are complemented and not in competition.

SUMMARY

Children with anxiety disorders manifest a wide variety of symptoms and severity ranging from mild worry and distress to overwhelming, incapacitating anxiety that can interfere significantly with functioning. These symptoms are also often associated with a variety of cognitive, behavioral, and social difficulties. Some children may overcome or outgrow their anxiety symptoms with little residual impairment, while others suffer remissions and exacerbations all their lives (Bernstein 1990). In a study on the chronic course of anxiety it was demonstrated that children with these disorders who do not receive treatment have a low rate of remission (Keller et al. 1992). It was estimated that 46 percent of children and adolescents with an anxiety disorder would still be ill eight years after the onset of the disorder. This suggests the probability that in many children, anxiety may be more chronic than previously thought.

Anxiolytics are largely underresearched in children and adolescents. While preliminary data in this population suggest possible uses, specific applications for their use and dosage are generally lacking. Medication should always be used to complement other therapeutic approaches, depending on the associated disturbances in each case (Reiter et al. 1992). When pharmacological treatment alleviates the symptoms of anxiety it allows the clinician to work with the child and family and improve the negative cognitive, behavioral, and familial dysfunctions. Interventions that help the active mastery of anxiety symptoms are also important to prevent the return of symptoms after the discontinuation of medication (AACAP 1993). The expanding variety of treatments and available medications increase the available treatment options, but also place more complex demands on the clinician. An important general issue in child and adolescent psychopharmacology is when and how to use medications, and how to develop the capacity for comprehensive diagnosis and the implementation of a treatment plan that considers and integrates available therapies (Robinowitz and Wiener 1990). Social and cultural factors are also often involved in the diagnosis and treatment of childhood anxiety disorders. Too often clinicians and parents seem reluctant to use medication when anxiety is manifested by children. However, following a comprehensive diagnostic assessment, when the disorder seriously interferes with the individual child's development, family, school, and social adjustments, the present state of medical knowledge and experience often mandates the judicious use of pharmacotherapy.

REFERENCES

AACAP Official Action (1993). Practice parameters for the assessment and treatment of anxiety disorders. *Journal of the American Academy of Child and Adolescent Psychiatry* 32:1089–1098.

Alessi, N., and Bos, T. (1991). Buspirone augmentation of fluoxetine in a depressed child with obsessive-compulsive disorder. *American Journal of Psychiatry* 148:1605–1606.

Ambrosini, P. J., Bianchi, M. D., Rabinovich, H., and Elia, J. (1993). Antidepressant treatments in children and adolescents. II: Anxiety, physical and behavioral disorders. *Journal of the American Academy of Child and Adolescent Psychiatry* 32:483–493.

Beitchman, J. H., Inglis, A., and Schachter, D. (1992a). Child psychiatry and early intervention: I. The aggregate burden of suffering. *Canadian Journal of Psychiatry* 37:230–233.

—— (1992b). Child psychiatry and early intervention: II. The internalizing disorders. *Canadian Journal of Psychiatry* 37:234–239.

Berney, T., Kolvin, I., Bhate, S. R., et al. (1981). School phobia: a therapeutic trial with clomipramine and short term outcome. *British Journal of Psychiatry* 138:110–118.

Bernstein, G. A. (1990). Anxiety disorders. In *Psychiatric Disorders in Children and*

Adolescents, ed. B. D. Garfinkel, G. A. Carlson, and E. B. Weller. Philadelphia, PA: W. B. Saunders.

Bernstein, G. A., Garfinkel, B. D., and Burchardt, C. M. (1990). Comparative studies of pharmacotherapy for school refusal. *Journal of the American Academy of Child and Adolescent Psychiatry* 29:773–781.

Biederman, J. (1987). Clonazepam in the treatment of prepubertal children with panic-like symptoms. *Journal of Clinical Psychiatry* 48:38–42.

——— (1990). The diagnosis and treatment of adolescent anxiety disorders. *Journal of Clinical Psychiatry* 51:20–26.

Bond, A. J., Lader, M., and Shrotriya, R. (1983). Comparative effects of a repeated dose regime of diazepam and buspirone on subjective ratings, psychological tests and the EEG. *European Journal of Clinical Pharmacology* 24:463–467.

Coffey, B. J. (1990). Anxiolytics for children and adolescents: traditional and new drugs. *Journal of Child and Adolescent Psychopharmacology* 1:57–83.

Connor, D. F. (1993). Beta blockers for aggression: a review of the pediatric experience. *Journal of Child and Adolescent Psychopharmacology* 3:99–114.

D'Amato, G. (1962). Chlordiazepoxide in the management of school phobia. *Diseases of the Nervous System* 23:292–295.

DeVeaugh-Geiss, J., Moroz, G., Biederman, J., et al. (1992). Clomipramine hydrochloride in childhood and adolescent obsessive-compulsive disorders – a multicenter trial. *Journal of the American Academy of Child and Adolescent Psychiatry* 31:45–49.

Diagnostic and Statistical Manual of Mental Disorders (1987). 3rd ed., revised. Washington, DC: American Psychiatric Association.

Famularo, R., Kinscherff, R., and Fenton, T. (1988). Propranolol treatment for childhood post traumatic stress disorder, acute type: a pilot study. *American Journal of Diseases of Children* 142:1244–1247.

Flament, M. F., Rapoport, J. L., Berg, C. Z., et al. (1985). Clomipramine treatment of childhood obsessive-compulsive disorder: a double-blind, controlled study. *Archives of General Psychiatry* 42:977–983.

Gadow, K. D. (1992). Pediatric psychopharmacology: a review of recent research. *Journal of Child Psychology and Psychiatry* 33:153–195.

Gittelman-Klein, R., and Klein, D. E. (1971). Controlled imipramine treatment of school phobia. *Archives of General Psychiatry* 25:204–207.

Hoehn-Saric, E., Maisami, M., and Weigand, D. (1987). Measurement of anxiety in children and adolescents using semi-structured interviews. *Journal of the American Academy of Child and Adolescent Psychiatry* 26:541–545.

Jenike, M. A., Buttolph, L., Baer, L., et al. (1989). Open trial of fluoxetine in obsessive-compulsive disorder. *American Journal of Psychiatry* 146:909–911.

Joorabchi, B. (1977). Expressions of the hyperventilation syndrome in childhood: studies in management, including an evaluation of the effectiveness of propranolol. *Clinical Pediatrics* 16:1110–1115.

Keller, M. B., Lavori, P. W., Wunder, J., et al. (1992). Chronic course of anxiety disorders in children and adolescents. *Journal of the American Academy of Child and Adolescent Psychiatry* 31:595–599.

Klein, R. G., Koplewicz, H. S., and Kanner, A. (1992). Imipramine treatment of children with separation anxiety disorder. *Journal of the American Academy of Child and Adolescent Psychiatry* 31:21–28.

Kraft, I. (1965). A clinical study of chlordiazepoxide used in psychiatric disorders of children. *International Journal of Neuropsychiatry* 1:433–437.

Kranzler, H. R. (1988). Use of buspirone in an adolescent with overanxious disorder. *Journal of the American Academy of Child and Adolescent Psychiatry* 27:789–790.

Kutcher, S. P., and Mackenzie, S. (1988). Successful clonazepam treatment of adolescents with panic disorder. *Journal of Clinical Psychopharmacology* 8:299–301.

_____ (1990). *High potency benzodiazepines in child and adolescent anxiety disorders.* Paper presented at the 29th annual meeting of the American College of Neuropsychopharmacology, Puerto Rico.

Kutcher, S. P., Reiter, S., Gardner, D. M., and Klein, R. G. (1992). The pharmacotherapy of anxiety disorders in children and adolescents. *Psychiatric Clinics of North America* 15:41–67.

Lader, M. (1987). Long-term anxiolytic therapy: the issue of drug withdrawal. *Journal of Clinical Psychiatry* 48:12–16.

Leonard, H. L., Swedo, S. E., Rapoport, J. L., et al. (1989). Treatment of obsessive compulsive disorder with clomipramine and desipramine in children and adolescents: a double-blind crossover trial. *Archives of General Psychiatry* 46:1088–1092.

Liebowitz, M. R., Hollander, E., Fairbanks, J., and Campeas, R. (1990). Fluoxetine for adolescents with obsessive-compulsive disorder. *American Journal of Psychiatry* 147:370–371.

Mattila, M. J., Aranko, K., and Seppala, T. (1982). Acute effects of buspirone and alcohol on psychomotor skills. *Journal of Clinical Psychiatry* 43:56–61.

Pfefferbaum, B., Overall, J. E., Boren, H. A., et al. (1987). Alprazolam in the treatment of anticipatory and acute situational anxiety in children with cancer. *Journal of the American Academy of Child and Adolescent Psychiatry* 26:532–535.

Popper, C. W. (1993). Psychopharmacologic treatment of anxiety disorders in adolescents and children. *Journal of Clinical Psychiatry* 54:52–63.

Popper, C. W., and Elliott, G. R. (1990). Sudden death and tricyclic antidepressants in clinical considerations for children. *Journal of Child and Adolescent Psychopharmacology* 1:125–132.

Realmuto, G. M., August, G. J., and Garfinkel, B. D. (1989). Clinical effect of buspirone in autistic children. *Journal of Clinical Psychopharmacology* 9:122–125.

Reiter, S., Kutcher, S., and Gardner, D. (1992). Anxiety disorders in children and adolescents: clinical and related issues in pharmacological treatment. *Canadian Journal of Psychiatry* 37:432–438.

Rickels, K., Schweizer, E., Csanalosi, I., et al. (1988). Long-term treatment of anxiety and risk of withdrawal: prospective comparison of clorazepate and buspirone. *Archives of General Psychiatry* 45:444-450.

Riddle, M. A., Nelson, J. C., Kleinman, C. S., et al. (1991). Sudden death in children receiving Norpramin: a review of three reported cases and commentary. *Journal of the American Academy of Child and Adolescent Psychiatry* 30:104-108.

Riddle, M. A., Scahill, L., King, R. A., et al. (1992). Double-blind, crossover trial of fluoxetine and placebo in children and adolescents with obsessive-compulsive disorder. *Journal of the American Academy of Child and Adolescent Psychiatry* 31:1062-1069.

Robinowitz, C. B., and Wiener, J. (1990). Learning about innovations in clinical treatment. *Journal of Child and Adolescent Psychopharmacology* 1:165-168.

Russo, R. M., Gururaj, V. J. and Allen, J. E. (1976). The effectiveness of diphenhydramine Hcl in pediatric sleep disorders. *Journal of Clinical Pharmacology* 16:284-288.

Saraf, K. R., Klein, D. F., Gittelman-Klein, R., and Groff, S. (1974). Imipramine side effects in children. *Psychopharmacologia* 37:265-274.

Simeon, J. G. (1989). Pediatric psychopharmacology. *Canadian Journal of Psychiatry* 34:115-122.

———— (1990). Child and adolescent psychopharmacology. In *Treatment Strategies in Child and Adolescent Psychiatry*, eds. J. G. Simeon and H. B. Ferguson. New York: Plenum.

———— (1991). Buspirone effects in adolescent psychiatric disorders. *European Neuropsychopharmacology* 1:421.

———— (1993). Use of anxiolytics in children. *L'Encephale* 19:71-74.

Simeon, J. G., and Ferguson, H. B. (1985). Recent developments in the use of antidepressant and anxiolytic medications. *Psychiatric Clinics of North America* 8:893-907.

———— (1987). Alprazolam effects in children with anxiety disorders. *Canadian Journal of Psychiatry* 32:570-574.

Simeon, J. G., Ferguson, H. B., Knott, V., et al. (1992). Clinical, cognitive and neurophysiological effects of alprazolam in children with overanxious and avoidant disorders. *Journal of the American Academy of Child and Adolescent Psychiatry* 31:29-33.

Simeon, J. G., Knott, V. J., Thatte, S., et al. (in press). Buspirone therapy in childhood anxiety disorders: a pilot study. *Journal of Child and Adolescent Psychopharmacology.*

Simeon, J. G., Thatte, S., and Wiggins, D. (1990). Treatment of adolescent obsessive-compulsive disorder with a clomipramine-fluoxetine combination. *Psychopharmacology Bulletin* 26:285-290.

Sussman, N. (1987). Treatment of anxiety with buspirone. *Psychiatric Annals* 17:114-117.

Part IV

FUTURE
DIRECTIONS

19

THE TREATMENT OF ANXIETY DISORDERS IN YOUTH

Philip C. Kendall
Jennifer P. MacDonald
Kimberli R. H. Treadwell

CHILDHOOD ANXIETY DISORDERS have been differentiated as separate diagnostic entities within *DSM-III-R*. The research that has been generated by this classification has contributed to our knowledge of anxious symptomatology and its treatment; however, this should be viewed as the beginning of our understanding of these phenomena in children and adolescents. This chapter focuses on things to come in this line of research. First the treatment of anxiety in its historical context will be reviewed. Next, the state of our knowledge regarding current focuses in mental health, the nature of anxiety, recommended treatments, and parental roles in treatment will be examined. Finally, future research goals, preventative measures, and diagnostic criteria in *DSM-IV* will be discussed in order to guide future investigations and clinical pursuits in childhood anxiety.

HISTORICAL PRECIS

Psychosocial treatments for childhood psychopathology have generally paralleled the models used in adult therapy; psychodynamic, humanistic, behavioral, and more recently, cognitive paradigms have guided psychological interventions. Anxiety, in particular, has historically been a central focus for psychodynamic and behavioral interventions (e.g., Wachtel 1977). For instance, the treatment of impairments caused by anxiety was a focus in early psychoanalytic therapy, as play therapy techniques were being defined. This trend was apparent from approximately 1950 to 1965, when play therapy was an oft-used treatment in child residential settings (Davids 1975).

The treatment of anxiety buttressed the introduction of behavior therapy in the mid-1960s to mid-1970s (Davids 1975). The celebrated classical conditioning of a young boy's fearful reaction to white rabbits provided early support for the behavioral paradigm. Success over the decades in such interventions as systematic desensitization and modeling for childhood fears and anxieties supported the behavioral paradigm. Other behavioral therapies, such as self-regulation and cognitive-behavioral therapy, can also be traced to the development of treatments for anxieties in children. In fact, it has been asserted that children's anxieties were a useful tool for promoting and exemplifying the attributes of behavioral theory and interventions (Barrios and O'Dell 1989).

Cognitive constructs impacted radical behaviorism, leading to cognitive social learning theory and, more recently, information-processing approaches (Kendall and Ingram 1989). A union of behaviorism and cognitive theory maintains the importance of environmental contingencies on performance, while underscoring the centrality of information-processing factors in the development and maintenance of psychopathology (Kendall 1985, 1991).

CURRENT TRENDS IN CHILD TREATMENT

It is only very recently that diagnosed cases of anxiety disorders in youth have received rigorous empirical attention in treatment outcome research. For many years "undercontrolled" behaviors, such as impulsiveness, ADHD, conduct disorder, and aggression, have received a greater amount of empirical attention (Francis 1988) and comprised the bulk of clinic referrals for children (McMahon and Wells 1989). These acting-out children are disruptive to school and family activities and thus are more likely candidates for referral and intervention. The distress that children with anxiety disorders suffer and the debilitating effects on daily functioning have increasingly come to the attention of mental health professionals. However, although more anxious youth are being identified as potential clients, anxiety disorders still do not dominate referrals for assessment or treatment (Cosper and Erikson 1983, Maag, et al. 1988, Ritter 1989, Sacco and Graves 1985). The accurate identification and referral of anxiety-disordered youth requires that teachers, coaches, school nurses, and other individuals spending time with children become aware of the symptoms of anxiety disorders and the centers that provide effective treatments.

A second focus in children's mental health treatment is the role of families. Two useful research methods for examining this topic are top-down and bottom-up designs. For instance, a top-down approach to addressing family concerns found that children of anxious parents had a greater incidence of *DSM-III* anxiety diagnoses and dysthymia (e.g., Turner et al. 1987). Empirical research following a bottom-up design reported that children in an inpatient unit who were suffering primarily from anxiety had relatives with high occurrence rates of affective illness and alcoholism (e.g., Livingston et al. 1985). These strategies can help address the extent to which the family contributes to children's anxiety symptoms (Brady and Kendall 1992) and can help to direct family-oriented interventions. The inclusion of the family in the treatment of childhood anxiety disorders is an area that deserves increased empirical and clinical attention and will be discussed in a later section.

THE NATURE OF CHILDHOOD ANXIETY AS IT INFORMS TREATMENT IMPLICATIONS

Only recently have clinicians and researchers begun to examine the nature of anxiety disorders in youth, and the resulting implications for treatment (Kendall et al. 1992b). Continuing research efforts will advance our understanding of childhood anxiety and maximally inform intervention methods.

Cognition

As recently as 1988, it was concluded that "no definitive statements about the cognitions of anxious children can be made" (Francis 1988, p. 276). A useful heuristic in characterizing cognitions involves distinguishing between cognitive distortions and cognitive deficiencies (Kendall 1985, 1991, Kendall and MacDonald 1993). *Cognitive deficiencies* are defined as a lack of cognitive activity in situations where mental activity would be useful or beneficial, such as an absence of problem solving, perspective taking, or planning. *Cognitive distortions*, on the other hand, refer to an active, but crooked, thinking process. The child attends to social or environmental cues but does so in a distorted or dysfunctional manner. Theoretically, anxious children's tendency to misperceive the environment, worry excessively, and exaggerate threats to the self would fall under the rubric of cognitive distortions.

The majority of empirical studies investigating cognition in anxious children involve nonclinical samples with specific fears, rather than samples of youth who have been diagnosed with an anxiety disorder. Nevertheless, this literature provides some helpful information; for example, test-anxious children evidenced negative distortions in their opinions of their abilities (Zatz and Chassin 1983, 1985), and children with extreme dental anxiety reported greater negative self-statements than children with lower dental anxiety (Prins 1986). The results of these studies and others indicate that anxiety involves distortions in cognitive processing, yet further study is needed to determine if these findings hold for the experience of children with diagnostic levels of anxiety disorders.

Methods of measurement are a concern. Using a thought-listing procedure, Kendall and Chansky (1991) found that clinic-referred anxious youth reported coping self-talk, yet the self-talk was not functional. The endorsement method (questionnaires) has shown promise. For example, a potentially useful instrument for the investigation of cognitions in clinically anxious children is the Negative Affectivity Self-Statement Questionnaire (NASSQ, Ronan et al. in press). The NASSQ assesses the frequency of anxious (and depressive) self-statements. Reliability and validity are supportive; the measure differentiated anxious from nonanxious clinic-referred children between the ages of 8 and 15 years old (Ronan et al. in press). Additional studies examining the nature of the cognitive processing in clinical cases of childhood anxiety are still needed to increase our understanding and inform our treatment programs.

Distinctions have been drawn between fear, anxiety, and phobia. Fear has been described as a discrete response to a circumscribed experience of threat. Anxiety is considered to be a more diverse response to more diffuse stimuli (Johnson and Melamed 1979), whereas phobias are fears that are severe, persistent behavioral patterns of avoidance (Barrios and Hartmann 1988, Miller et al. 1974, Morris and Kratochwill 1983). Anxiety is considered to be longer-standing and more disruptive than fears or phobias (Kendall et al. 1992a, Morris and Kratochwill 1991). Fears are part of the normal and healthy developmental sequence, emerging and receding throughout childhood and adolescence, whereas excessive anxiety and phobias are not common in healthy development. Increased knowledge of the nature and manifestations of disturbing anxiety (within the various childhood anxiety diagnoses) is needed. Fortunately, there are a growing number of research endeavors using diagnosed cases of anxiety-disordered youth.

PSYCHOSOCIAL TREATMENT

Illustrative Treatment Protocol

A psychosocial (cognitive-behavioral) protocol (Kendall et al. 1989) targeting childhood anxiety disorders has received initial empirical support (Kendall

1994). The protocol addresses the thinking, feeling, and behavior associated with distressing anxiety by incorporating behavioral techniques, such as relaxation training, with cognitive strategies, such as modifying self-statements, in a multicomponent intervention. The ultimate goal is for the child to develop a coping template—a functional way to view anxiety-provoking situations as manageable.

Participating children attend individual fifty- to sixty-minute sessions with their therapist. The treatment is divided into two segments: the first segment has an educational orientation and focuses on the cognitive skills necessary to alter anxious reactions to anxiety-provoking situations. The first segment of treatment culminates in the acronym FEAR, representing the first letter in each step of the coping plan. This acronym serves as a useful reminder to use the FEAR steps in anxious situations, as well as a guide to the correct order of steps. Children often make a poster and/or a wallet-size card illustrating the FEAR steps to carry with them as a reminder of their work thus far in treatment.

A focus on physiological arousal leads to the first FEAR step called "Feeling Frightened?" Children learn within the first few weeks to differentiate anxious arousal from other emotions and to reliably identify these feelings when they occur in a variety of situations. Physiological arousal serves as a signal of anxious distress—and becomes a cue to initiate coping strategies. Therapists teach relaxation skills, consisting of deep breathing and progressive muscle relaxation, to target the child's specific physiological response (e.g., butterflies in their stomach, tightened neck muscles), and cognitive imagery.

The next step is summarized by the phrase "Expecting Bad Things to Happen?" Children learn to identify and modify the anxious self-talk associated with the negative outcomes that they are anticipating. Through techniques such as examining the thought bubbles of favorite cartoon characters, children can become adept at identifying their own internal dialogue. Thought bubbles introduce the idea that thoughts run through people's minds and children can learn to fill in their own thought bubbles with "coping" self-talk. Children are encouraged to think of nonanxious self-talk that could also apply to the anxious situation and to challenge their own anxious cognitions. For instance, rather than think that "someone might laugh" when they give an oral book report, the child might also think that people might listen and that laughter isn't the end of the world, that they will do okay, that people will listen to them, that this is not the end of the world, and so on.

The phrase "Actions and Attitudes that Can Help" describes the next step. Children are taught problem-solving steps to develop behavioral plans to cope with anxiety-provoking situations. Therapists help the child to identify a number of alternative behaviors, to evaluate each behavioral option, and to choose the behavior that best accomplishes the goal in an appropriate, nonavoiding, and non-anxiety-provoking manner.

Self-evaluation and reward are the final step in the FEAR system ("Results and Rewards"). This step is particularly important for anxious youth, who often have perfectionistic tendencies, require reassurance from others, and worry about their competence. Children are helped to "Rate and Reward" the execution of their action plan and are encouraged to positively evaluate all successful approximations of coping behavior. Finally, the children learn to reward themselves for a job well done. A list of preferred items or activities is generated, such as playing a game or receiving stickers or a candy bar. Tangible rewards are often paired with social praise from the therapist to help teach the child to respond to social praise as a reinforcer as well.

The second treatment segment is practicing the newly acquired FEAR steps in both imaginal and real situations. The therapist designs anxiety-provoking situations that are specific to the child's anxieties and presents them in a hierarchical fashion. In general, the first several sessions focus on low-level anxiety situations. The child may be exposed to a situation imaginally, with the therapist guiding the child through the use of the FEAR steps. Next, the child participates in low-level distressing situations, after being prepared for the situation with the therapist. The child progresses to mastery of moderately arousing events, and finally manages highly arousing events. Thus, the child uses the FEAR steps in successively difficult situations. The child also practices using the FEAR steps during the week at home and in school.

A specific and crucial element of maintenance and generalization begins with the final sessions of therapy. These final sessions are geared toward consolidating successes and fine-tuning the child's coping skills. The child can begin to "show off" and demonstrate these coping strengths to others. A crucial part of this final aspect of treatment occurs in the very last session. During this final session, the child creates a video commercial to take home—a commercial in which the child gives advice to others about how to cope with anxiety. This provides the child a chance to organize the therapeutic experience, recognize his or her accomplishment, gain a sense of mastery by becoming the "expert" in the video, and demonstrate these new skills in a creative manner to others. The commercial also allows the child to put a personal signature on the FEAR steps, and as a result, this can help to strengthen the vital link between the learning of skills and their assimilation and generalization for use in everyday situations.

This intervention was evaluated in a randomized clinical treatment outcome study (Kendall 1994). Forty-seven children with a *DSM-III-R* diagnosis of overanxious disorder, separation anxiety disorder, or avoidant disorder were randomly assigned to a treatment or wait-list condition. Judged against wait-list, subjects participating in treatment showed significant gains on child-, parent-, and teacher-report measures, and child behavioral observations (Kendall 1994). Importantly, two-thirds of the children no longer met diagnostic criteria for an anxiety disorder at posttreatment. These improvements were maintained at one-year follow-up.

A second randomized clinical trial is currently under way at the CAADC, with a mid-treatment assessment that will permit an evaluation of the effects of each segment of treatment. In other words, the cognitive focus of the first segment will be compared to the addition of a behavioral focus during the second segment. Comorbidity as it relates to treatment outcome will also be addressed.

Future Trends in Intervention

Youth are known for their responsiveness to and concern about peers. What is surprising is that little research has addressed the role of peer behavior with regard to anxiety disorders. Peer nomination methods for study in acceptance and the use of peers as a part of intervention are examples of potentially beneficial peer involvement. Preliminary observations suggest that the use of anxious youth who are in treatment as peers for in vivo experiences of other in-treatment youth carries great potential. However, research has yet to separate the influence of the in vivo experience itself from the influence of the peer involvement. Certainly a worthwhile future study would be one that addresses this question.

Relatedly, there is an unfortunate absence of studies of the effects of treatments that use small groups of anxious youth. Recent studies in the adult anxiety literature suggest that group cognitive-behavioral treatments can be effective. A cognitive-behavioral treatment for social-phobic adults showed improvement over control subjects, and maintenance over three- and six-month follow-up periods (Heimberg et al. 1990). In addition, researchers are beginning to investigate the effectiveness of group treatments with depressed children (Clarke et al. 1992, Fine et al. 1991), and with anxiety-disordered children (Cadbury et al. 1990, see Ginsburg et al., this volume).

Due to the influence of behavioral approaches, and their empirical support, there is likely to be an increase in the use of in vivo exposure treatment. Also, due to the social nature of some of the anxiety disorders, there is likely to be an increase in the use of social in vivo experiences. That is, one can anticipate that there will be more therapists placing a prepared child in a situation with peers where the ongoing activity (behavioral, emotional, and cognitive) can be guided by the therapist.

With the trend toward manualized treatments that have empirical support, there is likely to be a reduction in the use of more psychoanalytic approaches, such as play therapy or psychodynamic child therapy. In the absence of a manualization of the procedures used by these approaches and a lack of research support of their effects, third party and other payers are inclined to steer toward other approaches.

PARENTAL AND FAMILIAL ROLES IN THE TREATMENT OF ANXIETY-DISORDERED YOUTH

Researchers and clinicians have long recognized the important and often crucial role that parents play in the treatment of their children's psychopathology. Many treatments, such as parent training and family therapy, include parents in the therapy process. Other treatments are child focused. Yet even when the treatment focuses on the identified child, parents and families can be an important asset in the assessment and treatment of their child's difficulties. Although a large body of literature documents the benefits of individual therapy for a variety of child disorders (Weisz et al. 1987), the degree to which a treatment generalizes to situations outside the therapeutic environment can vary greatly depending on the nature of the home setting. The child's social and interpersonal contexts are inextricably linked (Kendall 1985, 1991), and thus, not only are the child's expectations and attributions responses to the external social environment, but the child's context responds to the child's actions. Thus, a child who has learned a more adaptive way of coping with his or her environment will have more difficulty maintaining therapeutic gains when the environment has not adapted to the child's gains.

Parental participation in the treatment of youth with anxiety disorders can take various forms, with a wide range of involvement. As supportive consultants in a child-focused treatment, parents can be involved in their child's treatment from the outset. Parents' reports of their child's experiences at home are a valuable source of information for the therapist. Information-gathering from parents can be particularly useful when the child has difficulty discussing painful thoughts and feelings, or when the child has a tendency to deny or underestimate his or her anxious reactions. It can also be beneficial in understanding the environmental factors that may be contributing to the child's disorder, such as losses that the child may have experienced, the emotional and financial resources of the parents, and any current familial stressors. Therapists' observations of discussions with child and parents can provide information regarding the interaction patterns that contribute to or maintain child anxiety. For example, some parents are overly involved with the child and his or her activities and performance. Witnessing this pattern provides a target for treatment. Overall, parents as consultants for the child in individual therapy provide a wealth of information that is useful for diagnostic and treatment decisions.

Beyond the consultant role, caregivers can serve as coaches by participating in the in vivo exposure sessions and facilitating additional exposure experiences in the home setting. Relatedly, parents can serve as coping models for their child (Kendall et al. 1992a), demonstrating how to apply strategies that are appropriate for the management of anxiety.

Family involvement may include parents or caretakers directly in therapy with the child. Although the anxious child remains the focus of treatment, parents would participate in sessions by learning new parenting techniques and altering their expectations for the child and attributions about outcome to be consistent with developmental norms. As an illustration of the involvement of parents as co-clients, consider the multiple baseline design evaluation of treatment conducted with the family as a unit (Howard 1993). A modified version of the cognitive-behavioral treatment described earlier was effective in decreasing anxious symptomatology in the identified child client and awaits empirical comparison with individual cognitive-behavioral therapy for child anxiety disorders (Kendall 1994). The use of more traditional family therapy in the treatment of childhood anxiety disorders is largely unexplored (see Moen, this volume).

Historically, psychology has been prone to blame the mother for childhood psychopathology. Of the studies that address parental characteristics of children with disorders, far too many focus on mothers, and fathers are dramatically underrepresented in clinical child and adolescent research (Phares 1992). What is needed, in the anxiety disorders specifically and in child psychopathology in general, is systematic investigation of the role of paternal practices in the onset and maintenance of emotional and behavioral problems in youth. Preliminary studies indicate that there is substantial association between paternal characteristics and child and adolescent psychopathology, that the presence of paternal psychopathology is a sufficient but not necessary condition for psychopathology in youth, and that the degree of risk associated with paternal psychopathology is comparable to that associated with maternal psychopathology (Phares and Compas 1992). Regarding anxiety disorders specifically, studies of paternal characteristics are scarce. Both fathers and mothers of anxious and obsessive-compulsive adolescents were found to have more obsessional characteristics than parents of children in a nonclinical sample (Clark and Bolton 1985). Fathers of school phobic children reported clinically significant levels of family dysfunction in the father–child relationship (Bernstein et al. 1990). It appears that there is some evidence for greater disturbance in the fathers of anxious children than in the fathers of nonclinical children, but further research in this area is certainly needed.

Similarly, within the study of familial influences, literature focuses on parents and on the identified child, neglecting any examination of siblings within the same family. One wonders why it is one child, and not others within the family, who develops an anxiety disorder. Studies of the siblings of identified cases may help to untangle the role of family and parenting practices in childhood anxiety disorders.

DEVELOPMENTAL CONSIDERATIONS

The evaluation of psychotherapeutic treatments for children requires a clear understanding of the normal rates and courses of emotional and behavioral problems over different ages and developmental periods. It is crucial that researchers not fall prey to the uniformity myth about children (i.e., the idea that the term *children* designates a homogeneous group) in both the diagnosis and treatment of childhood disorders (Kendall 1984, Morris and Kratochwill 1983). Consideration was given in *DSM-III-R* (1987) to the differential manifestations of anxiety disorders in adults and children. For example, rather than receiving diagnoses similar to adults, as is the case with depression, there are anxiety diagnoses that are unique to children. However, additional attention to the characteristics of anxious children of varying ages and to the resulting treatment outcome effects is needed.

As fears are common in normal childhood populations, developmental factors are important both to distinguish common, developmentally appropriate childhood fears from maladaptive anxiety, and to understand the distinct forms that both clinical and nonclinical anxiety might take depending on a child's age. Assessing inappropriate fears for a child's developmental level is crucial in determining the severity of the disturbance and the potential need for intervention (Miller et al. 1974). In addition, as children's cognitive abilities develop, their fears begin to change in manifestation. For example, preliminary data suggest that the maturational content of children's fears appears to move from global, undifferentiated, and externalized fears to those that are increasingly differentiated, abstract, and internalized (Kendall and Ronan 1990). Several researchers have provided information regarding the organization of the content of children's fears through factor analyses (Miller et al. 1972, Ollendick et al. 1985). It also appears that the decrease in fears as children grow older is not as great as might be expected given the qualitative changes in children's fears. Developmental concerns are also relevant for diagnoses. Children presenting with separation anxiety disorder tended to be younger than children presenting with overanxious disorder (Last et al. 1987b). Panic disorder was not manifested until the onset of puberty and adolescence (Last and Strauss 1989). Thus, although some knowledge exists concerning developmental issues in both clinical and nonclinical childhood anxiety, there is a paucity of longitudinal research. Such questions as whether early forms of anxiety develop into difficulties later in the course of development remain virtually unanswered (Sroufe 1983).

Developmental issues must also be recognized and examined due to the possibility of differential treatment outcomes that can result given the age of the child in question. This area is relatively unexplored in outcome research. A small number of studies have evaluated age in an effort to integrate developmental differences into treatment research with disorders other than anxiety and have shown differential differences in outcome (e.g., Kolvin et al. 1981, Miller et al. 1972). What remains to be done is not necessarily an examination of the effect of age, per se, on treatment effects, but an examination, within specific treatment modalities, of developmental issues that may affect treatment outcome for that particular treatment. Different facets of development may be more relevant to certain interventions (Kazdin 1991), and this needs to be taken into account in both the design and analysis of treatments for disordered youth. For example, a cognitive-behavioral treatment for anxiety might be directed only to those children who have developed the cognitive capabilities that enable the child to grasp the cognitive skills presented in the treatment.

Social development may also be relevant for treatment of the anxious child, especially if anxious distress relates to social interaction or social evaluation. Developmentally, peer problems change with increasing social demands. Interventions for the younger client may address structured situations, whereas the older child needs to handle more ambiguous social contexts (Kendall et al. 1992a). Last, it remains to be answered whether earlier intervention in general has more beneficial effects. If this were the case, early detection and intervention would be crucial in treating anxious youth in order to prevent anxious children growing into anxious adults.

RESEARCH NEEDS

Comorbidity

This chapter, indeed this volume, deals with children with anxiety disorders. However, most children present not only with anxiety symptoms and difficulties, but with additional symptoms and/or comorbid diagnoses (see Kendall and Brady in press), often creating a potentially distinct clinical picture. Comorbidity with depression (Brady and Kendall 1992) occurs with sufficient regularity to be a concern for treatment planning. For example, children comorbid for anxiety and depression suffered greater peer impairments than children with anxiety disorders alone (Strauss et al. 1988a). Comorbidity of anxiety with other anxiety disorders, depression, and externalizing disorders will be reviewed in turn (see Perrin and Last, this volume, for full explication).

Comorbidity within the Anxiety Disorders

Comorbidity for anxious children often involves an additional anxiety disorder diagnosis (Kendall and Brady in press, Last et al. 1987b). Although the diagnostic validity, specificity, demographics, and pattern of comorbidity have begun to be delineated, further efforts are necessary (Last et al. 1987a, Last et al. 1987b, Last et al. 1987c, Last et al. 1992). Research is necessary to examine the effects on treatment outcome that result from various patterns of comorbidity within the childhood anxiety disorders.

Comorbidity with Depression

Current comorbidity estimates for anxiety and depression range from 15.9–61.9 percent (Brady and Kendall 1992). It is hypothesized that a unified mood-based personality construct, negative affectivity, best represents the relationship between anxiety and depression (King et al. 1991, Watson and Clark 1984, Wolfe et al. 1987). Understanding the nature of the relationship between anxiety and depression in childhood is crucial for diagnostic purposes, and also important in terms of the treatment of children with anxiety, depression, and comorbid mood and anxiety disorders. However, additional concerns arise in terms of creating, implementing, and evaluating treatment approaches for these children. One of the most important questions regarding treatment outcome is whether there are differential outcome effects for comorbid children versus children with only anxiety or depression. A range of interventions (largely cognitive-behavioral) has been developed separately to address anxiety and depression in children, yet there are currently no outcome data on the treatment of children comorbid for anxiety and depression. Some related empirical data exist, such as the finding that comorbid children are typically older and more severely disturbed (Strauss et al. 1988b), and that it is unusual to find depressed children without symptoms of anxiety, while anxiety alone in children does exist (Puig-Antich and Rabinovich 1986). It has been suggested that one approach to treating these comorbid children would be to shift away from diagnosis-based interventions and move toward treatments geared to meet the individual child's symptom pattern (Kendall et al. 1992b; see Eisen and Engler, this volume).

Comorbidity with Externalizing Disorders

Anxious children may also present with the diagnosis of an externalizing disorder, such as attention deficit hyperactivity disorder. In our clinic, 15 percent of anxiety-disordered youth (aged 9–11) also met criteria for ADHD (Kendall 1994). In general, studies investigating the overlap between anxiety disorders and externalizing disorders in children are scarce (Steingard et al. 1992). However, empirical investigation of anxiety-disordered children presenting with externalizing behaviors as well requires additional research efforts in terms of prevalence rates, diagnosis, and differential response to treatment.

The Effects of Cultural, Economic, and Ethnic Differences on Treatment

Our nation is increasingly culturally and economically diverse, and thus so too are the child clients requiring mental health services. Cultural and economic diversity becomes an important issue to our profession. In fact, we are called upon in the current *Guidelines for Providers of Psychological Services to Ethnic and Culturally Diverse Populations* to "recognize ethnicity and culture as significant parameters in understanding psychological process" (1990, p. 4). There is virtual unanimity among researchers and theorists that some degree of compatibility between culture and treatment is necessary (Tharp 1991). However, research on cultural issues in the clinical treatment of children is scant. In diagnosing children with anxiety disorders, cultural, ethnic, and socioeconomic differences may lead to distinct manifestations of anxiety and/or different concerns felt by the anxious children. For example, regarding socioeconomic status (SES), a child from a more socioeconomically advantaged background may worry about his or her performance on tests and in athletics, but a child from a lower status may have concerns about his or her safety when walking to school, or his or her family's financial well-being. Last and colleagues (1987b) found that children diagnosed with SAD came from a lower SES than did children diagnosed with OAD.

Future research efforts should be directed toward the study of the manifestation, treatment, and familial view of anxiety within specific ethnic groups. For example, Neal and Turner (1991) and Kashani and Orvaschel (1988) stress the paucity of research concerning anxiety in the African-American populations. Regarding anxiety in African-American children, a review of existing literature found no studies focusing on OCD, SAD, avoidant disorder of childhood, or GAD in African-American children, and only one study involving OAD-diagnosed African-American children (Neal and Turner 1991). Neal and Turner suggest that this scarcity of research may be affected by factors such as the small number of African-Americans conducting research, and a general disinterest in African-Americans in the research community. These authors also suggest that African-Americans (adults and children alike) may be less likely to seek help for psychological distress and may have a negative perception of research in general.

Interestingly, with respect to ethnicity, more similarities than differences have been noted between Caucasian and African-American children. Child-, parent- and teacher-report of children's anxiety and functioning, as well as diagnostic status, did not vary as a function of ethnicity (Treadwell et al. 1993). Contrary to previously held views, it appears that the fears of nonclinical samples of Caucasian and African-American children transcend ethnic differences and are more similar than dissimilar (Neal et al. 1993). Eight of the top eleven fears are the same for Caucasian and African-American children.

There are additional concerns regarding cultural and ethnic diversity that affect the treatment of anxious youth. Therapy should be adapted to fit the individual needs of the child, and thus it is important to give consideration to the child's cultural and economic background. Therapy of many modalities is language dependent, and there may be differences in language or colloquial speech between the therapist and the child client. In addition, the importance of forming a therapeutic relationship is recognized across treatment modalities. This may be more difficult if there are cultural and economic differences between the child and his or her therapist. Anxious children are often shy, fearful of adults, and overly aware of how they might be judged as different from others; thus it is particularly important with this population to be aware of differences resulting from the child's culture and to adapt whenever possible. Minority status itself has been described as a stressor, partially because of prejudice and hostility that often must be endured, and associated with ineffective coping styles (Moritsugu and Sue 1983, Tharp 1991). It would be important for the therapist of an anxious child to be aware of anxieties that may result from minority status and to assess the child's coping skills. Although these may be legitimate concerns, initial empirical research in this area suggests comparability in the effectiveness of a cognitive-behavioral treatment for Caucasian and for African-American youth (Treadwell et al. 1993).

ISSUES IN CLASSIFICATION: *DSM-IV*

The most fundamental change to the child anxiety disorders in *DSM-IV* is the elimination of OAD as a disorder. Instead, overanxious children can be classified as generalized anxiety disorder (GAD). The first criteria for GAD is persistent and excessive worry more days than not over a period of six months. The duration of symptoms that warrant a diagnosis of GAD is similar to *DSM-III-R* OAD; the child must display symptoms for a period of six months or longer. Several additions to the *DSM-III-R* GAD diagnosis include the criteria that the worry must be difficult to control, and that the worry or physical symptoms must cause clinically significant distress or impairment in functioning. Another significant alteration is that the eighteen physical symptoms listed in *DSM-III-R* have been reduced to six symptoms in *DSM-IV*. In accordance with this deletion, only three of the six symptoms must be present. These symptoms include restlessness, fatigue, difficulty in concentration, irritability, muscle tension, and sleep disturbance. Two differential criteria in *DSM-III-R* (i.e., GAD must not occur only during a mood or psychotic disorder and must not be due to organic factors) have been collapsed to a single criteria in *DSM-IV*.

The change from OAD to GAD holds several implications for overly anxious children. In *DSM-III-R*, children had to have four of seven symptoms, including excessive worries about the future, the past, or competence; somatic complaints; self-consciousness; a need for reassurance; and tension or an inability to relax. Technically, a child could qualify for OAD without the presence of excessive worries. In the new classification system, excessive worries occurring more days than not becomes a necessary criteria for diagnosis. In addition, *DSM-IV*'s GAD places no distinctions concerning the specific source of worry, as in *DSM-III-R*'s OAD. Another necessary criteria for the new GAD is that the child must display physical symptoms associated with worry, whereas in *DSM-III-R* physical symptoms could be present, but did not have to necessarily be present for diagnosis. Using the OAD classification, it was possible for a child to meet criteria for OAD without endorsement (by either parent or child) of any physiological symptoms. Some children may be unaware of the link between their physiological arousal and their anxiety, and in fact, helping them to understand this link is often a major component to therapy. Other children may disclose their physiological distress, such as children with irritable bowel syndrome whose physiological reactions are embarrassing. Thus, if the link between physiology and anxiety cannot be made at the time of diagnosis, children who may in fact possess clinical levels of anxious distress may not fit diagnostic criteria for an anxiety disorder. In summary, the shift to GAD from OAD will impact the samples of children studied in terms of worry and physical symptoms.

The decision to eliminate OAD as a diagnostic category will have unwanted effects on the empirical studies that have specifically focused on this disorder since its inception in 1980. To change diagnostic criteria now for a syndrome that can be reliably diagnosed and that carries some prognostic, demographic, and symptomatological patterns could render obsolete the empirical research that examined this childhood anxiety disorder. New efforts will be needed to examine familial, longitudinal, and comorbid topics using the GAD criteria.

Minor changes in diagnostic criteria for SAD in *DSM-IV* appear to increase the specificity of the diagnosis. Rather than discriminating realistic from unrealistic worries, as was the case for *DSM-III-R*, worries rather must be excessive to warrant diagnosis. The duration criterion has increased, with symptom duration of four weeks required for diagnosis of SAD in *DSM-IV*, as compared to two weeks in *DSM-III-R*. It is hoped that these changes will discriminate worries centering around attachment figures from worries about multiple sources.

The diagnosis of social phobia now includes references to children. For instance, if children display the persistent fear of one or more social situations, which is the primary symptom of social phobia, this fear must be present in peer situations, and the child must evidence a capacity for social relationships with familiar people. The physiological response of adults includes feelings that may mimic panic, but in children these symptoms may also be expressed as crying, tantrums, freezing, or withdrawal. Finally, adults must recognize that their social fear is excessive to warrant diagnosis, but children do not have to possess such recognition. Additionally, avoidant disorder of childhood is now eliminated. Under *DSM-III-R*, a child could not receive a diagnosis of both social phobia and avoidant disorder. Thus, the prevalence of the social phobia diagnosis may increase, despite minimal change in the characteristics of children being diagnosed.

The distinctiveness of the childhood anxiety disorders was unclear, since symptoms overlapped and anxiety disorders were often comorbid with other anxiety disorders (Last et al. 1987b). These concerns would support the changes noted in SAD and social phobia, which have changed wording to increase the specificity of each disorder and have clarified differential diagnoses.

As noted earlier, the high rate of comorbidity of anxiety and depression in children questions the specificity of each disorder. Are they distinct (Kendall and Watson 1989)? As in the adult literature, where some data support a mixed anxiety/depression syndrome (negative affectivity; Clark and Watson 1991, Katon and Roy-Byrne 1991), a review of the literature of the comorbidity of anxiety and depression in children and adolescents suggests that a similar syndrome may exist in children as well. Will future editions of *DSM* offer a diagnostic category for comorbid anxiety and depression—that is, negative affectivity?

Several perspectives are important in an attempt to differentiate anxiety and depression in youth. Both constructs have physiological, affective, behavioral, and cognitive components, and could be compared on any combination of these aspects (see Finch et al. 1989). For instance, a key cognitive component of anxiety is hypothesized to be an expectation of apprehension, whereas in depression cognitions focus on loss or failure (Kendall and Ingram 1989). The addition of positive affect was reported to be key in differentiating anxiety and depression in children: depressed children reported a combination of high negative affectivity and low positive affectivity, while anxious children reported high negative affectivity with positive affectivity being irrelevant (Finch et al. 1989). Another perspective concerns the level of analysis; one can examine anxiety and depression as individual symptoms, transitory states, enduring personality traits, or clinical syndromes. The overlap (and need for an additional diagnostic category) may differ depending on one's level of analysis (Kendall et al. 1987).

Research is needed to examine three populations: pure anxiety, pure depression, and mixed anxiety/depression. These populations may be distinguishable, and future research could determine the defining characteristics of each. Some evidence indicates that children with primary anxiety scored high for anxiety and lower on depression, whereas depressed children scored high on both anxiety and depression measures (Brady and Kendall 1992). In addition, children who evidenced a mixed symptomatology exhibited more diverse symptoms of both disorders than children with only one primary concern.

PREVENTION

Professionals from varying disciplines have expressed concern about the increasing numbers of young people at high risk for psychosocial and health-related problems (e.g., *Children in Need* 1987, Gans et al. 1990). In addition, it appears that traditional treatment approaches can address only a small portion of the youth in need of services (Tuma 1989, Weissberg et al. 1991). Yet the mental health community continues to direct the majority of its efforts toward the assessment, diagnosis, and treatment of disordered youth, rather than toward the development and evaluation of programs aimed at the prevention of psychological disturbance (Cowen et al. 1980, Weissberg et al. 1991). Recently, the field of prevention science has, with input from psychopathology, criminology, psychiatric epidemiology, human development and education (Coie et al. 1993) stressed the prevention of major human dysfunctions and the elimination or mitigation of the causes of disorders. Prevention science thus focuses on the systematic study of both risk factors and protective factors. Coie and colleagues emphasize the need for such a discipline and suggest various areas in which this type of research can be expanded and improved.

Regarding childhood anxiety specifically, there is little, if any, empirical data concerning preventive approaches. Earlier theorists believed that if left untreated, childhood anxiety disorders develop into adult anxiety disorders (e.g., Warren 1965, Weiss and Burke 1967), and they thus stressed the need for preventative measures. The prevention of adult anxiety disorders by treating anxiety-disordered youth has been discussed (Kendall 1992), yet there is need for greater study of the causes and precipitants of childhood anxiety as well as continued development of preventative techniques.

More knowledge about prevalence rates within certain populations would be a guide in establishing target samples of children at risk. Additional developmental information would have to be acquired and integrated as well, in order to establish an appropriate developmental level at which to begin preventative programs and/or activities. Perhaps a general program of problem-solving and coping skills training would assist in the prevention of a variety of child and adolescent difficulties, including anxiety. Last, the current incidence of anxiety in children may be historically and culturally related. If so, perhaps an additional role for individuals outside the mental health community would be open discussion with children about the stressors and difficulties of living in a fast-paced, achievement-oriented society.

WHAT CAN CLINICIANS AND RESEARCHERS EXPECT?

The manifestations of anxiety with which children will present will necessarily be affected by current factors in both the field of psychology and society in general. As mentioned earlier, the diagnostic changes within DSM-IV will lead to a slightly different population of anxious children in terms of diagnostic distribution.

The issues on the minds of parents change with the state of affairs in the local and world community. Therefore, in a society with steadily increasing rates of violence, crime, kidnapping, sexual abuse, and so forth, one might expect to see an increase in the prevalence of anxiety disorders in children. Treatments may need to shift more toward treating children in how to cope with realistic fears and less on reducing catastrophic thinking processes. Issues such as kidnapping are now more realistic worries for children, many more children spend time alone while both parents work, and fewer children are cared for by their extended families. Society's increasing use of the media to publicize unpleasant or frightening events and situations makes our children more vulnerable and knowledgeable about anxiety-provoking situations, which may also increase the number of children who become clinically anxious. Our already success-oriented society may be facing an economy in which academic and professional merit prove crucial in finding and keeping employment, and children's worries and anxieties may be increased as they pick up on this information from their parents and from the media. Last, with children becoming involved in mature behaviors such as sexual activity and substance use at earlier ages, the related responsibilities and concerns may manifest themselves through worry as well.

Clinicians' choice of treatment approach may also be affected by societal changes. Managed health care may necessitate the use of short-term, time-limited, and behavioral interventions. If overall mental health resources are reduced, the quieter internalizing children may once again be passed by in favor of treating the more disruptive externalizers. Health care changes may necessitate more work with training parents in how to prevent and/or parent anxious children. With present biological interests, there is likely to be a trend toward medication trials with anxiety-disordered children. Although medications have a favorable track record for certain childhood disorders (e.g., ADHD), there are other conditions (e.g., childhood depression) where medications have not received empirical support. Clearly, studies are needed to examine the potential merits and demerits of the use of antianxiety medications with children and adolescents.

REFERENCES

Barrios, B. A., and Hartmann, D. B. (1988). Fears and anxieties. In *Behavioral Assessment of Childhood Disorders*, ed. E. J. Mash and L. G. Terdal, 2nd ed., pp. 196–264. New York: Guilford.

Barrios, B. A., and O'Dell, S. L. (1989). Fears and anxieties. In *Treatment of Childhood Disorders*, ed. E. J. Mash and R. A. Barkley, pp. 167–221. New York: Guilford.

Bernstein, G. A., Svingen, P. H., and Garfinkel, B. D. (1990). School phobia: patterns of family functioning. *Journal of the American Academy of Child and Adolescent Psychiatry* 29:24–30.

Brady, E. U., and Kendall, P. C. (1992). Comorbidity of anxiety and depression in children and adolescents. *Psychological Bulletin* 111:244–255.

Cadbury, S., Childs-Clark, A., and Sandhu, S. (1990). Group anxiety management: effectiveness, perceived helpfulness, and follow-up. *British Journal of Clinical Psychology* 29:245–247.

Children in Need: Investment Strategies for the Educationally Disadvantaged (1987). New York: Committee for Economic Development.

Clark, D. A., and Bolton, D. (1985). Obsessive-compulsive adolescents and their parents: a psychometric study. *Journal of Child Psychology and Psychiatry* 26:267–276.

Clark, L. A., and Watson, D. (1991). Tripartite model of anxiety and depression: psychometric evidence and taxonomic implications. *Journal of Abnormal Psychology* 100:316–336.

Clarke, G., Hops, H., Lewinsohn, P. M., et al. (1992). Cognitive-behavioral group treatment of adolescent depression: prediction of outcome. *Behavior Therapy* 23:341–354.

Coie, J. D., Watt, N. F., West, S. G., et al. (1993). The science of prevention: a conceptual framework and some directions for a national research program. *American Psychologist* 48:1013–1034.

Cosper, M. R., and Erikson, M. T. (1983). Relationships among observed classroom behavior and three types of teacher ratings. *Behavioral Disorders* 9:189–195.

Cowen, E. L., Gesten, E. L., and Weissberg, R. P. (1980). An interrelated network of preventively oriented school-based health approaches. In *Evaluation and Action in the Community Context*, ed. R. H. Price and P. Politzer, pp. 173–210. New York: Academic Press.

Davids, A. (1975). Therapeutic approaches to children in residential treatments: changes from the mid 1950's to the mid 1970's. *American Psychologist*, 30:809–814.

Diagnostic and Statistical Manual of Mental Disorders (1987). 3rd ed. revised. Washington, DC: American Psychiatric Association.

_____ (1994). 4th ed. Washington, DC: American Psychiatric Association.

Fauber, R. L., and Long, N. (1991). Children in context: the role of the family in child psychotherapy. *Journal of Consulting and Clinical Psychology* 59:813–820.

Finch, A. J., Lipovsky, J. A., and Casat, C. D. (1989). Anxiety and depression in children and adolescents: negative affectivity or separate constructs? In *Anxiety and Depression: Distinctive and Overlapping Features*, ed. P. C. Kendall and D. Watson, pp. 171–202. San Diego, CA: Academic Press.

Fine, S., Forth, A., Gilbert, M., and Haley, G. (1991). Group therapy for adolescent depressive disorder: a comparison of social skills and therapeutic support. *Journal of the American Academy of Child and Adolescent Psychiatry* 30:79–85.

Francis, G. (1988). Assessing cognitions in anxious children. *Behavior Modification* 12:267–281.

Gans, J. E., Blyth, D. A., Elster A. B., and Gaveras, L. L. (1990). *America's Adolescents: How Healthy Are They?* Chicago: American Medical Association.

Guidelines for Providers of Psychological Services to Ethnic and Culturally Diverse Populations (1990). Washington, DC: American Psychological Association.

Heimberg, R. G., Dodge, C. S., Hope, D. A., et al. (1990). Cognitive-behavioral group treatment for social phobia: comparison with a credible placebo control. *Cognitive Therapy and Research* 14:1–23.

Howard, B. (1993). *A family cognitive-behavioral therapy for anxiety disordered youth.* Unpublished manuscript, Temple University.

Johnson, S. B., and Melamed, B. G. (1979). The assessment and treatment of children's fears. In *Advances in Clinical Child Psychology*, vol. 2, ed. B. B. Lahey and A. E. Kazdin, pp. 107–139. New York: Plenum.

Kashani, J. H., and Orvaschel, H. (1988). Anxiety disorders in mid-adolescence: a community sample. *American Journal of Psychiatry* 145:960–964.

Katon, W., and Roy-Byrne, P. P. (1991). Mixed anxiety and depression. *Journal of Abnormal Psychology* 100:337–345.

Kazdin, A. E. (1991). Effectiveness of psychotherapy with children and adolescents. *Journal of Consulting and Clinical Psychology* 59:785–798.

Kendall, P. C. (1984). Social cognition and problem-solving: a development and child-clinical interface. In *Applications of Cognitive-Developmental Theory*, ed. B. Gholson and T. Rosenthal, pp. 115–148. New York: Academic Press.

_____ (1985). Toward a cognitive-behavioral model of child psychopathology and a critique of related interventions. *Journal of Abnormal Psychology* 13:357–372.

_____ (1991). Guiding theory for therapy with children and adolescents. In *Child and Adolescent Therapy: Cognitive-Behavioral Procedures*, ed. P. C. Kendall, pp. 3–22. New York: Guilford.

_____ (1992). Childhood coping: avoiding a lifetime of anxiety. *Behavioural Change* 9:1–8.

_____ (1994). Treating anxiety disorders in youth: results of a randomized clinical trial. *Journal of Consulting and Clinical Psychology* 62:100–110.

Kendall, P. C., and Brady, E. U. (in press). Comorbidity in the anxiety disorders of childhood: implications for validity and clinical significance. In *Anxiety and Depression in Adults and Children*, ed. K. B. Craig and K. S. Dobson. Newbury Park, CA: Sage.

Kendall, P. C., and Chansky, T. E. (1991). Considering cognition in anxiety-disordered children. *Journal of Anxiety Disorders* 5:167–185.

Kendall, P. C., Chansky, T. E., Kane, M. T., et al. (1992a). *Anxiety Disorders in Youth: Cognitive-Behavioral Interventions*. Boston: Allyn & Bacon.

Kendall, P. C., and Dobson, K. S. (1993). On the nature of cognition and its role in psychopathology. In *Psychopathology and Cognition*, ed. K. S. Dobson and P. C. Kendall. San Diego, CA: Academic Press.

Kendall, P. C., Hollon, S. D., Beck, A. T., et al. (1987). Issues and recommendation regarding the use of the Beck Depression Inventory. *Cognitive Therapy and Research* 11:523–536.

Kendall, P. C., and Ingram, R. (1989). Cognitive-behavioral perspectives: theory and research on depression and anxiety. In *Anxiety and Depression: Distinctive and Overlapping Features*, ed. P. C. Kendall and D. Watson. New York: Academic Press.

Kendall, P. C., Kane, M., Howard, B., and Siqueland, L. (1989). *Cognitive-Behavioral Therapy for Anxious Children: Treatment Manual*. Available from the author, Department of Psychology, Temple University, Philadelphia, PA 19122.

Kendall, P. C., Kortlander, E., Chansky, T. E., and Brady, E. U. (1992b). Co-morbidity of anxiety and depression in youth: treatment implications. *Journal of Consulting and Clinical Psychology* 60:869–880.

Kendall, P. C., and MacDonald, J. P. (1993). Cognition in the psychopathology of youth, and implications for treatment. In *Psychopathology and Cognition*, ed. K. S. Dobson and P. C. Kendall. San Diego, CA: Academic Press.

Kendall, P. C., and Ronan, K. R. (1990). Assessment of children's anxieties, fears and phobias: cognitive-behavioral models and methods. In *Handbook of Psychological and Educational Assessment of Children*, ed. C. R. Reynolds and R. W. Kamphaus, pp. 223–244. New York: Guilford.

Kendall, P. C., and Watson, D., eds. (1989). *Anxiety and Depression: Distinctive and Overlapping Features*. San Diego, CA: Academic Press.

King, N. J., Ollendick, T. H., and Gullone, E. (1991). Negative affectivity in children and adolescents: relations between anxiety and depression. *Clinical Psychology Review* 11:441–459.

Kolvin, I., Garside, R. F., Nicol, A. R., et al. (1981). *Help Starts Here: The Maladjusted Child in the Ordinary School*. London: Tavistock.

Last, C. G., Francis, G., Hersen, M., et al. (1987a). Separation anxiety and school phobia: a comparison using *DSM-III* criteria. *American Journal of Psychiatry* 144:653–657.

Last, C. G., Hersen, M., Kazdin, A. E., et al. (1987b). Comparison of *DSM-III* separation anxiety and overanxious disorders: demographic characteristics and patterns of comorbidity. *Journal of the American Academy of Child and Adolescent Psychiatry* 26:527-531.

Last, C. G., Perrin, S., Hersen, M., and Kazdin, A. E. (1992). DSM-III-R anxiety disorders in children: socio-demographic and clinical characteristics. *Journal of the American Academy of Child and Adolescent Psychiatry* 31:1070-1076.

Last, C. G., and Strauss, C. C. (1989). Panic disorder in children and adolescents. *Journal of Anxiety Disorders* 3:87-95.

Last, C. G., Strauss, C. C., and Francis, G. (1987c). Comorbidity among childhood anxiety disorders. *Journal of Nervous and Mental Disease* 175:726-730.

Livingston, R., Nugent, H., Rader, L., and Smith, G. R. (1985). Family histories of depressed and severely anxious children. *American Journal of Psychiatry* 142:1497-1499.

Maag, J. W., Rutherford, R. B., and Parks, B. T. (1988). Secondary school professionals' ability to identify depression in adolescents. *Adolescence* 23:73-82.

McMahon, R. J., and Wells, K. C. (1989). Conduct disorders. In *Treatment of Childhood Disorders*, ed. E. J. Mash and R. A. Barkley, pp. 73-132. New York: Guilford.

Miller, L. G., Barrett, C. L., and Hampe, E. (1974). Phobias of childhood in a prescientific era. In *Child Personality and Psychotherapy: Current Topics*, ed. A. Davids. New York: Wiley.

Miller, L. G., Barrett, C. L., Hampe, E., and Noble, H. (1972). Factor structure of childhood fears. *Journal of Consulting and Clinical Psychology* 39:264-268.

Moritsugu, L., and Sue, S. (1983). Minority status as a stressor. In *Preventative Psychology: Theory, Research and Practice*, ed. R. D. Felner, L. A. Jason, and S. S. Farber, pp. 162-174. Elmsford, NY: Pergamon.

Morris, R. J., and Kratochwill, T. R. (1983). *Treating Children's Fears and Phobias: A Behavioral Approach*. Elmsford, NY: Pergamon.

——— (1991). Childhood fears and phobias. In *The Practice of Child Therapy*, ed. T. R. Kratochwill and R. J. Morris, 2nd ed., pp.76-114. New York: Pergamon.

Neal, A. M., Lilly, R. S., and Zakis, S. (1993). What are African American children afraid of? *Journal of Anxiety Disorders* 7:129-139.

Neal, A. M., and Turner, S. M. (1991). Anxiety disorders research with African Americans: current status. *Psychological Bulletin* 109:400-410.

Ollendick, T. H., Matson, J. L. and Helsel, W. J. (1985). Fears in children and adolescents: Normative data. *Behavior Research and Therapy* 23:465-467.

Phares, V. (1992). Where's Poppa? The relative lack of attention to the role of fathers in child and adolescent psychopathology. *American Psychologist* 47:656-664.

Phares, V., and Compas, B. C. (1992). The role of fathers in child and adolescent psychopathology: make room for Daddy. *Psychological Bulletin* 111:387-412.

Prins, P. J. (1986). Children's self-speech and self-regulation during a fear-provoking behavioral test. *Behaviour Research and Therapy* 24:181-191.

Puig-Antich, J., and Rabinovich, H. (1986). Relationship between affective and anxiety disorders in childhood. In *Anxiety Disorders of Childhood*, ed. R. Gittelman. New York: Guilford.

Ritter, D. R. (1989). Teachers' perceptions of problem behaviors in general and special education. *Exceptional Children* 55:559–564.

Ronan, K., Kendall, P. C., and Rowe, M. (in press). Negative affectivity in children: development and validation of a self-statement questionnaire. *Cognitive Therapy and Research*.

Sacco, S. P., and Graves, D. J. (1985). Correspondence between teacher ratings of childhood depression and child self-ratings. *Journal of Clinical Child Psychology* 14:353–355.

Sroufe, L. A. (1983). Infant caregiver attachment and patterns of adaptation in preschool: the roots of maladaptation and competence. In *Minnesota Symposium on Child Psychology*, vol. 16, ed. M. Perlmutter. Minneapolis: University of Minnesota Press.

Steingard, R., Biederman, J., Doyle, A., and Sprich-Buckminster, S. (1992). Psychiatric comorbidity in Attention Deficit Disorder: impact on the interpretation of the Child Behavior Checklist. *Journal of the American Academy of Child and Adolescent Psychiatry* 31:449–454.

Strauss, C. C., Lahey, B. B., Frick, P., et al. (1988a). Peer social status of children with anxiety disorders. *Journal of Consulting and Clinical Psychology* 56:137–141.

Strauss, C. C., Last, C. G., Hersen, M., and Kazdin, A. E. (1988b). Association between anxiety and depression in children and adolescents with anxiety disorders. *Journal of Abnormal Child Psychology* 16:57–68.

Tharp, R. G. (1991). Cultural diversity and treatment of children. *Journal of Consulting and Clinical Psychology* 59:799–812.

Treadwell, K. R. H., Flannery, E. C., Kendall, P. C., and Ichii, M. (1993). *Ethnicity and gender in clinic-referred children: adaptive functioning, diagnostic status, and treatment outcome.* Poster presented at the convention of the Association for the Advancement of Behavior Therapy, Atlanta, GA, November.

Tuma, J. (1989). Mental health services for children: the state of the art. *American Psychologist* 44:188–189.

Turner, S. M., Beidel, D. C., and Costello, A. (1987). Psychopathology in the offspring of anxiety disorder patients. *Journal of Consulting and Clinical Psychology* 55:229–235.

Wachtel, P. L. (1977). *Psychoanalysis and Behavior Therapy.* New York: Basic Books.

Warren, W. (1965). A study of adolescent psychiatric inpatients and the outcome six or more years later. II: The follow-up study. *Journal of Child Psychology and Psychiatry* 6:141–160.

Watson, D., and Clark, L. A. (1984). Negative affectivity: the disposition to experience aversive emotional states. *Psychological Bulletin* 96:465–490.

Weiss, M., and Burke, A. G. (1967). A five- to ten-year follow up of hospitalized school phobic children and adolescents. *American Journal of Orthopsychiatry* 37:294–295.

Weissberg, R. P., Caplan, M., and Harwood, R. L. (1991). Promoting competent young people in competence-enhancing environments: a systems-based perspective on primary prevention. *Journal of Consulting and Clinical Psychology* 59:830–841.

Weisz, J. R., Weiss, B., Alicke, M. D., and Klotz, M. L. (1987). Effectiveness of psychotherapy with children and adolescents: a meta-analysis for clinicians. *Journal of Consulting and Clinical Psychology* 55:542–549.

Wolfe, V. V., Finch, A. J., Jr., Saylor, C. F., et al. (1987). Negative affectivity in children: a multitrait-multimethod investigation. *Journal of Consulting and Clinical Psychology* 55:245–250.

Zatz, S., and Chassin, L. (1983). Cognitions of test anxious children. *Journal of Consulting and Clinical Psychology* 51:526–534.

Zatz, S., and Chassin, L. (1985). Cognitions of test anxious children under naturalistic test-taking conditions. *Journal of Consulting and Clinical Psychology* 53:393–401.

SUBJECT INDEX